OCCUPATIONAL SAFETY and HEALTH POLICY

Melvin L. Myers, MPA

Melvin L. Myers, MPA

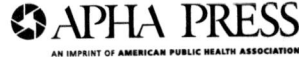

WASHINGTON, D.C. • 2015

American Public Health Association
800 I Street, NW
Washington, DC 20001-3710
www.apha.org

© 2015 by the American Public Health Association

All rights reserved. No part of this publication may be reproduced, stored in a retrieval system, or transmitted in any form or by any means, electronic, mechanical, photocopying, recording, scanning, or otherwise, except as permitted under Sections 107 and 108 of the 1976 United States Copyright Act, without either the prior written permission of the Publisher or authorization through payment of the appropriate per-copy fee to the Copyright Clearance Center [222 Rosewood Drive, Danvers, MA 01923, (978) 750-8400, fax (978) 646-8600, www.copyright.com]. Requests to the Publisher for permission should be addressed to the Permissions Department, American Public Health Association, 800 I Street, NW, Washington, DC 20001-3710; fax (202) 777-2531.

DISCLAIMER: The views expressed in the publications of the American Public Health Association are those of the authors and do not necessarily reflect the views of the American Public Health Association, or its staff, advisory panels, officers, or members of the Association's Executive Board.

Georges C. Benjamin, MD, FACP, FACEP (Emeritus), Executive Director

Printed and bound in the United States of America
Book Production Editor: Maya Ribault
Typesetting: The Charlesworth Group
Cover Design: Mazin Abdelgader
Printing and Binding: Sheridan Press Books, Inc.

Library of Congress Cataloging-in-Publication Data

Myers, Melvin L., author.
 Occupational safety and health policy / Melvin L. Myers.
    p. ; cm.
 Includes bibliographical references and index.
 Summary: "Compilation of historical information for occupational safety and health professionals and advocates regarding policy formulation and implementation"–Provided by publisher.
 ISBN 978-0-87553-271-4 (pbk.)
 I. American Public Health Association, publisher. II. Title.
 [DNLM: 1. Health Policy–United States. 2. Occupational Health–legislation & jurisprudence–United States. 3. History, 19th Century–United States. 4. History, 20th Century–United States. 5. Occupational Health–history–United States. 6. Occupational Health–standards–United States. WA 33 AA1]
 RC967
 363.11–dc23
                                                                            2014020856

TABLE OF CONTENTS

Preface		vii
1.	Introduction	1
PART I. PRECEPTS OF POLICY		**13**
2.	Occupational Safety and Health as Public Health	15
3.	Occupational Safety and Health as Environmental Health	35
4.	Law and Governance	51
5.	History of Occupational Safety and Health Policy	83
6.	Policy Advocacy Through Argument	125
PART II. IMPLEMENTATION OF POLICY		**167**
7.	Standards and the Occupational Safety and Health Act	169
8.	Enforcement and the Occupational Safety and Health Act	211
9.	Research and the Occupational Safety and Health Act	257
10.	The Mine Safety and Health Act	311
11.	Other Worker Protections and Exclusions	365
12.	International Policy	395

PART III. INSTRUMENTS OF POLICY 465

13.	Workers' Compensation and Work as an Economic Activity	467
14.	Right-to-Know and Privacy	527
15.	Leadership and Ethics	565
16.	Occupational Safety and Health Policy Analysis	599

Appendix. Occupational Safety and Health Act of 1970   671

Index   727

Preface

Government is the means by which all the people acting together do for themselves those things that people cannot do one-by-one. That is the great principle of government. The things that government must do have changed as society has changed, but that principle remains the same.

—Hubert H. Humphrey[1]

Writing this book came about as a result of teaching an occupational and environmental health policy class for 23 years at the Emory University Rollins School of Public Health in Atlanta, Georgia. The primary focus of this book is to describe the premises of occupational safety and health policy (occupational safety and health as public and environmental health, law, history, and advocacy), the implementation of this policy (the Occupational Safety and Health Act, mine safety, other protection policies, and international affairs), and instruments of policy (economics, right-to-know, leadership, and policy analysis). The purpose of this book is to compile information useful for occupational safety and health professionals and advocates regarding policy formulation and implementation. Historical information is the foundation for this purpose, as precedent is important regarding relevant laws and incrementalism is an important aspect for policy evolution.

For the contents of this book, I wish to thank the more than 500 students whom I taught. Their questions in class and their answers revealed in essays, theme papers, and oral presentations, including mock trials, helped shape the book. Most were candidates for a master of public health degree. I also acknowledge co-teachers in the class. Marcia Owens taught with me in the 1990s. She was then an environmental attorney with the City of Atlanta and formerly an attorney with the U.S. Environmental Protection Agency. She is currently on the faculty with the School of the Environment at the Florida Agricultural and Mechanical University. Barry Johnson, a co-teacher from 2000 to 2011, is the former assistant administrator of the Agency for Toxic Substances and Disease Registry. Johnson and I served together in the U.S. Public Health Service's National Air Pollution Control Administration prior to the creation of the EPA in 1970, and we later served together at the National Institute for Occupational Safety and Health.

I thank both Owens and Johnson for insights that informed me in writing this book. Owens brought hands-on knowledge regarding environmental law to the class that we taught, and Johnson filled conceptional gaps in our teaching. He defined the term "policy" for our class: "a definite course of action selected from among alternatives with regard to certain conditions to guide and determine present and future actions."

I wrote parts of this book more than 10 years ago as handouts for my students, and the actual writing of the book began in summer 2011 and was completed in spring 2013. This book is best read from start to finish, as the information that it presents builds on information presented earlier, but it is also designed as a reference source regarding occupational safety and health policy and advocacy.

—Melvin L. Myers, MPA

REFERENCE

1. Caouette M. Hubert H. Humphrey: the art of the possible. South Hill Films. 2010. Available at: http://www.hhh.umn.edu/news_events/Centennial/pdf/ArtofthePossibleTranscript.pdf. Accessed September 17, 2014.

1

Introduction

I wouldn't give you two cents for all your fancy rules if, behind them, they didn't have a little bit of plain, ordinary, everyday kindness and a little looking out for the other fella, too.

—Jefferson Smith in *Mr. Smith Goes to Washington*[1]

THE ERGONOMICS NARRATIVE

In the early 1990s, the Occupational Safety and Health Administration (OSHA) and the National Institute for Occupational Safety and Health (NIOSH) investigated an epidemic of carpal tunnel syndrome cases in the meatpacking industry.[2,3] The problem of musculoskeletal disorders was so open and obvious that opposition to correcting the causes of these disorders was muted or nil. However, the musculoskeletal disorder problem was prevalent across a much broader range of U.S. workplaces.[3a] Indeed, its traditional designation as sprains and strains was not only the most frequently reported of injury cases in the United States, but sprains and strains were the most costly of overall claims to workers' compensation systems. Consequently, OSHA proposed an ergonomics standard that would reduce musculoskeletal disorders across all industries.[4] This standard turned the world upside down for employers, requiring the job to be designed for the worker rather than making the worker conform to the job. In the face of overwhelming scientific and factual evidence in support of the standard, a broad-based industry-supported lobby mounted a massive effort in 2000 that prolonged the promulgation of the final regulation into the waning months of President Bill Clinton's administration.[5] However, with the election of President George W. Bush and a Republican-controlled Congress, special interest lobbying efforts successfully thwarted the regulation in early 2001 when Congress dissolved the standard.[6,7]

- Was this standard good public policy?
- With overwhelming scientific and factual evidence of this insidious public health problem, why and how did politics extinguish this policy?

Answers to these two questions are core lessons of this book. The lessons include not only descriptions of occupational safety and health policy but also the concept of critical thinking and evidence-based argumentation as necessary in advocating policy. These lessons are revealed within a historical context, as policies build incrementally over time and narratives are a necessary part of advocacy.

1.1. THE OCCUPATIONAL SAFETY AND HEALTH ACT OF 1970

Individual judgment and choice are replaced by governmental action that automatically wards off evils before they manifest themselves.
—Sanford Weiner and Aaron Wildavsky[8]

In 1970, Congress enacted the Occupational Safety and Health Act (OSHAct; see Appendix) as a remarkable piece of social legislation based on a command-and-control approach and a milestone in public health policy. Its promise for U.S. policy was "to assure so far as possible every working man and woman in the Nation safe and healthful working conditions." This book examines this promise as a benchmark for public policy in protecting American workers—indeed, workers worldwide—from occupational diseases and injuries; and lest one forget, another phrase in this promise in the OSHAct was "to preserve our human resources." The OSHAct is reproduced in full in the Appendix.[9]

The OSHAct and its creation, OSHA, were contentious. As an example, Senator Steve Symms (R) of Idaho proposed a bill annually throughout the 1980s to abolish OSHA. Moreover, contention between labor unions and business interests was manifest in the passage of the OSHAct (Chapters 5 and 6) and in challenging regulations and enforcement actions after the passage of the OSHAct (Chapters 7 and 8), and these and other special interests advocated reforms to the OSHAct with stark polar positions in the mid-1990s (Chapter 16). Nevertheless, OSHA persevered and, over time, OSHA has become a fixed institution in American society but with a challenge to OSHA's command-and-control approach vis-à-vis its role as a consultative agency.[10]

While a clue to a policy claim is the inclusion of the words "should" or "aught,"[11] policy is viewed as a high-level plan that embraces the general goals and acceptable procedures in governmental action. Policy prescribes a definite course of action selected from among alternatives with regard to certain conditions to guide and determine present and future actions.[12] Furthermore, implementation by people as well as the resources that they use to effect policies is part of policy. Moreover, balancing those who benefit from the policy with those who pay for or are regulated by the policy brings into play the realm of politics.[13] The derivation of the word "policy" is closely related to "police," and policy typically relates to government or regulation.[14] The World Health Organization (WHO) defines health as "a state of complete physical, mental, and social well-being and not merely the absence of disease or infirmity."[15]

1.2. THE OCCUPATIONAL SAFETY AND HEALTH PROBLEM

The International Labour Organization estimates that among the world's 2.7 billion workers, at least 2 million deaths per year are associated with occupational diseases and injuries, but the WHO has only identified 40% of the causes of these deaths.[16] Nonfatal injuries and illnesses add to this tragedy, but because data for estimating nonfatal injuries and illnesses are unavailable for most of the world, the magnitude of the problem is unknown.[17]

During 1972, the first full year of the federal statistics collected in the United States after the enactment of the OSHAct, the Bureau of Labor Statistics (BLS) reported 5.7 million occupational injuries in the private sector—mostly cuts and bruises—and 1.7 million of these injured workers missed at least one day of work. In that year, the BLS reported 11,000 occupational fatalities.[18]

Occupational fatalities decreased by more than half this amount by 2011, but the promise of the OSHAct has a long way to go to assure safe and healthful working conditions in the nation's workplaces. A total of 4,693 fatal work injuries were recorded in the United States in 2011, and the rate at which fatal work injuries occurred that year was 3.5 per 100,000 full-time equivalent (FTE) workers as reported by BLS from the Census of Fatal Occupational Injuries.[19] Figure 1-1 shows the decline from 6,217 deaths in 1992 and a high of 6,632 deaths in 1994 to a low of 4,547 deaths in 2010. From 1992 to 2011, the fatality rate steadily declined from 5.0 to a low of 3.5 deaths per 100,000 FTE workers.

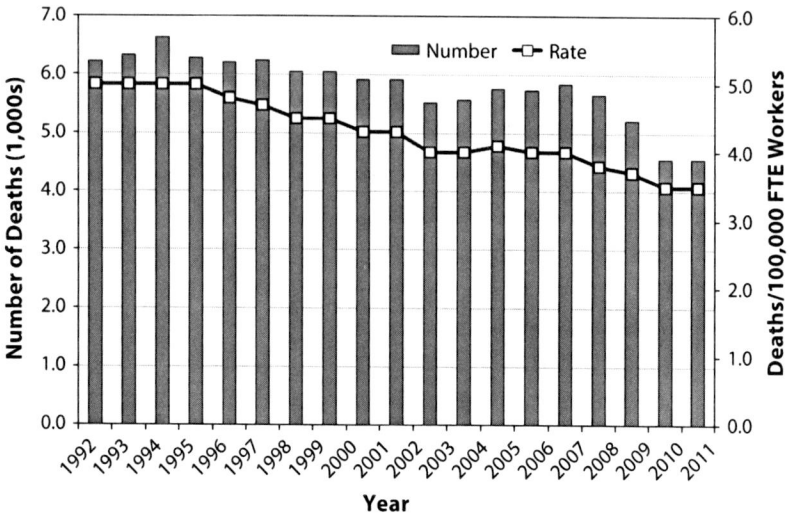

Source: Bureau of Labor Standards.[19]
Note: FTE = full-time equivalent. The sample size was *n* = 114,954 deaths.
Figure 1-1. Occupational fatality frequency and rate per 100,000 workers in the United States, 1992-2011.

Data indicate marked differences in both the frequency and rate of occupational fatalities between industry categories in 2011. The highest frequencies in order of the number of deaths occurred in transportation and warehousing (733); construction (721); agriculture, forestry, and hunting (557); and government (495). The order is different when measured by rate. Four industries stood out above all others in 2011. These were, in order of the annual fatality rate at deaths per 100,000 FTE workers, agriculture, forestry, and hunting (24.9); mining (15.9); transportation and warehousing (15.3); and construction (9.1).[19]

Both the frequency and rate of nonfatal injuries have declined since 1997, but these injuries and illnesses have been prevalent in specific workplaces as shown in Figure 1-2, as classified by the North American Industry Classification System.[20] However, occupational diseases of long latency have been and continue to be undercounted. As far back as 1978, the U.S. Department of Labor (DoL) estimated that about 1.9 million people were severely or partially disabled from occupationally related diseases.[21] Nationally, 350,000 new cases of occupational illnesses occur each year and cause an estimated 50,000

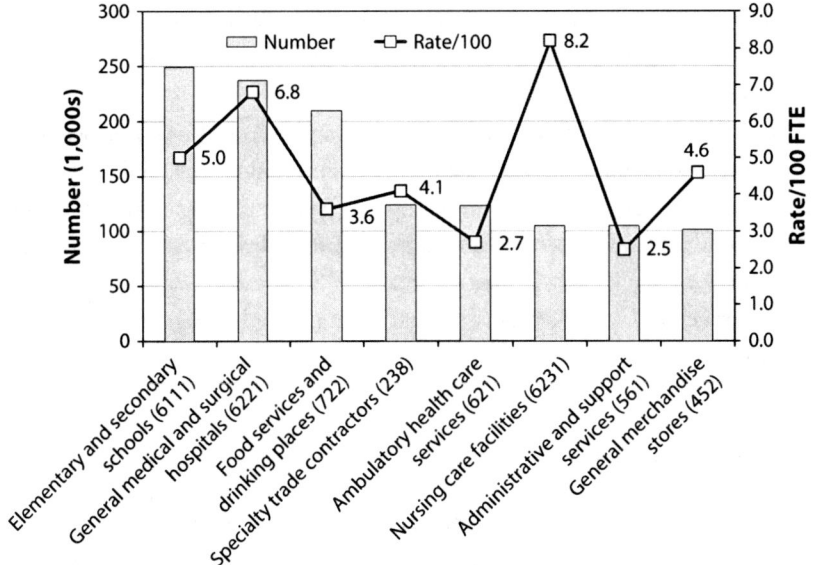

Source: Bureau of Labor Standards.[20]
Note: FTE = full-time equivalent. The sample size was n = 1,252,900.

Figure 1-2. Number of cases and incidence rate of nonfatal occupational injuries and illnesses for industries (North American Industry Classification System) with 100,000 or more cases, 2011.

deaths.[22] NIOSH currently estimates that about 20,000 cancer deaths and 40,000 new cases of cancer each year in the United States are attributable to occupation.[23] Moreover, as the population ages, the number and rate of diseases of long latency are expected to increase because a longer life span gives additional time for these diseases to manifest.[24]

An occupational disease may be described as an ill-health condition caused by a person's exposure to a work activity. In England, the more serious diseases are subject to a legal requirement to report to the Health and Safety Executive.[25] In the United States, the states establish occupational reportable diseases that are reported in each state to the health department by physicians, healthcare facilities, and clinical laboratories. As an example, the state of New York requires the reporting of 26 different occupational lung diseases by physicians to the state health department within 10 days of diagnosis. Other occupation-related conditions that are reportable in New York include heavy metals in blood or urine, pesticide poisoning, radiation illness, and congenital malformations.[26]

An estimated 100 million occupational injuries and 11 million occupational diseases occur worldwide each year.[27] These estimates include 800,000 work-related deaths per year, comprising 100,000 fatal injuries and 700,000 deaths from diseases. Much of what is learned regarding intervention strategies to prevent work-related diseases and injuries in industrialized countries is fully applicable to the 80% of the world's workforce that lives in developing countries.[16]

1.3. OVERVIEW

In politics there are no right answers, none, only a continuing flow of compromises among groups resulting in a changing, cloudy and ambiguous series of public decisions where appetite and ambition compete openly with knowledge and wisdom. That's all there is.

—Former Senator Alan K. Simpson (R) of Wyoming[28]

The purpose of this book is to (1) offer occupational safety and health professionals a scholarly update of the state of occupational safety and health policy, (2) provide students with a working familiarity with all major federal occupational health statutes and examples of state and local statutes as well as international efforts to promote occupational safety and health, (3) convey historical and contemporary occupational health policy information to policy makers to help them understand the possible consequences of their actions, and (4) inform the public to empower them with knowledge about the politics, economics, and ethics of policy development and options for dealing with work-related health risk. The book also presents advice for policy advocacy. The Institute of Medicine has described a public health framework to guide local and national governments in their policy efforts, as shown in Figure 1-3, and the elements of the OSHAct are mapped against that process: research as assessment, standards as policy development, enforcement as assurance, and surveillance as evaluation.[29] This book uses this framework.

This book comprises 3 parts and 16 chapters. It presents the environment of workers in the context of occupational safety and health policy as being influenced by many factors, including biology, economics, ethics, politics, law,

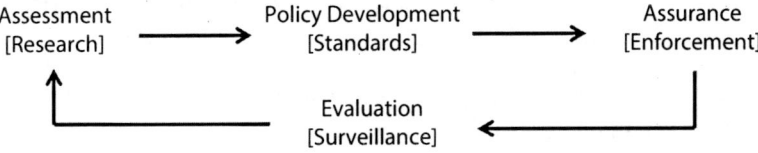

Source: Institute of Medicine.[29]

Figure 1-3. The Occupational Safety and Health Act sections mapped against the government's role in protecting health.

and technology. Furthermore, this book aims to provide the student of occupational safety and health with a fundamental knowledge, not only of policy and its creation, but also of ways to cope with policies as they exist and change. In addition, because a measure of empathy for the potential victims of occupational injuries and diseases is an important part of any caring profession, including the profession of occupational safety and health, the book acknowledges empathy as it discusses occupational safety and health policy. Following this introductory chapter, the remainder of the book is organized into three parts, which are described below.

In Part I (Chapters 2–6), I address precepts of policy with descriptions of occupational safety and health policy as part of public health policy, and more specifically as part of environmental safety and health policy. In these chapters, I explain law as an instrument of policy and describe a precedent-setting debate in the passage of the OSHAct as well as approaches to policy advocacy. Regarding advocacy, it is not enough to understand the stimulation of change through mass media or social marketing; one must also comprehend how arguments are made with an understanding of claims, evidence, and fallacies.

In Part II (Chapters 7–12), I address implementation of policy. In these chapters, I cover the OSHAct and its relationship to standard-setting, enforcement of standards, and research activities, respectively. In addition, I describe the Federal Mine Safety and Health Act, other laws that protect workers, and the plight of workers who are unprotected by legislation. I also address international policies regarding occupational safety and health.

In Part III (Chapters 13–16), I address instruments of policy. In these chapters, I present the policy implications of work as an economic activity, hazard communication, and leadership and ethics. I also examine informal leadership from within organizations in which many professionals serve as employees themselves. In the final chapter, through the lens of policy analysis, I address past and current reforms in occupational safety and health policy. The learning objectives for students who use this book as a text are as follows:

- To explain general principles of occupational health policy and apply them to human health.
- To identify and explain approaches to the prevention and control of major occupational risks to human health.
- To identify key issues in the management of occupational health programs, such as legal and ethical challenges.
- To explain major policy issues in occupational health such as regulatory and economic frameworks that guide employers and others in compliance.
- To describe advocacy approaches using techniques of argument, leadership, and evidence.

Each chapter begins and ends with a narrative. I chose this structure because true stories add a human dimension to policy writings and also highlight why policy is so important. In a complex, uncertain, and polarized world, memorable stories drive policy. They represent a crucial aspect of occupational safety and health policy advocacy, adding meaning to claims and evidence and helping to clarify cloudy and ambiguous public policy decisions.[28]

THE RIGHT-TO-KNOW NARRATIVE

The opening paragraph tells briefly about the rise and fall of the ergonomics standard. Another OSHA standard was catalyzed in a California baseball field in 1979. Men—members of the Oil, Chemical, and Atomic Workers Union (OCAW)—were playing ball as their wives observed them from the bleachers. As the women chatted about their lives, they all discovered that their attempts to conceive children were futile. This discovery led the union to ask the California Department of Public Health to investigate the problem and to request NIOSH to perform a Health Hazard Evaluation of the reproductive status of the workers. State and NIOSH investigators found that this cohort of workers was sterile, with a very low or no sperm count, resulting from exposure to dibromochloropropane (DBCP), an ingredient in the manufacture at their plant of a nematicide used as a soil fumigant; moreover, DBCP was known to cause sterility in test animals. OSHA issued an emergency temporary standard followed by a permanent standard for the control of exposure to DBCP, but this is not the end of the story.[30,31]

OCAW questioned the lack of information provided to the workforce about the toxicity of DBCP: How about other chemical exposures? Any national regulation was unlikely, since with his election as president in 1980, President Ronald Reagan was committed to eliminating regulations and not instituting new ones. As a result, OCAW and other advocates launched a systematic but disparate nationwide campaign at state and local levels of government to promulgate "right-to-know" laws to inform workers of potential chemical hazards. These state and local laws required labeling chemicals, providing information sheets, and training to notify workers of the potential hazards and their control. These laws required a variety of standards across the nation for chemical industry compliance. Labels and Material Safety Data Sheets differed based upon where the chemicals were sold or used. Moreover, some laws went beyond the workplace and required informing the local public of the hazards. The chemical industry was desperate for standardization and asked the federal government to establish a hazard communication standard, and a business-friendly administration complied with OSHA's promulgation of the Hazard Communication Standard (HazCom Standard) in 1983.[32] However, this standard only applied narrowly to the chemical industry. How about other industries where the chemical was used? An answer came in a later court ruling that extended the protection of this standard to all workers nationwide, which applied to all chemicals that might present an occupational hazard (i.e., potential to harm).[33]

- Would OSHA have successfully promulgated the HazCom Standard if it initially targeted all workplaces? The answer is that it would likely not have been successful if it had initially applied also to workers beyond the chemical industry.
- What lesson is apparent from the success of the HazCom Standard in contrast to the failure of the ergonomics standard? The answer is that for the policy to be successful, it may need to focus first on a segment of an industry in which there is no dispute regarding the hazard (e.g., the meatpacking industry) rather than all industries.

REFERENCES

1. Weschler R. Mr. Smith goes to Washington. 2002. Available at: http://www.eslnotes.com/movies/pdf/Mr-Smith-Goes-to-Washington.pdf. Accessed November 11, 2011.

2. Occupational Safety and Health Administration (OSHA). *Ergonomics Program Management Guidelines for Meatpacking Plants.* Washington, DC: U.S. Government Printing Office;1993. OSHA Publication No. 3123.

3. Steven L, Johnson SL. Chapter 41. Meatpacking operations. In: Marras WS, Karwowski W, eds. *Interventions, Controls, and Applications in Occupational Ergonomics.* Boca Raton, FL: CRC Press;2006:41-1–41-9.

3a. Centers for Disease Control and Prevention. Perspectives in disease prevention and health promotion leading work-related diseases and injuries—United States. *MMWR Morb Mortal Wkly Rep.* 1983;32(14):189–191.

4. Kome P. *Wounded Workers: The Politics of Musculoskeletal Injuries.* Toronto, ON: University of Toronto Press;1998:177–189.

5. Maraniss D, Weisskopf M. *"Tell Newt to Shut Up!"* New York, NY: Simon and Schuster;1996:60–64.

6. Biddle J, Roberts K. More evidence of the need for an ergonomic standard. *Am J Indust Med.* 2004;45(4):329–337.

7. Shapiro S. The role of procedural controls in OSHA's ergonomics rulemaking. *Public Admin Rev.* 2007;67(4):688–701.

8. Weiner S, Wildavsky A. The prophylactic presidency. In: Lipset SM, ed. *The Third Century: America as a Post-industrial Society.* Chicago, IL: The University of Chicago Press;1979:79–108.

9. Occupational Safety and Health Act of 1970 as amended, Pub L No. 91-596, 84 Stat 1590. Available at: https://www.osha.gov/pls/oshaweb/owadisp.show_document?p_table=oshact&p_id=274. Accessed May 22, 2014.

10. Pedersen DH. Industrial responses to constrained OSHA regulation. *AIHA J.* 2000;61:381–387.

11. Zarefsky D. *Argumentation: The Study of Effective Reasoning.* 2nd ed. Chantilly, VA: The Teaching Company;2005:2, 72.

12. Johnson BL. *Environmental Policy and Public Health.* Boca Raton, FL: CRC Press;2007:1.

13. Birkland TA. *An Introduction to the Policy Process: Theories, Concepts, and Models of Public Policy Making.* Armonk, NY: M.E. Sharpe;2001:20.

14. Hunter D. *The Diseases of Occupations.* London, UK: Hodder and Stoughton;1975.

15. World Health Organization. *Preamble to the Constitution of the World Health Organization as Adopted by the International Health Conference.* Geneva, Switzerland: World Health Organization;1948.

16. Rosenstock L, Cullen M, Fingerhut M. Occupational health. In: Jamison DT, Breman JG, Measham AR, et al., eds. *Disease Control Priorities in Developing Countries.* New York, NY: The International Bank for Reconstruction and Development/The World Bank;2006:1128–1145.

17. Driscoll T, Takala J, Steenland K, et al. Review of estimates of the global burden of injury and illness due to occupational exposures. *Am J Indust Med.* 2005; 48(6):491–502.

18. Kelman S. Occupational Safety and Health Administration. In: Wilson JQ, ed. *The Politics of Regulation.* New York, NY: Basic Books;1980:236–266.

19. Bureau of Labor Statistics. Revisions to the 2011 census of fatal occupational injuries (CFOI) counts. Available at: http://www.bls.gov/iif/oshwc/cfoi/cfoi_revised11.pdf. Accessed July 9, 2013.

20. Bureau of Labor Statistics. 2011 Survey of occupational injuries and illnesses summary estimates charts package. October 25, 2012. Available at: http://www.bls.gov/iif/oshwc/osh/os/osch0046.pdf. Accessed July 9, 2013.

21. Freund E, Seligman PJ, Chorba TL, et al. Mandatory reporting of occupational diseases by clinicians. *MMWR Recomm Rep.* June 22, 1990;39(RR-9): 19–23.

22. Kaufman JD, Alden K, Henderson AK. Occupational disease reporting: a step toward safer workplaces. *Washington Public Health.* 1996:14. Available at: http://www.nwpublichealth.org/docs/wph/occdis.html. Accessed December 1, 2006.

23. National Institute for Occupational Safety and Health. Safety and health topic: occupational cancer. Available at: http://www.cdc.gov/niosh/topics/cancer. Accessed December 1, 2006.

24. Breysse PN, Herbstman J. *Emerging Technology Literature Review.* Baltimore, MD;April 31, 2005. Report prepared by Johns Hopkins Bloomberg School of Public Health.

25. University of the West of England. Safety guidance note. Occupational disease and accident reporting. Available at: http://imp.uwe.ac.uk/imp_public/displayEntry.asp?URN=2038&rp=listEntry.asp. Accessed December 1, 2006.

26. New York Department of Health. Reportable diseases and conditions. Available at: http://www.health.state.ny.us/nysdoh/reportable_conditions/reportable_conditions.htm. Accessed December 2, 2006.

27. Leigh J, Macaskill P, Kuosma E, et al. Global burden of disease and injury due to occupational factors. *Epidemiology.* 1999;10(5):626–631.

28. Simpson AK, Theodore H. White lecture on press and politics. Shorenstein Center on Media, Politics and Public Policy, Harvard Kennedy School. 2013. Available at: http://shorensteincenter.org/wp-content/uploads/2012/02/THWhite2013_Lecture_Seminar.pdf. Accessed July 22, 2014.

29. Institute of Medicine. *The Future of Public Health.* Washington, DC: National Academy Press;1988:43.

30. Robinson JC. *Toil and Toxics: Workplace Struggles and Political Strategies for Occupational Health.* Berkeley, CA: University of California Press;1991:xiii–xviii.

31. Regenstein L. *America the Poisoned: How Deadly Chemicals Are Destroying Our Environment, Our Wildlife, Ourselves and How We Can Survive!* Washington, DC: Acropolis Books Ltd.;1982:316–325.

32. Morse T. Dying to know: A historical analysis of the right-to-know movement. *New Solutions.* 1998;8(1):117–145.

33. Ashford NA, Caldart CC. *Technology, Law, and the Working Environment.* Washington, DC: Island Press;1996:322–330.

I. PRECEPTS OF POLICY

In Part I, I describe cultural drivers for actions to protect occupational safety and health. In Chapter 2, I address occupational safety and health as public health. Public health policy has emerged as an important part of modern society. It takes a broad look at populations, not just individual care. The health of populations of workers has always been an important part of public health. In Chapter 3, I focus on occupational safety and health as environmental health, that aspect of public health that addresses the protection of populations from insults to health (including injuries) beyond the control of individuals. A key change in recent decades has been the move of environmental health policy from public health agencies to protection agencies, such as the Occupational Safety and Health Administration.

In Chapter 4, I address the law. I offer a lesson in civics, describing the sources of law: common, constitutional, statutory, and administrative law. Beyond public health law, other legal domains for the protection of workers' safety and health include labor, environmental, and transportation laws. History is a driver that informs occupational safety and health and is the subject of Chapter 5. In this chapter, I describe the pioneers who advanced occupational safety and health policy, the importance of the labor movement in the evolution of this field, and the policies that preceded and informed the emergence of the Occupational Safety and Health Act of 1970 (OSHAct; see Appendix).

In Chapter 6, I address the role of advocacy and argument in advancing occupational safety and health policy. Persuasion is a key element in this advance. Moreover, occupational safety and health policy is controversial, and argument is inherent in advancing this policy. Argument is composed of claims, inference, and evidence in order to arrive at resolution of controversy. The argument process is described by way of politics in the creation and passage of the OSHAct. In addition, I discuss differences between inductive and abductive reasoning and the framing of arguments. I also touch on fallacies and enemies of prevention.

2

Occupational Safety and Health as Public Health

Hygeia guarded health by prescribing self-discipline and a good environment, and Panacea used drugs and various hands-on actions to heal.

—Heather Menzies[1]

THE NOTIFIABLE DISEASE NARRATIVE

The first two great public health threats when the U.S. Public Health Service (USPHS) was created in 1912 were infectious and occupational diseases. One year later, the USPHS recommended a model law for a system of notifiable diseases and injuries that included infectious diseases, occupational diseases and injuries, and miscellaneous diseases such as cancer and pellagra. The model law listed the following occupational diseases and injuries: poisonings by arsenic, brass, carbon monoxide, lead, mercury, natural gas, phosphorus, wood alcohol, naphtha, bisulfide of carbon, and dinitrobenzene, as well as caisson disease (compressed-air illness) and any other disease or disability contracted as a result of a person's employment. Silicosis was added later, as was silico-tuberculosis.[2] Limited to primarily infectious diseases but including silicosis, the list of notifiable diseases today is reported to the Centers for Disease Control and Prevention (CDC).[3] States report incidences of these diseases to the CDC, which publishes their occurrence in the *Mortality and Morbidity Weekly Report*. While some states such as New York maintain reporting of occupational diseases such as lung diseases (e.g., metal fume fever, silicosis), metal poisoning, and pesticide poisoning, the legacy of national occupational disease reports has diminished over time while reports of infectious diseases remain.[4]

2.1. INTRODUCTION

This chapter reviews public health policy in the context of occupational and environmental health. It explains the health fields model and its influence on the USPHS's "Objectives for the Nation," including the difference between the "health fields terms," health protection, health promotion, and public health services. The chapter describes the occupational health problem, centered on injuries and diseases, and the broader issues of global health and health disparities. The chapter also introduces several prevention models, including the surveillance-containment model, the prevention spectrum, the agent-environment-host model and its relationship to the Haddon Matrix, and the hierarchy of controls.

2.2. PUBLIC HEALTH

The ideal is a skillful and loyal civil service free from political interference and dedicated to the implementation and efficient administration of politically mandated programs according to sound principles of management.
—David L. Weimer and Aidan R. Vining[5]

In 1988, the Institute of Medicine (IOM) identified the goal "of public health as protecting the community against the hazards engendered by group life," which was quoted from a 1984 article.[6] Public health is concerned with the health of the community as a whole and focuses on entire populations rather than on individual patients. Over time, public health organizations and agencies have emerged to intervene against threats to public safety and health. While health was defined in Chapter 1, safety is defined as "an assessment of the level and acceptability of risk of adverse outcomes that occur as a result of a prevention technique in the context of a specific prevention strategy and disease or injury outcome."[7] Historically, two factors have determined public health policies:[8]

1. The level of scientific and technical knowledge has changed public health measures with advances in the understanding of the causes and control of diseases and injuries.
2. Public values and popular opinions have been affected by beliefs about illness and injuries and by attitudes regarding appropriate governmental action.

The IOM defined four core public health policy functions, as previously shown in Figure 1-3. The first is the assessment and monitoring of the health of at-risk populations to identify health problems and priorities. The second function is the formulation of public policies designed to solve local and national health problems and priorities. The third is to assure that all populations have access to appropriate and cost-effective health protection, promotion, and care services. The fourth is an evaluation of the effectiveness of those services. As described in Chapter 1, this framework can be mapped on the occupational safety and health policy guidelines from the Occupational Safety and Health Act (OSHAct; see Appendix), with (1) assessment as the research function, (2) formulation of policy as the standard-setting function, (3) assurance as the enforcement function, and (4) evaluation as the surveillance function (e.g., Bureau of Labor Statistics).

Public health agencies are organized into three levels in the United States. First is the national government, which is in partnership with the second level of state governments—together named the federal system. The third level is local governments (creations of state governments), which include city and county governments.[8] The U.S. Department of Health and Human Services (DHHS) contains national public health agencies, whereas states have established state health departments and local governments have established county and municipal health departments. Yet many health protection agencies have emerged outside of the public health agency system, including the U.S. Environmental Protection Agency (EPA) and the Occupational Safety and Health Administration (OSHA) within the U.S. Department of Labor (DoL).

The CDC, a DHHS agency and home for the OSHAct-created National Institute for Occupational Safety and Health (NIOSH), selected safer workplaces as one of the 10 great public health achievements gained in the United States between 1900 and 1999. Work-related health problems, such as coal workers' pneumoconiosis (black lung) and silicosis, have come under better control. Severe injuries and deaths related to high-hazard industries that included mining, manufacturing, construction, and transportation have also decreased. Since 1980, safer workplaces have led to about a 40% reduction in the rate of fatal occupational injuries.[9]

Public health professionals approach three stages of intervention—primary, secondary, and tertiary—in a cascade fashion to prevent disease or injury.[7] Intervention at the earliest stage is the most effective:

- Primary prevention: An intervention implemented before there is evidence of a disease or injury. This strategy can reduce or eliminate causative risk

factors (risk reduction) for a health problem. It includes the reduction of risk factors, such as ambient lead exposures to prevent intellectual impairment, and health service interventions, such as vaccinations.
- Secondary prevention: An intervention implemented after a disease has begun but before it is symptomatic (screening and treatment). Secondary prevention involves early detection and treatment, such as measuring lead presence in the blood so that interventions can be taken to reduce exposure or to chelate the metal from the body. The focus is on cure.
- Tertiary prevention: An intervention implemented after a disease or injury is established. This strategy can prevent sequelae. Tertiary prevention involves providing appropriate supportive and rehabilitative services to minimize morbidity and maximize quality of life, such as rehabilitation from injuries. It includes preventing secondary complications among individuals with disabilities, such as muscle atrophy linked to nonactivity. The focus is on care.

Whereas healthcare systems become involved in secondary or tertiary prevention cases, they also serve two important functions in the first stage (primary prevention). First, cases of injury or disease signal new or emerging problems as sentinels for preventive action within a population at risk. Second, a health care intervention such as vaccinations can act to prevent an illness. As an example, the Veterans Administration (VA) hospital system has patients for life, and it provides preventive health services that last over a lifetime, including the promotion of healthy behaviors. Thus, through prevention, the VA is able to maintain an average cost per patient of $5,000 per year, as contrasted with the average annual cost per patient of $6,500 paid by Medicare to private institutions.[10]

2.3. HEALTH FIELDS

As a society, when we posit "health policy," we typically think of "healthcare policy." However, contemporary public health policy in the United States has its roots in a health fields model formulated in 1974 by Marc Lalonde, the Canadian Minister of National Health and Welfare. He proposed a way to classify Canada's federal budget into four general determinants that interact in their effect on public health. These health fields, or determinants of health, were termed "human biology," "environment," "lifestyle," and "healthcare organization," as shown in Figure 2-1.[7,11]

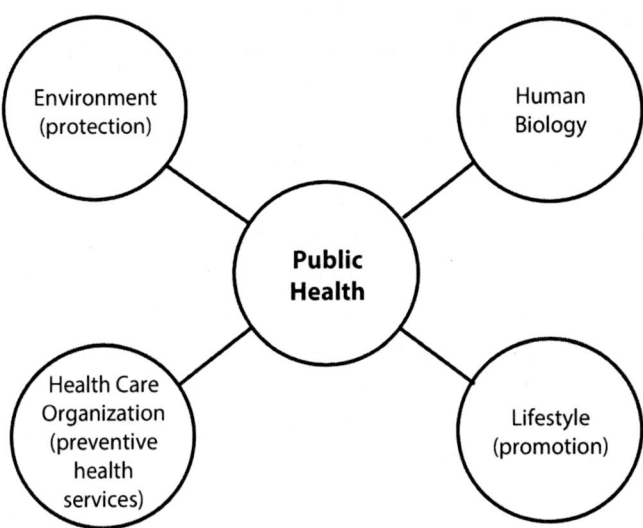

Figure 2-1. The relationship of the determinants of public health.

The USPHS, part of the DHHS, initiated a process in 1980 that applied the health fields model to a national strategy for improving the health of the U.S. population.[12] At that time, biology was viewed as inherent and insusceptible to intervention. Thus, the strategy focused interventions on the other three determinants of health, as shown parenthetically in Figure 2-1:

- Health protection. This intervention strategy was aimed at the environment field, which was a community concern and required regulatory action to alter an individual's surroundings (environmental); occupational safety and health was included as a priority in this strategy.
- Health promotion. The intervention strategy for the lifestyle field relied upon individual behavior change and individual responsibility (behavioral).
- Preventive health services. Last, the strategy for the healthcare organization depended upon provider-to-patient interaction (clinical).

These three strategies can interact. For example, exposures to both workplace noise (a health protection issue) and recreational sound (a health promotion issue) can combine to create noise-induced hearing loss.[12a] Furthermore, preventive health services can, for example, protect healthcare workers from contracting communicable diseases by providing vaccinations.[12b] Each decade after 1980, the

USPHS has published intervention strategies in its *Healthy People* report, with corresponding preventive healthcare "Objectives for the Nation." These strategies include focusing on occupational safety and health as a national priority area.[13-17]

Consistent with the World Health Organization (WHO) definition of health, *Healthy People 2010* expanded the environmental determinant of health to include both physical and social environments. Moreover, policies and interventions were important factors that affected these two newly classified environment types.[16] Not only is occupational health affected by the physical environment of the workplace but also by the social environment—that is, working conditions, particularly the legal, economic, and technological concerns continuing to evolve across all industries. The social environment in its different but interrelated dimensions is addressed throughout this text.

The Healthy People Objectives for 2020 are listed below.[17] Each objective is quantified and has baseline data. The objective may have subobjectives, such as by industry or worker age.

1. Reduce deaths from work-related injuries.
2. Reduce nonfatal work-related injuries.
3. Reduce the rate of injury and illness cases involving days away from work due to overexertion or repetitive motion.
4. Reduce pneumoconiosis deaths.
5. Reduce deaths from work-related homicides.
6. Reduce work-related assaults.
7. Reduce the proportion of persons who have elevated blood lead concentrations from work exposures.
8. Reduce occupational skin diseases or disorders among full-time workers.
9. Increase the proportion of employees who have access to workplace programs that prevent or reduce employee stress.
10. Reduce new cases of work-related, noise-induced hearing loss.

Sometimes diseases associated with work are affected by nonwork exposures. An example is a smoker who is exposed to asbestos at work and the effect of this combined exposure on lung cancer. In combination, smoking and asbestos exposures increase the risk of lung cancer fivefold over either exposure alone.[18]

2.4. HEALTH DISPARITIES AND GLOBAL HEALTH

2.4.1. Health Disparities

The International Labour Organization (ILO) estimates that the average hours of a work year vary in a disparate way from country to country: 1,467 hours per work year in Germany; 1,821 hours per work year in the United States; and 2,447 hours per work year in Korea. Worldwide, the nature of work changes as the world's economies change.[19] A variety of labor, economic, and social policies potentially affect occupational health disparities.[20]

Several groups of workers have been excluded from labor protections. Both agricultural and domestic workers across the United States are largely unprotected by the labor provisions afforded many other workers, which significantly contributes to occupational health disparities. Farm workers represent just 3% of the total labor force in the United States but account for 13% of all workplace fatalities. Unregulated and unsafe workplaces worsen preventable health disparities, increase cost-shifting from employers to individual workers and social safety nets, and tempt employers to cut corners by violating protective standards to maintain economic viability.[19]

In the United States, fear of deportation and the risks involved with reentering the country creates disincentives for illegal immigrants to report workplace safety violations, request access to training and protective equipment, and seek medical attention. Furthermore, only one workplace fatality for every 3,000 cases has been prosecuted. In 2009, the average penalty resulting from an OSHA investigation for fatalities was $6,750, and for a serious violation, it was $965.[19] That year, OSHA conducted 797 fatality investigations and 67,668 serious violation investigations.[21]

Disparity is apparent for uninsured people who have worse health and die sooner than people with health insurance. Barriers in workers' compensation systems affect occupational health disparities through disparate mechanisms that are supposed to ensure timely, adequate, and appropriate provision of occupational medical services. For example, workers' compensation systems inadequately compensate workers who have contracted chronic occupational diseases due to hazardous workplace exposures. Furthermore, there are increasing numbers of workers who are not covered at all under workers' compensation because they are considered self-employed or independent contractors.[19]

2.4.2. Global Occupational Health

Workers in developing countries face occupational health problems along with other endemic health risks such as infectious and parasitic diseases, malnutrition, and lack of health care. Workers in the informal sector (not counted in the economy, such as day laborers), migrant workers, female workers, and child laborers are at high risk of occupational diseases and injuries. The nature of work life depends upon the stage of economic development in the country. By one measure, 99% of acute pesticide poisoning in the world occurs in developing economies.[22]

The ILO estimates that among the 2.7 billion workers worldwide, 2 million die each year of occupational diseases and injuries. Moreover, the WHO estimates that 9% of all cancers of the lung, trachea, and bronchus and about 2% of all leukemias are work-related.[20]

Globalization has moved national industries into international companies and a global workplace. These companies have sophisticated occupational health infrastructures, and trade agreements offer the potential to incorporate industrialized nations' rules regarding occupational safety and health in developing countries. Indeed, these companies have high-quality services and training that can enhance workers' awareness and promote other industries in the region to conform to safety standards.[20,22,23] However, multinational companies may create an occupational safety and health "caste system," providing a high level of care and service for their international managers and for technical support staff members while offering local, possibly inferior, sources of care for indigenous workers.[20]

The host countries often resist rules, perceiving them as trade restrictions. As long as the labor is plentiful and the direct illness and injury costs to employers are low, the competitive advantage goes to those companies with a lower investment in health and safety. Thus, there is pressure to minimize or reduce the intensity and quality of occupational safety and health protection.[20,22,23]

For example, the health and safety language in the North American Free Trade Agreement is much less demanding than rules in the United States. Some multinational companies abandon the stricter rules as they seek broad economic relief and thus move across borders.[23]

As in the industrial world, high injury fatality rates in the developing world are clustered in disparate sectors, including agriculture, construction, oil and gas extraction, and mining.[20] WHO has noted that temporary, insecure, and low-income jobs are associated with more hazardous working conditions and increased social income inequality. In many developing countries, the informal economy that includes street vendors and immigrant labor offers fewer rights than to local laborers.[24]

2.5. PREVENTION MODELS

Prevention emphasizes the development and assessment of community or population-based interventions. It is concerned with the study of effective preventive interventions within systems, including systems of employment and work.

2.5.1. Surveillance–Containment Model

An important public health model for the prevention of diseases is the surveillance–containment model. This model was created and implemented in 1966 when Dr. William Foege was serving as a medical missionary in Nigeria. Smallpox, a contagious virus that kills about a third of its victims, had been eliminated in Western Europe, North America, and Japan, but it was still claiming more than two million lives a year worldwide in such places as India and Africa. Even though the strategy was to vaccinate everyone, Foege's clinic received a limited shipment of smallpox vaccine. He was told over his ham radio that more vaccines were on the way (ham radios were part of a network among missionaries for their personal safety). Before the next shipment could arrive, however, he got word of a smallpox outbreak in a remote region of the country. Foege needed to act quickly to prevent an epidemic but lacked enough vaccine to inoculate 100% of the population. He knew he had to get to susceptible people before the virus spread. Foege enlisted the help of local missionaries and, using maps and radios, divided up the area around the outbreak and sent runners to the surrounding villages.[25]

Within 24 hours, Foege and his colleagues had isolated all cases of the disease and the contacts of the diseased patients with other people in which disease transfer could occur. Next, they traced routes where those who were infected had lived, shopped, and gathered, targeting those villages and markets with vaccinations to create a buffer zone of immunity around the epidemic's epicenter. Four weeks later, there were no new smallpox cases in the area. This strategy of surveillance and containment eliminated smallpox in West Africa in three and a half years. It has since become the standard for

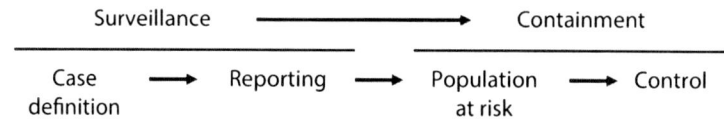

Figure 2-2. The surveillance-containment model.

infectious disease eradication. In 1979, WHO announced the end of the effort to eradicate smallpox.[25] Rather than "eradication," the term "elimination" is used to indicate that a disease is terminated at the national level.

The surveillance–containment model as shown in Figure 2-2 is similar in concept to the operational model of industrial hygienists. The industrial hygiene model is process-driven, starting with recognition and reporting of the problem (surveillance), following with an evaluation of the problem (population at risk), and culminating in the control of the problem (containment). In recent years, the industrial hygiene profession has added another step to the front end of its model: "anticipation" of the problem, which aims to be proactive before health effects are manifested from an occupational hazard.

2.5.2. The Spectrum of Prevention

The spectrum of prevention couples comprehensive strategy development with interdisciplinary collaboration as a way to solve complex problems. It emerged in 1983 from the clinical work of Dr. Marshall Swift of Hahnemann College in the United Kingdom as a tool for addressing developmental disability problems that moved from a practice of focusing only on education to six sequentially expanding action levels:[26]

1. Strengthening individual knowledge and skills that transfer information and know-how to increase an individual's resources and capacity for preventing injury or disease. An example is safe lifting technique training for firefighters.[27]
2. Promoting community education; mass media campaigns notify individuals about new health and safety information as well as build support and political will for healthier behavior, norms, and policy change. As an example, media campaigns have warned the public to drink a lot of water when working outside in hot weather.[28]
3. Educating providers results in influencing peers and informing patients, clients, and colleagues to improve their understanding of prevention.

Moreover, the providers can be effective advocates for policy changes related to work safety. As an example, educating physicians and nurses about occupational safety and health builds a cadre of expertise that can advocate for prevention practices within organizations as well as in public bodies.[29]
4. Fostering coalitions and networks. This is vital in successful public health movements for prevention. Coalitions are useful for accomplishing a broad range of goals that reach beyond the capacity of any individual member organization. As an example, the Council of Occupational Safety and Health, a nationwide federation of 21 local and statewide groups established in 1971, comprises private, nonprofit coalitions of labor unions, health and technical professionals, and others interested in promoting and advocating for worker health and safety.[30]
5. Changing organizational practices. This has much potential by effecting internal regulations and norms to improve the health and safety of its workers with side benefits for the people they serve. As an example, infection prevention policies in hospitals protect the workers as well as the patients and their visitors.[31]
6. Influencing policy and legislation. This has the potential for broad improvement in health outcomes. As an example, banning smoking in all public places has reduced heart attack incident rates.[32]

2.5.3. Haddon Matrix

Public health regarding infectious diseases is part of environmental health and when associated with work is part of occupational health.[33] In the development of causal relationships of infectious diseases, an epidemiological model was created to explain the temporal relationship between the human host of the disease, the causal agent of the disease, and the environment whether special or general. Wade Hampton Frost developed and used this model in the early 1900s as an example of circumstantial evidence for what he called "the epidemiological argument." Frost had initiated waterborne disease investigations for the USPHS in 1914, and in 1921, he became the first professor of epidemiology in the United States at John Hopkins University.[34]

In 1968, William Haddon Jr., a public health physician with the New York State Health Department, developed a matrix of categories using the epidemiological model to assist researchers trying to systematically address injury prevention by identifying major modifiable factors that lead to unhealthy outcomes. The idea was to look at injuries associated with causal and

Table 2-1. Analysis of Features of Commercial Fishing Injury Events in Alaska, Using the Haddon Matrix

Phase	Host/Human	Agent/Vehicle/Vector	Environment
Pre-event	Captain and crew fatigue, stress	Unstable vessel	High winds
		Unstable work platform	Large waves
	Prescription or illegal drugs/ alcohol	Complex machinery and operations	Icing
			Short daylight
	Inadequate training/ exposure		Limited fishing seasons
			Vessels far apart
Event	Captain and crew reaction to emergency	Listing or capsized vessel	High winds
		Delayed abandonment	Large waves
	Personal flotation devices unavailable or not working	Emergency circumstance misunderstood	Darkness
			Poor radio communications
		Man overboard (MOB)	Cold water
Post-event	Hypothermia	Vessel sinking	High winds
	Drowning	Poor crew response to MOB	Large waves
	Lost at sea		Cold water
	Poor use of available emergency equipment		

Source: National Institute for Occupational Safety and Health.[36]

contributing factors and not just to adopt a descriptive approach. The matrix classified these factors into "human" factors, "agent or vehicle" factors, and "environment" factors (physical and social environment).[35]

Each factor was then considered in a pre-event phase, an event phase, and a post-event phase. Although this matrix has typically been used only in epidemiologic studies, it serves as a framework to investigate the circumstances of traumatic deaths. As shown in Table 2-1, the matrix consists of three rows representing time phases and three columns representing characteristics and circumstances of the injured person, the vehicle or vector, and the environment. The matrix in Table 2-1 is an adaptation of the analytical tool to occupational injury circumstances, characteristics of, and countermeasures for Alaska commercial fishing injury events.[36] In other cases, the matrix has been expanded by adding the social environment.

2.5.4. Hierarchy of Controls

The essence of setting priorities for the protection of workers against hazards is that control at the source is most preferable, control along the pathway between the source and the potential victim is secondary, and control by the potential victim is least preferable. Many professional principles support this doctrine for protecting occupational safety and health. One of these, established by the Organisation for Economic Co-operation and Development in 1973, is the "polluter pays principle," as opposed to the "victim pays principle."[36a] Another is the "compensation principle," whereby "employers and entrepreneurs who enjoy the economic benefits of businesses should ultimately bear the cost of the injuries and deaths that are incident to the manufacture, preparation, and distribution of goods and services."[37]

Lucian Chaney at the DoL created this approach upon completion of a safety study in 1917, using the term "engineering revision." He claimed the engineering approach would no longer depend on workers' vigilance to ensure their own safety and could result in the "entire elimination of fatalities." This revision expressed a cultural shift from blaming the worker for carelessness to an emphasis on the cause of the injury and its prevention. The new safety engineering profession ardently accepted the revision.[38] Table 2-2 shows different elements of the hierarchy of controls.

Table 2-2. Different Elements of Hierarchy of Controls in Priority Order

ANSI/AIHA[42]	Description	Industrial Hygiene[41]	Engineering Design[40]	Control[39]
1. Elimination	Consider methods to eliminate the hazard		Eliminate the hazard (and risk)	Prevent exposure: 1-3 (passive control)
2. Substitution	Substitute a less hazardous method or process	Substitution		
3. Engineering controls	Consider controls such as machine guards or ventilation systems	Isolation	Guard against the hazard	
4. Warnings	Include audible or visual warning technologies or labels or symbols		Warn against the hazard	Mitigate exposure: 4-6 (active control)
5. Administrative control	Training or limiting exposure such as through job rotation	Administrative control		
6. Personal protective equipment		Personal protective equipment		

Note: ANSI/AIHA = American National Standards Institute/American Industrial Hygiene Association.

Haddon developed a two-level hierarchy of controls—passive and active—in which preferred passive controls required no personal intervention by the potential victim of an injury (e.g., air bags), whereas active controls required a personal intervention (e.g., fastening seat belts).[39] Along similar lines, professional safety engineers established a hierarchy of controls for protecting workers from injury. The hierarchy has three steps, from the most to the least protective:[40]

- Eliminate the hazard. An example is burying electric power lines underground to eliminate construction cranes' contact with electricity.
- Control the hazard. An example is the ventilation of fumes away from a worksite.
- Warn of the hazard. An example is warning workers to shield themselves from solar radiation while working outside.

The hierarchy of controls from the industrial hygiene perspective also follows the logic of controlling the hazards first at the source.[41] This hierarchy is listed below:

- Substitution involves replacing a hazardous substance, machinery, or work process with a nonhazardous or less hazardous one. Examples of substitution are using a nonflammable solvent in place of a flammable one, using chemicals in pellet or paste form instead of dusty powders, or replacing an unstable chair with a stable one.
- Isolation. If a hazard cannot be eliminated or substituted, the next preferred measure is to control the risk. Engineering controls may include modification of tools and equipment, using enclosures, guarding, local exhaust ventilation, or automation.
- Administrative control. Where a health and safety risk cannot be eliminated or controlled by engineering, administrative controls should be used. Administrative controls introduce work practices that reduce risk, and they limit the exposure of the employee to the hazard. They include measures such as rotating jobs, adopting purchasing policies that take account of health and safety, following special measures for using hazardous chemicals or processes, and using lockout procedures.
- Personal protective equipment (PPE) should only be used where other measures are not practicable. Efforts to remove health and safety risks using the above measures should continue. In general, protective clothing

and equipment should only be used for short-term or emergency procedures, or as additional protection when other control measures do not provide sufficient exposure control. The reason for limiting the use of PPE is that it is difficult to fully protect employees with PPE or equipment. In addition, compliance with usage may be challenging. PPE can fall into disuse if it is uncomfortable or hinders movement, if supervision is not undertaken, or if adequate training and instruction are not given. Where protective clothing or equipment must be used, the employer should ensure that it is appropriate for the job, that it fits the operator correctly, that training is provided in its need and use, and that it is cleaned and maintained regularly.

In 2005, the American National Standards Institute (ANSI) approved a consensus standard that merged safety and the industrial hierarchy of controls, in the ANSI/American Industrial Hygiene Association (AIHA) Z10, Occupational Health and Safety Management Systems.[42] The ANSI/AIHA standard adopted a six-level hierarchy with the following precedence: (1) elimination, (2) substitution, (3) engineering controls, (4) warnings, (5) administrative control, and (6) PPE.

Training is the most popular method used to control hazards. Indeed, training is very important because it is an effective way to diffuse information about hazards and hazard controls across large numbers of workers. However, training lacks success when it is the only method used. This is because important factors covering hazards may have been ignored. To be effective, training must support the other control measures discussed above. One should remember, however, that training not only supports other control methods, but it is also a legal requirement.

THE COMMAND-AND-CONTROL NARRATIVE

Wolfgang Thomas Rau created the term "medical police" in 1764 in the German states, giving birth to a governmental medical policy implemented through administrative regulation. The concept was applied to major health problems of the period and gained widespread popularity. The popularity spread to another physician, Peter Frank, who in 1766 conceived of writing regulations on the measures to be taken by government to protect the public health. He wrote six volumes of code, published from 1779 to 1817. His code covered public health comprehensively, addressing the spectrum of "womb to tomb" health, including the health of a variety of occupational groups. In his fourth and fifth volumes, he turned his attention to the problem of preventing injuries.[43] Frank's code set the precedent for national governmental command-and-control policies to protect the public health, which is prominent today in occupational safety and health policies.

REFERENCES

1. Menzies H. *No Time: Stress and the Crisis of Modern Life.* Vancouver, BC: Douglas & McIntyre Publishing Group;1995:122.

2. Trask JW. Section XII: Vital statistics. In: Rosenau MJ, ed. *Preventive Medicine and Hygiene.* New York, NY: D. Appleton-Century;1935:1191–1192.

3. Centers for Disease Control and Prevention (CDC). *2012 Case Definitions: Nationally Notifiable Conditions, Infectious and Non-Infectious Cases.* Atlanta, GA: CDC;2012.

4. New York State Department of Health. When is a disease considered "occupational"? Available at: http://www.health.ny.gov/environmental/workplace/lung_disease_registry/docs/lungreg.pdf. Accessed May 02, 2012.

5. Weimer DL, Vining AR. *Policy Analysis: Concepts and Practice.* Upper Saddle River, NJ: Prentice Hall;1998:33.

6. Ellencweig AY, Yoshpe RB. Definition of public health. *Public Health Rev.* 1984;12(1):65–78.

7. Teutsch SM. A framework for assessing the effectiveness of disease and injury prevention. *MMWR Recomm Rep.* 1992;41(RR-3):1–12.

8. Institute of Medicine. *The Future of Public Health.* Washington, DC: National Academy Press;1988:7, 42–47, 56–57.

9. Centers for Disease Control and Prevention. Ten great public health achievements—United States, 1900-1999. *MMWR Morb Mortal Wkly Rep.* 1999;48(12):241–243.

10. Waller D. How VA hospitals became the best. *Time.* September 4, 2006;168(10):36–37.

11. Morgan RW. *Prospects for Preventive Medicine.* Toronto, ON: Ontario Economic Council;1977. Occasional Paper 2.

12. Surgeon General of the U.S. Public Health Service. *Healthy People: The Surgeon General's Report on Health Promotion and Disease Prevention.* Washington, DC: U.S. Government Printing Office;1979.

12a. Rabinowitz PM. Noise-induced hearing loss. *Am Fam Physician.* 2000;61(9): 2749-2756.

12b. Shefer A, Atkinson W, Friedman C, et al. Immunization of health-care personnel: recommendations of the Advisory Committee on Immunization Practices (ACIP). *MMWR Recommendations and Reports.* November 25, 2011/60(RR07);1-45.

13. Millar JD, Myers ML. Occupational safety and health: Progress toward the 1990 objectives for the nation. *Public Health Rep.* 1983;98(4):324-336.

14. U.S. Department of Health and Human Services. *Healthy People 1990: Promoting Health/Preventing Disease: Objectives for the Nation.* Washington, DC: U.S. Government Printing Office;1980.

15. U.S. Department of Health and Human Services. *Healthy People 2000: National Health Promotion and Disease Prevention Objectives.* Washington, DC: U.S. Government Printing Office;1990.

16. U.S. Department of Health and Human Services. *Healthy People 2010: National Health Promotion and Disease Prevention Objectives.* Washington, DC: U.S. Government Printing Office;2000.

17. U.S. Department of Health and Human Services. *Healthy People 2020.* Washington, DC: U.S. Government Printing Office;2010. ODPHP Publication No. B0132.

18. Fairbanks J, Wiese WH. *The Public Health Primer.* London, UK: Sage Publications;1998:56.

19. Siqueira CE, Gaydo M, Monforton C, et al. Effects of social, economic, and labor policies on occupational health disparities. Paper presented at: Eliminating Health and Safety Disparities at Work Conference; September 14-15, 2011; Chicago, IL.

20. Rosenstock L, Cullen M, Fingerhut M. Occupational health. In: Jamison DT, Breman JG, Measham AR, et al., eds. *Disease Control Priorities in Developing Countries.* New York, NY: The International Bank for Reconstruction and Development/The World Bank;2006:1128-1145.

21. Occupational Safety and Health Administration. *OSHA Enforcement: Ensuring Safe and Healthy Workplaces.* Washington, DC: U.S. Department of Labor. Available at: https://www.osha.gov/dep/2009_enforcement_summary.html. Accessed May 21, 2014.

22. Reich MR, Okubo T. Workers and health in the third world. In: Reich MR, Okubo T, eds. *Protecting Workers' Health in the Third World: National and International Strategies.* New York, NY: Auburn House;1992:1-11.

23. Frumkin H. Across the water and down the ladder: Workers in the global economy. *Occup Med*. 1999;14(3):637–663.

24. Perry M, Hu H. Workplace health and safety. In: Frumkin H, ed. *Environmental Health From Global to Local*. San Francisco, CA: Jossey-Bass;2005:648–682.

25. Loftus MJ. Health for all. *Emory Magazine*. 2002;77(4). Available at: http://www.emory.edu/EMORY_MAGAZINE/winter2002/foege.html. Accessed November 30, 2006.

26. Cohen L, Swift S. The spectrum of prevention: developing a comprehensive approach to injury prevention. *Inj Prev*. 1999;5(3):203–207.

27. Peate WF, Bates G, Lunda K, Francis S, Bellamy K. Core strength: A new model for injury prediction and prevention. *J Occup Med Toxicol*. 2007;2(3). Available at: http://www.occup-med.com/content/pdf/1745-6673-2-3.pdf. Accessed March 9, 2012.

28. National Institute for Occupational Safety and Health. *Working in Hot Environments*. Cincinnati, OH: NIOSH;1986. NIOSH Publication No. 86-112.

29. LaDou J. The rise and fall of occupational medicine in the United States. *Am J Prev Med*. 2002;22(4):285–295.

30. Council of Occupational Safety and Health. Committees (or coalitions) on occupational safety and health. 2009. Available at: http://www.coshnetwork.org. Accessed April 3, 2012.

31. Uchida M, Stone PW, Conway LJ, Pogorzelska M, Larson EL, Raveis VH. Exploring infection prevention: policy implications from a qualitative study. *Policy Polit Nurs Pract*. 2011;12(2):82–89.

32. Meyers DG, Neuberger JS, He J. Cardiovascular effect of bans on smoking in public places: a systematic review and meta-analysis. *J Am Coll Cardiol*. 2009;54(14):1249–1255.

33. Susser M. *Causal Thinking in the Health Sciences: Concepts and Strategies of Epidemiology*. New York, NY: Oxford University Press;1973:27–29.

34. Stolley PD, Lasky T. *Investigating Disease Patterns: The Science of Epidemiology*. New York, NY: Scientific American Library;1995.

35. Conroy C, Fowler J. The Haddon Matrix: applying an epidemiologic research tool as a framework for death investigation. *Am J Forensic Med Pathol*. 2000;21(4):339–342.

36. National Institute for Occupational Safety and Health. *Commercial Fishing Fatalities in Alaska: Risk Factors and Prevention Strategies*. Cincinnati, OH: National

Institute for Occupational Safety and Health;1997. Current Intelligence Bulletin 58, DHHS (NIOSH) Publication No. 97-163.

36a. Mirovitskaya N, Ascher WL, eds. *Guide to Sustainable Development and Environmental Policy*. Durham, NC: Duke University Press;2002:194–195.

37. Little JW, Eaton TA, Smith GR. *Cases and Materials on Workers' Compensation*. St. Paul, MN: West Publishing Co.;1993.

38. Aldrich, M. *Safety First: Technology, Labor, and Business in the Building of American Work Safety 1870-1939*. Baltimore, MD: The John Hopkins University Press;1997:115–117.

39. Haddon W. Jr. Strategy in preventive medicine: passive vs. active approaches to reducing human wastage. *J Trauma*. 1974;14(4):353–354.

40. Wogalter MS. Purposes and scope of warnings. In: Wogalter MS, ed. *Handbook of Warnings*. Mahwah, NJ: Lawrence Erlbaum Associates;2006:3–10.

41. Weinberg JL, Bunin LJ, Das R. Application of the industrial hygiene hierarchy of controls to prioritize and promote safer methods of pest control: A case study. *Public Health Rep*. 2009;124(suppl 1):53–62.

42. Manuele FA. ANSI/AIHA Z10-2005: The new benchmark for safety management systems. *The Compass*. 2011;(special issue):5–14. Available at: http://www.asse.org/practicespecialties/docs/Z10SpecialIssue.pdf. Accessed September 29, 2011.

43. Rosen G. *A History of Public Health*. Baltimore, MD: The Johns Hopkins University Press;1993:137–142.

3

Occupational Safety and Health as Environmental Health

Environmental law attempts to build foresight into the human decisional system, along with an awareness of costs and values that are typically invisible because, though real, they exist outside the formal market economy.
—Plater, Abrams, and Goldfarb[1]

KEPONE: THE WORKER NARRATIVE

When the Occupational Safety and Health Administration (OSHA) first set up a complaint policy, informal complaints did not always lead to workplace inspections, and typically formal written complaints were evaluated without employers contacting complainants to determine whether there were "reasonable grounds to believe" if a hazard existed, as required by the Occupational Safety and Health Act (OSHAct; see Appendix). In late 1974, a former worker at Life Science Products (LSP) Company had lodged a complaint with OSHA claiming that he had been fired for refusing to work in a dangerous Kepone-laden work setting. Kepone was a trade name for an insecticide. In response, OSHA sent an inquiry to LSP, but LSP claimed that the former worker was a disgruntled employee. Unfortunately mollified, OSHA closed the file without making an on-site inspection.[2] In 1975, doctors in Virginia started to get suspicious about the unusual symptoms they observed in LSP employees, which included uncontrollable shaking, loss of vision, joint pain, chest pain and heart palpitations, and other neurological and liver problems. It also seemed possible that Kepone could be a carcinogen. The blood of one of the workers was sent to the Centers for Disease Control and Prevention (CDC) in Atlanta for tests, which revealed extremely high levels of Kepone in his blood. Further tests revealed that most of the other workers did too. On July 25, 1975, the state Department of Health closed the plant. The presence of Kepone at LSP eventually led to the hospitalization of 29 employees. As a result, OSHA's complaint policy changed in 1976 by giving top priority to on-site inspections in response to complaints received. OSHA issued four citations to the two owners of LSP, carrying a $16,500 total penalty.[3]

3.1. INTRODUCTION

Effective action is dependent upon knowledge, much of which does not yet exist and much of which, while existing, has never been marshaled into applicable relationships.

—Lynton K. Caldwell[4]

In the late 1960s and early 1970s, environmental consciousness erupted upon the American scene, driven by two events: one occupational, the other environmental.[5] On November 20, 1968, 78 miners were killed by a coal mine explosion in Farmington, West Virginia. On January 28, 1969, an oil rig explosion created a massive oil spill off the coast of Santa Barbara, California, polluting 13 miles of ocean beach. These incidents were covered extensively by national news organizations, stimulating an outrage that fed urgency for governmental action.

The previous chapter introduced the health fields model, an element of which was environmental health protection. A consistent movement within the occupational safety and health field has encouraged classifying occupational safety and health as part of environmental health. Five issues emerge regarding this movement. First, nearly all of the environmental health issues that involve respiratory or dermal exposures are preceded by occupational exposures (e.g., pesticides). Second, the safety aspect of occupational health introduces injury prevention as an environmental concern. Third, chemical safety associated with catastrophic events such as explosions affects workers as well as bystanders. Fourth, a toxics use reduction movement has as its aim to protect both workers and the public beyond the workplace. Fifth, efforts among researchers, business, scientists, and regulators to collaborate have been mounted in the past regarding chemical agents such as the Interagency Regulatory Liaison Group (IRLG), to be described later in this chapter. The chapter concludes with an explanation of the emergence of the "protection" agencies from the U.S. Public Health Service: the National Highway Traffic Safety Administration (NHTSA), OSHA, the U.S. Environmental Protection Agency (EPA), and the Consumer Product Safety Commission (CPSC).

3.2. OCCUPATIONAL EXPOSURES IN THE VANGUARD

The work environment may entail exposures experienced in the general environment but with a higher intensity of exposure. Occupational safety and health policy may be envisioned as a micro-environment within the context of environmental health.

Much of Rachel Carson's landmark book, *Silent Spring*, was founded on studies of pesticide exposures to workers.[6] Industrial hygiene work regarding air contaminants spawned studies within the environmental sciences concerning air pollution effects and control as well as health physics. Moreover, with the passage of the Toxic Substances Control Act of 1976,[6a] the initial list of substances that EPA used under that statute came from the Registry of Toxic Effects of Chemical Substances established by the National Institute for Occupational Safety and Health (NIOSH) under the OSHAct. In addition, as noted later, the risk assessment approach has its genesis from a Supreme Court ruling regarding an OSHA regulation on benzene. Many consumer safety innovations also had their origin with occupational safety policies such as the use of personal protective equipment (e.g., safety helmets, hearing protectors) or guards on machines.

Indeed, many examples indicate that occupational health policy is in the vanguard of environmental health policy, yet it is environmental health policy, which brings saliency to the issues, that results in the broader control of recognized hazards. The following is a short list to illustrate this policy synergism:

- The science of the effects of exposure to radon decay progeny on uranium miners[7] became the foundation for establishing environmental standards for radon progeny emissions from the ground into indoor environments and implementation of the Indoor Radon Abatement Act of 1988.
- Intensive occupational health studies of the causes of mesothelioma, lung cancer, and asbestosis led to the more general recognition of asbestos-related health effects in the general population and action by EPA to control the exposures.[8]

- It was after secondhand smoke from cigarettes was identified as an occupational hazard[9] that a sea change in cigarette smoke (indoor air pollution) control was implemented.
- A NIOSH investigation of the effects of asbestos in schools on teachers led to the broader concern of exposures to schoolchildren by EPA and parents and the passage of the Asbestos Hazard Emergency Response Act of 1986.[10,10a]
- Workers exposed to lead fumes in the manufacture of tetraethyl lead were the original victims of lead poisoning, but it was not until EPA phased out lead in gasoline as a health risk under the Clean Air Act that its elimination was accomplished.[11,11a]
- Studies of mad hatter's disease that resulted from hat manufacturing established the science for governmental action to reduce exposure to mercury in the general environment.[12,13]
- The discovery of the effects (angiosarcoma) of vinyl chloride monomer (VCM) on chemical workers led to the removal of VCM as a propellant from hair sprays.[14,15]
- The NIOSH investigation of the effects of computer workstation design on the musculoskeletal system (e.g., carpal tunnel syndrome) led to the ergonomic redesign of computer workstations that are now prevalent throughout society.[16]
- NIOSH employees investigating workers' potential radiation exposure from airport security machines observed children riding the conveyers through the ground-level X-ray machines, which led to raising the conveyors above ground level.[17]
- Safety devices such as rollover protective structures on commercial tractors became more common on residential tractors.[18]
- The OSHA Hazard Communication Standard of 1983 informed the EPA Emergency Planning and Community Right-to-Know Act of 1986.[18a]

3.3. INJURY PREVENTION

Injuries escape consideration in environmental health policies, but they are a principal driver for occupational health policy. Nonetheless, injuries are a public health problem. In 1949, JE Gordon claimed that from 1900 to 1946, injuries advanced from sixth to third place as a cause of death in the United States and were a public health problem.[19] He identified the physical, biologic, and socioeconomic environments as causative factors for injuries.

Table 3-1. Energy Transfer Methods and Associated Injuries

Energy	Injury	Event
Mechanical	Fracture, crushing injury	Fall from elevation, vehicle overturn
Thermal	Burn, hypothermia	Hot metal splatter, fall overboard into cold water
Chemical	Burn, asphyxiation	Battery explosion, ammonia leak, oxygen deficiency
Electrical	Burn, heart fibrillation	Electrical shock
Ionizing radiation	Cerebral edema, gastroenteritis	Nuclear power plant breach

A 1985 study by the Institute of Medicine reported that the potential life-years lost from injuries (40.8%) were greater than those lost from cancer (18.0%), heart disease (16.4%), or all other diseases (24.8%). That report recognized that most of the attention in previous research and policies had focused on the role of people in initiating injury events, whereas environmental factors had been identified as important in the prevention of injuries. Environments that include products and vehicles contribute to injury events, and these man-made environments cover transportation, the workplace, and recreation.[20]

Injuries are defined as the end result of a transfer of energy, usually sudden, above or below certain limits of human tissue, causing physical damage to tissue or death.[20] Table 3-1 lists some of the methods of energy transfer that may cause damage to human tissue and gives examples of some specific injuries that may result, as well as the event that caused them. Little distinguishes occupational from environmental injuries in the event examples provided.

3.4. CHEMICAL SAFETY

The Occupational Safety and Health Administration's (OSHA's) experience with process safety began in the 1980s, when a series of oil refinery explosions occurred, such as the one at Philips Petroleum refinery in Pasadena, Texas, that resulted in 23 deaths and 132 injuries in 1989. OSHA investigations of these incidents helped shape the OSHA Process Safety Management of Highly Hazardous Chemicals (PSM) standard, which was promulgated in 1992.[21] This action by OSHA was mandated by Congress under Section 304 of the Clean Air Act Amendments (CAAA) of 1990, but EPA was also mandated under Section 112 of the CAAA to publish regulations and guidance for chemical incident prevention at facilities using substances that posed the greatest risk of harm from chemical incident releases. EPA published its risk management plan regulations in 1996 consistent with OSHA's PSM standard that aimed to prevent incidents of substance releases and enhance awareness of the dangers regarding handling and storing hazardous chemicals.[22]

Section 112(r) of the CAAA encompasses a general duty clause stating that "owners and operators of stationary sources producing, processing, handling and storing extremely hazardous substances have a general duty to identify hazards associated with an accidental release, design and maintain a safe facility, and minimize consequences of accidental releases that occur."[23,24] This general duty is remarkable as a generic standard that places the burden on the potential polluter rather than the government to protect the public. This duty under the CAAA is similar to the general duty clause under the 1970 OSHAct that places the burden on employers to protect their workers from "recognized" hazards.

In the aftermath of the refinery explosion, Section 302 of the CAAA also established the independent Chemical Safety and Hazard Investigation Board to investigate, determine, and report to the public in writing the facts, conditions, circumstances, and cause or probable cause of any unintentional release resulting in a fatality, serious injury, or substantial property damages. These reports include recommendations to EPA and OSHA. The board is required to cooperate with the National Transportation Safety Board and OSHA in their investigations.

3.5. TOXICS USE REDUCTION AND POLLUTION PREVENTION

Arguments have pitted environmental interests against labor interests, such as pollution regulations that are alleged job killers, but policies have been established to protect both workers and the environment from toxic chemical exposures. In 1989, the state of Massachusetts enacted the Toxics Use Reduction Act to eliminate or reduce exposures of workers and the environment to hazardous chemicals. State officials and stakeholders determine policies and which chemicals to reduce. Toxics reduction policies emphasize reducing chemical use by companies at the source so that exposures both inside and outside the workplace are prevented, thus protecting public health, the environment, and workers' health while helping businesses to become more competitive. In 2009, an Administrative Council consisting of three state agencies was set up to establish policies for toxics use reduction.[25] However, signaling a priority for general environmental protection rather than worker protection, the Massachusetts Department of Environmental Protection was represented on the council, while the Massachusetts Department of Labor and Workforce Development was not.

At the behest of EPA, the 1989 Massachusetts law led Congress to enact the Pollution Prevention Act (PPA) of 1990. The act affirms a hierarchical policy approach for pollution prevention, that is, toxics use reduction:

> The Congress hereby declares it to be the national policy of the United States that pollution should be prevented or reduced at the source whenever feasible; pollution that cannot be prevented should be recycled in an environmentally safe manner, whenever feasible; pollution that cannot be prevented or recycled should be treated in an environmentally safe manner whenever feasible; and disposal or other release into the environment should be employed only as a last resort and should be conducted in an environmentally safe manner.[26]

Because EPA was the only advocate for the PPA, an overt focus on toxics reduction to protect workers was lost. Nonetheless, if EPA reduces toxic substances as an input into processes, then workers are protected as well.[5]

3.6. NATIONAL ENVIRONMENTAL POLICY ACT

The National Environmental Policy Act of 1970 (NEPA) is a short, simple, and comprehensive declaration of policy.[26a] It has action-forcing provisions to protect the human environment that are broad enough to address the work environment. Its purpose is "to foster and promote the general welfare, to create and maintain conditions under which man and nature can exist in productive harmony, and fulfill the social, economic, and other requirements of present and future generations of Americans." In addition, NEPA created the Council on Environmental Quality (CEQ) and required that environmental impact statements (EIS) be prepared for federal actions that significantly affect the environment. The CEQ has played a major environmental policy and education role and acts as the caretaker of the EIS process. The implication of this act is that there is not one environment; there are as many environments as there are living things in the world. The act applies to federal agency jurisdictions, whether domestic or international, and to federal economic policies as they affect the environment.[27]

The EIS is NEPA's action-forcing tool. The principle behind this action is learning and, moreover, teaching how to live and survive within limits. The act is meant to transform society from a pioneer to a custodial and caring ethos. Rapidly expanding technological innovation and economic development have led to unforeseen and unwanted consequences for which many assessment techniques have emerged, such as comparative risk assessment and cost-benefit analysis. However, the EIS is an assessment technique that anticipates the environmental consequences of governmental plans, programs, and decisions. The EIS provides a procedure and learning process for anticipating the potential environmental consequences of federal agency actions.[27] EPA is tasked with reviewing these actions as reported in the EIS process.

By the mid-1970s, environmental concerns were routinely included in government actions. Environmental and citizen groups used NEPA to sue a host of federal agencies for noncompliance. The courts generally came down on their side. The courts interpreted NEPA to cover not only direct impacts but also indirect effects from federal projects and activities, which might include increased traffic or secondary development from projects. The NEPA process has been replicated to varying degrees in 23 states.[28] However, even with the broad NEPA mandate, little attention has been given to the work environment up to now.

3.7. INTERAGENCY REGULATORY LIAISON GROUP

In its attempt to regulate interstate commerce of chemicals within the United States, Congress created five regulatory agencies responsible for overseeing various aspects of that trade: EPA, CPSC, OSHA, the U.S. Food and Drug Administration (FDA), and the U.S. Department of Agriculture's Food Safety and Inspection Service (FSIS). Because each of these agencies arose through different enabling legislation and is concerned with a different use of chemicals, it is likely that any one chemical will be independently regulated by two or more of those agencies.

In October 1977, at the urging of the executive branch, the agency heads of EPA, CPSC, FDA, and OSHA formally announced the creation of the IRLG. FSIS joined IRLG later. The stated goal of the IRLG was "to increase the public health and protect the environment by sharing information, avoiding duplication of effort, and developing consistent regulatory policy while reducing the burden on those regulated and the agencies themselves."[29]

Each of the agency heads agreed to recommend those specific areas in which interagency cooperation would be beneficial to all the agencies.[29] Much effort went into forging an interagency cancer policy, but when President Ronald Reagan took office in 1980, agency leaders were replaced and the president disbanded the IRLG. Nevertheless, the IRLG had demonstrated the common ground between environmental, consumer, and occupational health protection agencies.[30]

3.8. THE PROTECTION AGENCIES

When we are dealing with the possible harmful effects of the byproducts of industry and the wastes of nuclear technology, our goal is not conquest but containment.
—U.S. Surgeon General Luther L. Burney, 1958[31]

Laws are not enough. They must be implemented, and their implementation by agencies is strongly wedded to politics. The implementation of each individual environmental law tells a distinct story,[32] but a pattern has been manifest in the creation of health protection agencies as offshoots of public health agencies over the past 50 years. This pattern is linked to special interest perceptions of foot-dragging by the public health agencies, leading to the genesis of four health protection agencies as described below and shown in Figure 3-1. Foremost among these special interests was American lawyer Ralph Nader,

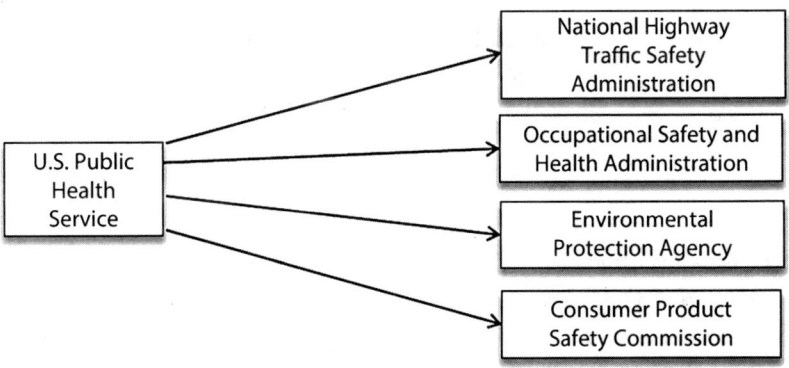

Figure 3-1. A flowchart showing an example of the movement from public health agencies to health protection agencies in the United States.

who founded the Center for the Study of Responsive Law in 1969, to expose corporate safety neglect and governmental failure to protect consumers. Nader and his consumer advocate team's writings were replete with criticism of the USPHS as a "get along, go along" entity.

Several programs affected by the creation of EPA and OSHA in 1970 and CPSC in 1972 were originally part of the USPHS Consumer Protection and Environmental Health Service, established in 1970. This agency contained three units: the National Air Pollution Control Administration (NAPCA), the FDA, and the Environmental Control Administration. The Environmental Control Administration comprised (1) the Bureau of Community Environment Management, (2) the Bureau of Occupational Safety and Health, (3) the Bureau of Solid Waste Management, (4) the Bureau of Water Hygiene, and (5) the Bureau of Radiological Health.[33] A pesticides research program to be transferred to EPA was based in the CDC's Bureau of Disease Prevention and Environmental Control.

3.8.1. The National Highway Traffic Safety Administration

In 1957, then-Senator Lyndon B. Johnson had proposed an automobile and highway safety division in the U.S. Department of Health, Education, and Welfare where USPHS was based. Nader wrote the landmark work *Unsafe at Any Speed* in 1965, a major accusation of inadequate automobile safety standards for consumers. This book was partly responsible for the passage of the National Traffic and Motor Vehicle Safety Act of 1966,[33a] which created organizations that later became the National Highway Traffic Safety Administration. Nader accused the USPHS Division of Accident Prevention of doing nothing regarding vehicle hazards and only focusing on human factors and alleged that the division's director was influenced by the interests of the automobile industry.[34]

Dr. William J. Haddon Jr. was named the head of the National Traffic Safety Bureau, which began operations in the Department of Commerce in 1966. Like Nader, Haddon was frustrated with the behavior-modification approach of the Division of Accident Prevention and was successful at transferring the division's highway safety activities to the new National Highway Safety Bureau. The division ceased to exist with the creation of CPSC in 1972.[35]

3.8.2. The Occupational Safety and Health Administration

Page and O'Brien[33] of Nader's team wrote the results of their investigation of worker safety and health policies after the creation of OSHA. Their investigation was critical of the USPHS, stating that it kowtowed to industry in its studies of occupational health,[33] but the genesis of the 1970 OSHAct was in the USPHS's Bureau of Occupational Safety and Health, from which the OSHAct created NIOSH (see Chapters 5 and 6). Title IV of the Social Security Act of 1936 had provided for federal funding to state health departments for occupational health (industrial hygiene) programs.[36] With the creation of OSHA in the DoL, a tremendous shift of occupational health programs occurred at state levels from health departments to labor agencies.

3.8.3. The Environmental Protection Agency

Esposito[37] from Nader's team investigated implementation efforts by the USPHS under the Air Quality Act of 1967, and Zwick and Benstock[38] (also from Nader's team) reported on their investigation of governmental programs to clean up the nation's water. In 1970, Nader's team claimed that NAPCA was a "disorganized band of government officials acting out a pollution control charade."[37] President Richard Nixon, with the concurrence of Congress, created EPA by Reorganization Plan Number 3 in December 1970. The reorganization shifted NAPCA and much of the Environmental Control Administration to EPA. Moreover, the Federal Water Quality Administration (FWQA) was transferred to EPA from the U.S. Department of the Interior (DoI). The FWQA was previously the Federal Water Pollution Control Administration in the USPHS, created by the Water Quality Act of 1965 and transferred to DoI by Reorganization Plan Number 2 of 1966. The USPHS program dates back to the Division of Water Supply and Pollution Control, which administered the Water Pollution Control Act of 1948. An aggressive stance was delimited by this early USPHS water pollution control program with a focus on complementing state-level programs or interstate agencies.[39]

3.8.4. The Consumer Product Safety Commission

The Consumer Product Safety Act of 1972[39a] created the independent agency, CPSC, which absorbed programs that were based in the FDA: the National

Injury Surveillance System (NISS), the Bureau of Product Safety (the remnant of the Division of Accident Prevention), and the National Clearinghouse of Poison Control Centers. CPSC merged two separate data-collection programs: NISS and the Hospital Emergency Room Injury Reporting System set up by the former National Commission on Product Safety into the National Electronic Injury Surveillance System.[40] The Bureau of Product Safety had enforced the Refrigerator Safety Act of 1956 and the Federal Hazardous Substances Labeling Act of 1960, and the National Clearinghouse of Poison Control Centers enforced the Poison Prevention Packaging Act of 1970.

KEPONE: THE REFUSE NARRATIVE

Ironically, the poisoning of a Virginia factory worker in 1975 from Kepone led to the control of the chemical through state and federal environmental laws and not the OSHAct.[1] An environmental law had lingered on the books for decades before it was resurrected in 1970: the Refuse Act of 1899, in which Congress authorized the U.S. Army Corps of Engineers to make it criminally unlawful to discharge refuse into any navigable waters or tributaries of those waters.[1] In violation of this statute, Allied Chemical discharged Kepone process wastes through three pipes into a tributary to the James River, a navigable waterway, from 1966 to 1974 without informing the federal government. With the Federal Water Pollution Control Act Amendments of 1972 (Clean Water Act), the permitting system was transferred from the Corps to EPA. In 1973, LSP was incorporated and took over the production of Kepone, while Allied maintained ownership of the material used in the process. LSP commenced operations in 1974 by way of an agreement with the City of Hopewell, Virginia, to discharge waste into the municipal treatment plant, but only after the waste was pretreated. LSP violated the Clean Water Act by polluting the wastewater treatment facility.[1] Over the years, approximately 200,000 pounds of Kepone had been released into the environment through atmospheric emissions, wastewater discharge, and bulk waste disposal. Anywhere from 20,000 to 40,000 pounds of Kepone went into the James River, which resulted in a ban on fishing. In 1976, a federal grand jury indicted Allied Chemical, LSP, the city of Hopewell, and several individuals on 1,097 counts of violating federal antipollution laws. EPA fined the indicted companies $13.2 million, $8.2 million of which went to form the Virginia Environmental Endowment.[41]

REFERENCES

1. Plater ZJB, Abrams RH, Goldfarb W. *Environmental Law and Policy: Nature, Law, and Society.* St. Paul, MN: West Publishing Co.;1992.

2. Plater ZJB. Facing a time of counter-revolution—the Kepone incident and a review of first principles. *Univ Richmond Law Rev.* 1995;29:657–713.

3. *Hearing Before the Occupational Safety and Health Review Commission. Life Science Products Company, a Corporation; Virgil A. Hundtofte and W. P. Moore, Individually and as Co-Partners Doing Business as Life Science Products Company.* OSHRC Docket No. 14910. November 11, 1977. Available at: http://www.oshrc.gov/decisions/html_1977/14910.html. Accessed January 4, 2012.

4. Caldwell LK. *Defense of Earth: International Protection of the Biosphere.* Bloomington, IN: Indiana University Press;1972.

5. Ashford NA, Caldart CC. *Technology, Law, and the Working Environment.* Washington, DC: Island Press;1996.

6. Carson R. *Silent Spring.* New York, NY: Fawcett Crest;1962.

6a. Toxic Substances Control Act, 15 U.S.C. § 2601 et seq. (1976).

7. National Institute for Occupational Safety and Health. *Radon Daughters.* Cincinnati, OH: NIOSH; 1976. Current Intelligence Bulletin 10, U.S. Department of Health and Human Services (NIOSH) Publication No. 78-127.

8. Selikoff IJ, Hammond EC, Seidman H. Cancer risk of insulation workers in the United States. In: Proceedings of the International Conference on the Biological Effects of Asbestos; October 2–5, 1972; Lyon, France: International Agency for Research on Cancer;1973:1–20.

9. National Institute for Occupational Safety and Health. *Environmental Tobacco Smoke in the Workplace: Lung Cancer and Other Health Effects.* Cincinnati, OH: NIOSH;1991. Current Intelligence Bulletin 54, DHHS (NIOSH) Publication No. 91-108.

10. Roberts DR. *Asbestos Analysis Report for Reading Community Schools, Ceiling Insulating Material.* Cincinnati, OH: National Institute for Occupational Safety and Health, U.S. Department of Health and Human Services;1980. Report No. IWS-127-16.

10a. Asbestos Hazard Emergency Response Act, 15 U.S.C. § 2651 (1986).

11. Kovarik W. Ethyl-leaded gasoline: how a classic occupational disease became an international public health disaster. *Int J Occup Environ Health.* 2005;11(4): 384–397.

11a. Clean Air Act, 42 U.S.C. § 7401 et seq. (1970).

12. Wedeen RP. Were the hatters of New Jersey "mad"? *Am J Ind Med.* 1989;16(2): 225–233.

13. U.S. Environmental Protection Agency. *Mercury Study Report to Congress, Vol. 1: Executive Summary.* 1997. EPA-452/R-97-003.

14. Key MM. Statement on proposed permanent standard for vinyl chloride. Paper presented at: OSHA Hearing, U.S. Department of Labor; June 25, 1974:55–60.

15. Moyers B. Trade secrets: a Moyers Report program transcript. Available at: http://www.pbs.org/tradesecrets/transcript.html. Accessed January 15, 2012.

16. National Institute for Occupational Safety and Health. Select research reports on health issues in video display terminal operations. Cincinnati, OH: NIOSH, U.S. Department of Health and Human Services;1981.

17. Larsen LB. *An Occupational Health Survey of Selected Airports.* Cincinnati, OH: National Institute of Occupational Safety and Health, U.S. Department of Health and Human Services;1974. NIOSH 74-123.

18. Myers ML. Avocational farmers and the tractor overturn hazard. Paper presented at: National Symposium on Agriculture, Forestry, and Fishing Health and Safety; Boise, ID; June 30, 2011.

18a. Emergency Planning and Community Right-to-Know Act, 42 U.S.C. § 11001–11050 (1986).

19. Gordon JE. The epidemiology of accidents. *Am J Pub Health.* 1949;39(4):504–515.

20. Institute of Medicine. *Injury in America: A Continuing Public Health Problem.* Washington, DC: National Academy Press;1985:48, 53.

21. Long LA. History of process safety at OSHA. *Process Safety Prog.* 2009;28(2): 128–130.

22. Roughton JE, Buchalter DS. OSHA's process safety management standard vs. EPA's risk management plan: A comparison of requirements. *Prof Safety.* 1997; 42(1):36–41.

23. U.S. Environmental Protection Agency. The General Duty Clause, Section 112(r)(1) of Clean Air Act, 42 U.S.C. § 7412(r) (1990). Available at: http://www.epa.gov/oem/docs/chem/gdc-fact.pdf. Accessed May 22, 2014.

24. Clean Air Act, 42 U.S.C. § 7401 et seq. (1970). Available at: http://www2.epa.gov/laws-regulations/summary-clean-air-act. Accessed May 22, 2014.

25. Massey R, Eliason P, Harriman E, et al. *Massachusetts Toxics Use Reduction Act Program Assessment*. Lowell, MA;2009. TURI Methods and Policy Report No. 26, Toxics Use Reduction Institute, University of Massachusetts-Lowell.

26. Pollution Prevention Act, 42 U.S.C. § 13101 et seq. (1990). Available at: http://www.epa.gov/p2/pubs/p2policy/act1990.htm. Accessed May 22, 2014.

26a. National Environmental Policy Act, 42 U.S.C. § 4321 et seq. (1969).

27. Caldwell LK. *The National Environmental Policy Act: An Agenda for the Future*. Bloomington, IN: Indiana University Press;1998.

28. Alm AL. NEPA: past, present, and future. *EPA J.* 1988(1–2):14. Available at: http://www.epa.gov/aboutepa/history/topics/nepa/01.html. Accessed March 21, 2012.

29. Johns PA. Interagency Regulatory Liaison Group role in phthalates. *Environ Health Perspect*. 1982;45:145–147.

30. Landy MK, Roberts MJ, Thomas SR. *The Environmental Protection Agency: Asking the Wrong Questions from Nixon to Clinton*. New York, NY: Oxford University Press;1994.

31. Mullan F. *Plagues and Politics: The Story of the United States Public Health Service*. New York: Basic Books, Inc.;1989:145.

32. Scheberle D. *Federalism and Environmental Policy: Trust and the Politics of Implementation*. Washington, DC: Georgetown University Press;2004.

33. Page JA, O'Brien M-W. *Bitter Wages: The Report on Disease and Injury on the Job*. New York, NY: Grossman;1973.

33a. National Traffic and Motor Vehicle Safety Act, 49 U.S.C. § 30101 et seq. (1966).

34. Nader R. *Unsafe at Any Speed: The Designed-in Dangers of the American Automobile*. New York, NY: Grossman;1965.

35. Waller JA. Reflections on a half century of injury control. *Am J Pub Health*. 1994;84(4):664–670.

36. Rosner D, Markowitz G. Research or advocacy: Federal occupational safety and health polices during the New Deal. *J Soc Hist*. 1985;18(3):365–381.

37. Esposito JC. *Vanishing Air: Ralph Nader's Study Group Report on Air Pollution*. New York, NY: Grossman;1970.

38. Zwick D, Benstock M. *Water Wasteland: The Report on Water Pollution*. New York, NY: Grossman;1971.

39. Hollis MD, McCallum GE. Federal water pollution control legislation. *Sewage and Industrial Waste.* 1956;28(3):306–310.

39a. 15 U.S.C. § 2051 et seq. (1972).

40. Broussalian VL. Risk measurement and safety standards in consumer products. In: Terleckyj NE, ed. *Household Production and Consumption.* New York, NY: National Bureau of Economic Research;1976:491–525.

41. Wilson SS. Kepone's legacy. *Hopewell News and Patriot.* June 13, 2011. Available at: http://www.hopewellnews.com/article_3468.shtml. Accessed January 13, 2012.

4

Law and Governance

The life of the law has not been logic, it has been experience. The study of law is still to a large extent the study of history.

—Oliver Wendell Holmes[1]

THE HAMMURABI NARRATIVE

Hammurabi was the ruler of the world's first metropolis, Babylon, and reigned from 1795 to 1750 BC. He proclaimed publicly to his people and in writing (preserved in stone), the earliest-known example of an entire body of laws. Although by today's standards, the Code of Hammurabi was harsh in its punishment and in its slave culture, it was remarkable, for it was the first body of laws under which the king was also held accountable: a rule of law, not of men. The code had 282 laws that addressed all aspects of life, both criminal and civil. Hammurabi looked to a higher power under a social contract, which was reflected four millennia later in the U.S. Declaration of Independence as truths that are self-evident. All people live under the same law, whether king or those for hire. We live today under the principle of the rule of law, not the whim of the ruler. Hammurabi invented and placed in stone the concept that no one is above the law.[2]

4.1. INTRODUCTION

In the early 1960s, Lon L. Fuller wrote that "Law is the enterprise of subjecting of human behavior to the governance of norms."[3] Law is an array of rules of human conduct—in the Anglo American system of law—that are enforced by the state. In the long run, rules of law survive if they remain in substantial accord with the community's concepts of justice.[4] Law has become an important component of public health intervention as well as occupational safety and health policy. Furthermore, occupational health involves a social dimension, the master-servant relationship between employer and employee, which presents unique conditions regarding exposure to hazards that involve the twin concepts of rights and duties.

Law is a complex matter, and its sources are many. One source is common law; another source is constitutional law, while a third is statutory law (laws enacted by law-making bodies, e.g., legislators, county commissioners). International law is based upon custom, or customary law, a form of common law that evolves through the courts. There are many categories of statutory law that apply to occupational safety and health. These categories include labor law, public health law, and environmental law. Under these laws, the regulatory approach predominates in the United States, and this approach has its own set of laws to govern the procedures that regulatory agencies must follow in fulfilling their statutory mandates. This set of laws is known as administrative law. Each of these sources of law is described in this chapter. At the base of these laws is common law, as shown in Figure 4-1.

The parliamentary system is an alternative to constitutional law, which is used in the United States where the president is elected by the people. The

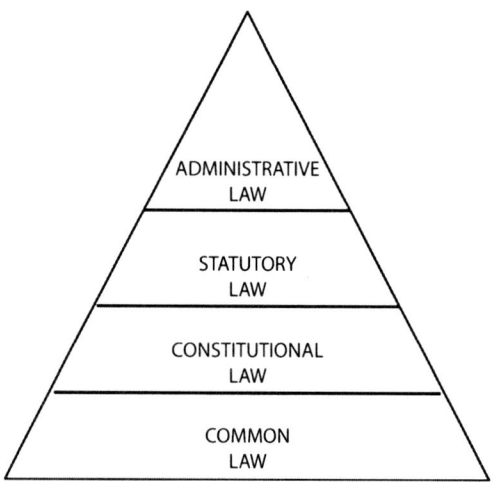

Note: International law as customary law falls under the rubric of common law.

Figure 4-1. Sources of law built on a foundation of common law.

parliament is a democratically elected law-making body, and it elects the prime minister and ministers of the government.

The term "civil law" is used in the United States to differentiate it from criminal law, which is prosecuted by the state to protect society from harm, while civil law involves resolving issues between citizens regarding rights. Criminal law can result in imprisoning the defendant, and civil law does not. The government can also act as a party in a civil case. The term "civil law" is also used as a general term for the Napoleonic Code, which is described further below.

4.2. COMMON LAW

Its roots strike deep into the soil of national ideas and institutions.
— Sir Carleton Kemp Allen[5]

One source of law in the United States is common law, a body of legal principles based upon judicial decisions rather than upon legislation.[6] Common law's obligation of duty of care is applicable to everyone to ensure that the outcome of one's actions or interactions does not affect others negatively. People have the right to expect and ensure an adequate level of control over those environmental factors that affect their state of health. Members of a community should have the right to drink safe water, breathe safe air, eat safe food, live in safe shelter, and have a safe workplace in which to earn an income and a safe community in which to live.[7] The common law method of adjudication—the doctrine of judicial precedent—is fundamental to the protection of rights and the prevention of arbitrary determinations.

When law is not based upon common law, it is described as civil law, and through custom it is called the Napoleonic Code. Most of the world uses civil law, while former British colonies typically use common law. Islamic law is another legal foundation used in some countries. The common law tradition is based upon the principle that one person should not be judged differently than another over time. The origin of civil law is ancient Roman law from which the Napoleonic Code was drawn. Civil law places more reliance on judges than on juries and on statutes rather than precedence. The state of Louisiana, for example, bases its legal system on civil law because of its Spanish and French history, whereas the rest of the United States has common law as its legal foundation. Quebec uses civil law for civil cases, but it goes along with the rest of Canada in using common law as the foundation for criminal cases.

The word "common law" is used in the present context to describe the body of legal principles and concepts that evolved over many centuries by judges in the English courts of law. At the start of the 20th century, common law was the existing recourse in the United States for dealing with occupational injuries.

4.2.1. Common Law Defenses

At the turn of the last century, the probability of death among U.S. railroad workers was staggering. One commentator of that era observed that "a brakeman's chances of dying a natural death in 1888 [was] 1 to 47," and the "average life expectancy of a switchman in 1893 [was] seven years."[8] The need for a fair and equitable system of workers' compensation evolved out of the Industrial Revolution. As economic and industrial activities flourished, the number of work injuries also grew. The increasing use of machinery, new concepts of producing goods, and the pressure of increased demand for products resulted in more injury problems without solutions for employers and employees. For the most part, workers who were injured on the job had no recourse other than to sue their employers at common law, an expensive and time-consuming process. The court system was crowded, causing long delays. Compensation for injuries was usually insufficient and uncertain. Employees sometimes were forced to bear the expense of injury or had to throw themselves on the mercy of welfare.

When suing under common law, employees had the burden to prove that their injuries were caused by employer negligence. Workers could be deterred from suing for several reasons. With the burden of proof on the worker, he or she had to show that (1) the employer was negligent, (2) the injury was work-related, and (3) the negligence caused the injury. In addition, the worker would need to shoulder the cost of hiring an attorney, and proving the case would likely involve the testimony of other workers, who along with the plaintiff could be easily fired. Moreover, employers had three strong defenses—effective in two-thirds of the cases brought—against negligence suits that were used when a judge determined by any one of the defenses that an employer be held not liable:[9]

1. The fellow-servant rule—A fellow employee's actions were found to have contributed the injury. This defense had its origin in an 1837 case in England where an injured employee brought suit against an employer for the "vicarious" act of a fellow servant who had overloaded a van that

broke down and threw the plaintiff to the ground with resulting injury. The judge held as absurd the holding of an employer liable for the actions of a fellow servant.[10]
2. Assumption of risk—Injuries were caused by common or unusual hazards about which the employees were aware. This assumption of risk was tied to the idea that employers owed no duty of care to their employees regarding recognized risks.[9]
3. Contributory negligence—The employees contributed to their own injuries in any way. This defense was less effective than the other two defenses, especially when a supervisor had ordered an employee to encounter a recognized risk or assured the employee that there was no danger.[9]

Civil liability in common law has its roots in the concept of trespass, wherein parties had to prove in the King's Court in England that they had sustained physical contact on their person or property as a result of the actions of another.[11] However, the modern tort law system in the United States emerged from a history of contract law that protected the producer of a dangerous product by the assumption of risk but moved to a doctrine of enterprise liability in the early 1960s. According to this doctrine—strict liability (see Chapter 13)—business enterprises were held responsible for the safety of products that they introduced into commerce because society would benefit by internalizing the costs to the manufacturer to encourage the prevention of or insurance against injuries.[12]

4.2.2. Employment-at-Will Doctrine

Prior to the advent of statutory law, employees who were injured on the job in the United States were only able to pursue their employer through civil or tort law. A tort is a negligent or intentional civil wrong not arising out of a contract or statute. In some countries like England, this was difficult due to the legal view of employment as a master-servant relationship. Proof of employer malice or negligence was usually required but difficult for an employee to attain. Although employers' liability was unlimited, courts usually awarded in favor of the employer and paid little attention to the full losses experienced by workers: medical costs, lost wages, and damages for loss of future earning capacity.

The employment-at-will doctrine is founded on English contract law, but the United States diverged from England in its application. In England, hiring a servant by a master was interpreted as a contract for at least a year through the four seasons. This interpretation assured a wage for the servant through productive months as well as the unproductive months that are no fault of the servant (e.g., during winter). This policy was extended beyond the agrarian environment to all work. Termination notice to a servant was held to be at least one month.[13]

In the United States, the employment-at-will doctrine was adapted to day laborers, for whom the contract was presumed to be hour-to-hour, and by 1870, reliance upon English law precedent was dissolved. The adoption of the doctrine in the United States, absent proof by the employees, was that the term of employment was indefinite and employment could be dissolved at any time at the will of either party. This departure followed the amendment to the U.S. Constitution that made involuntary servitude illegal; thus, an employee had the right to terminate employment at any time regardless of the contract.[13] Throughout the 20th century, this doctrine was not negated, but the courts found that it could be modified by state and federal action—principally arising from union activity.[14]

4.2.3. Law of Nations

While the Founding Fathers recognized in the Declaration of Independence that the new United States was to take its place among the nations by respecting the laws of nature, the role of the federal government regarding the law of nations fell to the courts. The Supreme Court found that since the United States took its place among the nations of the earth, it was answerable to the law of nations. In 1804, the court found that Congress should never violate the law of nations; treaties had the power of statutes under the law, and in the absence of a treaty, executive authority, or judicial decision, customary law among the nations must rule.[15]

Customary law is similar to common law (among nations), but it differs in one important way: Statutes do not negate it. Moreover, nations represent subordinate governments as one in relations with other nations or international organizations. In contemporary usage, "international law" has taken the place of the term "the law of nations." Customary law is the result of deliberations between nations, but in the modern global economy, deliberations are numerous between so many nations and happen quickly when compared with the past. Consensus is not quick and easy, but some human rights norms have achieved recognition as customary law, including no slavery or torture. Moreover, since World War II, starting with the Nuremberg Charter, the United States has successfully pressed for holding individuals culpable for human rights crimes. Nevertheless, the courts in the United States will rule on international law regardless of disagreements by either the executive or legislative branches of government.[16]

In the realm of international law, labor standards are a continually contentious area regarding global trade. Common international labor standards remain an important policy concern, and foremost among the issues is child labor, which has captured much attention.[17] And in the United States, the Alien Tort Statute of 1789 has been used by foreigners to bring tort suits against companies in the United States.[18]

4.3. THE CONSTITUTIONAL SYSTEM

Our Constitution works. We are a nation of laws, not men. Here the people rule.
—President Gerald R. Ford[19]

Another source of law is the U.S. Constitution. The framers of the Constitution established the federal system of government that distributes power among the national government and state governments. The Constitution provides for the delegation of specific powers to the national government; powers not delegated specifically to the federal government reside with the states. The states create local governments, including city and county or parish governments. This three-level system of federal, state, and local governments includes more than 80,000 units of government. The states have held a pivotal role in public health, for the Constitution fails to specify public health as a function of the federal government.[20,21] Table 4-1 shows this relationship of the three branches and three levels of government in the United States.

A chief justice of the King's Bench of England wrote a text published in 1714, *On the Governance of the Kingdom of England,* in which he described two types of rule. One type was rule by edict of the king, and the other type was the making of laws by the ruled through a parliament.[22] The latter type of rule is demanded in American society, which has bridled governmental action so as to not impinge upon individual freedoms. This societal demand has built a legacy of policy restraint in the United States, and its history can be divided

Table 4-1. Branches and Levels of Government in the U.S. Federal System

Level	Legislative	Executive	Judicial
National	Congress	President and administrative agencies	Supreme Court and other federal courts
State	State Legislature	Governor and administrative agencies	State courts
County or city	Council or commission	Mayor and administrative agencies	County or city courts

Note: The branches and levels of government interact horizontally and vertically in fulfilling their functions.

into four eras as listed below—a testament to the flexibility and stability of the U.S. constitutional system:[23]

- A period of divided power (1787–1870) in which power was divided between the states and the national government yet with strong limits on the national government.
- An era of state activism (1870s–1933) when the country experienced a shift from an agrarian to an industrial economy, and states exercised control over monopolies, diseases, mass uprisings, labor strife, and industrial disasters. The national government followed the tenets of laissez-faire economics in which it allowed states and individuals to conduct business without government intrusion.
- An era of national activism (1933–1961) when demands were placed upon the national government by the Great Depression, and the national government created the modern system of regulatory bodies, public support systems such as Social Security and the GI Bill, and Cold War initiatives such as the space program and the interstate highway system.
- An era of national standards (1961–present) inaugurated by the civil rights movement and continuing to deal with poverty, pollution, highway deaths, and workplace safety—all driven by the national government establishing standards in the pursuit of national goals.

Drafted in secret by delegates to the Constitutional Convention during summer 1787, the four-page Constitution, signed on September 17, 1787, established the government of the United States. The framers of the Constitution created a strong federal government resting on the concept of "separation of powers." This concept provided for checks and balances between three branches of government: the legislative, executive, and judicial, which is a key feature of the U.S. government's success. The preamble to the Constitution of the United States follows:[24]

> We the people of the United States, in order to form a more perfect union, establish justice, insure domestic tranquility, provide for the common defense, promote the general welfare, and secure the blessings of liberty to ourselves and our posterity, do ordain and establish this Constitution for the United States of America.

The Constitution grants powers to the federal government, but the government's powers cannot go beyond what is provided in the Constitution. Thus, any federal law that applies to the protection of workers from hazards, for example, must be justified by the Constitution.

4.3.1. Legislative Branch

Article I of the Constitution created the legislative branch to make laws.[25] The legislative branch of the federal government is the Congress, which is divided into two chambers: the Senate and the House of Representatives. Each member of Congress is elected by the people of his or her state. The creation of these two chambers provides for further checks and balances between immediate concerns expressed in the House and longer-term concerns expressed in the Senate.

The Senate is composed of 100 members, two from each state. The term of office is six years, and one-third of the total membership of the Senate is elected every second year. The terms of both senators from a state do not terminate at the same time. Each senator has one vote.[25]

The House of Representatives is composed of 435 members elected every two years from among the 50 states, apportioned to their total populations. The Constitution requires that "as nearly as is practicable one man's vote in a congressional election is to be worth as much as another's." Each representative has one vote.[25]

Each house of Congress comprises committees that are responsible for authoring new or amended legislation and conducting oversight of the agencies responsible for implementing the legislation. Each house also has an appropriations committee with subcommittees responsible for funding agencies authorized under federal statutes. Table 4-2 lists the authorizing committees and

Table 4-2. Authorizing and Appropriations Committees With Jurisdiction Over the Occupational Safety and Health Act

Committee Role	House of Representatives	Senate
Authorizing and oversight	Subcommittee on Workforce Protections, Committee on Education and the Workforce	Subcommittee on Employment and Workplace Safety, and Subcommittee on Bioterrorism Preparedness and Public Health Committee on Health, Education, Labor, and Pensions
Appropriations	Subcommittee on Labor, Health and Human Services Education, and Related Agencies	Subcommittee on Labor Health and Human Services, Education, and Related Agencies

Source: U.S. Congress.[26]

subcommittees and appropriations subcommittees that have jurisdiction over the Occupational Safety and Health Act (OSH Act; see Appendix) and its associated agencies: the Occupational Safety and Health Administration (OSHA) and the National Institute for Occupational Safety and Health (NIOSH).[26] When a bill is passed in one house, it also needs a companion bill in the other house to be passed as well. To resolve conflicts between the two bills, a conference committee is created that negotiates on the differences. The conferees make their recommendations to both houses for a final vote.[25] Congress appropriates funds annually by fiscal year, which is October through September.

The U.S. Government Accountability Office (GAO) is an independent, nonpartisan agency that works for Congress. The office investigates how the federal government spends taxpayer dollars and gathers information to help Congress determine how well executive branch agencies are doing their jobs. In its work, GAO routinely answers questions such as whether government programs are meeting their objectives or providing good service to the public. The office provides senators and representatives with materials to inform their policy decisions for improved accountability to the American people. The following is an example of the report titles resulting from GAO investigations:

- *Black Lung Benefits Program: Administrative and Structural Changes Could Improve Miners' Ability to Pursue Claims.* Washington, DC: U.S. Government Accountability Office;2009. GAO-10-7.
- *OSHA Worksite Safety and Health Programs Show Promise.* Washington, DC: U.S. Government Accountability Office;1992. HRD-92-68.

- *OSHA Action Needed to Improve Compliance With Hazard Communication Standard.* Washington, DC: U.S. Government Accountability Office; 1991. HRD-92-8.
- *OSHA Policy Changes Needed to Confirm That Employers Abate Serious Hazards.* Washington, DC: U.S. Government Accountability Office;1991. HRD-91-35.
- *OSHA Assuring Accuracy in Employer Injury and Illness Records.* Washington, DC: U.S. Government Accountability Office;1988. HRD-89-23.
- *Coast Guard and Interior Could Improve Their Offshore Energy Inspection Programs.* Washington, DC: U.S. Government Accountability Office;2011. GAO-12-203T.
- *Workplace Safety and Health: Multiple Challenges Lengthen OSHA's Standard-Setting.* Washington, DC: U.S. Government Accountability Office;2012. GAO-12-330.

During its 23-year history, the congressional Office of Technology Assessment (OTA) provided congressional members and committees with objective and authoritative analysis of the complex scientific and technical issues of the late 20th century. It was a leader in practicing and encouraging delivery of public services in innovative and inexpensive ways, including distribution of government documents through electronic publishing. The OTA closed on September 29, 1995. During its existence, the OTA produced the following reports related to occupational safety and health:[27]

- *Preventing Illness and Injury in the Workplace.* Washington, DC: U.S. Congress, Office of Technology Assessment;1985.
- *Reproductive Health Hazards in the Workplace: Selected Aspects of Reproductive Health Hazards Regulations.* Washington, DC: U.S. Congress, Office of Technology Assessment;1985.
- *Reproductive Health Hazards in the Workplace.* Washington, DC: U.S. Congress, Office of Technology Assessment;1985.
- *Passive Smoking in the Workplace: Selected Issues.* Washington, DC: U.S. Congress, Office of Technology Assessment;1986.
- *Gauging Control Technology and Regulatory Impacts in Occupational Safety and Health: An Appraisal of OSHA's Analytic Approach.* Washington, DC: U.S. Congress, Office of Technology Assessment;1995.

4.3.2. Executive Branch

Every bill passed by Congress is presented to the president. The bill becomes law either if the president signs it or, without signing it, does not return the bill within 10 days. The president can veto a bill, which does not become law unless a two-thirds affirmative vote is made in each house to pass the bill, which overrides the president's veto.[25]

The power of the executive branch is vested in the president, who also serves as commander-in-chief of the armed forces and the principal officer of the executive branch. The president appoints the cabinet and oversees the various agencies and departments of the federal government including OSHA and NIOSH, respectively, located in the cabinet-level Departments of Labor and Health and Human Services. To qualify to become president, a candidate must be a natural-born citizen of the United States, be at least 35 years old, and have resided in the United States for at least 14 years. Once elected, the president serves a term of four years and may be re-elected once, but no more. The president also appoints federal judges with the advice and consent of the Senate.

Within the Executive Office of the president, the Office of Management and Budget (OMB) assists the president in overseeing the preparation of the federal budget and supervising its administration in executive branch agencies. OMB ensures that agency reports, rules, testimony, and proposed legislation are consistent with the president's budget and with administration policies.

The president, a governor, or some administrative authority such as county and city executives issues executive orders as a rule or regulation that has the force of law. The chief executive uses executive orders to implement and give administrative effect to the Constitution or statutes. These orders may create or modify organizations or procedures within administrative agencies.[21]

The centralized review of draft regulations has been accepted since President Nixon's "Quality of Life" review—established by a 1971 memorandum from Director George Shultz of OMB to executive department heads—as the first mechanism to require agencies to conduct cost-benefit analyses of proposed rules and to submit their regulations to OMB prior to their publication in the *Federal Register*. This policy was established as a result of business complaints regarding fear of U.S. Environmental Protection Agency (EPA) regulations under the Clean Air Act.[28] Cost-benefit analysis was first used during the 1930s to guide flood control efforts and during the 1960s for defense planning

Table 4-3. Executive Orders That Placed Controls on Regulatory Agencies

President	Executive Order	Requirement
Ford	No. 11821 in 1974, No. 11949 in 1977	Prepare inflation/economic impact statements
Carter	No. 12044 in 1978	Improving government regulations: cost-impact analyses, elimination of unnecessary regulation, and regulatory analyses
Reagan	No. 12291 in 1981	Regulatory impact analysis: show that the benefits of the regulation outweigh the costs
	No. 12498 in 1986	Regulatory planning process: publish upcoming regulation list after paperwork reduction review
Clinton	No. 12866 in 1993	Regulatory planning and review: show that the benefits of the regulation justify the costs; assess both the costs and the benefits of the intended regulation, recognize that some costs and benefits are difficult to quantify, propose or adopt a regulation only upon a reasoned determination that the benefits of the intended regulation justify its costs
Bush	No. 13272 in 2002	*Proper Consideration of Small Entities in Agency Rulemaking*: consider the potential impact of rules on small businesses, governmental jurisdictions, and organizations during rule development
Obama	No. 13563 in 2011, No. 13579 in 2011	*Improving Regulation and Regulatory Review and Regulation* and *Independent Regulatory Agencies*: Facilitate the periodic review of existing significant regulations: promote retrospective analysis of rules that may be outmoded, ineffective, insufficient, or excessively burdensome, and modify, streamline, expand, or repeal them

Source: National Archives.[29]
Note: Executive orders are official documents and are numbered consecutively.

and budgeting. Such policies continued as presidents issued executive orders to provide operational guidance to executive agencies, as shown in Table 4-3.[29]

Since the early 1980s, OMB has performed an extensive review of new OSHA standards, often sending them back to the agency for additional documentation. OMB has an important role to play in assessing the overall burden of a new standard and ensuring regulatory consistency between different federal agencies. However, a 1993 study of OSHA by the Administrative Conference of the United States strongly criticized "the tendency of OMB economists to range beyond their technical competence," and stated that "OMB's constant interventions have made a slow OSHA decision-making process even slower."[30]

4.3.3. Judicial Branch

The Constitution provides that the judicial power of the United States shall be vested in one Supreme Court and in such inferior Courts as the Congress may from time to time ordain and establish. The Supreme Court was organized on February 2, 1790. Congress has "conferred upon the Supreme Court power to prescribe rules of procedure to be followed by the lower courts of the United States."[25] As an example, courts are obligated to two types of judicial notice. One type of notice is "matter of fact," meaning a matter of common knowledge requiring no proof (e.g., the sun rises every morning), and the other type is "matter of law," which is what the court administers (e.g., a state court would take notice of the U.S. government).

Power to nominate the justices is vested in the president, and appointments are made with the advice and consent of the Senate. Appointees to the federal bench serve for life. The number of justices is determined by Congress rather than the Constitution, and since 1869, the Supreme Court has been composed of one chief justice and eight associate justices. The Supreme Court hears cases that may begin in the federal or state courts, and they usually involve important questions about the Constitution or federal law.[14]

Judicial interpretations are important in policy formulations. These interpretations deal with many issues including agency jurisdiction, constitutional authority, inconsistencies in the law, and the application of the law. Judicial interpretations of particular statutes affect occupational safety and health legislation including environmental (e.g., the Toxic Substances Control Act [TSCA] of 1976), labor, and civil rights laws. Statutory inclusion of public access to law through the courts is provided for in the OSHAct.[14]

Federal courts can get involved in occupational safety and health litigation in several ways. An employer can bring a case to a court of appeals after a ruling of the Occupational Safety and Health Review Commission (OSHRC). In addition, under Section 6(d) of the OSHAct, any person with standing (affected or harmed by) can challenge a rule by OSHA within 60 days after its promulgation. The government can bring criminal charges against an employer under Section 17 of the OSHAct.[14]

The judicial time line is important, for a previous case becomes a precedent for later cases. Cases come to the Supreme Court on appeal as a writ of certiorari, which the high court can either accept or deny. Certiorari means a proceeding in which a losing party files a writ with the Supreme Court asking it to review the decision of a lower court.[14]

In court cases, the name of the case is based on the plaintiff's name first, followed by the defendant's name. The conjunction between the plaintiff's and defendant's names is "versus" (v). In an appeal, the names may be reversed if the defendant in the original case becomes the plaintiff.

The court of appeals for the federal circuit is organized into 12 regional circuits plus the District of Columbia Circuit Court and has nationwide jurisdiction to hear appeals in specialized cases. A court of appeals hears appeals from the district courts located within its circuit, as well as appeals from decisions of federal administrative agencies. In addition, the court of appeals for the federal circuit has nationwide jurisdiction to hear appeals in specialized cases, such as those involving international trade.[14]

The district courts are the trial courts of the federal court system. They have jurisdiction to hear federal cases, including both civil and criminal matters. There are 94 federal judicial districts, including at least one district in each state, the District of Columbia, and Puerto Rico. Three territories of the United States—the Virgin Islands, Guam, and the Northern Mariana Islands—have district courts that hear federal cases. Every day hundreds of people across the nation are selected for jury duty and help decide some of these cases.[14]

4.4. STATUTORY LAW

Congress is empowered to enact statutes (e.g., the OSHAct). Statutory (law-making) authorities have a legal and binding duty to control those factors posing an unacceptable risk to the community, which can override the common laws established by judges.[31] Historically, the courts have provided wide latitude for statutory authority to protect the public health. For example, statutes have authorized the control of white phosphorus match production using the tax authority of the Constitution, extended workday restrictions to the protection of children and women in certain occupations or underground mines, and made it possible for public health officials to exercise extensive police powers, principally regarding communicable diseases such as smallpox, tuberculosis, zoonotic diseases, and food-borne diseases.[4]

4.5. ADMINISTRATIVE LAW

Administrative law is established by statute: The Administrative Procedures Act (APA) of 1946 governs the way that administrative agencies make and implement decisions.[14] These decisions, as they affect the public, are regulations.

Typically, the legislative branch creates administrative agencies, the executive branch manages the agencies, and the judicial branch vets and interprets the actions of the agencies as cases arise based either on the Constitution or a statute and its legislative history.

An originating statute (enabling legislation) gives an agency a substantive mandate that may provide the administrative procedure for the agency. When the substantive mandate provides for regulatory procedure, it takes precedence over the APA—which is the case with both the OSHAct and the Federal Mine Safety and Health Act of 1977 (Mine Act). If the substantive mandate lacks these procedures, then compliance with the APA is required.[14]

4.5.1. Administrative Procedures Act of 1946

In 1946, Congress passed the APA, which provides due process requirements for all federal actions. The APA applies to any federal agency that engages in rule making and, when the agency is so doing, it must publish a general notice of proposed rule making in the *Federal Register*. APA provides procedures for formal and informal rule making as described in Table 4-4. Formal rule making is rare and occurs primarily if a statute requires it. The OSHAct provides procedures for

Table 4-4. Formal and Informal Rulemaking Under the Administrative Procedure Act and Hybrid Rulemaking Under the Occupational Safety and Health Act

Formal Rulemaking	Hybrid Rulemaking	Informal Rulemaking
• Only if specified by Congress • Trial-type hearing • Evidence presented • Cross-examination of witnesses • Decision made on the record • Verbatim record made • Agency action must be supported by substantial evidence as a whole	• Informal notice and comment • No trial-type hearing required • Agency action must be supported by substantial evidence as a whole • Informal public hearing • Cross-examining of witnesses* • Advisory committees can provide input but do not supplant the agency's power	• To be used unless specified otherwise by the statute • Called notice and comment rulemaking • Give notice of opportunity for comment in the Federal Register • Give opportunity for interested parties to submit data, views, or arguments in writing or orally • No hearing required • Information outside of the record can be considered • Cannot be arbitrary or capricious

Source: Ashford et al.[14]
*Not required by the OSHAct but provided by the Occupational Safety and Health Administration as a matter of policy; however, the Toxic Substances Control Act, for example, requires cross-examination.

rule making, shown in Table 4-4 as "hybrid rule-making," a blend of formal and informal rule making.[14] The APA also requires that all federal executive orders be published in the *Federal Register*.[21] When a statute prescribes a procedure for rule making, it supersedes the procedures required in the APA.

4.5.2. Administrative Law Judges

Federal administrative law judges (ALJs) are certified by the Office of Personnel Management and appointed by the president at the federal level. These judges, at either the state or federal level, ensure that citizens have fair, impartial, and independent opportunities to be heard before a state or federal agency acts against them. They preside over hearings, determine facts, and issue a decision while providing a neutral, fair forum and prompt and objective hearings for any person affected by the actions of any state or federal administrative agency. The authority of an ALJ is functionally comparable to a judge. These judges can issue subpoenas, rule on evidence, examine the facts of a case, apply law, and recommend or make decisions regarding a case. Their findings are often preliminary and are sent out for review. Every state and the District of Columbia have ALJs, though their number and frequency of use vary.

The OSHAct and the Mine Act provide for the OSHRC and the Mine Safety and Health Review Commission, respectively. These commissions can appoint ALJs independent from the U.S. Department of Labor (DoL), where OSHA and the Mine Safety and Health Administration (MSHA) are located.

4.5.3. Other U.S. Administrative Law Acts

Administrative laws over the years have placed requirements on federal agencies to follow specified procedures. Additional administrative laws are described below and are summarized in Table 4-5.

4.5.4. Freedom of Information Act of 1966

Like all federal agencies, OSHA is required under the Freedom of Information Act (FOIA) to disclose records requested in writing by any person. However, agencies may withhold information pursuant to nine exemptions and three exclusions contained in the statute. FOIA applies only to federal agencies and does not create a right of access to records held by Congress, the courts, or state

Table 4-5. Administrative Laws Enacted in the United States

Administrative Act	Responsibilities of Federal Agencies
Administrative Procedures Act of 1946	Provides due process requirements for all federal regulatory actions.
Freedom of Information Act of 1966	Requires disclosure of records requested in writing by any person.
National Environmental Policy Act of 1969	Requires preparation of environmental impact statements when the agency's actions significantly affect the quality of the human environment.
Federal Advisory Committee Act of 1973	Requires a charter for each advisory committee and that it meet in public.
Regulatory Flexibility Act of 1980	Requires publication of a notice of proposed rule making and its availability for public comment; a regulatory flexibility analysis must describe the impact of the proposed rule on small entities.
Negotiated Rulemaking Act of 1990	Can choose to use negotiated rule making for informal rule making through a negotiated rule-making committee that derives consensus on the wording of a proposed rule.
Paperwork Reduction Act of 1995	Requires OMB approval before requesting most types of information from the public.
Unfunded Mandates Reform Act of 1995	Curbs the practice of imposing unfunded 68 federal mandates on states and local governments.
Congressional Review Act of 1996	Before a rule can take effect, it must be submitted to each house of Congress and to the Comptroller General, upon which 60 days later the rule takes effect unless overridden by congressional action.
Small Business Regulatory Enforcement Fairness Act of 1996	Requires a regulatory flexibility analysis when a final rule will have a significant impact on a substantial number of small entities.
Government Paperwork Elimination Act of 1998	Must give the option to submit required information electronically, when practicable, to the government.
Information Quality Act of 2000	Requires data quality to maximize the quality, objectivity, utility, and integrity of information prior to dissemination; allows affected individuals to seek and obtain correction of information; and requires reporting the number and nature of complaints received regarding agency compliance to OMB.

Note: OMB = Office of Management and Budget.

or local governmental agencies.[32] Each state has its own public access laws that should be consulted for access to state and local records. The FOIA mandates that every federal agency maintain a FOIA web page.

4.5.5. National Environmental Policy Act of 1969

The National Environmental Policy Act[32a] requires that environmental impact statements (EISs) be prepared by any federal agency when its action would significantly affect the quality of the human environment. This requirement applies to safety and health standards promulgated by OSHA, which must make an initial determination as to whether a statement is required. For example, OSHA has issued an EIS on its Standard on Coke Oven Emissions.[33] If the Council on Environmental Quality recommends that a statement be made, but OSHA disagrees, then a statement of reasons must be presented to the public for comment.

4.5.6. Federal Advisory Committee Act of 1973

The Federal Advisory Committee Act (FACA) established uniform standards for committees, boards, and other groups of nongovernment professionals that provide advice to the executive branch. At the time there were as many as 5,000 committees, and concerns were raised that many of them were acting without sufficient review, supervision, or accountability. FACA set up basic rules, including that each committee must have a charter and meet in public.[34] OSHA is authorized to appoint ad hoc advisory committees in developing specific workplace regulations.

4.5.7. Regulatory Flexibility Act of 1980

The Regulatory Flexibility Act requires an agency to publish a general notice of proposed rule making for any anticipated rule and prepare and make available for public comment an initial regulatory flexibility analysis. This analysis must describe the impact of the proposed rule on small entities. Prior to 1980, American small businesses were forced to adhere to the same regulations as far larger companies, even though they did not have nearly the same resources to bring to bear to comply with the rules.[35] Entrepreneurs and directors of nonprofit organizations had charged that when regulations put forth by EPA, OSHA, and other agencies were applied evenly, without regard to the size of the enterprises affected, they sometimes did serious damage to smaller organizations. Such regulations had to do with taxes, workplace safety, and the environment, among other issues.

4.5.8. Negotiated Rulemaking Act of 1990

In 1990, Congress amended the APA with the Negotiated Rulemaking Act with procedures for an agency to follow if it chooses to use negotiated rule making for informal rule making. In the public interest, an agency can decide whether to proceed with negotiated rule making. If an agency does choose to proceed, it first must identify interests that would be significantly affected by a proposed rule for which a negotiated rule making committee that represents these interests plus a representative of the federal agency is established. The task for the committee is to derive consensus on the wording of such a proposed rule.[14] As an example, OSHA used the negotiated rule making process and convened the Cranes and Derricks Negotiated Rulemaking Advisory Committee, about which John Henshaw, assistant secretary of labor for Occupational Safety and Health, said in 2004, "The members of this committee were tasked with a formidable challenge—to develop and reach consensus on a revised cranes and derricks standard in one year—and they achieved that ambitious task."[36]

4.5.9. Paperwork Reduction Act of 1995

The Paperwork Reduction Act requires agencies to obtain OMB approval before requesting most types of information from the public. The focus of this act is to limit the redundancy in the federal government's collection of information from the public.

4.5.10. Unfunded Mandates Reform Act of 1995

This act discourages the federal government from imposing mandates on state, local, and tribal governments or the private sector without paying the costs of those mandates by increasing the amount of information available to Congress and the executive branch agencies about the impact of the mandates. It encourages policy makers to take that information into account when developing laws and regulations.

4.5.11. Congressional Review Act of 1996

This act provides that before a rule can take effect, the federal agency that is promulgating a "major" rule must submit a report to each house of Congress and to the Comptroller General. A major rule is defined as one that will result in $100 million or more of an economic impact. After Congress receives the report, the rule takes effect unless Congress passes a joint resolution of disapproval within

60 days. If a rule is disapproved by a joint resolution of Congress, the agency cannot propose new, similar standards unless authorized to do so by Congress.[37] The OSHA Ergonomics Standard was terminated by this procedure in 2001.

4.5.12. Small Business Regulatory Enforcement Fairness Act of 1996

The Small Business Regulatory Enforcement Fairness Act was designed to create a more cooperative regulatory environment between agencies and small businesses. It provides for the development of a Regulatory Fairness (RegFair) Program by agencies whose enforcement and compliance activities impact small businesses, and it furnishes a mechanism through which small businesses may comment on the enforcement and compliance activities of the federal agencies that regulate them.

4.5.13. Government Paperwork Elimination Act of 1998

The focus of this act is to promote electronic submission of information to the government. Under this act, persons required to submit information to the government, or maintain governmental information, must be given the option to do so electronically when practicable.

4.5.14. Information Quality Act of 2000

The Information Quality Act (IQA) was passed as a two-sentence rider that was concealed in the Treasury and General Government Appropriations Act for fiscal year 2000 with neither hearings nor recorded debate on the law. It requires OMB to issue data quality guidelines to federal agencies by September 30, 2001. All agencies subject to the IQA are required to establish and follow data quality guidelines that ensure and maximize the quality, objectivity, utility, and integrity of information including statistical information prior to dissemination; to allow affected individuals and/or organizations to seek and obtain the correction of information maintained and disseminated by the agency; and to report to OMB regarding the number and nature of complaints received by the agency regarding compliance with OMB guidelines.[38]

The IQA is clearly a covert strategy aimed at delaying agency decision making or limiting public awareness of an issue that potentially affects public or environmental health. It raises the level of uncertainty about science by placing a high burden of proof on the government with no burden in making the claim. Such barriers for governmental action, including warnings to the public, have been referred to as "paralysis by analysis."[39] Two examples of the results of this strategy that impact worker safety and health follow.[40]

- With no disclosed client, the law firm Morgan, Lewis, and Bockius filed an IQA petition on August 19, 2003, with EPA, challenging its 1986 publication "Guidance for Preventing Asbestos Disease Among Auto Mechanics."[40] The law firm claimed that the publication, known as EPA's Gold Book, failed to comply with EPA's data quality standards of "objectivity" and "utility" because it relied on inadequate and inappropriate data; was outdated; contradictory studies had since been published; and verification of its origins, preparations, funding, review, and approval were unknown or not possible. The 1986 Gold Book began with the phrase "preventing asbestos disease among auto mechanics," indicating to readers that its foremost purpose was disease prevention. EPA's response approved most of the petition, explaining that a new brochure would be available in spring 2004 for public comment, but until that time, EPA would add a note to the Gold Book explaining that the material was being updated. Even though NIOSH, in collaboration with EPA, issued a report in 1989 on the industrial hygiene practices used to control workers' exposure to asbestos during vehicle brake drum service, few peer-reviewed articles were published on the specific population of brake drum workers, since overwhelming evidence had already shown that asbestos was a known carcinogen among factory and construction workers. This is an example of where "matter of law" overrules "matter of fact." In effect, like regulations, public information strategies can be channeled into a quasi-rule-making process. Indeed, regarding this issue, David Michaels (the current OSHA administrator) and Celeste Monforton wrote in 2007, "The risk of disease in humans associated with asbestos exposure has already been demonstrated, confirmed and reconfirmed in many and varied occupations and industries."[40]
- A coalition of mining companies and trade associations appears to have used the IQA to derail an MSHA proposed rule published September 7, 2005, that would protect miners from harmful particulate matter in diesel exhaust. The challenge did not raise actual objections to data quality;

instead, it couched industry's disagreements with the rule in data quality language. However, the tactic appears to have succeeded in impelling the agency to publish a modification to the rule that weakens the mine worker protections. Meanwhile, NIOSH has determined that diesel exhaust is a potential human carcinogen. In addition, acute exposures to diesel exhaust have been linked to health problems such as eye and nose irritation, headaches, nausea, and asthma.[41]

4.6. REGULATIONS

In the occupational safety and health arena, regulations protect workers from risks by intervening in work environments where occupational health may be at risk. The rudiments of regulation can be understood from the field of cybernetics, which deals with the regulation of systems as shown in Figure 4-2.[42] Cybernetics regulates the complexity involved with occupational safety and health by creating a negative feedback loop to restrain unsafe actions and environments.

"Regulation" is a term used in cybernetics that assures that a system does not go out of control and stays within acceptable limits. However, in society, regulations are creatures of law and more specifically, creations from legislation. Regulatory agencies are relatively recent phenomena of law to deal with the complexity of economic activity that exceeds the legislative body's ability to cope. Regulators bring their knowledge, experience, and expertise to bear on complex problems that overwhelm the diffuse and larger ambit of the legislative process. Regulations carry the force of law and are promulgated to protect the public against hazards, while the regulators' discretion is limited by the power of the legislature and the courts.[43]

When a federal agency promulgates a proposed or final regulation, it is published in the *Federal Register*. A final regulation is then published in the *Code of Federal Regulations* as part of the body of the law of the land.[14]

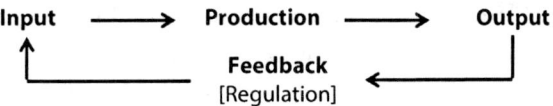

Figure 4-2. A cybernetic flowchart regarding the function of regulation.

4.7. A WORD ABOUT PERSONS AND TRANSNATIONAL LAW

Corporations have been enthroned and an era of corruption in high places will follow, and the money power of the country will endeavor to prolong its reign by working upon the prejudices of the people until all wealth is aggregated in a few hands and the Republic is destroyed.

—Abraham Lincoln[44]

A corporation is an artificial being, invisible, intangible. It possesses only those properties which the charter of its creation confers upon it.

—Chief Justice John Marshall[45]

[A corporation is] *a collection of many individuals united into one body, under a special denomination, having perpetual succession under an artificial form, and vested, by policy of the law, with the capacity of acting, in several respects, as an individual.*

—Stewart Kyd[46]

A characteristic of governments is sovereign immunity, whereby governments cannot be sued for damages. In the United States, the federal government forfeited sovereign immunity when Congress enacted the Federal Tort Claims Act of 1946 that provided rights for an individual to sue the government under common law. However, the federal and state governments can place exceptions on such cases such as lack of performance (e.g., omissions by OSHA compliance officers). From an international perspective, Congress had previously enacted the Alien Tort Claims Act of 1789 that allowed aliens to sue "individuals" in federal court for violations of international laws or treaties of the United States. The law was passed originally regarding the protection of foreign diplomats in the United States and piracy at sea but lay dormant until 1979. It had the potential for application to individuals for human rights violations that could be construed to apply to workers.[47]

In 2012, the Supreme Court heard argument on the legal issue as to whether the Alien Tort Claims Act (in conjunction with the Torture Victim Protection Act of 1991) permitted corporations and other organizations (as opposed to "individuals," as named in the laws) to be held liable for aiding and abetting violations of international law. Plaintiffs compared the term "individual" to the term "person," which the Supreme Court had read to extend legal rights to corporations. The court found that Congress intended only to hold flesh-and-blood torturers liable, not the organizations or corporations to which they belonged. In its finding for the defendant, the court determined that "person" has often been recognized to have a broader meaning in the law than "individual."[47] Indeed, the OSHAct defines "person" as one or more individuals, partnerships, associations, corporations, business trusts, or legal representatives, or any organized group of persons.[48]

The Supreme Court took another direction in 2013, by holding in a 9-0 decision that the Alien Tort Claims Act is presumed not to apply to conduct in foreign countries, such that noncitizens are not authorized to sue "individuals" in U.S. courts over violations of international law for wrongs committed overseas. The court was concerned that affirming such liability would make U.S. courts a magnet for aggrieved foreign plaintiffs bringing claims for acts unrelated to the United States and could invite foreign courts to encourage judging U.S. corporations for actions outside U.S. borders.[48]

As the world has become increasingly global in its political economy, transnational corporations play an ever larger role in international occupational safety and health and the law. Corporations are sanctioned by the state. For centuries, the law considered corporations as beings separate from human beings, including their owners. However, they shared some human attributes such as making contracts and owning property. Their legal powers traditionally were limited to specific functions spelled out in their charters. Then a court reporter recorded Chief Justice Morrison Waite's instructions to attorneys in the case of *Southern Pacific Railroad v. State of California* to skip over the 14th Amendment, stating that "The court does not wish to hear argument on the question whether the provision in the Fourteenth Amendment to the Constitution, which forbids a State to deny to any person within its jurisdiction the equal protection of the laws, applies to these corporations. We are all of the opinion that it does." This statement, made in 1886 during the Industrial Revolution, was meant to shield business activity from taxes, regulation, and legislative initiatives.[49]

Justice Sonia Sotomayor recently commented on corporation rights under the First Amendment regarding political spending limits that judges had "created corporations as persons. There could be an argument made that that was the court's error to start with a creature of the state with human characteristics." Conversely, Justice Anthony Kennedy stated, "Corporations have lots of knowledge about environment, transportation issues, and you are silencing them during the election." Nonetheless, Justice Ruth Bader

Ginsburg, evoking the Declaration of Independence, stated, "A corporation, after all, is not endowed by its creator with inalienable rights."[49] In a 1928 case, the Supreme Court struck down a Pennsylvania tax on corporations because taxicab drivers were exempt from the tax—the court ruled and Justice Pierce Butler opined that corporations get the same protection as natural persons. However, in 1973, Justice William O. Douglas challenged the Butler opinion as "a relic" that second-guessed the legislature's decision to tax corporations differently than humans. Today corporate rights are in a state of confusion, augmented by then–Associate Justice William Rehnquist's dissenting opinion in 1979 regarding a Massachusetts law to restrict corporate spending on referendums because corporations benefit from related legal or tax benefits. He stated that "it might reasonably be concluded that those properties, so beneficial in the economic sphere, pose dangers in the political sphere."[49]

In 2008, the Organisation for Economic Co-operation and Development established a code of conduct and guidelines for multinational companies. This code created a set of standards for business conduct in a variety of areas including employment and industrial relations, human rights, and the environment. The code included the following verbatim standards selected from a list in a section entitled "Employment and Industrial Relations":[50]

- Respect the right of their employees to be represented by trade unions and other bona fide representatives of employees, and engage in constructive negotiations, either individually or through employers' associations, with such representatives with a view to reaching agreements on employment conditions.
- Contribute to the effective abolition of child labor and the elimination of all forms of forced or compulsory labor.
- Observe standards of employment and industrial relations not less favorable than those observed by comparable employers in the host country.
- Take adequate steps to ensure occupational health and safety in their operations.
- Consistent with the scientific and technical understanding of the risks, where there are threats of serious damage to the environment, taking also into account human health and safety, not use the lack of full scientific certainty as a reason for postponing cost-effective measures to prevent or minimize such damage.

THE PHOSPHORUS NECROSIS NARRATIVE

Diseases that have been eradicated by worldwide action are rare. Rarer still are examples of occupational diseases that have been eradicated. Phosphorus necrosis, also known as "phossy jaw," was associated with the manufacture of matches during the late 19th century. Phossy jaw, or necrosis of the bone, was caused by toxic fumes from phosphorus. The whole side of the face would turn green and then black, discharging foul-smelling pus and resulting in eventual death. International action to overcome this disease was seen as necessary so that one nation would not have a competitive cost advantage over another resulting from the elimination of white phosphorus in the manufacture of matches but with safer yet higher-priced matches. In the United States, the tax power of the federal government was used as the control measure. Following passage of the White Phosphorus Matches Prohibition Act of 1912 by Congress, the United States joined other nations in eliminating the dreaded disease from its population.[51]

Two decades earlier, the Salvation Army in England was particularly concerned about women making matches. Not only were these women earning very little for working a 16-hour day, but they were also risking their health when they dipped their match heads in the phosphorus supplied by manufacturers such as Bryant & May. A large number of these women suffered from phossy jaw.

In 1891, the Salvation Army opened its own match factory in Old Ford, East London. Only using harmless red phosphorus, the workers were soon producing six million boxes a year. In addition, the Salvation Army paid its employees twice the amount that Bryant & May paid its workers. Salvation Army creator William Booth organized conducted tours for members of Parliament and journalists around this "model" factory (see Chapter 5).[52,53]

In the United States, President William Howard Taft recommended a tax on the use of white phosphorus in the manufacture of matches in a 1910 message to Congress.[54] Representative John J. Esch (R) of Wisconsin introduced the bill on June 3, 1910.[55] The "Esch Act" established a prohibitive tax on each box of matches made with white phosphorus;[56] white phosphorus matches then ceased to exist, as did phossy jaw. The feasibility for eradicating this exposure was enhanced by the availability of an innocuous substitute, sesquisulfide. The Diamond Match Company held the patent to this substitute and agreed to assign its patent to three trustees: Professor E.R.A. Seligman of Columbia University, Attorney Jackson Ralston of the American Federation of Labor, and Commissioner Charles P. Neill of the U.S. Bureau of Labor, a predecessor agency to the DoL. At the request of these trustees and with the concurrence of President Taft, the owners cancelled the patent to "allay suspicion of monopoly" so that any manufacturer could produce sesquisulfide. The trust held that universal use of this substitute was necessary "in order that phossy jaw might be abolished." Furthermore, the USPHS, then a component of the Treasury Department, was responsible for inspecting match factories for any remaining use of white phosphorus.[51]

REFERENCES

1. George RP. What is law? A century of arguments. *First Things*. 2001;112: 23–29.

2. Fears JR. *The World Was Never the Same: Events That Changed the World.* Chantilly, VA: The Teaching Company;2010. The Great Courses, Course No. 3890.

3. Fuller L. *The Morality of Law.* New Haven, CT: Yale University Press;1964:30.

4. Clark GL. *Summary of American Law.* Rochester, NY: The Lawyers Cooperative Publishing Company;1947.

5. Allen CK. *Law in the Making.* New York, NY: Oxford University Press;1964:71.

6. Boden LI. Workers' compensation. In: Levy BS, Wegman DH, eds. *Occupational Health: Recognizing and Preventing Work-Related Disease.* Boston: Little, Brown and Co.;1988:149–162.

7. Sadleir B. Environmental and occupational health issues in hospitals. 2010. Available at: http://www.tropmed.org/rreh/vol1_2.htm. Accessed January 7, 2012.

8. Little JW, Eaton TA, Smith GR. *Cases and Materials on Workers' Compensation.* St. Paul, MN: West Publishing Co.;1993.

9. Boden LI. Workers' compensation. In: Levy BS, Wegman DH, eds. *Occupational Health: Recognizing and Prevention Work-Related Disease and Injury.* Philadelphia, PA: Lippincott, Williams & Wilkins;2000:237–256.

10. *Priestley v. Fowler,* 18370 3 M & W 1, 150 Eng. Rep. 1030 (1837).

11. Posner RA. A theory of negligence. *J Legal Stud.*1972;1:29–34, 36–48.

12. Priest GL. The invention of enterprise liability: a critical history of the intellectual foundations of modern tort law. *J Legal Stud.* 1985;14:461–465, 505–512, 518–521, 527.

13. Feinman JM. The development of the employment-at-will rule. *Am J Legal Hist.* 1976;20(2):118–120.

14. Ashford NA, Caldart CC. *Technology, Law, and the Working Environment.* Washington, DC: Island Press;1996.

15. Blackmun HA. The Supreme Court and the law of nations. *Yale Law J.* 1994;104(1):39–49.

16. Stephens B. The law of our land: customary international law as federal law after Erie. *Fordham L. Rev.* 1997;66. Available at: http://ir.lawnet.fordham.edu/flr/vol66/iss2/6. Accessed April 4, 2012.

17. Brown DK. Labor standards: where do they belong on the international trade agenda? *J Econ Perspect.* 2001;15(3):89–112.

18. Casto WR. The new federal common law of tort remedies for violations of international law. *Rutgers Law J.* 2006;37:635–669.

19. Ford GR. Remarks upon being sworn in as President of the United States, August 9, 1974. Available at: http://www.fordlibrarymuseum.gov/grf/quotes.asp. Accessed April 3, 2012.

20. Institute of Medicine. *The Future of Public Health.* Washington, DC: National Academy Press;1988:47–51.

21. Klinger DE. *Public Administration: A Management Approach.* Boston, MA: Houghton Mifflin Co.;1983:354.

22. Crick B. *Democracy: A Very Short Introduction.* New York, NY: Oxford University Press;2002.

23. Birkland TA. *An Introduction to the Policy Process: Theories, Concepts, and Models of Public Policy Making.* Armonk, NY: ME Sharpe;2001.

24. U.S. Constitution. Available at: http://www.archives.gov/exhibits/charters/constitution_transcript.html. Accessed January 15, 2012.

25. Sullivan JV. *How Our Laws Are Made.* Washington, DC: U.S. Government Printing Office;2007. U.S. House of Representatives Document No. 110-47. Available at: http://www.gpo.gov/fdsys/pkg/CDOC-110hdoc49/pdf/CDOC-110hdoc49.pdf. Accessed January 15, 2012.

26. U.S. Congress. Committees of the U.S. Congress. Congress.gov. Available at: https://beta.congress.gov/committees. Accessed July 23, 2014.

27. Bimber B. *The Politics of Expertise in Congress: The Rise and Fall of the Office of Technology Assessment.* Albany, NY: State University of New York;1996.

28. Conley JG. Environmentalism contained: a history of corporate responses to the new environmentalism [dissertation]. Princeton, NJ: Princeton University; 2006.

29. National Archives. Executive orders disposition tables index. *Federal Register.* Available at: http://www.archives.gov/federal-register/executive-orders/disposition.html. Accessed July 23, 2014.

30. McGarity TO, Shapiro SA. *Workers at Risk: The Failed Promise of the Occupational Safety and Health Administration.* Westport, CT: Praeger;1993: 229–243.

31. Gostin LO. *Public Health Law: Power, Duty, Restraint.* Berkeley, CA: University of California Press;2000.

32. U.S. Department of Labor. Freedom of Information Act (FOIA). Available at: http://www.dol.gov/dol/foia/main.htm. Accessed April 10, 2012.

32a. National Environmental Policy Act, 42 U.S.C. § 4321 et seq. (1969).

33. Savelson D. *Occupational Safety and Health Law.* New York, NY: Practicing Law Institute;1978.

34. Ginsberg WR. *Federal Advisory Committees: An Overview.* Washington, DC: U.S. Congress;2009. Congressional Research Service Report No. 7-5700.

35. Dear JA. Statement before the Small Business Committee of the U.S. House of Representatives. July 26, 1995. Available at: https://www.osha.gov/pls/oshaweb/owadisp.show_document?p_table=TESTIMONIES&p_id=80. Accessed July 22, 2014.

36. Occupational Safety and Health Administration. Consensus reached on recommendation for OSHA cranes and derricks standard [news release]. July 13, 2004. Available at: https://www.osha.gov/pls/oshaweb/owadisp.show_document?p_table=NEWS_RELEASES&p_id=10938. Accessed May 22, 2014.

37. Anonymous. The mysteries of the Congressional Review Act. *Harvard Law Rev.* 2009;122(8):2162–2184.

38. Shapiro SA. The Information Quality Act and environmental protection: the perils of reform by appropriations rider. *Wm Mary Environ Law Policy Rev.* 2004;28(2):339–374.

39. Johnson BL. *Environmental Policy and Public Health.* Boca Raton, FL: CRC Press;2007:1.

40. Michaels D, Monforton C. How litigation shapes the scientific literature: asbestos and disease among automobile mechanics. *J Law Policy.* 2007;15:1137–1169.

41. OMB Watch. Industry derails labor safety rule with data quality challenge. 2005. Available at: http://www.ombwatch.org/node/766. Accessed April 10, 2012.

42. Beer S. *Cybernetics and Management.* New York, NY: John Wiley & Sons;1959: 28–38.

43. Green HP. The role of law in determining acceptability of risk. *Ann N Y Acad Sci.* 1981;363:1–12.

44. Sun P. From a 21 November 1864, letter to Col. William F. Elkins. Quoted in Shaw AH. *The Lincoln Encyclopedia.* New York, NY: Macmillan;1950:40. Available at: http://www.patriciasun.com/html/abraham_lincoln.html. Accessed January 16, 2012.

45. Wataugawatch. American corporate power and the U.S. Supreme Court. September 29, 2009. Available at: http://blog.wataugawatch.net/2009/09/american-corporate-power-us-supreme.html. Accessed January 15, 2012.

46. Kyd SA. *Treatise on the Law of Corporations.* Vol. 1. London, UK: J. Butterworth; 1794:13.

47. Bravin J. Corporations may be persons, but they're not individuals. *Wall Street J.* April 18, 2012. Available at: http://blogs.wsj.com/law/2012/04/18/corporations-may-be-persons-but-theyre-not-individuals. Accessed August 25, 2013.

48. Bravin J. Justices probe "Alien Tort" law. *Wall Street J.* October 1, 2012. Available at: http://online.wsj.com/article/SB10000872396390443862604578030790341573044.html. Accessed August 25, 2013.

49. Bravin J. Sotomayor issues challenge to a century of corporate law. *Wall Street J.* September 17, 2009:A19.

50. Organisation for Economic Co-operation and Development. *OECD Guidelines for Multinational Enterprises.* Paris: OECD;2008. Available at: http://www.oecd.org/corporate/mne/1922428.pdf. Accessed August 25, 2013.

51. Myers ML, McGlothlin JD. Matchmakers' "phossy jaw" eradicated. *Am Ind Hyg Assoc J.* 1996;57(4):330–332.

52. Marx RE. Uncovering the cause of "phossy jaw" circa 1858 to 1906: oral and maxillofacial surgery closed case files? case closed. *J Oral Maxillofac Surg.* 2008; 66(11):2356–2363.

53. Aronson SM. The Salvation Army and phossy jaw. *Med Health R I*. 1997;80(10): 315–316.

54. Goldberg JP, Moye WT. *The First Hundred Years of the Bureau of Labor Statistics.* Washington, DC; U.S. Government Printing Office;1985.

55. Alton LR. The eradication of phossy jaw: A unique development of federal police power. *The Historian*. 1966;29(1):1–24.

56. Wolf S, Bruhn JG, Goodell H. *Occupational Health as Human Ecology.* Springfield, IL: Charles C. Thomas Publishers;1978.

5

History of Occupational Safety and Health Policy

We get wisdom from history. We get wisdom from what works.
— Daniel N. Robinson[1]

"LIFE AMONG THE LOWLY" NARRATIVE

To Harriet Beecher Stowe, President Abraham Lincoln said, "So this is the little lady who started this great war [Civil War]."[2] Lincoln's statement, appearing for the first time posthumously in 1893, confirmed to many the role that literature can play in social change. Lincoln was referring to Stowe's novel *Uncle Tom's Cabin*, the subtitle of which was *Life Among the Lowly*. Stowe was active in the underground railway that helped chattel slaves escape their bondage in the South. With the passage of the Fugitive Slave Act in 1850 that required all American citizens, North and South, to return runaway slaves as property to their owners, she decided to write *Uncle Tom's Cabin*. She wrote to her editor, "I shall show the best side of the thing, and something faintly approaching the worst." Her novel, exposing the plight of the slave population and human trafficking for the degrading and dangerous work that slaves were ordered to do, ran as a serial novel in 1851 and 1852 and was published in book form in 1852. She wrote "either from observation, incidents which have occurred in the sphere of my personal knowledge, or in the knowledge of my friends," according to her letter to her editor. She told the story of slaves' lives, their struggles to escape slavery, and, most compelling in her motivation to write the novel, how children were sold off from their families. Stowe's husband told the publisher that he hoped the book was successful enough that

Stowe could buy "a good black dress." *Uncle Tom's Cabin* sold 10,000 copies in the first week of publication, 300,000 copies in the first year, and after the Bible, more copies than any other book in the century.[3] The abolition of slavery drove an enlightened social change, setting the course for freed men and women from chattel labor in the United States.

5.1. INTRODUCTION

History is not static. Yesterday's actions are today's history.
—Cynthia McGuire Dunn and Gary Chawick[4]

History is important for two reasons: (1) tragic events lead to policy formulation, and (2) policy formulation is incremental, informed by previous policies and legal precedents. Pioneers in occupational safety and health revealed the plight of the working population, and information collected about this population revealed more of their troubles, fueling salience for action to protect workers from hazards and blame. Implementing solutions has been a struggle for laborers as their attitudes changed from espousing fatalism to exercising unified action for sustenance and their safety and health. In the United States for more than a century, state-level safety and health policies evolved into a patchwork of protections, mostly minimal. In the face of the Industrial Revolution, Great Britain preceded the United States in providing protection for workers; slowly, national policies emerged in the United States to protect the safety and health of workers, culminating in the Occupational Safety and Health Act of 1970 (OSHAct; see Appendix).

5.2. PIONEERS OF OCCUPATIONAL SAFETY AND HEALTH

The many distressing accidents which of late have occurred in that portion of our navigation carried on by the use of steam power, deserve the immediate and unremitting attention of the constituted authorities of the country. The fact that the number of those fatal disasters is constantly increasing, notwithstanding the great improvements which are everywhere made in the machinery employed, and in the rapid advances which have been made in that branch of science, show very clearly that they are in a great degree the result of criminal negligence on the part of those by whom the vessels are navigated, and to whose care and attention the lives and property of our citizens are so extensively entrusted. That these

evils may be greatly lessened, if not substantially removed, by means of precautionary and penal legislation, seems to be highly probable . . .
    —President Andrew Jackson, State of the Union address to Congress[5]

Circa 370 B.C., Hippocrates described what may have been hookworm that was likely contracted in unsanitary mines. He described other diseases that related to metallurgists, fullers, tailors, horse handlers, farmers, and fish catchers. In describing the unhealthy condition of the metal worker, he observed him as pale, livid, and having difficulty breathing, a distended and hard abdomen, a large spleen, and a swollen right hypochondrium. He correctly described a lead poisoning case, but it would not have even occurred to him to prescribe hygiene to manual laborers.[6,7]

During 23–70 A.D., Plinius Secundus, also called Pliny the Elder, wrote about the use of a bladder as a protective mask that blocked the inhalation of dust and was transparent enough to allow the worker to see. The bladder was placed over the face to stop breathing in poisonous dusts and vapors. The mask was recommended for use by cinnabar grinders and workers exposed to lead fumes. He also described lead, mercury, zinc, and sulfur poisoning.[6–8]

In 1556, Georgius Agricola's book *De Re Metallica* was published three years after his death. Agricola studied medicine and the natural sciences in Italy and practiced medicine in a small mining town. His book is a classic in metallurgy, but the last section describes diseases and injuries prevalent among miners and means for preventing them. He described hand bellows and fans for ventilation and pumps for removing water from the mines. It was commonly thought, in Agricola's day, that miners crossed paths with demons in the mines. Agricola wrote of how to expel evil demons, although many of these demons were believed to be jolly and kind. These demons were later interpreted as dwarfs in the woods who befriended the children who were persecuted by work in the mines. Walt Disney adapted this story into his film, *Snow White and the Seven Dwarfs*.[6–8]

In 1700, Bernardino Ramazzini published his *De Morbis Artificum Diatriba* (*Discourse on the Diseases of Workers*). He identified diseases that were linked to the hazards of occupations, and he laid the foundation for occupational medicine and hygiene. Ramazzini built upon the contributions to medicine made by Hippocrates by adding a question to the physician's inquiry into the cause of disease, "What trade he is of?"[9]

Table 5-1. Occupations for Which Ramazzini Described Diseases Incidental to Their Work

Discourse on the Diseases of Workers (1700)

miners and gilders	bakers and millers	sulfur workers
goldsmiths	corn sifters	Jews: diseases incident to rag-picking and
apothecaries	copper and tin founders	other inferior occupations forced upon
surgeons administering mercury	salt makers	them in the Middle Ages
to syphilitics	couriers	those whose work strains the eyes
glass blowers and mirror	stone cutters	fishermen
makers	washer women	soldiers
wet-nurses	bath keepers	orators and singers
chemists	horsemen	flax and oakum pickers and silk spinners
scavengers	porters	painters
tobacconists	those who work standing	midwives
oil men, tanners, grave diggers,	those who work sitting	
butchers, fish handlers, and	wrestlers	
cheese mongers	farmers	

Diseases of Workers (1713)

printers	scribes and notaries	hunters
weavers	confectioners	carpenters and cabinet makers
grinders	brassfounders	cutlers and knife grinders
well diggers	brick makers	sailors and galley hands

Source: Hunter;[9] Rosen.[11]
Note: The text in this table is reproduced verbatim.

Ramazzini earned the position of "father of industrial medicine."[10] In addition to diseases of scholars and literary men, his discourse covered 40 different occupations, as shown in Table 5-1. In 1713, Ramazzini published a second edition of his work, *De Morbis Artificum* (*Diseases of Workers*), to which he added 12 more occupations, also shown in Table 5-1.[11]

Percival Pott, a distinguished surgeon at St. Bartholomew's Hospital in London, brought attention to soot as the cause of scrotal cancer among chimney sweeps in 1775. He was the first person ever to describe an occupational cancer.[8]

Charles Turner Thackrah, also an English physician, published a 220-page treatise in 1832: *The Effects of Arts, Trades, and Professions, and of Civic States and Habits of Living, on Health and Longevity*. He revealed that in the industrial city of Leeds, where there were 128 different trades, there was one death per 55 inhabitants in 1821, while in a neighboring rural area there was one death per 74 inhabitants that year. He concluded that an additional 450 people died in Leeds because of the "artificial state of society." He extrapolated from this number of excess deaths to observe "that 50,000 persons die annually in Great Britain from the effects of manufactures, civic states, and the intemperance connected with these states and occupations." His work attracted social reformers and men of medicine.[8,12]

The public health movement began in England with Edwin Chadwick's publication of *The Sanitary Condition of the Labouring Population of Britain* in 1842. Chadwick was the Secretary to the Poor Law Commission in London. He believed that pauperism was caused by preventable illness and that public health money should be spent on paupers. His report established the basis for environmental sanitation as a public health program and inspired similar reports in New York, Boston, and elsewhere.[9]

Previously, Chadwick had successfully insisted in 1839 that William Farr be appointed as the compiler of abstracts in the new General Register Office in London. In 1851, Farr's work led to the publication of England and Wales's first *Occupational Mortality Supplement by the Registrar General*. This register of occupational mortality, based on death certificates, was tabulated every 10 years thereafter.[9]

British women Catherine Booth and Annie Besant started a crusade to wipe out phossy jaw,[12a] which Colonel James Barker continued after Booth's death in 1840. He led tours of news reporters and legislators into the homes of factory workers who were exposed to white phosphorus. He provided a climax for the tour by dimming the gas lamp in the home to display the greenish-white glow of the victim's jaw, blouse, and hands. The creator of the Salvation Army and Booth's widower, General William Booth, opened an airy, well-lit model match factory in London in 1891, following an investigation by Barker. With 120 workers, the Salvation Army manufactured matches from the harmless red phosphorus to demonstrate that a safe, but more expensive, substitute for the white phosphorus that was in common use was available. At its peak, this factory produced six million boxes of matches in one year.[9]

Congress passed the "coupler bill" (the Safety Appliance Act of 1893), with support from the Interstate Commerce Commission (ICC) and labor unions. This bill regulated the railroad industry by banning the use of the hazardous link-and-pin method of coupling cars.[13] It also required the testing of safety devices, and if these tests indicated an advance in safety then they were mandatory safety "appliances" for the industry. This was the federal government's first major intervention into occupational safety. Much of the credit for its passage goes to a Civil War preacher, Lorenzo A. Coffin, who dedicated years of his life to the prevention of amputations and other injuries through the substitution of safer appliances, such as the Westinghouse air brake.[14]

Alice Hamilton, the first physician in the United States to dedicate her career to occupational medicine, was one of nine investigators appointed to the Illinois Commission on Occupational Diseases in 1908. In 1909, the commission reported a list of industries that likely exposed thousands of workers to diseases. At its recommendation, the state legislature funded an investigation of industrial diseases by medical experts. Hamilton was named the lead medical investigator for this survey in 1910. The survey found problems related to lead, arsenic, brass, and zinc manufacturing; zinc smelting; carbon monoxide; cyanide; and turpentine, as well as caisson disease, deafness, and miner's nystagmus.[15]

In 1910, Crystal Eastman's *Work-Accidents and the Law* reinforced a movement to compensate workers for injury. The Russell Sage Foundation funded Eastman, an attorney, to investigate working conditions in a Pittsburgh survey.[16] In the resulting monograph, she documented 455 on-the-job fatalities—71 of which were mine-related—in one year in Allegheny County, Pennsylvania.[7] She maintained a Death Calendar, marking each daily death with a red X on it.[17]

On March 25, 1911, Frances Perkins witnessed a fire at the Triangle Shirtwaist Company in New York City that trapped workers in a loft. The factory was on notice for lack of fire egress. Workers, mostly immigrant women, leaped to their death or were trapped by the fire, resulting in 146 deaths.[8] On that same day, the state supreme court declared the New York law to compensate workers for injuries unconstitutional as a violation of property rights. Since 1910, Perkins was active in public service.[18] She was later named Secretary of Labor in 1933, the first female cabinet member in the U.S. government. In 1935, Secretary Perkins was instrumental in developing federal legislation for improving working conditions. She led the way in the preparation of proposed legislation for the Social Security Act of 1935, which included public health grants that would establish industrial hygiene programs at the state level across the country. In addition, she campaigned for national legislation for worker safety and health, which led to the Fair Labor Standards Act of 1938 that banned exploitative child labor and provided federal power to ban workers under age 18 from dangerous occupations, and the Walsh-Healey Public Contracts Act of 1936.

This act provided a foundation for a national occupational safety and health program, albeit limited to work under federal contracts.[13]

In the 1930s, DuPont employee Wilhelm C. Hueper became the principal critic of cancer-causing chemicals during the rise of the chemical revolution before and after World War II. DuPont fired him, but he went on to found the Environmental Cancer Section of the National Cancer Institute. Hueper published his 896-page "magnus opus" in 1942, *Occupational Tumors and Allied Diseases*. Because it was published during the war, it received little immediate attention, but later Rachel Carson's book *Silent Spring* gave heavy weight to his work.[19]

Alice Hamilton invited Harriet L. Hardy to coauthor an update of her 1934 textbook, *Industrial Toxicology*. Hardy was then a physician employed by the Massachusetts Division of Occupational Hygiene. Their revised textbook was published in 1949. Three more editions were published up to 1983. Hardy was known for her research on beryllium poisoning in the manufacture of fluorescent lamps. She identified beryllium as the cause of chronic respiratory disease in 1946, and in 1952, she established the National Beryllium Registry, one of the first registries to collect long-term data on a chronic disorder. Furthermore, she was on the frontier of recognizing the connection between asbestos and cancer. Hardy's studies covered a diversity of occupational health problems, including these poisonings and diseases: anthrax, arsenic, asbestosis, benzene, beryllium, cadmium, carbon tetrachloride, coal workers' lung disease, cyanide, lead, mercury, mesothelioma, pesticides, and radiation.[15,20,21]

Donald Hunter, a London Hospital physician, published *Diseases of Occupations* in 1955 with other editions to follow. His writing was of prime importance to clinicians for identifying occupational diseases with a classification of hazards. In his book, he compiled an extensive history of the interaction of work with disease in Great Britain. Hunter was also the founding editor of the *British Journal of Industrial Medicine*.[22]

In the 1960s, Dr. Irving J. Selikoff at Mount Sinai Hospital in New York City cared for asbestos workers, who had a high death rate from lung cancer. He launched a study of 17,000 insulation workers and confirmed that asbestos was associated with mesothelioma and lung cancer. His research was a driver for the Occupational Safety and Health Administration (OSHA) to regulate workers' exposure to asbestos and for the U.S. Environmental Protection Agency (EPA) to attempt to ban its use in the United States.[23]

5.3. THE HISTORICAL IMPERATIVE

The job safety law of 1970: its passage was perilous.

—Judson MacLaury[13]

In 1908, when the working population in the United States numbered 30 million, a journalist estimated that 35,000 workers were killed and 536,000 were injured annually. For the period 1911 through 1914, a study in New York State found that the most significant cause of nonfatal injuries was powered machinery. The number of industrial injuries during the period 1926 through 1929 was twice of that during the period 1950 to 1970, even as the working population had increased.[24]

During the Depression years, the number of injuries decreased as employment dropped. During the first three years of World War II, the number of workers killed and injured at work exceeded the number of Americans killed in the military.[24] From 1961 to 1970, the incidence of occupational injuries increased by 29%.[25] Injury rates rose sharply in the industries supporting the Vietnam War and doubled in the ordnance industries.[26]

The principal predictor of the occupational injury rate was the business cycle, for as industrial growth increased, the injury rate also increased, but as growth slowed the rate would decrease.[24] Starting in 1966, the injury rate rose faster than could be related to the business cycle, which was explained in part by the increase in the pace of work as employers faced declining profits.[27]

Injuries were not the only calamity to visit workers in the United States in the early 1900s. Stone cutters were struck with "consumption," later known as silicosis or tuberculosilicosis, tobacco workers suffered from heart and respiratory illness, hat makers contracted "mad hatter's disease" from mercury exposure, and woman employed to paint clock faces with radium died of radiation poisoning.[24] A physician at the 1936 United Auto Workers convention reported 13,000 lead poisonings in automobile factories since 1926.[27]

Many silent epidemics that were latent in the post–World War II era became visible with the passage of time.[24] The introduction of continuous mining technology after World War II increased productivity and reduced employment levels in coal mines while increasing coal mine dust levels. An epidemic of coal workers' pneumoconiosis emerged. The demand for uranium increased, which placed miners at risk of radon progeny exposures and led to an epidemic of lung cancer. The increase in petrochemical production posed a variety of new occupational hazards. In 1961, rubber workers experienced respiratory illness from a new vulcanizing process. During the 1960s, asbestos was found to be the source of an epidemic of lung cancer, asbestosis, and mesothelioma. Also in the 1960s, coke oven workers at steel plants experienced high rates of cancer.[28]

By 1970, the occupational safety and health problem had become a public health crisis.[24] While 21 million employees, such as miners and atomic energy workers, received protection under some type of federal law, 67 of 88 million workers had no legislation that protected their safety and health prior to 1970. To address the crisis of work-related diseases and injuries, the U.S. Department of Labor (DoL) issued standards in 1968 under the Walsh-Healey Public Contracts Act, basing standards on the American Conference of Governmental Industrial Hygienists' threshold limit values. Congress passed the Coal Mine Health and Safety Act of 1969 on December 30, 1969, and President Nixon signed the OSHAct on December 29, 1970, which became effective on April 29, 1971.[29]

During 1972, the first full year of federal statistics collected after the enactment of the OSHAct, the Bureau of Labor Statistics (BLS) reported 11,000 occupational fatalities and 5.7 million occupational injuries in the private sector—mostly cuts and bruises—but 1.7 million of these injured workers missed at least one day of work.[30]

5.4. THE LABOR AND SAFETY MOVEMENTS

The very act of congregating is an exceptionally powerful stimulant. Once the individuals are gathered together, a sort of electricity is generated from their closeness and an extraordinary height of exaltation.

—Émile Durkheim[31]

Labor organization is a collective reaction to some type of grievance, which includes economic and working conditions. To appreciate occupational safety and health policy, one must understand the history of the labor movement. Notwithstanding that a union of Pennsylvania cordwainers struck in 1806 for higher pay,[32] the labor movement in the United States was born in 1827 at first as a reaction against industrialization. Later, the movement became part of the antislavery movement.[33] Initially, unions organized around trades as protection against intrusions of changes in work organization. Trade workers held ideals and customs of independent action that included work habits and beliefs, traditions of self-organization and community development, and radical politics.[34] Low wages were a common complaint, and strikes emerged. Early on, managers countered with the common law instrument against conspiracies to unite to raise wages.[33]

The emergence of the labor movement parallels the rise of capitalism and covers two centuries of "toil and trouble," as Thomas Brooks put it in his history of the labor movement.[33] The safety movement came later, starting to emerge in 1870 as detailed by Mark Aldrich in his account *Safety First*.[35] While labor fought for a livable wage, in the shadow of this fight were the death and disability—and the wear and tear—that came with manual work. The following is a brief synopsis of this history through the prisms of the widespread rise of mutual aid societies, strikes to reduce the length of the workday, battles for livable wages, and development of the Safety First movement. It is a history associated with the suppression of labor organization.

5.4.1. Mutual Aid Societies

While there were incidents as early as 1853 of workers walking off their jobs because of deteriorating working conditions,[36] the labor movement arose initially in the United States as mutual aid societies. Mutual dependence helped workers cope with their shared struggles and misfortunes and thereby build strong bonds with each other. The major factor influencing the aid societies was crippling and fatal injuries as well as debilitating diseases.[34] The Brotherhood of Locomotive Engineers, formed in 1863 by the union locals of the failed remnants of the National Protective Association of Locomotive Engineers, had as its major function a mutual aid society providing insurance for injury, death, and burial.[36]

Two other fraternal organizations of railroad workers also formed as benevolent societies. The Conductors Union, formed in 1868 and renamed the Order of Railroad Conductors of America in 1878, established a life insurance program for its members. The Brotherhood of Locomotive Firemen was founded in 1873, establishing a life insurance program with a policy of $1,000 financed with member payments of 50¢ per month. This organization later became an active trade union under the leadership of a young fireman named Eugene Victor Debs.[36]

The first major industrial union was the Workingman's Benevolent Association of anthracite miners, organized in 1868.[37] For rescues in the mines, miners were the only ones who were there to help, and many times they jeopardized their own lives and sometimes paid with their lives as rescuers. Mutual aid societies were prevalent among Western unions representing hard rock miners, prominently the Coeur d'Alene Miners' Union Hospital in Idaho in 1891.[33] Another union that later wielded power was the Knights of Labor, organized by nine garment cutters in 1869 with the motto "An injury to one is the concern of all."[38]

Mutual aid still exists today. Because fishers in Alaska work beyond the territorial waters of the state and the reach of the workers' compensation system, they participate in the Alaska Fishermen's Fund. This fund was established in 1952, and in 1994, it provided $2,500 per work-related injury.[39]

5.4.2. Sunrise to Sunset

A workday in early factories was set during daylight hours, perhaps as a remnant of farm work but also necessary for natural lighting. As an example, in mills in Lowell, Massachusetts, the workday prior to 1912 averaged 12 hours and 13 minutes, or a 6-day workweek equal to 73.5 hours per worker. A workday during the winter months of December and January averaged 11 hours and 24 minutes, whereas by April, the workday was 13 hours and 31 minutes.[32] Since the 1830s, reform societies advocated first a 10-hour workday, drawn from an 1830 proposal by Robert Owen in Great Britain, then later an 8-hour workday.[22,38]

In 1840, President Martin Van Buren, a friend of labor, established a 10-hour workday for federal employees.[33] Then in 1868, Congress passed an act that established an 8-hour day for federal workers.[40]

The Federation of Organized Trades and Labor Unions launched an 8-hour workday advocacy movement in 1884 with this goal: "[e]ight hours shall constitute a legal day's work from and after May 1, 1886." Despite contrary views by the national leadership of the Knights of Labor, which favored cooperative approaches to advance the labor agenda over a perceived anarchy as a means for achieving this agenda, local assemblies organized an "Eight Hour League" that local trade unions quickly joined in February 1886.[38] Word-of-mouth and sermons from the pulpit spread the news and support of the league. Skilled and unskilled workers, including both men and women, offered money and time for the movement.[38] Moreover, Samuel Gompers, the president of the newly formed American Federation of Labor (AFL), supported the movement.[40]

The league made its demands known to employers to no avail, which sparked a general May Day strike by 8,000 workers that reached across industries. By the next day, 14,000 workers were on strike. Some employers consequently granted an 8-hour day, which encouraged other workers across the nation that success was possible. Some workers used a tactic to show up for work at 8:00 and leave at 5:00. Strikes flared across the nation, in Connecticut, Illinois, Kentucky, Maine, Maryland, Massachusetts, Michigan, Missouri, New Jersey, New York, Pennsylvania, Rhode Island, Texas, and Washington, DC.[38]

Employers countered with contract law, standing on their right to manage their business and the workers' right to sell their time and labor.[38] Furthermore, employers who allowed an 8-hour day were at a disadvantage compared with the cutthroat methods of competitors.[22] At the core of this dispute was determining who had the power to determine wages, working conditions, and the length of the workday.[38]

While many employers made concessions to the strikers, other employers organized into associations in a massive battle between management and labor. The associations fought to check and crush the union movement, aided by the public perception of violence attributed to labor such as the bombing of employers' property. By September 1886, firings, lockouts, blacklisting, and "yellow dog contracts" (oaths not to join a union) had quashed this union movement.[38]

In the wake of later strikes, in such workplaces as Carnegie's Homestead Works in Pittsburgh, where the 8-hour workday was established in 1892, workdays reverted to 12-hour days by 1907. In 1894, some Colorado mine owners attempted to change the workday from 8 to 10 hours, which resulted in a union organized across many mines. The miners walked out on strike at the largest mines. One hundred armed men marched to the mine at Cripple Creek to face off with an army of deputies in support of the mine owner. Only by the governor's intervention was conflict averted and agreement reached. The 8-hour day was preserved—for the time being.[38]

In 1919, against union orders, 120,000 textile workers across New England struck for an 8-hour day with no reduction in daily pay; 30,000 New Jersey silk workers arrived at 8:00 rather than 7:00 to begin work. In addition, female workers in the feathers and artificial flowers industry in New York City struck for a 44-hour workweek and the abolition of homework,[38] which involved middlemen contracting piecework in private households for women to produce through sewing, needlework, or binding (e.g., cigars), and likely involved child labor as well.[22]

The fight for the 8-hour day in the United States continued into the Great Depression, but with the claim that a shorter workday could stimulate more employment. In 1936, the AFL proposed "minimum wage legislation for women and children but not for men" and, in addition, that year Congress enacted the Walsh-Healey Public Contracts Act, which included a provision for federal contractors for an 8-hour workday and a 40-hour workweek, with time-and-a-half for overtime. Congress passed the Fair Labor Standards Act in 1938, which set the workweek at 44 hours, to be reduced by two hours per year until a 40-hour workweek was established. The act also provided for child labor protections.[40]

5.4.3. "Wage Slavery"

Mutual aid and shorter workdays only went so far. In his 1907 novel *The Jungle*, Upton Sinclair described the plight of workers employed in factories as wage slavery.[41] Reflective of this plight, the treasurer of the Pacific Mill in Lawrence, Massachusetts, said in 1882, "I believe the operatives (workers) would not strike if they were starving."[42]

Current events in other parts of the world provide a perspective on the issue of wage slavery. In August 2012, 28,000 miners mounted a wildcat strike in Marikana, South Africa, at the Lonmin platinum mine. Hundreds of rock drillers led the strike with demands for a minimum wage to be increased from $688 to $1,560 per month. Many earned less than the minimum wage, at about $490 (4,000 rand in local currency) per month or even less by other reports at $300 per month, and some lived on less than $2 per day. The strike was reported as illegal, likely because a union contract (but where competing unions were a factor) was in place that may have set the minimum wage. Poor working conditions were cited, and many workers lived in "tin box" shacks at the edge of the mine with neither running water nor electricity. Ten deaths were attributed to the strike, two of whom were police officers hacked to death by machetes.

Then a week into the strike, police shot and killed 34 striking miners and injured another 78 strikers. The miners, with sticks and machetes, were reportedly charging a literal cauldron of police officers 540 strong. The police arrested 259 strikers, charging many with the murder of their shot comrades.

Three days after the shooting, mine management set an ultimatum for the miners to return to work or be fired but with no response to the wage demands. One-third of the workers reported to work on the appointed day, not enough to resume production. One stockholder in the company offered $250,000 to pay for the funerals of the dead workers.[43,44] A month later, the strike remained unresolved and had spread to other mines in South Africa.[45] An agreement was reached after more than a month on September 21; the miners had secured a 22% raise in wages.

Back to pre-modernity: In 1806, the Federal Society of Journeymen Cordwainers—a 12-year-old union of Philadelphia shoemakers—went on strike to demand higher wages. In a response, instigated and paid for by the employers, the Commonwealth of Pennsylvania charged the strikers as a "criminal conspiracy" that used unlawful coercion to achieve its economic goals. The government won, the union was broken, and its leaders were fined.[32,46]

In the post–Civil War years, called the "Gilded Age" by Mark Twain and Charles Dudley Warner, great fortunes were made by a few.[47] During this time, an 1864 congressional authorization allowed employers to import foreign workers and indenture them under contract law to pay off the price of their passage to the United States. Immigration was a cheap source of labor; 28.5 million people immigrated to the United States between 1860 and 1929.[38] Wages below subsistence levels and poor working conditions pervaded the Gilded Age, when economic depressions and unemployment were common.

The Baltimore and Ohio Railroad cut wages in 1877, which sparked a strike by the workers with overwhelming support by the local West Virginia community. The state militia was called, followed by the shooting death of a soldier, and the shooter in turn was shot dead. This local strike ignited a national railroad strike known as the Great Upheaval. Not led by a central authority of a union, unity in the strike emerged spontaneously from the frustration of the individual workers driven by the slogan of "bread and blood." A wage of 95¢ per day would not sustain a family, work-related injury or death was a constant threat, and workers had little time at home with their families. The strike was joined by thousands across the nation and became increasingly general beyond the railroads. Companies hired special police to quell the strikes, state militias were called, and finally the U.S. military intervened, thus defeating the Great Upheaval.[38]

Hundreds of strikes followed over the years on the issue of subsistence pay. Famous are the Haymarket strike (Chicago) in 1886, the Homestead Works

(Pittsburgh) and Coeur d'Alene (Idaho) mine strikes of 1892, the Pullman strike (near Chicago) by the American Railway Union of 1894 led by Eugene V. Debs, and the 1912 "Bread and Roses" strike in the Lawrence, Massachusetts, textile mills. According to Elizabeth Shapleigh, a Lawrence physician at the time of the strike, "A considerable number of the boys and girls [children worked in the mills] die within the first two or three years after beginning work." She reported that 36% of all men and women who worked in the mills died by the time they were 25 years old.[48]

In Lawrence, a new Massachusetts law reduced the workweek from 56 to 54 hours; the employers had cut pay proportionally and consequently workers walked out in January 1912. As many as 20,000 workers were on a strike that lasted for months. The Industrial Workers of the World (known as the Wobblies) took the lead for organizing the spontaneous strike, stressing nonviolence. Nonetheless, the labor leaders were jailed.[38]

The Wobblies were publicity masters who generated widespread sympathy for the strike. This sympathy moved to a congressional hearing attended by First Lady Helen Taft. At the hearing a weaver, Samuel Lipson, said employees were charged at work for drinking water and named children that the police had thrown into a wagon so that they could not escape the stricken city, and he told of soup kitchens serving thousands and his own hearing loss from the machines at the mills. Then children testified. One girl displayed where a machine had entangled her hair and removed her scalp from the back of her head. A boy said he survived on bread and water a few days each week. Female witnesses spoke of beatings by police and malnourished children.[38]

For an opposing version of events, Reverend Clark Carter testified that the striker parades were mobs, referring to some workers as blundering, untrained, and "foreign-tongued" individuals. He saw nothing wrong with child labor at 14 years of age, as children "needed to be occupied at something profitable lest they not amount to much." He added that it was "better to be congenial in the mills rather than uncongenial in the schools," admitting that even a 10-hour day might be too severe in some cases.[38] After going up against undercover detectives, the planting of bombs at workers' homes , physical intimidation, and fear-mongering, the strike was finally successful in restoring daily wages.

Seven years later, the great strike of 1919 was less successful. Preceding 1919, during World War I, the federal government controlled prices and wages and cooperated with the AFL, which agreed to oppose strikes during the war. This policy legitimized trade unions, whereas prior to the war employers had fought trade unions, preferring to deal with workers individually. When price controls ended after the war, inflation doubled over the wage rate, effectively reducing pay by half, but labor had experienced the power of unified action.[38]

Against these factors, employers were driven to hysteria from a fear of Bolshevism emerging in the United States, at a time when the government no longer intervened to halt union busting. Industrial conflict was imminent. While the AFL comprised the skilled trades, the larger worker population found unity with the Wobblies, who aimed to organize all workers across an industry into one union. The militant Wobblies mounted a general strike in Seattle in 1919 with sympathy strikes elsewhere, which spontaneously grew into strikes nationwide across trades and industries, involving thousands of workers. Many died in outright battle. Nonetheless, state and federal intervention eventually extinguished the strikes under President Warren Harding in 1920.[38] Tactics of divide-and-conquer, fear-mongering, and military suppression effectively ended the union movement until the Great Depression.

During the Great Depression, wages and employment fell. Strikes rose in great number, challenged by vigilantes and the National Guard. A great strike wave in 1933 and 1934 included citywide general strikes and factory takeovers. Violent confrontations occurred between workers trying to form unions and the police and private security forces defending the interests of antiunion employers. Some companies shortened the workweek so as to keep more workers employed, while the Wobblies had been discredited because of ties to Communism. Populism and unrest spread like the wind.[38] Change was imminent.

In 1934, the National Labor Relations Act limited employer reactions to workers who (1) create labor unions, (2) engage in collective bargaining, and (3) take part in strikes and concerted activity in support of their demands. In the same year, President Franklin D. Roosevelt issued an executive order for the National Labor Relations Board to conduct elections for labor union representation and investigate and remedy unfair labor practices. The Congress of Industrial Organizations (CIO) emerged in 1938 as a federation of industrial unions. Later, in 1955, the AFL-CIO merged into one federation of unions.[33]

5.4.4. Safety

Trade societies were the first to recognize the need for worker safety, starting with the Federal Society of Journeymen Cordwainers, formed in 1794. The problem of safety was inherently personal, dating back eons, but with the advent of the Industrial Revolution, the problem of safety became an integral part of industry for both workers and employers. Two solutions were employed. One was applied science, depending on the gathering and application of knowledge, and the other was engineering, depending on controlling the forces of nature for human benefit. Engineers became responsible for eliminating or controlling the hazards inherent with working with machines.[49]

The industrial safety movement initially addressed property protection. This changed when applied science associated the statistics of injuries with working conditions according to the type of industry. The public was astounded when publicity of the numbers revealed the lethal result of poor working conditions, and mounting public pressure modified the relationship between workers and their employers in the early 1900s. In 1907, working conditions killed 3,242 coal miners and 4,534 railroad workers. In 1908, Frederick Hoffman of the BLS estimated that 25,000 workers were killed on the job each year.[35] In reaction to the tragedy of work-related deaths, engineers became responsible for controlling the hazards inherent with working with machines.

Three public policy approaches to address worker safety were emerging beginning in the mid-1800s: (1) regulations, (2) volunteerism, and (3) financial incentives,[35] and in 1906, the Safety First movement emerged. This movement promoted not only reengineering for safety but also joint labor-management safety committees.[50]

5.4.5. State Regulations

After 1850, the labor movement advocated state legislation to protect the safety of workers, much of which was directed at the mining and railroad industries.[51] Regarding industrial injuries, the Knights of Labor called for safety legislation in 1885.[38] States initially set as a priority relieving the exploitation of women and children.[22] In 1836, Massachusetts enacted a child labor law followed by the establishment of a state Bureau of Labor Statistics in 1869, which was emulated by eight other states in short order. Massachusetts enacted the first job safety law in the United States in 1867.[52] In 1877, Massachusetts passed the first factory inspection law with state-paid inspectors. Wisconsin passed a similar bill in that year.[50]

Pennsylvania enacted the first law that provided for coal mine inspections in 1869, followed by similar acts in other states in 1890 and 1891. By 1890,

21 states had passed laws to protect workers by regulating ventilation, heating, lighting, and fire safety. Later in the decade, states passed laws to control sweatshop working conditions in tenements, concentrating on the exploitation of children and women. Ohio passed a law in 1890 that placed a general duty on the employer to "make suitable provision to prevent injury to persons who may come in contact with" specified machinery.[51]

A 1902 Massachusetts law required that half-hour meal breaks be allowed for women and children working 16 hours or more. Other states followed with 45- or 60-minute meal breaks for all workers. Five states established laws to provide places for meal breaks free from noxious fumes or poisonous substances. A 1906 Maryland law required the sprinkling of water on the floor in shirt factories to keep cotton dust down.[51]

In 1908, Governor Charles S. Deneen (R) of Illinois appointed a nine-member team of investigators that included Alice Hamilton as the lead investigator to the Illinois Commission on Occupational Diseases. In 1911, the commission presented its results of the Illinois survey to the governor in which Hamilton had identified 578 cases of lead poisoning.[15] The state then enacted an occupational health law, which required monthly physical examinations of workers exposed to lead, zinc, arsenic, brass, mercury, or phosphorus.[53] Likewise, an occupational disease law followed in six other states. The laws required safety measures and medical examinations backed by factory inspections and prosecutions of violators.[15]

President Theodore Roosevelt lauded a 1911 Wisconsin bill to create a state industrial commission with the aim to regulate occupational safety and health. The bill passed and became a triumph of regulatory governance that served as a laboratory for reform. Also in 1911, labor economist John R. Commons of Wisconsin led the way to establish the Industrial Commission of Wisconsin to make rules to protect occupational safety and health rather than legislating piecemeal factory laws. State-sponsored administrative rule-making bodies replaced limited laws regarding child labor, the protection of women, factory inspection, mine safety, and workers' compensation. Commons's other innovation was tripartite committees that were composed of workers, employers, and experts (nominated by groups represented by employers, labor, and the public). These two ideas produced effective, scientific, and state-of-the-art rules supported by both labor and business.[54]

After 1920, states began using safety standards developed by the American Standards Association,[51] and by 1931, 19 states emulated the governmental powers assigned by the Wisconsin plan.[54] Nonetheless, state laws varied greatly, and many did little to protect workers. Prior to 1935, several states—Connecticut, Maryland, Massachusetts, Mississippi, New York, Ohio, and Rhode Island—had taken measures to protect the health of workers with industrial hygiene programs through their health and labor departments. The Social Security Act of 1935 provided funding for states through the U.S. Public Health Service (USPHS) for industrial hygiene programs. As a result, 26 states had industrial hygiene units by 1938.[55] Even though the Walsh-Healey Public Contracts Act was passed in June 1936, it depended upon state laws where they existed, and it applied only to employers involved in government contracts that exceeded $10,000 in value.[55a]

5.4.6. Volunteerism

Volunteerism initially emphasized company actions to reduce disasters (and the aftermath of negative publicity), aimed principally at railroads, to protect passengers from harm in the event of a train wreck, and at mining companies, to prevent fires and explosions in underground mines.[35] To improve fire safety, the insurance industry was responsible for creating the National Board of Fire Underwriters in 1866 and the National Fire Protection Association in 1896. The voluntary safety movement was marked by what followed with a focus on job safety programs and education.[51]

In 1907, the Association of Iron and Steel Electrical Engineers was formed and called for a national conference in 1911. As a result, the First Cooperative Safety Congress met in Milwaukee, Wisconsin, in 1912. In the following year, a second meeting led to the creation by industry of the National Council for Industrial Safety, which was soon renamed the National Safety Council. From this action, the safety movement was born. Its purpose was to establish safety standards with a focus on communications and solve common problems within an industry. Following a national survey by the council in 1917, and working with the National Bureau of Standards in the U.S. Department of Commerce, a joint conference was convened in 1919 that led to the creation of the American Standards Association, which became the American National Standards Institute (ANSI) in 1928. ANSI addressed "things" of safety such as personal protective equipment and machine guards, while the National Safety Council placed its emphasis on "people" issues.[56] The focus on people was stated by a National Safety Council official later in 1933: "Safety can never be legislated and enforced to individuals. Safety must be sold and taught to individuals."[57]

Congress created the Bureau of Mines (BoM) in 1910, premised on business-government cooperation rather than on governmental coercion. In the absence of economic incentives or regulation, BoM's effectiveness was limited to research into politically popular issues such as mine explosions. Volunteerism had its best success among large companies and instilling cooperation within strong trade associations. These companies sought favorable publicity and were able to garner cost savings from safety programs. Moreover, their trade associations spread intervention information among the companies so as to share solutions to safety problems.[35]

In 1915, the American Association of Industrial Physicians was organized, which became the Industrial Medical Association in 1959 and the American Occupational Medical Association in 1977. In 1959, the association published its first issue of the *Journal of Occupational Medicine*. Dr. Robert A. Kehoe was closely aligned with the publication. As far back as 1925, as a consultant for the lead industry, he had advocated a philosophy of industry volunteerism (i.e., self-regulation). This philosophy led to a "cascading uncertainty rule" by blending uncertainty with a skewed cost-benefit analysis. This rule balanced the near-term worth of tetraethyl lead additives weighted against future human health hazards. Some company physicians appeared to place the interest of employers ahead of their employee patients, and the conflict of interest was inherent in this pattern of volunteerism of "company first." There are more examples.[58]

5.4.7. Financial Incentives

Occupational injuries kindled public demands for preventive action. In 1903, 1,066 railroad workers were injured, and an average of 328 workers were killed each year from 1888 to 1908. The estimate for all industries during that period was 536,000 injured and 35,000 killed. Because of defenses available to employers, only an estimated 15% of injured workers were able to receive compensation under tort law.[59] Employers were successful at defending against liability cases regarding occupational injury with the common law defenses of the fellow servant rule, contributory negligence, and assumption of risk. However, reforms in England in 1880 and 1884 greatly limited the fellow servant defense that employers used in liability suits.[35] Attitudes were also adjusting in U.S. courts along this line, and businesses were increasingly threatened not only by negative publicity but also by rising liability cost.

Prussia originated the workers' compensation system by statute in 1854, which required employers' payments to go into a fund that would pay injured workers for lost wages. The fund was changed into compulsory payments for a mutual aid system that was not tied to employer culpability. In 1880, the British Parliament passed the Employers Liability Act, providing that a worker could recover up to three years of lost wages because of an injury, and an amendment in 1897 adopted the concept of employer liability.[60] In the United States, Congress enacted the Federal Employers Liability Act in 1908, which modified the tort doctrine by eliminating the assumption of risk defense when a safety violation was involved.[61]

The 1908 statute stimulated industry coalitions to move toward a no-fault system patterned after the British system. The National Civic Association (NCA) was one of these coalitions, which big business organized while facing rising threats of violent strikes. NCA was conceived as a tripartite organization made up of business, labor, and government. AFL President Samuel Gompers was invited into this organization and became its vice-president, but the Wobblies were excluded as too radical and socialist. Within NCA, big business encouraged reforms and advocated workers' compensation, but Samuel Gompers resisted, favoring weakened employer defenses in liability laws, until a reform organization, the American Association for Labor Legislation, endorsed the compensation idea. In 1911, Washington and Wisconsin were the first states to pass a workers' compensation law, and California expanded its law in 1917 to cover occupational diseases.[62] By 1920, 20 states had passed these laws. Mississippi was the last state to pass a workers' compensation law in 1948.[35,59,63]

Workers' compensation laws were considered no-fault, in which injured workers were assured of coverage of medical expenses to treat the injury and a percentage of wage loss that resulted from the injury. In return, the employer bore the cost of insurance for the workers, and they were held free of liability under tort law.[35,59]

5.5. THE EVOLUTION OF NATIONAL PROTECTIVE LEGISLATION

5.5.1. British History

The Act of 1842 marked the beginning of a new era in mining by establishing the principles of Government inspection and State interference in the conduct of the industry.

—Donald Hunter[9]

After the Great Fire of London in 1666, tall chimneys became common, and the chimneys needed to be cleaned of the soot created by burnt coal. The job of sweeping the chimneys went to the climbing boys. These boys had to be small to negotiate the 7-inch-diameter chimneys. Exploitation of small boys as apprentices began when they were either sold by or kidnapped from their parents. The Futile Act of 1814 banned the climbing of chimneys by children, but it had little effect as climbing boy employment increased through the 1860s. Many met their death from the chimney sweeps' cancer of the scrotum. Another act was passed in 1834 that forbade the apprenticeship of boys younger than 10. In that same year, the Chimney Sweepers Act of 1834 was passed, which required the chimney to be 12 inches in diameter or rectangular measuring 14 by nine inches. This act aimed to reduce the danger of suffocation or getting jammed in the chimney. With the passage of the Chimney Sweepers Act of 1875, police were empowered to enforce the earlier acts and to license the chimney sweeps annually. Any violation would result in denial of the license.[9]

More broadly, the British Parliament enacted the Health and Morals Act in 1802. This act came about as a result of child servitude in the cotton and woolen factories. The act limited work hours to a 12-hour day, banned night work, required rooms to be ventilated, and ordered walls to be washed at least twice per year, but it made no limitation on age. The Factory Act of 1819 set the minimum age of employment at nine years.[9]

The Factory Act of 1833 followed with the longer title, "An Act to Regulate the Labor of Children in the Mills and Factories of the United Kingdom." It applied to textile factories, banned night work for employees younger than 18, and restricted the workday to 12 hours and a workweek to 69 hours. The minimum age of employment was set at nine years, and factory schools were required for children younger than 13.[9]

Rising publicity about the squalid and degrading conditions in mines led to public outrage. Children as young as six or seven years old worked in the coal pits 12 hours at a time. Children and naked women were harnessed to coal carts as they hauled the coal out of the mines on all fours. The drawings for these conditions fueled further public outrage. Six-year-old girls were found carrying 50-lb. baskets of coal on their backs up ladders. Some children worked double or triple shifts, adding up to as long as 36 continuous hours in the mines.[9]

Public indignation led the parliament to pass the Mines Act of 1842 despite spirited opposition by the coal owners in the House of Lords. The act prohibited the employment of women and girls underground, and boys' age of employment was set at 15. The act did not allow the inspection of mines but only the examination of the employees working in the mines. However, this limitation stirred seven successive Mine Regulation Acts through 1911, which gave birth to the "principle of government inspection" as the rights of the miners to safety, health, and well-being gained salience.[9]

Sweating refers to underpaid and overworked labor in which middlemen (the "factor," the origin of the term "factory") profited from the sweat of the workers and not from the manufacturer. The practice emerged by contracting with immigrants with few skills to do the work at a lower wage than the trades. An outcry against the sweating system starting in 1843 led to the passage of the Consolidating Factories and Workshops Act of 1878, which regulated this practice in factories and workshops but applied only to hired labor. However, many sweatshops in which work was farmed out as piecework to individual or whole families who worked in nothing more than rooms in homes escaped the regulation because those workers were not employees. The Trade Boards Act of 1909 closed some of the loopholes.[9]

The Print Works Act of 1845 moved government interventions beyond the textile industry, and the Factories and Workshops Act of 1867 brought regulations to control the hazards in the dangerous trades. The Factories Act of 1883 aimed to control the problem of lead poisoning.[9] In the early 20th century, laws focused on the notification to the government of occupational diseases and workers' compensation.[21]

5.5.2. United States History

While the disease (byssinosis) may not have been as prevalent in the United States as in England, ample evidence exists that American cotton mill workers suffered its effects in substantial numbers. What accounts for this lag in science and the lack of attention to workers' health in the United States?
—Charles Levenstein, Dianne Platamura, William Mass[64]

Early federal legislation focused on job safety and not occupational health when Congress established a Bureau of Labor in 1884 within the U.S. Department of the Interior (DoI), but in 1888, the bureau became an independent agency (subcabinet-level) through the Department of Labor Act. Then in 1903, it was absorbed into the new U.S. Department of Commerce and Labor, and re-created again as the Bureau of Labor. In 1910, the bureau launched a program on injury-rate calculations for the iron and steel industry. Until 1910, the bureau made the iron and steel injury data available only to the industry; it then published a bulletin, *The Safety Movement in the Iron and Steel Industry*, followed with another bulletin, *Causes and Prevention of Accidents in the Iron and Steel Industry*, in 1922. With the creation of the DoL in 1913, the bureau became the BLS.[65]

In 1931, Herbert W. Heinrich brought attention to the issue of occupational safety and published his landmark book, *Industrial Accident Prevention: A Scientific Approach*, followed by three more editions. The last edition was published in 1959.[66] He added concepts to the field of safety such as the injury pyramid, which is helpful in understanding the distribution of injuries by severity (ratios are useful in generalizing to larger populations).[67] However, his work generated two myths that have been recognized as having no place in professional safety. These myths are: (1) "unsafe acts of workers are the principal causes of occupational accidents," and (2) "reducing accident frequency will equivalently reduce severe injuries." The first myth is blaming the victim for "unsafe acts" rather than taking an approach for eliminating "unsafe conditions." The blaming-the-victim approach runs counter to the hierarchy of controls approach described in Chapter 2. The second myth goes back to the injury pyramid, which does not address different causes of injuries by severity; thus, resources may be diverted from serious injuries to close calls with the premise of like causes, but the close calls may have no relationship to fatal events.[66] Moreover, the use of the word "accident" implies a chance event resulting from carelessness (i.e., an unsafe act). A better term is "incident" or something more precise, such as "crash" or "fall from elevation."

In 1934, Secretary of Labor Perkins established the Office of Labor Standards, which later became the Bureau of Labor Standards and was a foundation for the eventual establishment of OSHA. In 1946, in order to protect returning World War II veterans, the DoL mounted a nationwide safety campaign culminating in an annual President's Conference on Occupational Safety.[65]

President Harry S. Truman initiated conferences on industrial safety in 1948 that continued through the Eisenhower administration. In 1951, Senator Hubert Humphrey (D) introduced a bill that called for uniform national safety and health standards and enforcement, which Congress never passed. However, health and safety provisions were included in the McNamara-O'Hara Public Service Contract Act of 1965 and the National Foundation on Arts and

Humanities Act of 1965. The first major federal occupational safety and health legislation came with the passage of the Federal Coal Mine Health and Safety Act of 1969 (Coal Act), which protected a small part of the nation's workforce.[68] Some early statutes that have affected occupational safety and health policy are described in Table 5-2.[14,53,69–72]

Table 5-2. Early U.S. Laws Affecting Occupational Safety and Health

Statute	Description
Bureau of Labor Act of 1884	Established the Bureau of Labor in the DoL to collect information about employment and labor.
Department of Labor Act of 1888	The Bureau of Labor became an independent (subcabinet) department called the Department of Labor until it was incorporated into the new Department of Commerce and Labor, reverting to the name Bureau of Labor.
Safety Appliance Act of 1893 (coupler bill)	In 1887, Congress created the ICC. Part of the reason for its establishment was the need to prevent the large number of deaths and injuries among railroad workers. Six years later, Congress passed the "coupler bill" to be implemented by the ICC.
Organic Act of 1910	Congress established the Bureau of Mines within the DoL. The bureau was charged with the responsibility to conduct research and to reduce accidents in the coal mining industry, but with no inspection authority.
Public Health Service Act of 1912	This act established the USPHS, which authorized investigations into human diseases. A major effort within the new USPHS was the investigation of industrial diseases. The Office of Industrial Hygiene was established pursuant to this act in 1914, which was the eventual predecessor of the National Institute for Occupational Safety and Health (NIOSH).
White Phosphorus Matches Prohibition Act of 1912 ("Esch" Act)	Congress used its power to tax to eliminate the dreaded disease phossy jaw among match makers. Representative John J. Esch of Wisconsin introduced the bill in 1910. It established a prohibitive tax on each box of matches made with white phosphorus, and white phosphorus matches then ceased to exist in the United States.
Railway Labor Act of 1926	This act, as amended in 1934 to prohibit "yellow dog" contracts and to establish a permanent National Mediation Board, sought to substitute bargaining, arbitration, and mediation for strikes as a means of resolving labor disputes in the railway industries. It was amended in 1936 to also apply to the airline industry.
National Labor Relations Act of 1935 (Wagner Act) and of 1947 (Taft-Hartley Act)	This act guaranteed workers the right to join unions without fear of management reprisal. It created the National Labor Relations Board to enforce this right. Opponents of organized labor countered in 1947 with the passage of the Taft-Hartley Act, which added provisions that allowed unions to be prosecuted, enjoined, and sued for a variety of activities, including mass picketing and secondary boycotts. The Landrum-Griffin Act of 1959 imposed further restrictions on unions.

(Continued)

Table 5-2. (Continued)

Statute	Description
Contract Work Hours and Safety Standards Act of 1936 (Walsh-Healey Public Contracts Act) and of 1969 (Construction Safety Act)	For work conducted under federal contract, this act established an overtime rate for hours worked in excess of eight hours per day or 40 hours per week, established the minimum wage as the prevailing wage, and set standards for child labor and on-the-job safety. A 1969 amendment, the Construction Safety Act, significantly strengthened employee protection by providing for occupational safety and health standards for employees of the building trades and construction industry in federal projects. The Secretary of Labor issued safety and health regulations for construction in 1971, days before the OSHAct became effective.
Fair Labor Standards Act of 1938 (Wages and Hours Act)	The act banned the interstate shipment of goods produced by employees who were paid less than a minimum wage or who had worked more than 44 hours a week without overtime pay.
Federal Coal Mine Safety Act of 1952	This act provided for annual inspections in certain underground coal mines and gave the Bureau of Mines limited enforcement authority to issue violation notices and imminent danger withdrawal orders. The act also authorized the assessment of civil penalties against mine operators for noncompliance with withdrawal orders or for refusing to give inspectors access to mine property.
McNamara-O'Hara Public Service Contract Act of 1965	This act protected employees of contractors performing maintenance work for federal agencies. For contracts of more than $2,500, the contactor had to comply with minimum wage laws, and for prime contracts in excess of $100,000, contractors and subcontractors had to comply with the Contract Work Hours and Safety Standards Act of 1962 (an amendment to the Walsh-Healey Public Contracts Act of 1936).
Federal Metal and Nonmetallic Mine Safety Act of 1966	The act provided for the promulgation of standards and for inspections and investigations but with minimal enforcement authority.
Federal Coal Mine Health and Safety Act of 1969	Referred to as the Coal Act, it included surface as well as underground coal mines within its scope, required two annual inspections of every surface coal mine and four at every underground coal mine, dramatically increased federal enforcement powers in coal mines, and provided for black lung compensation.

Note: DoI = U.S. Department of the Interior; ICC = Interstate Commerce Commission; USPHS = U.S. Public Health Service; OSHAct = Occupational Safety and Health Act.

5.5.3. Constitutional Intervention

The labor of a human being is not a commodity or article of commerce.
—Louis D. Brandeis[73]

Progress in worker protection was challenged by interpretations of three parts of the Constitution. One part was the interpretation of the interstate commerce clause in Section 8—"The Congress shall have Power . . . [t]o regulate

Commerce with foreign Nations, and among the several States, and with the Indian Tribes."[74] The 14th Amendment, ratified on July 9, 1868, states, "nor shall any State deprive any person of life, liberty, or property, without due process of law"[75]—building on the due process clause in the 5th Amendment that applies to the federal government.[76] The third interpretation restricted state legislators by Article I, Section 10, Clause 1, called the "contract clause," from providing private relief to those under contract.[77] This clause was originally targeted at wealthy citizens who found relief within the state legislature from debts incurred under contract. However, the contract clause was later used for decisions regarding the employee-employer contract.

Constitutional law in the United States has had its own paradigm shifts over time. Up through the Civil War, the Supreme Court restricted its decisions to procedural due process issues. The 14th Amendment extended due process judicial review to laws passed by the states. This was accompanied by a shift to substantive due process reinterpretations of constitutional text. Substantive review reinterpreted the "liberty of contract" and "private property" to protect economic interests, most notoriously demonstrated by the *Lochner v. New York* case as described in Table 5-3.[78] Another judicial review paradigm shift to judicial review defenses of social welfare programs using the due process clause occurred during the Great Depression. Another shift occurred in the 1960s regarding privacy issues and civil rights, with an emphasis on personal freedoms.[79,80]

With a landmark decision in 1819 regarding taxation of the Bank of the United States by a state (*McCulloch v. Maryland*), the Supreme Court established two principles: (1) the Constitution grants to Congress incidental and implied powers for a practical and functional government, and (2) state action may not impede valid constitutional exercises of power by the federal government. This decision laid the foundation for expanded federal involvement in public health under the Commerce Clause in the Constitution.[81]

Five years later, the Supreme Court struck down a New York law in the case of *Gibbons v. Ogden* that created a steamship monopoly for traffic between New York and New Jersey based on the Commerce Clause.[71] The principal constraint in applying the Commerce Clause has been in its definition.[82] The clause was intended to make a free-trade zone across the United States.[71] Commerce has always been construed to include the transportation of goods and persons across state lines.[82] Accordingly, the decision of the Supreme Court laid down the principle that the national government has jurisdiction over

Table 5-3. Supreme Court Decisions Regarding State and Federal Enacted Laws Related to the Commerce Clause and the Tax Power Under the Constitution

Statute	Decision
New York Bakeshop Act of 1895	A state law restricting the hours employees could work in the baking industry to 60 hours per week, but in 1905, the court struck it down as a violation of the freedom of contract guaranteed by the Due Process Clause. In this case (*Lochner v. New York*), the court interpreted the Due Process Clause to protect certain economic and property interests, such as the right of employers and employees to determine the terms and conditions of their employment relationship free from governmental intrusion. The "Lochner era" continued until 1937, when the court moved from an emphasis on property to private rights.[78]
Federal Employers' Liability Act of 1906	This act required a railroad company to compensate for an occupational death or injury of an employee if proven that the employer was partially culpable, but the Supreme Court ruled it unconstitutional because it failed to specify only interstate commerce. In 1908, a revamped law was upheld with improved wording under the Commerce Clause.
Federal Child Labor Act of 1916	In an attempt to reduce the abuse of child labor, this act barred the interstate shipment of products that were made by children under age 14 or between ages 14 and 16 who worked more than eight hours a day, more than six days a week, or at night. The court found that the act did not regulate transportation among the states, but aimed to standardize the ages at which children could be employed in mining and manufacturing within the states and held that this law exceeded Congress's constitutional authority. Again in 1918, the court struck down a prohibition on the interstate shipment of goods produced in plants using child labor.
Child Labor Tax Act of 1919	This act imposed an excise tax of 10% on the net profits of a company that employed children. The law defined child labor as employing a child "under the age of sixteen in any mine or quarry, and under the age of fourteen in any mill, cannery, workshop, factory, or manufacturing establishment." In 1922, the court ruled that the law was unconstitutional as an improper use of taxes meant for revenue by Congress to penalize employers using child labor. Chief Justice Taft delivered the opinion, which countered the logic of the earlier tax on matches for which he advocated and signed as president.
National Industrial Recovery Act of 1935	This act was the first effort of the administration of Franklin D. Roosevelt to address the unemployment of nearly 13 million American men and women caused by the Great Depression. On May 27, 1935, the court declared it unconstitutional. Within a month, the Senate began considering a bill proposed by Secretary of Labor Perkins to address the same problems on a less sweeping scale, which became the Walsh-Healey Public Contracts Act of 1936.
National Labor Relations Act of 1935	The court upheld this act, which compelled employers to engage in collective bargaining, holding that the Commerce Clause subsumed those things "affecting commerce." In this particular case, the court said that the phrase meant "tending to lead to a labor dispute burdening or obstructing commerce." The idea behind the ruling was that unfair actions by businesses caused strikes and other actions by workers that hindered the flow of interstate commerce.

Table 5-3. (Continued)

Statute	Decision
Civil Rights Act of 1964	The fundamental change in policy toward a more liberal interpretation of the Commerce Clause came when the court found that the Civil Rights Act of 1964, which banned racial discrimination in public accommodations, was constitutional under its commerce power. The court held that it should not second-guess Congress when it sees a connection to interstate commerce. Thus, once a person who wished to eat in a restaurant could not be discriminated against—based upon the Commerce Clause—a number of public safety, environmental, and occupational health and safety laws were enacted and were likewise held to be constitutional.

issues that involve interstate commerce. While this decision dealt with the trafficking of goods between states, it excluded the manufacture of the goods.[71]

Because boiler explosions plagued the steamboat industry in the early 1800s, Congress enacted two groundbreaking pieces of legislation under its commerce powers—one in the Steamboat Inspection Act of 1838 and the other in the Steamboat Act of 1852. In 1870, the Supreme Court upheld federal authority under the 1852 act regarding the inspection of steam passenger vessels that remained within a single state but carried goods shipped between states.[83]

The Safety Appliance Act of 1893 established the Commerce Clause as the vehicle for future comprehensive protection of workers from the hazards of work among several states, notwithstanding the congressional power to tax, embodied in the White Phosphorus Matches Prohibition Act of 1912. The clause was later applied to the telegraph and correspondence schools, followed later by the insurance business. Nevertheless, courts continued to confine the Commerce Clause power to the movement of goods and not the production of goods, thus excluding agriculture, mining, fishing, and manufacturing.[82] Descriptions of some Supreme Court decisions regarding related legislation are shown in Table 5-3.[52,69,78,84,85]

5.6. THE RISE OF THE OCCUPATIONAL SAFETY AND HEALTH ACT

Mr. Chairman and members of the Committee (Senate Subcommittee on Labor), while we sit here talking, from now until noon, 17 American men and women will be killed on their jobs. Every minute we talk, 18 to 20 people will be hurt severely enough to have to leave their jobs—some of them never to work again. In the time these two sentences have taken, another 20 people—one every second—have been injured on the job—less seriously, but in most cases needlessly. Today's industrial casualty list—like yesterday's—and tomorrow's—and every working day's week after month after year—will be 55 dead, 8,500 disabled, over 27,200 hurt. The figures for the year will be 14,000 to 15,000 dead, over 2 million disabled, over 7 million hurt.

—Willard Wirtz[86]

5.6.1. The Executive Branch as Initiator of Policy

The emergence of the idea of an occupational safety and health act came from the executive branch and not from Congress or interest groups. Thus, it was an idiosyncratic initiative, and it was founded upon a "good cause" as part of President Lyndon B. Johnson's "Quality of Life" initiative.

The DoL included a proposal for a federal occupational safety and health bill to the White House in 1967. The seed for the emergence of this bill went back to Jack Hardesty at the Bureau of Occupational Safety and Health (BOSH)—the predecessor agency to NIOSH—who lobbied with his brother and speechwriter for President Johnson, Robert Hardesty, to place references in the president's speeches to occupational safety and health.[87] This proposal emerged from these references and from concerns by Assistant Secretary of Labor Esther Peterson regarding the high incidence of lung cancer among uranium miners. The president included the DoL draft among his ideas—written by Robert Hardesty—in his 1968 Manpower Message.[30] On January 23, 1968, President Johnson proposed to Congress "the nation's first comprehensive Occupational Health and Safety Program" and included a bill to protect every worker while on the job in his 1968 legislative program.[52]

The bill contained provisions for research in the Department of Health, Education, and Welfare (DHEW) to develop occupational safety and health standards, and the Secretary of Labor was empowered to promulgate and enforce the standards and to provide federal assistance to the states to improve their occupational safety and health programs.

Following the president's 1968 message, he introduced the draft bill to Congress. The House subcommittee of the Education and Labor Committee began hearings on the bill on February 1, 1968. Congressional committees convened hearings on the proposed bill that degenerated into confrontation between trade unions and business groups. Several representatives of organized labor testified for the bill, including AFL-CIO President George Meany.[13,57]

Business interests led by the U.S. Chamber of Commerce, the National Association of Manufacturers, the American Iron and Steel Institute, and the Manufacturing Chemists Association opposed any federal enforcement for occupational safety and health. The Chamber of Commerce and the National Association of Manufacturers testified that the legislation was unnecessary because most "accidents" were due to human error or negligence.[30]

Events of 1968 rendered the proposal a low priority. The president announced that he would not run for reelection, both Martin Luther King Jr. and Robert F. Kennedy were assassinated, and demonstrators at the Democratic Convention met violent confrontation by the Chicago police. Action on the bill stalled.

5.6.2. Public Opinion Aroused

Nonetheless, several Democratic representatives introduced occupational health and safety legislation in 1969. Buffeted by mounting public opinion for protecting workers following the 1968 mine disaster in Farmington, West Virginia, in which 78 miners died, the Democrats reintroduced the bill in 1969. If a proposed bill had not already been available, it is likely that the momentum for passage of the OSHAct would have been absent in the aftermath of the Farmington disaster.[13]

There was a rush for stricter coal mine safety laws, while a grassroots movement had emerged to compensate victims of coal workers' pneumoconiosis (CWP), commonly called black lung. The black lung movement led to several wildcat strikes and a march on the state capital in Charleston, West Virginia. Ralph Nader participated in this movement, and Gary Sellers, who had worked on the coal mine bill at the Office of Management and Budget, joined Nader in crafting proposed safety and health legislation. Both the United Mine Workers of America and the United Steelworkers of America represented the miners, and the steelworkers wanted legislation to help the cancer victims that worked in coke oven plants at the steel mills.[57]

In 1970, organized labor made an occupational safety and health act its top priority. The new head of the AFL-CIO's Industrial Union Department, Iorwith Wilber Abel, led this initiative. Abel had been the steelworkers' president and had experience in influencing the passage of the Coal Act of 1969. The steelworkers' chief lobbyist and advisor to Abel was Jack Sheehan, who was intense in his pursuit for passage of an occupational health and safety act.[57]

Sellers worked with Nader and with Representative Phillip Burton (D) of California and teamed up with Daniel Kravit, the counsel for the Select Subcommittee on Labor, which was responsible for occupational safety and health bills under the chairmanship of Domenick Daniels (D) of New Jersey. The subcommittee crafted legislation that was much more sweeping than was considered in earlier hearings. The subcommittee drew from the Coal Act, the steelworkers' suggestions, and the Nader network to draft safety and health legislation.[57]

Among the changes from earlier bills was a system of citations based upon a violation rather than upon failure to correct a violation, the burden of appeal placed upon the violator, and penalties made mandatory. The legislation also established procedures for informing workers and establishing standards not only on permissible exposure levels but also on prescriptions for personal protective equipment, medical examinations, and environmental monitoring.

The subcommittee reported the "Daniels bill" to the House Education and Labor Committee in March 1970, which approved it in June. As a result, the Senate Labor and Public Welfare Committee, chaired by Senator Harrison Williams (D) of New Jersey, adopted most of the Daniels bill in September, and with the White House's involvement, Representative William A. Steiger (R) of Wisconsin helped champion the movement with a bill that differed from the Daniels bill. The Steiger bill aimed to set up an independent board to establish standards and another board to hear appeals, while the DoL would be relegated to the role of conducting inspections—a diminished role opposed by labor.[13,57]

5.6.3. Congressional Politics

For years, Harold Lasswell had provided the lay definition of politics in the title of his 1936 book, *Politics: Who Gets What, When, How.*[88] More recent insights into the definition of political behavior capture the idea of coalitions, in which politics can be defined as the coalition of human activity (through the distribution of power) in the pursuit of value-laden goals. Some coalitions act to gain goals, and other coalitions can obstruct or neutralize these actions. Coalitions were important in the passage of the OSHAct.[89]

Newly elected President Nixon countered with a bill of his own in an attempt to draw the blue collar "hard-hats" from the Democratic Party, but with no sympathy for unions.[30] This marked the start of a political battle between a coalition supporting business interests and a Congress controlled by Democrats who supported labor's interests.

The Nixon bill was proposed by Senator Jacob Javits (R) of New York and Representative William Ayers (R) of Ohio, and when Ayers was not reelected, he was supplanted by Representative Steiger as the cosponsor of the Nixon bill. The Republican bill (i.e., the Nixon proposal) added votes for the passage of an act with the backing of business while it energized the unions to lambast the president. It differed from the Democratic bill in many ways, including the establishment of an independent rule-making commission rather than a regulatory agency within the DoL. The AFL-CIO placed the passage of the Democratic version of the bill as a priority for its lobbying in 1969 and 1970.[13,57]

In the hearings on the bills, the Republicans focused their efforts on procedural issues rather than the substance of the bills, attempting to protect against the threat to employers' self-interest. The testimony at hearings emphasized the infinite value of human life and that a single injury or death related to work was too much, and thus the cost of implementation was avoided in testimony. Indeed, the cost issue was avoided by the bill's proponents under the imprecise term "feasibility." Even though most legislators from both parties thought cost was an issue, they wished to avoid it so as to pass the bill. In addition, business groups and Republican legislators sought to avoid the stigma of "putting a price tag on life." They were driven by the need to be portrayed as people as concerned about safety as anyone else. Raising the cost issue would compromise that image.[57]

Another part of crafting these bills was the creation of NIOSH (Marcus Key, oral communication, April 1996). Dr. Marcus Key, director of BOSH, had testified for the passage of the Coal Act. Now he joined covertly with Sheehan and other labor lobbyists—notably George Taylor—in crafting the different versions of the occupational safety and health bills. The bills placed much responsibility upon NIOSH to conduct research and training and propose standards as well as to possess the right of entry into workplaces and access to records like that given to the Labor Department.

Key recalled an incident in which the secretary of his department, Nixon appointee Casper W. Weinberger, walked by in the Senate halls to a room to give testimony where he, Sheehan, and Taylor sat on the floor with their backs to the wall outside a committee hearing room. Sitting on the floor next to them, Key raised up his newspaper to conceal his face from the secretary as he walked into the room.

The Democrats controlled both the House of Representatives and the Senate. The House subcommittee of the Education and Labor Committee moved to report the bill out to the full committee, but the Republicans on the subcommittee boycotted the sessions to stop a quorum and this action by the subcommittee. Only when the chairman of the full committee attended a session as an ex-officio member could a quorum be established and the bill reported out to the full committee. Contention followed the bills to the floors of both the House and Senate. Amendments modifying the bills as reported to the floor of both houses were made with partisan votes swaying the compromises of the bill one way or another. Nevertheless, the final bill reflected more of the Democratic version than the Republican version.

In the full House, the Steiger bill passed over the Daniels bill by a vote of 220 to 172. Meanwhile, the Senate passed a bill that resembled the Daniels bill that left most of the functions in the Labor Department except for a modification by Senator Javits, wherein an independent Occupational Safety and Health Review Commission was established to hear appeals. The Conference Committee resolved most of the issues in favor of the Senate bill. The Williams-Steiger Act passed overwhelmingly, with the Senate voting 83–3 and the House voting 384–5 for passage. Some special interests encouraged President Nixon to veto the bill, but as he had placed it on his agenda and had vetoed another labor bill regarding public jobs earlier in the month, he now felt compelled to sign the bill. President Nixon signed the OSHAct on December 29, 1970.[30] With the overwhelming vote in both houses, a veto would be futile because it could be easily overridden by Congress.[52] A more detailed account of the arguments regarding passage of the OSHAct is provided in Section 6.3 in the next chapter.

THE JUNGLE NARRATIVE

Upton Sinclair published exposés of the terrible working conditions faced by employees during his career. One was the novel *The Jungle*,[41] first published in 1905, and another novel entitled *King Coal* was published in 1917.[90] *The Jungle* revealed the scandalous working conditions in meatpacking plants. It also told of poor working conditions in canneries and fertilizer mills and of economic savagery: the poor living conditions of workers and their families, the struggles of organized labor, wage slavery, and jail time of family breadwinners. Sinclair's exposé of working conditions held little traction with the public, but people were outraged with how meat was produced in the slaughterhouses and the graft that tempered the vigilance of elected meat inspectors. His novel led to official investigations and the passage of the Federal Pure Food and Drug Act and the Meat Inspection Act in 1906. A year before his death, Sinclair was invited to the White House to witness President Johnson signing the Wholesome Meat Act of 1967.[91] Food affected the many, thus action was taken; but working conditions affected the scattered few, and the struggle for protection continued.

REFERENCES

1. Robinson DN. *American Ideals: Founding a "Republic of Virtue."* Chantilly, VA: The Teaching Company;2004. Lecture No. 11: With Liberty and Justice for All.

2. Winship M. Uncle Tom's Cabin: history of the book in the 19th-century United States. Presented at: Uncle Tom's Cabin in the Web of Culture conference, sponsored by the National Endowment for the Humanities, presented by the Harriet Beecher Stowe Center (Hartford, CT) and the Uncle Tom's Cabin and American Culture Project; June 2007; University of Virginia. Available at: http://utc.iath.virginia.edu/interpret/exhibits/winship/winship.html. Accessed January 15, 2012.

3. Claybaugh A. Introduction and notes. In: Stowe, HB. *Uncle Tom's Cabin.* New York, NY: Barnes & Nobles Classics;2003.

4. Dunn CM, Chawick G. *Protecting Study Volunteers in Research: A Manual for Investigative Sites.* Boston, MA: CenterWatch;1999.

5. Jackson A. State of the Union address. December 3, 1833. In: Jackson A. *State of the Union Addresses by United States Presidents.* Available at: http://www2.hn.psu.edu/faculty/jmanis/poldocs/uspressu/SUaddressAJackson.pdf. Accessed May 26, 2014.

6. Sigerist HE. The Wesley M. Carpenter Lecture: historical background of industrial and occupational diseases. *Bull N Y Acad Med.* 1936;12(11):597–609.

7. Wampler FJ. *The Principles and Practice of Industrial Medicine.* Baltimore, MD: The Williams and Wilkins Co.;1943.

8. Felton JS, Newman JP, Read DL. *Man, Medicine, and Work: Historic Events in Occupational Medicine*. Washington, DC: U.S. Government Printing Office;1964. U.S. Public Health Service Publication No. 1044.

9. Hunter D. *The Diseases of Occupations*. London, UK: Hodder and Stoughton; 1975.

10. Hazlett, TL. *Introduction to Industrial Medicine*. Chicago, IL: Industrial Medicine Publishing Co.;1947.

11. Rosen G. Introduction. In: Ramazzini B, Wright WC, trans. *De Morbis Artificum [Diseases of Workers]*. Trans. and reprint ed.;1713. New York, NY: Hafner Publishing Co.;1964:v–ix.

12. Hunter D. *The Diseases of Occupations*. London, UK: Hodder and Stoughton; 1978.

12a. Peytavi C. Anne Besant and the 1888 London matchgirls strike. Université Paris Ouest. October 11, 2003. Available at: http://anglais.u-paris10.fr/spip.php?article84. Accessed January 30, 2015.

13. MacLaury J. The job safety law of 1970: its passage was perilous. *Monthly Labor Rev.* 1981;104:18–24.

14. Holbrook SH. *Let Them Live*. New York, NY: The Macmillan Co.;1939.

15. Sicherman B. *Alice Hamilton: A Life in Letters*. Cambridge, MA: Harvard University Press;1984.

16. Eastman C. Work accidents and the law. In: Kellogg PU, ed. *The Pittsburgh Survey: Findings in Six Volumes*. New York, NY: Russell Sage Foundation;1910.

17. Lubove R. *20th-Century Pittsburgh: Government Business, and Environmental Change*. New York, NY: John Wiley and Sons, Inc.;1969.

18. Adler MJ, ed. 1929-1939: The Great Depression. *The Annals of American History*. Vol. 15. Chicago, IL: William Benton;1968.

19. Proctor RN. *Cancer Wars: How Politics Shapes What We Know and Don't Know About Cancer*. New York, NY: Basic Books;1995.

20. Salerno D, Feitshans I. Harriet L. Hardy, MD. Fighting man-made disease. *J Epidemiol Community Health*. 2003;57(12):924.

21. Hardy HL. Foreword. In: Finkel AJ, Hamilton A, Hardy HL, eds. *Hamilton and Hardy's Industrial Toxicology*. 4th ed. Boston, MA: John Wright-PSG Inc.; 1983.

22. Raffle PAB, Lee WR, McCallum RI, Murray R, eds. *Hunter's Diseases of Occupations*. Boston, MA: Little, Brown & Co.;1987.

23. Johnson BL. *Legacy of Hope: Stories of Lives Saved and Disabilities Prevented*. Atlanta, GA: Emory University;2011. Monograph, Department of Environmental Health, Rollins School of Public Health.

24. Ashford NA, Caldart CC. *Technology, Law, and the Working Environment*. New York, NY: Van Nostrand Reinhold;1991.

25. Ashford NA. *Crisis in the Workplace: Occupational Disease and Injury*. Cambridge, MA: MIT Press;1976.

26. Noble C. *Liberalism at Work: the Rise and Fall of OSHA*. Philadelphia, PA: Temple University Press;1986.

27. Bowles S, Gordon D, Weisskopf T. *Beyond the Wasteland*. Garden City, NY: Anchor Press;1983.

28. Kazis R, Grossman RL. *Fear at Work*. New York, NY: Pilgrim Press;1982.

29. Ferguson JS. Objectives of occupational health. In: *Introduction to Occupational Health*. Cincinnati, OH: National Institute for Occupational Safety and Health; 1979;509.

30. Kelman S. Occupational Safety and Health Administration. In: Wilson JQ, ed. *The Politics of Regulation*. New York, NY: Basic Books, Inc.;1980:236–266.

31. Durkheim E. *The Elementary Forms of Religious Life*. New York, NY: Free Press; 1995.

32. Morris RB, ed. *The U.S. Department of Labor History of the American Worker*. Washington, DC: U.S. Government Printing Office;1977.

33. Brooks TR. *Toil and Trouble: A History of American Labor*. New York, NY: Dell Publishing;1964.

34. Derickson A. *Workers' Health, Workers' Democracy: The Western Miners' Struggle, 1891-1925*. Ithaca, NY: Cornell University Press;1988.

35. Aldrich M. *Safety First: Technology, Labor, and Business of American Work Safety 1870–1939*. Baltimore, MD: The John Hopkins University Press;1997.

36. Light W. *Working for the Railroad: The Organization of Work in the Nineteenth Century*. Princeton, NJ: Princeton University Press;1983.

37. Schlegel MW. The Workingmen's Benevolent Association: first union of anthracite miners. *Pa Hist*. 1943;10(4):243–267.

38. Brecher J. *Strike!* Greenwich, CT: Fawcett Premier Book;1972.

39. Trapp PS. Non-fatal injuries in the Alaska commercial fishing industry. In: Myers ML, Klatt ML, eds. *Proceedings of the National Fishing Industry Safety and Health Workshop.* Cincinnati, OH: National Institute for Occupational Safety and Health (NIOSH);1994:45–47. NIOSH Publication No. 94-109.

40. Samuel HD. Troubled passage: the labor movement and the Fair Labor Standards Act. *Monthly Labor Rev.* 2000;127(12):32–37.

41. Sinclair U. *The Jungle.* New York, NY: Bantam Books;1981.

42. Watson B. *Bread and Roses: Mills, Migrants, and the Struggle for the American Dream.* New York, NY: Penguin Books;2006.

43. Drake A. Lonmin to SAfrica strikers: work Monday or fired. Associated Press. 2012. Available at: http://bigstory.ap.org/article/lonmin-safrica-strikers-work-monday-or-fired. Accessed February 21, 2015.

44. Maylie D. Shootings weigh on South Africa's leaders. *Wall Street Journal.* 2012; 260(41):A6.

45. Maylie D. Mine strikes spread in South Africa. *Wall Street Journal.* 2012;260(60):B3.

46. Foner PS. *History of the Labor Movement in the United States.* Vol. 1. New York, NY: International Publishers;1947.

47. Twain M, Warner CD. *The Gilded Age.* New York, NY: Oxford University Press;1996.

48. Lawrence History Center. Bread and Roses centennial exhibit. Bread and Roses Centennial Committee and the Lawrence History Center. Available at: http://exhibit.breadandrosescentennial.org/node/4. Accessed August 20, 2012.

49. Palmer LR. History of the safety movement. *Ann Am Acad Pol Soc Sci.* 1926; 123:9–19.

50. Taksa L. Intended or unintended consequences? A critical reappraisal of the Safety First movement and its non-union safety committees. *Econ Ind Democr.* 2009;30(1):9.

51. Rabinowitz RS, ed. *Occupational Safety and Health Law.* Washington, DC: Bureau of National Affairs;2002.

52. Ashford NA, Caldart CC. *Technology, Law, and the Working Environment.* Washington, DC: Island Press;1996.

53. Wolf S, Bruhn JG, Goodell H. *Occupational Health as Human Ecology.* Springfield, IL: Charles C. Thomas Publisher;1978.

54. Rogers DW. *Making Capitalism Safe: Work Safety and Health Regulation in America, 1880-1940.* Champaign, IL: University of Illinois Press;2010.

55. Corn JK. *Protecting the Health of Workers: The American Conference of Governmental Industrial Hygienists, 1938-1988.* Cincinnati, OH: American Conference of Governmental Industrial Hygienists;1989.

55a. Walsh-Healey Public Contracts Act, 41 U.S.C. 35-45 (1936).

56. National Safety Council. *Accident Prevention Manual for Industrial Operations: Administration and Programs.* Chicago, IL: National Safety Council;1988.

57. Page JA, O'Brien M-W. *Bitter Wages.* New York, NY: Grossman Publishers; 1973.

58. Ladou J, Teitelbaum DT, Egilman DS, et al. American College of Occupational and Environment Medicine (ACOEM): A professional association in service to industry. *Int J Occup Environ Health.* 2007;13(4):404-426.

59. Weinstein J. *The Corporate Ideal in the Liberal State, 1900-1916.* Boston, MA: Beacon Press;1968.

60. Carr JD. Workers' compensation systems: purpose and mandate. *Occup Med State Art Rev.* 1998;13(2):417-438.

61. Little JW, Eaton TA, Smith GR. *Workers' Compensation: Cases and Materials.* St. Paul, MN: West Publishing Co.;1993.

62. Barth PS, Hunt HA. *Workers' Compensation and Work-Related Illnesses and Diseases.* Cambridge, MA: MIT Press;1980.

63. Boden LI. Workers' compensation. In: Levy BS, Wegman DH, eds. *Occupational Health: Recognizing and Preventing Work-Related Disease.* Boston, MA: Little, Brown and Co.;1988:149-162.

64. Levenstein C, Platamura D, Mass W. Labor and Byssinosis, 1941-1969. In: Rosner D, Markowitz G, eds. *Dying for Work: Workers' Safety and Health in Twentieth-Century America.* Bloomington, IN: Indiana University Press;1987:208-223.

65. Clague E. *The Bureau of Labor Statistics.* New York, NY: Frederick A. Praeger Publishers;1968.

66. Manuele FA. Reviewing Heinrich: dislodging two myths from the practice of safety. *Prof Saf.* 2011;57(10):52-61.

67. Myers ML, Cole HP, Mazur JM. Cost effectiveness of wearing head protection on all-terrain vehicles. *J Agromed.* 2009;14(3):312-323.

68. Savelson DW. Legal aspects of the Occupational Safety and Health Act of 1970: Revised and supplemental course manual and outline. Cincinnati, OH: National Institute for Occupational Safety and Health;1978.

69. Myers ML, McGlothlin JD. Matchmakers' "phossy jaw" eradicated. *Am Ind Hyg Assoc J*. 1996;57(4):330–332.

70. Alton LR. The eradication of phossy jaw: a unique development of federal police power. *The Historian*. 1966;24:1–24.

71. Richmond S. The Commerce Clause: route to omnipotent government. Available at: http://www.fff.org/freedom/0895g.asp. Accessed September 7, 2006.

72. Mine Safety and Health Administration. History of mine safety and health legislation. Available at: http://www.msha.gov/mshainfo/mshainf2.htm. Accessed September 14, 2012.

73. Douglas WO. *Go East, Young Man: The Early Years, The Autobiography of William O. Douglas*. New York, NY: Delta Book;1974:453.

74. U.S. Const. art I, § 8, cl 3.

75. U.S. Const. amend. XIV, § 1.

76. U.S. Const. amend. V.

77. U.S. Const., art I, § 10, cl 1.

78. *Lochner v. New York*, 198 U.S. 45, 25 S. Ct. 539, 49 L. Ed. 937 (1905). Available at: http://legal-dictionary.thefreedictionary.com/Lochner+v+New+York. Accessed September 15, 2012.

79. White GW. *Oliver Wendell Holmes: Sage of the Supreme Court*. New York, NY: Oxford University Press;2000.

80. Koterski J. *Natural Law and Human Nature*. Chantilly, VA: The Teaching Company;2002. Course Guidebook.

81. Institute of Medicine. *The Future of Public Health*. Washington, DC: National Academy Press;1988.

82. Clark GL. Introduction. In: Clark GL. *Summary of American Law*. Rochester, NY: The Lawyers Cooperative Publishing Company;1947:486.

83. Sandukas GP. *How Exploding Steamboat Boilers in the 19th Century Ignited Federal Public Welfare Regulation* [third-year paper]. Redacted version. Cambridge, MA: Harvard Law School;2002. Available at: http://leda.law.harvard.edu/leda/data/530/Sandukas_redacted.pdf. Accessed March 30, 2012.

84. Rodell F. 1955. *Nine Men*. New York, NY: Random House;1947.
85. *Bailey v. Drexel Furniture Co.* 259 U.S. 20 (1922). Available at: http://law2.umkc.edu/faculty/projects/ftrials/conlaw/drexel.html. Accessed September 21, 2012.
86. Lemen RA, Mazzuckelli LF, Niemeier RW, Ahlers HW. Occupational safety and health standards. *Ann N Y Acad Sci*. 1989;572:100–106.
87. Sullivan P. Public health publicist Jack Hardesty. *Washington Post*. June 8, 2006:B07.
88. Lasswell HD. *Politics: Who Gets What, When, How*. New York, NY: Whittlesey House;1936.
89. Hanley J. What is politics? December 21, 2010. Available at: http://ordinary-gentlemen.com/blog/2010/12/21/what-is-politics. Accessed May 26, 2014.
90. Sinclair U. *King Cole*. New York, NY: Bantam Books;1994.
91. Dickerson M. Introduction. In: Sinclair U. *The Jungle*. New York, NY: Bantam Books;1981:xvii.

6

Policy Advocacy Through Argument

Critical thinking means being able to evaluate evidence, to tell fact from opinion, to see holes in an argument, to tell whether cause and effect has been established to spot illogic.

—D. Alan Bensley[1]

THE WILDFIRE NARRATIVE

The U.S. Forest Service implemented its smokejumper program in 1939 with the aim of parachuting firefighters into remote mountainous terrain to put out fires. The first jump occurred in 1940. Nine years later, on the afternoon of August 5, 1949, 15 elite smokejumpers parachuted into Mann Gulch, an isolated ravine near the Missouri River in Montana, to control and extinguish a forest fire ignited by lightning the night before. "Wag" Dodge was the crew foreman. Another firefighter already on the ground joined the crew. Wag was experienced, but he had not worked with this crew before. The fire crept along the ground higher up along one side of the ravine. It appeared to be a routine firefight and easy to control, so the crew paused to eat lunch. Then Wag led them down the forested gulch on the right side of the fire toward the river where they could fight it from an upwind position, but a high wind materialized and burst the fire into a blowup that reached into the tree canopy. This crown fire launched burning pine needles and pinecones called firebrands high into the air ahead of the crew, igniting a wall of flames between the crew and the river. The fire swept up the slope toward the men. Seeing that they were in a death trap, Wag immediately reversed the men back up the steep gulch toward the safety of the ridge. Now alarmed, he ordered the men to drop their tools and run. The crew emerged from the forest onto a grassy hillside, but the wind was even stronger away from the trees. It was truly a death trap now; Wag saw that the fire would overrun them. He reached down and intuitively started what would later be called an escape fire in the tall dry grass, which quickly burned off a small clearing. He yelled to the men, "Up this way!" The men either did not hear him or thought him crazy. Their intuition was to run. None followed Wag as he lay face down in the burned-out clearing. The fire passed around Wag. Two men made it to the safety of a rocky area at the top of the ridge, but the other 13 men died from the fire, two of whom died later from their burns. Some of the dead still held their tools in their hands. Wag failed as a leader because none of the crew followed him; he had not previously worked with the crew to build team confidence. The 13 victims' intuition to run cost them their lives, but Wag's intuition to ignite the escape fire saved his life. In this situation there was no time for critical thinking—intuition ruled. Following this incident, firefighters remembered Wag's innovation to "run for the black," as with good reason that is where the ground is devoid of fuel for the fire.[2-4]

6.1. INTRODUCTION

How can a defensible compromise be reached between the protection of health and counteracting factors such as economic, technological, or political feasibility?

—Sven Ove Hansson[5]

Policy is nothing unless moved to action. Accordingly, the next section of this chapter addresses advocacy and critical thinking and its close ally, argumentation. For advocacy, persuasion differentiates issues from the past. It entails gaining public support for a particular policy. Indeed, it is a responsibility of public health professionals.[6] Advocates can advance reason-based policies for occupational safety and health using techniques of argument. Arguments make claims based upon issues, which is a technique for both reasoned judgment and persuasive influence and is applicable for advancing occupational safety and health policy.[7]

In the third section, the foundation for the structure and analysis of the different types of arguments is demonstrated through a description of the congressional debate for the passage of the Occupational Safety and Health Act (OSHAct; see Appendix). While the argumentation approach is based on inductive reasoning that depends upon empirical information, the fourth section in this chapter describes abductive reasoning (hypothesis generation), which is at the core of the precautionary principle. The fifth section addresses agenda-setting and framing an argument, which affects successful advocacy whether publicly or within organizations. The final section of this chapter describes some fallacies in arguments and enemies of prevention.

6.2. THE OCCUPATIONAL SAFETY AND HEALTH PROFESSIONAL AS ADVOCATE

Advocacy is a strategy for blending science and politics with social justice values with an orientation to make the system work better, particularly with those with the least resources.

—Lawrence M. Wallack, Lora Dorfman,
David H. Jernigan, Makani Themba-Nixon[8]

The advocate must deal with power players of politics and engage in controversies with interest groups so as to resolve issues and claims though reasoning. Reasoning applies critical thinking to a decision of what to believe or to do and determines if the claims and conclusions are justified.[9,10] Argumentation is a technique used in critical thinking. Advocacy and controversy are discussed herein, as is constructing an issue statement that drives an argument. In addition, the structure of an argument is described, which involves a claim and the evidence and inferences that support the claim. Finally, the importance of addressing policy change in increments is noted.

6.2.1. Advocacy

An occupational safety and health advocate will face the task of convincing others of policy claims and contend with a plethora of disciplines and special interests in the presence of uncertainty. Advocacy is defined as a set of skills used to create a shift in public opinion and mobilize the necessary resources and forces to support an issue, policy, or constituency.[8] A public health advocate's armamentarium includes understanding sound strategy in promoting a policy position and defending quality research under conditions of uncertainty while encouraging precaution. Characteristics of advocacy are listed below:[11]

- People have rights that are enforceable.
- Advocacy needs to be specific and clear and focus different interests on common ground.
- It concerns the rights of communities that may represent health disparity.
- It is also concerned with ensuring that institutions work as they should, including legal and ethical behavior.

The great challenge for the advocate is to establish that injury or illness is likely under conditions of uncertainty. Public health is "essentially" political,[8] and public health advocacy may depend upon political and mass media battles. Advocacy can proceed either against entrenched beliefs and dogma or through reasoning in which argument is used to inform each side of an issue, leading to resolution. Advocacy against dogma entails political conflict with interest groups in efforts to change public opinion.[12]

Two well-organized advocacy coalitions historically have faced off regarding occupational safety and health. The business coalition includes the Business Round Table, the National Association of Manufacturers, the Chemical Manufacturers Association, and the U.S. Chamber of Commerce. These entities hardened into well-organized interest groups based on economic interests,[13] and they as well as individual companies are large campaign contributors and contributors to political action committees. Academic economists, especially those in business schools, tend to support business interests, and the business coalition generally pushes for weaker occupational safety and health policies or no regulation. This coalition has many advantages, including effective interest group articulation, resources, prestige and status, and knowledge about the system (e.g., lobbying Congress).[14] As an example, a business coalition was successful at defeating the ergonomics standard in 2001 after it was promulgated, as described in the leading narrative in Chapter 1.

The other advocacy coalition is organized labor, which increased its power from the 1930s to the 1960s.[13] This coalition advocates for occupational safety and health and is supported by public health professionals and the consumer safety advocacy organization Public Citizen, which has joined unions in the struggle to improve working conditions in the United States. Using the courts, organized labor has sued the government for its failure to protect workers. An exemplar of this tactic is its submission of a petition to the 3rd Circuit

Court of Appeals (Philadelphia, PA) to order the Occupational Safety and Health Administration (OSHA) to initiate rule making to protect workers from the adverse health effects of hexavalent chromium, which the court granted in 2002. It ordered OSHA to promulgate a standard, finding that it had unreasonably delayed taking action to protect workers from this dangerous substance, a danger that was popularized in the 2000 movie, *Erin Brockovich*.[15,16]

Argumentation is reasoning tested by doubt. It deals with giving reasons for our beliefs and actions under uncertainty, where the correct belief or action is not obvious. Arguments involve claims and evidence connected by inference based upon warrants. Arguments may be governed by institutional forums such as technical meetings, rule-making processes, giving testimony, or courtroom testimony, or they may occur in small groups or one-on-one dialogue.[17]

6.2.2. Controversy

Arguments arise out of five preconditions. First, there is a disagreement—a controversy—between people. Second, the disagreement is not trivial; it is serious. Third, the advocate desires assent by the other party. Fourth, if convinced, the other party's assent is freely given, and fifth, there is no easier way to resolve the disagreement than through argument.[12]

Policies are advocated and established by claims from which controversies begin. These claims involve action and address the question, "What should or ought we do?"[12] As an example, in 1973, the National Institute for Occupational Safety and Health (NIOSH) went beyond the use of blood-lead levels as the measure of safety for exposed workers and argued that monitoring for lead in the air should be the standard. The lead industry argued the converse: that measuring blood-lead levels was the only significant measure of lead toxicity. The NIOSH recommendation fueled a heated debate through the rest of the 1970s.[18] Resolution evolved with air monitoring for lead becoming the standard but with monitoring of blood-lead levels as a backup strategy.

Public health professionals are educated in a broad range of technical fields, including epidemiology, toxicology, infectious disease control, engineering, and injury prevention, which expertise is used to formulate policy claims. Support for these claims requires convincing decision makers of their necessity, sometimes against strong economic or value-laden interests. Moreover, the burden of proof will likely lie upon their shoulders; thus, formulating

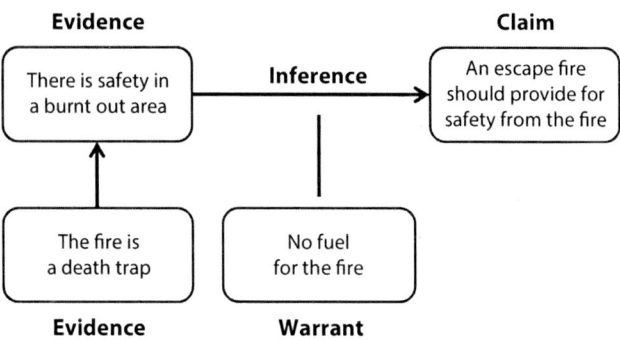

Figure 6-1. Simple argument diagram related to "The Wildfire Narrative."

a strategy for supporting their claims with reason-based evidence becomes crucial. It is also vital to recognize bad arguments, for they can drive out good arguments.

A critical thinking method from the field of argumentation offers a policy analysis approach for the advocate to engage issues for public policy. Policy analysis enables one to understand what is going on in an argument. Policy analysis is addressed more broadly in the final chapter of this book.

Developing sequentially as in a conversation, simple arguments deal with single claims. Arguments can be described in three segments: one is the claim, another is evidence, and third is the inference that links the evidence to the claim. Different types of arguments are examined in Section 6-3. The general model for this examination is shown in Figure 6-1, which is a simple argument, based upon "The Wildfire Narrative" above.[12] Claims emerge from stated issues or questions to be answered.

6.2.3. Issue Statement

A statement of an occupational safety and health issue is a clear articulation of the problem to be solved, potential solutions, data sources, and health outcomes. A typical outline for an issue statement includes background and data, policy questions, potential solutions, and potential outcomes. Issue statements may address objectives of an anticipated action, they may respond to a question from an elected or appointed public official, or they may result from an agency's needs assessment of a particular problem. The health needs and

Table 6-1. Types of Claims, Their Characteristics, Proof Requirements, and Topoi

Type	Characteristic	Proof Requirement	Topoi (used to define the issue)
Definition	Meaning, interpretation	Neutral source	Is the interpretation relevant? Is the interpretation fair? How do we choose among competing interpretations?
Fact	Description	Independent of arguers	How will we know if the statement is true—that is, what are the criteria? Are the criteria satisfied?
Value	Judgment of good or bad	Standards, criteria	Is the alleged condition good or bad? Has the value been properly applied to the situation? How do we choose among competing values?
Policy	Action	Deliberation	Is there a problem? Where is the credit or blame for the problem due? Will the proposal solve the problem? On balance, will things be better off with the proposal?

Source: Based on Zarefsky.[12]

desires of a population lead to an issue statement based upon a needs assessment. A needs assessment typically relies upon extant secondary data, which saves time and money, rather than on primary data collected by an advocate.[19]

The description of an issue is typical in the evidence-based public health approach, which is broad and imprecise. More precision is needed in defining the issue for an advocate to defend claims. More precisely, an issue statement is the question inherent in the controversy and necessary for resolution of the controversy.[12]

An aid to identifying issues is their categorization by *topoi*, which means "place," and in argumentation, metaphorical places of the mind.[12] Topoi are used to identify issues related to resolutions and claims. They are shortcuts packaged as questions for writing issue statements and are shown in Table 6-1 associated with different types of claims, which are described in Section 6.2.5. An example of an issue statement regarding a policy claim follows:

> On February 7, 2008, an explosion and fire occurred at the Imperial Sugar refinery near Savannah, Georgia, that resulted in 14 occupational fatalities and 38 nonfatal injuries to workers, 14 of which were life-threatening burns. The explosion was fueled by an accumulation of combustible sugar dust in

the sugar packaging building. In September 2009, the independent U.S. Chemical Safety Board called on OSHA to "proceed expeditiously" on an earlier 2006 recommendation to promulgate a new combustible dust standard for general industry. The board expressed a belief that such a standard is necessary to reduce or eliminate hazards from fires and explosions from a variety of combustible powders and dust.[20]

6.2.4. The Policy Network

Policy networks are important in resolving issues, and the network can be small. For example, based on personal experience, after the 1988 presidential election, when Congress received the president's budget but had not yet vetted the nominees for cabinet posts, the budget as prepared by the Office of Management and Budget (OMB) had eliminated an agency's funding for agricultural safety and health research by millions of dollars. An agency advocate interacted with a former agency director to resolve how to restore the funding in the budget. The plan was to prepare a set of questions to raise the issue to a high level during the Senate confirmation hearings of four different candidates nominated by the new president. The advocate and the former director wrote a set of questions that embedded the elements of an issue statement to be asked of the nominees. The former director gave the set of questions to a union contact, who in turn gave it to a Senate staffer. The staffer called the OMB examiner responsible for the agency's budget and told him of the questions to be asked unless the budget was restored. This was a minor but potentially embarrassing issue for the administration, so the budget was restored in the president's proposal. This action only involved five individuals, as shown in Figure 6-2, without members of the network knowing some of the other members, yet was an effective policy network that resulted in successful advocacy and change in policy. The irony was that a nationwide policy coalition of stakeholders of the affected program was formed, and as a result, congressional intervention added even more funds to the budget.

6.2.5. Claims and Resolution

While the controversy poses the question, the resolution answers the question that an advocate defends.[12] The resolution is the major claim. A claim is a declarative statement that a listener is asked to accept, supported by reasons if

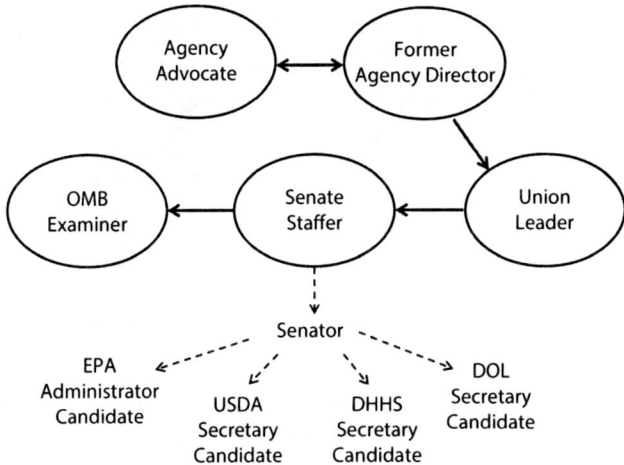

Note: EPA = U.S. Environmental Protection Agency; USDA = U.S. Department of Agriculture; DHHS = U.S. Department of Health and Human Services; DoL = U.S. Department of Labor; OMB = Office of Management and Budget.

Figure 6-2. Logic diagram of an effective policy network.

needed. In the world of uncertainty, when speaking or writing to the public, an advocate makes claims that must stand up against challenges. There are four types of claims: definition, fact, value, and policy. Each type of claim has a different requirement for proof, as shown in Table 6-1 and as described as follows.

6.2.5.1. *Definition.* Claims of definition are based upon meaning or interpretation.[12] Definitions can be controversial, as demonstrated in the benzene case to be described in Chapter 7. In that case, "in promulgating standards dealing with toxic materials or harmful physical agents," § 6(c)(5) of the OSHAct requires "that no employee will suffer material impairment of health or functional capacity."[21] This part of the act placed a priority first on health, followed by finding feasible approaches to protect impairment of health. However, § 3(8) of the OSHAct defines a standard as reasonably necessary or appropriate to provide safe or healthful employment and places of employment.[22] This part of the act focused on the need for balancing reasons for protecting health before a standard is issued. The Supreme Court resolved the inconsistency between these two definitions with an interpretation that defined significant risk, which led to risk assessment as a requirement in rule making.

6.2.5.2. Fact. Claims of fact depend upon description, which can be verified independently of the advocate.[12] Claims of fact relate to the past, present, or future; they have a high degree of consensus once verified, but the facts differ with different perspectives. The claim of facts exists when an advocate argues in favor of accepting a statement as true based upon facts that have been, are, or will be shown to be true. For example, a fact-based claim is "Asbestos is a carcinogen."

6.2.5.3. Value. A value-based claim can be powerful. It is based upon judgment between opposites such as good or bad and right or wrong.[12] This judgment draws from an evaluation or appraisal based upon standards or criteria. A claim of value may be absolute or comparative, or it may be terminal or instrumental. An example of a claim with an absolute value is "Climbing a ladder is unsafe." An example of a claim with a comparative value is "Water-based paints are safer than solvent-based paints." A terminal claim of value refers to ends such as "Saving lives is good," whereas an instrumental claim of value refers to means such as "Needlesticks are dangerous."

6.2.5.4. Policy. Claims of policy state what should or ought to be done and evolve from deliberations of formal bodies such as Congress or from decisions among groups. More arguments occur regarding policy claims than the other three types of claims because they involve the questions "What should we do?" or "What ought we do?"[12] An example of a policy claim, as suggested previously in the issue statement informed by the Chemical Safety Board in 2006, is "OSHA should promulgate a new combustible dust standard for general industry."

6.2.6. Evidence, Inference, and Warrants

In arguments, claims are supported and inferred by evidence. Evidence answers the question "How do you know?" or "What do you have to go on?"[12] If a claim is accepted, there is no further argument, but if not, the advocate will need to support the claim with evidence. If the truth of the evidence (its quality) is not accepted, then that evidence becomes a claim and a separate argument ensues about the veracity of the evidence. Alternatively, the truth of the evidence may not be disputed, but its connection to the claim may be in dispute. When this connection is disputed, one or more warrants must be presented that support the inference made for the connection between the claim and evidence.

A warrant is a license to make an inference. The inferences that link the evidence to the claim are useful to both the one making an argument and to an opponent that challenges the claim. There are six types of inferences: example, cause, sign, analogy, narrative, and form. However, the warrants may not be accepted, and then an argument emerges regarding the veracity of the warrant.[12]

Whereas evidence-based medicine depends upon a lot of evidence from experimental studies, an immediate intervention by licensed personnel, and a single decision maker, evidence-based public health depends upon observational or quasi-experimental studies with little evidence and a long-term intervention by a multidisciplinary professional team. Evidence-based public health aims to develop, implement, and evaluate effective programs and policies by applying principles of scientific reasoning, behavioral science theory, and program planning models.[19]

Evidence involves "the available body of facts or information indicating whether a belief or proposition is true or valid."[19] Much effort may be needed to understand the evidence—particularly unpublished information or fugitive (not peer-reviewed) literature.

Scientific evidence is a form of objective data, as shown in Table 6-2. It develops incrementally, based upon a series of research studies (e.g., the weight of the evidence). Science-based policies that rely upon a single study are rare. The strength of the evidence may be suggestive but inconclusive. Nonetheless, policy makers need to decide upon a course of action even though the evidence remains equivocal. They need to consider how serious the consequences are of either acting or not acting. Another consideration is to understand whether the action will reduce the frequency or severity of a negative health effect, or if there are few adverse effects of the action, and if the action is inexpensive and cost-effective.[19] Acceptability of evidence must meet the perspective of an audience.

Many issues of policy depend upon informal logic in which reasoning lacks certainty, so a range of evidence types as listed in Table 6-2 may be needed to support a claim. In addition to statistics, other forms of evidence that can support the advocate's claims under conditions of uncertainty include examples (anecdotal evidence), tangible objects such as photographs, testimony of fact or opinion from a credible expert, and social consensus (e.g., general beliefs that are treated as fact).[10]

Table 6-2. Types of Evidence

Type	Description
Objective data (two forms)	1. Facts that are descriptive of events, objects, persons, or places, which can be empirically verified. This form depends upon observations. 2. Statistics, which consist of quantification of events, persons, places, or other phenomena. Statistics depend upon numbers that can indicate quantity, relationships, trends, or changes. Misuse of statistics is easy when people do not know how they are gathered, interpreted, or should be used.
Examples	Brief or expanded stories used to build a generalization. Sometimes hypothetical or, conversely, literal, but must be true to be accepted (e.g., "The Wildfire Narrative"). At times examples are nothing more than a brief mention.
Tangible Objects	Actual things or pictures of things. An appropriate adage is "a picture is worth a thousand words." The objects may be artifacts from the past or material that caused a sickness or injury.
Testimony	An opinion expressed by an expert who judges or interprets events, objects, persons, or places. Evidence from testimony may be secondhand, in which a person quotes or paraphrases a quote of an expert. Testimony regarding interpretations explains what happened, and testimony regarding judgment presents a value determination.
Social consensus	Common knowledge is a type of social consensus or shared historical understandings. Social consensus relates to beliefs that are generally accepted as facts. A lawyer may claim that a hazard is "open and obvious" when countering claims of liability regarding a product, such as the sharp blade of a knife.

Source: Adapted from Verlinden.[10]

Evidence varies in quality (e.g., the search for the truth). The following six-level hierarchy spans from the lowest to the highest level of quality.[23]

1. Assertion (worst): Outright assertions as evidence may lack validity, such as blaming the victim, which is common in product liability trials.
2. Common knowledge: It is common knowledge that a knife blade can cut a finger; this is applied in law as being "open and obvious."
3. Lay opinion: A witness at a trial may say, "It was an accident waiting to happen."
4. Expert opinion: Experts may employ principles such as the hierarchy of controls.
5. Empirical study: Results from a study may be proffered at a legal hearing, such as "Benzene exposure has been found to be associated with leukemia."
6. Consensus of studies (best): A claim may be supported with evidence from multiple studies such as, "Many studies show that mesothelioma is caused by asbestos inhalation."

6.2.7. Incrementalism

The advocate needs to understand the concept of incrementalism in arguing for government programs or funding in the face of complexity. Evidence-based policy making for the most part is established in increments.[24] In 1959, Charles Lindblom published an article famous in political science circles entitled *The Science of Muddling Through*. This article explained how policy makers contend with complexity by simplifying their decision-making process.[25] According to Lindblom, history and prior decisions are of paramount importance. The process of simplification is achieved in two ways:

1. Policy makers limit comparisons to those policies that differ in a small degree from present policies.
2. Policy makers ignore consequences of possible policies as well as values attached to these consequences, a lesson that was proved regarding the complexity of policy comprehension that preceded the nuclear power disaster at Three Mile Island.[26]

According to Lindblom, policy is made and remade endlessly and is "not made once and for all." Policies are made through successive approximations with an aim toward desired objectives, yet these objectives continue to change as reconsideration occurs. The strongest measure of this behavior is the incrementalism in agency budgeting in which increments are added to existing programs and wholesale changes within agencies are rare.[25]

6.3. ARGUMENTS FOR THE OCCUPATIONAL SAFETY AND HEALTH ACT

Despite the many letters I have received from businessmen in St. Louis expressing alarm over aspects of the bill, I believe the weight of the evidence clearly establishes that the legislation is urgently needed and should be passed.

—Leonor K. Sullivan[27]

It is important as a lesson in advocacy to appreciate the political and historical context of how the OSHAct came about. Representative Leonor K. Sullivan (D) of Missouri had long recognized that in most industrial operations, safety standards were either completely voluntary or state-imposed yet were not often enforced. In the late 1950s, she learned of the deaths of several workers after exposure to carbon tetrachloride. They had not been provided with guidance or warned of the hazard of exposure. When she investigated protective standards regarding carbon tetrachloride, she found that the Bureau of Labor Standards (BLS) had issued many guidelines and warnings regarding working with the chemical but had no mandate to issue or enforce standards. Sullivan asked Secretary of Labor James Mitchell (under President Dwight Eisenhower) to draft a bill for establishing mandatory safety standards for working with hazardous chemicals in industry. Secretary Mitchell declined to act on Sullivan's request, explaining that the problem was not serious enough to warrant federal legislation.

Later, a group of workers in a St. Louis plant asked Sullivan to find out why so many of them had developed skin diseases. Local and state officials were unable to find the cause of the diseases. Sullivan asked the U.S. Public Health Service (USPHS) to investigate. The investigators found the cause was the result of a change in the composition of a chemical used in production so subtle that the plant manager was unaware of the change. The hazardous ingredient was removed, but some workers had gone on to develop liver disease and other serious side effects associated with the exposure.

In 1965, Sullivan introduced a bill in the 89th Congress (HR 1179) for safety regarding industrial hazardous materials. A diagram of her claim is shown in Figure 6-3. She asked Secretary of Labor Willard W. Wirtz (under President Lyndon Johnson) to examine her bill. Secretary Wirtz set up a task force under Assistant Secretary Esther Peterson, which prepared the DoL for later work on the OSHAct. Nonetheless, Secretary Wirtz did not back Sullivan's bill, the Hazardous Materials Safety Act, which she thought could

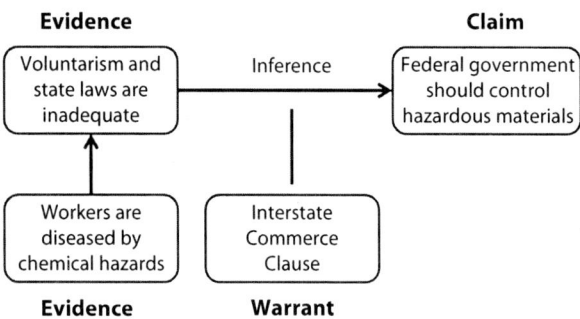

Figure 6-3. Simple argument diagram, as applied to the Sullivan bill.

have easily passed with administration support and with little controversy. Sullivan reintroduced her bill in the 90th Congress in 1966 and the 91st Congress in 1967.[27]

In 1965, the USPHS produced a report entitled *Protecting the Health of Eighty Million Americans,* which outlined recently found technological dangers in the workplace.[28] It noted that a new chemical entered the workplace every 20 minutes, that evidence now showed a strong link between cancer and the workplace, and that old problems were far from being eliminated. The report recommended a major national occupational health program centered in the USPHS. The American Federation of Labor-Congress of Industrial Organizations (AFL-CIO) urged President Johnson to support the report's recommendations.

6.3.1. The Johnson Proposal

In that same year, President Johnson told a meeting of labor reporters that "the time has ... come to do something about the effects of a workingman's job on his health." The DoL and the U.S. Department of Health, Education, and Welfare (DHEW) convened a joint task force to combine both departments' ideas and propose legislation to the president. However, turf intervened when the two departments could not agree on which department would control a national program, resulting in the dissolution of the task force.[29,30]

Nevertheless (see Chapter 5), in January 1968, President Johnson proposed a bill for a job safety and health law to address the workplace safety problem, stating that it was "the shame of a modern industrial nation." He referred to the 1965 USPHS report that each year more than 14,000 workers were killed and 2.2 million more were injured on the job.[29] Citing inadequate standards, lagging research, poor enforcement of laws, shortages of safety and health personnel, and a patchwork of ineffective federal laws, President Johnson argued that a comprehensive new law was needed. President Johnson's proposal included the following elements:

- The DoL had the responsibility for setting and enforcing standards to protect 50 million workers.
- A general duty clause required employers to "furnish employment and place of employment which are safe and healthful."

- Inspectors were given legal authority to enter workplaces without management's permission or prior notice.
- Violators could be fined or jailed, and the DoL secretary could blacklist transgressors who held government contracts.
- The DoL could help interested states develop their own programs in lieu of the federal program.
- DHEW could provide DoL with scientific material for new safety and health standards.

Representative James O'Hara (D) of Michigan and Senator Ralph Yarborough (D) of Texas introduced the Johnson proposal in the House and Senate, respectively. Congressional committee hearings began in February 1968, where Secretary of Labor Wirtz led off with testimony before the House Education and Labor Subcommittee and the Senate Subcommittee on Labor of the Committee on Labor and Public Welfare. Organized labor supported the bill, with AFL-CIO president George Meany heading a long list of union witnesses at the hearings. Both Irving R. Selikoff of the Mount Sinai School of Medicine and consumer advocate Ralph Nader testified in support of the bill.[29,30]

However, industry, led by the U.S. Chamber of Commerce, vehemently opposed the broad powers proposed for the Secretary of Labor. Industry campaigned intensely against a "crash program" that would undermine states' rights.[30] The controversy provides an example of the series structure of argument in the struggle for the creation of the OSHAct in regard to the issue of state versus federal primacy in protective interventions, as shown in the diagram in Figure 6-4.

The bill's opponents claimed that states should have primacy in regulating occupational safety and health protections, framing the discussion as a states' rights issue. However, supporters of the bill presented evidence for a counterclaim that the federal government should have primacy for

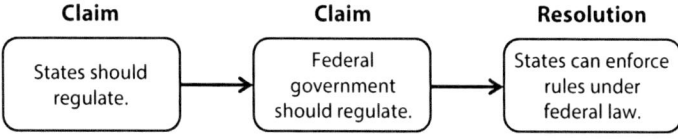

Figure 6-4. Complex series argument diagram applied to state versus federal primacy.

occupational safety and health interventions, as warranted by the Commerce Clause:

- Records of the states in protecting occupational safety and health had been poor.
- States lacked the capability to tackle the more severe and prevalent occupational health problems.
- Management organizations were relatively more powerful than unions at exercising influence at the state level.

The next claim by opponents was that states should have the option of enforcing the standards under the OSHAct with programs approved by the federal government. The bill never came to a vote in this Congress.

6.3.2. The Nixon Proposal

The 1968 mine explosion that caused 78 deaths in Farmington, West Virginia, led Congress to pass the Coal Mine Health and Safety Act of 1969 with enforcement powers residing in the Department of the Interior.[29] At the OMB, Gary Sellers worked on drafting the Coal Mine Act for the administration, but he then became an aide to Representative Phillip Burton (D) of California and worked closely with Ralph Nader to establish penalties for violations. Their work on compensation for black lung raised public salience of the high cost of occupational diseases and of inaction in preventing dangerous exposures.[30,31] This issue was quite prominent, as it resonated among the public as "an affront to community values."[32]

Early in 1969, Representative O'Hara and Senator Harrison Williams Jr. (D) of New Jersey reintroduced bills that were similar to the Johnson proposal of 1968. Meanwhile, newly elected President Nixon asked his cabinet departments to review his campaign speeches for election-year promises and report to him on what they were doing to meet pledges that he had made. Undersecretary of Labor James D. Hodgson learned that, in a speech in Cincinnati, the president had called for federal action on workplace safety and health. To counter the O'Hara-Williams bills, the White House asked Hodgson to prepare a bill, and he began work immediately, consulting extensively with labor and management.[29] The progress of this "perilous fight" for the OSHAct can be followed with reference to the flowchart in Figure 6-5.

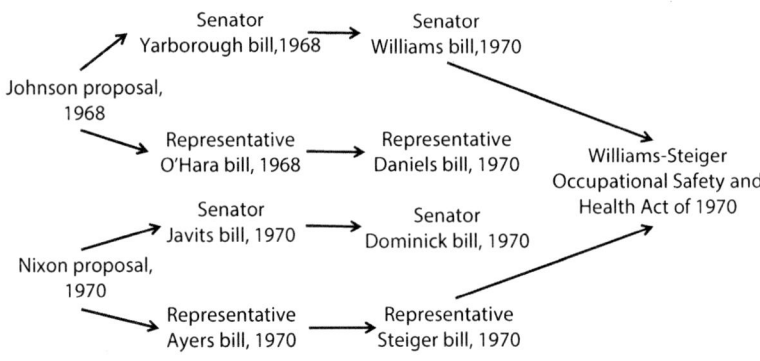

Figure 6-5. Flowchart depicting the legislative history of the OSHAct.

To answer businesses fears of increased powers within the DoL, the Nixon administration's proposal gave an independent five-person board named by the president the power to set and enforce job safety and health standards. The DoL would be limited to inspecting workplaces, and DHEW would conduct research. The federal concern would emphasize research, education, and training. Direct regulation was deemphasized, with an adoption of voluntary efforts by private industry and existing programs of state governments.[29]

President Nixon's action marked a critical change in the argument for federal legislation. That change was a new norm in which some kind of safety and health law was inevitable, even though the idea of federal regulation of conditions in the workplace was abhorrent to business. While the Chamber of Commerce had led the fight against President Johnson's proposal, it now came out in favor of President Nixon's bill, as did the National Association of Manufacturers and other industry groups. Industry also appreciated the administration listening to them in drafting the proposed legislation.[29]

President Nixon's proposed legislation was introduced in Congress in August 1969 by Representative William H. Ayers (R) of Ohio and Senator Jacob Javits (R) of New York, but Javits had reservations. He did not agree with the bill's proposal that board members would be appointed by the president rather than by the Secretary of Labor.[30]

Hundreds of witnesses from labor, industry, government, and the safety and health community gave thousands of pages of oral and written testimony. In addition to hearings in Washington, there were field hearings around the country at which rank-and-file workers in steel mills, automobile plants, and other industries testified. The United Steelworkers, which had worked with the United Mine Workers of America on passage of the Coal Mine Act, was ready to move toward a comprehensive occupational safety and health bill. Organized labor made an alternative bill modeled after President Johnson's proposal their top priority.[29,30]

Democratic representatives, and some Republicans, raised strong objections to the Ayers-Javits bill. Many felt that, with two departments already involved, a safety board would create administrative confusion. Rather than a board, labor unions argued for programs lodged in the DoL and against the proposed enforcement scheme because it only penalized willful, flagrant violators. They claimed that this would take away much of the deterrent effect, because employers would be tempted to ignore federal safety and health standards until after they were inspected. Exemptions of small employers, a three-year delay in the bill's effective date, and a reliance on "consensus" standards devised by industry groups also drew Democratic opposition.[30]

In addition to the steelworkers, Sellers and Nader teamed up with the counsel of the House Select Committee on Labor to create a bill in March 1970 that was much tougher than any considered so far. Named after Representative Domenick V. Daniels (D) of New Jersey, the Daniels bill included a policy of citations much like traffic citations to address violations, and the burden of appeal was placed on the violator. The bill made penalties for serious violations mandatory, and it expanded the concept of standards beyond exposure limits to also include rules for personal protective equipment use and medical exams and monitoring.[29]

While organized labor enthusiastically backed the Daniels bill, it completely opposed the Nixon proposal. Unions advocated for that primacy over safety and health to reside in the DoL and for strong action to deal with workplace hazards, especially dangers related to new chemicals. By November 1970, one month before the ultimate passage of the act, two bills were in play: the Williams bill from the Senate, and the Daniels bill from the House of Representatives.[30]

Despite Republican efforts to hold the bills in committee, the Daniels and Williams bills and not the Nixon bills were introduced on the floors of the House and Senate shortly before the 1970 congressional elections. Opponents succeeded in delaying consideration of these labor-backed measures until after the election, in hopes that it would prevent passage. The strategy was partially successful.

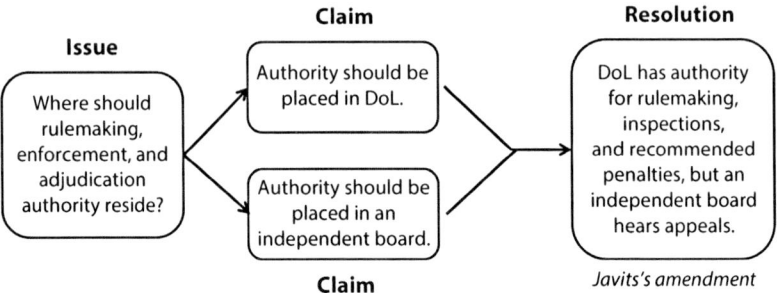

Note: DoL = U.S. Department of Labor.
Figure 6-6. Diagram of the resolution by a convergent argument regarding an independent board.

In the post-election "lame duck" session in November 1970, Senator Peter Dominick (R) of Colorado moved that his bill be substituted for the Williams bill in the full Senate, but his motion failed by just two votes. Senator Javits offered an amendment under which the Secretary of Labor would set safety and health standards and a separate commission would oversee DoL enforcement, serving as a court of appeals for parties to contest the secretary's decisions. Senate Democrats and the Nixon administration supported the compromise, and the Senate passed the Williams bill. Otherwise, the Williams bill as amended by Senator Javits in the Senate was essentially as introduced in the Johnson administration[33] and is shown as an example of a convergent argument in Figure 6-6.

In the House a week later, the Daniels bill was voted out of subcommittee and then out of the Education and Labor Committee. A grassroots effort that the Chamber of Commerce waged against the Daniels bill during the election campaign drained off some support. In a substitute bill that emerged to replace the Republican O'Hara bill, Representative William R. Steiger (R) of Wisconsin had introduced a bill earlier in the year that supported President Nixon's proposal and mirrored a companion bill introduced by Senator Dominick. It would place standard-setting and enforcement powers in independent boards with the DoL limited to conducting inspections. In a major defeat for labor, which had stoutly resisted any efforts at compromise, the Steiger bill passed easily in a vote of 220 to 172 in the full House, replacing the Daniels bill.[31] Thus, in essence the Senate passed the Johnson proposal of 1968, and the House passed the Nixon proposal of 1970. The difference needed to be resolved in a congressional conference committee.

6.3.3. Resolution

A House-Senate conference committee met to resolve the differences between the two bills, one passed in the Senate and the other in the House (Williams and Steiger bills). The conference committee members reflected the liberal views of the Democratic House and Senate committee chairmen who selected them.

The arguments up to and including the committee deliberations were complex, involving multiple claims, some supporting other claims—many at issue at the same time—and changing responses by lawmakers that were difficult to gauge. This complexity is shown in only a skeleton format in Figure 6-5.

There are three basic patterns of complex argument: the series structure, depending upon a chain of claims where each depends upon the former (Figure 6-4); the convergent structure, where each claim is independent but they all merge to support the resolution (Figure 6-6); and the parallel structure, where each claim is independent but any one of the claims can support the resolution (Figure 6-7). In the latter example, the deliberation over health standards demonstrated a parallel structure in setting standards. Three claims were in the argument: first, no employee should suffer material impairment of health or functional capacity even if such an employee had regular exposure to the hazard for the period of his or her working life; second, the latest available scientific data in the field should be considered; and third, consideration should be given to the feasibility of the standards. There was little dispute

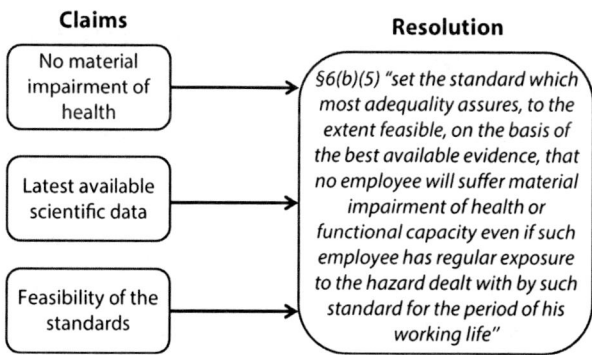

Source: Occupational Safety and Health Act.

Figure 6-7. Complex parallel argument diagram regarding standards development.

in bringing together the consideration of health protection, scientific, and feasibility criteria (these became § 6(b)(5) of the OSH Act).

In the conference committee, the most contentious part between the two bills was whether the authority for rule making, enforcement, and adjudication should be vested in an independent "board" either outside or within DoL. The Williams bill in the Senate—supported by organized labor as introduced in the Johnson administration—would house these three key functions within the DoL.

The deliberations in the conference committee converged again around the Javits amendment. The resolution was that standards were to be set by the Secretary of Labor and that an independent quasi-judicial Occupational Safety and Health Review Commission was established to consider appeals from employers regarding citations issued by DoL, as shown in Figure 6-6 consistent with the Javits amendment regarding an independent appeals board concerning penalties.[33,34] Figure 6-8 shows the relationship in these deliberations among controversies, resolutions, issues, and claims.

While the locus of standard setting, enforcement, and adjudication was the most controversial issue in the conference committee deliberations, other issues were discussed as well. The Williams bill as based on the Johnson proposal included a general duty that employers provide a workplace "free from recognized hazards," but the Steiger bill replaced this bill in a vote on the floor. The Steiger bill included much narrower language that used the term "readily

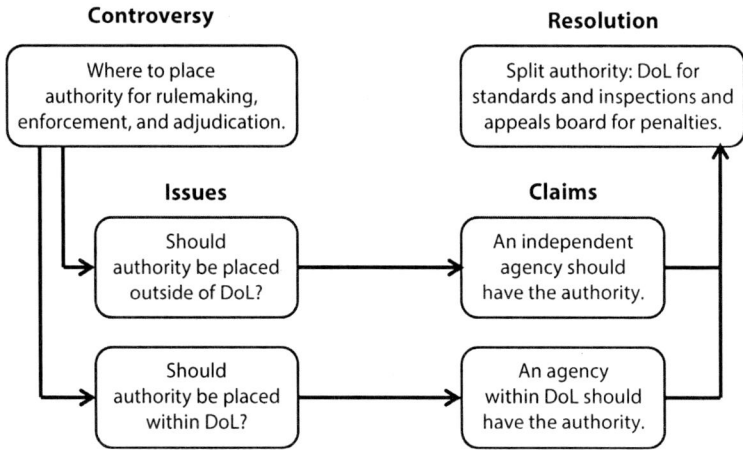

Note: DoL = U.S. Department of Labor.

Figure 6-8. Diagram of the relationship among controversies, resolutions, issues, and claims regarding an independent board versus a board under U.S. Department of Labor authority.

apparent" rather than a "recognized" hazard and moderated penalties regarding the clause. The Democrats on the conference committee argued successfully for the broader language of "recognized" hazard but compromised on penalties associated with the clause.[33,34]

Another issue was about whether formal rule making would be used as established in the Administrative Procedures Act. The committee resolved in favor of informal rule making, as specified within the act. However, in applying the procedure at a later time, OSHA used a hybrid by reference to the record of the deliberations, which is discussed in more detail in the next chapter.[33,34]

On a third issue, the only significant point on which the Senate yielded was deletion of a provision allowing the Secretary of Labor to close down a plant under conditions of imminent danger. An additional issue was whether the DoL could enforce standards in places that were under the jurisdiction of other agencies such as mines. The resolution was that action under the proposed OSHAct would defer to other agencies with statutory jurisdiction and standards to protect a population of workers from occupational hazards.

Another issue was resolved by making it a misdemeanor for any person to give advance notice of an impending inspection.[33,34] However, this part of the act eventually became moot because of a court case that required a search warrant if requested by an employer prior to an inspection. This case is discussed in Chapter 8. The issues addressed by the conference committee are summarized in Figure 6-9 and serve as an example of a complex parallel argument for the passage of the OSHAct.

When the conferees met in December 1970, they adopted the more liberal Senate bill almost unchanged.[29] The Senate immediately approved the measure and sent it on to the House. When Secretary of Labor Hodgson announced that President Nixon had approved of the bill, Republican opponents in the House abandoned plans to fight the conference committee version, and it passed easily. All sides praised the final bill. Appealing to blue collar workers, President Nixon lauded it as a significant piece of social legislation. Although he disagreed with specific provisions, he believed that it would help attain "the goal we all want to achieve"—the protection of Americans on the job. The Chamber of Commerce termed it "a substantial victory" for those in industry seeking a fair yet effective law. AFL-CIO President Meany called it "a long step . . . toward a safe and healthy workplace."[29]

President Nixon signed the milestone OSHAct of 1970 in a ceremony at the DoL. Meany and other labor figures, business community leaders, and prominent members of Congress were present. The ceremony ended

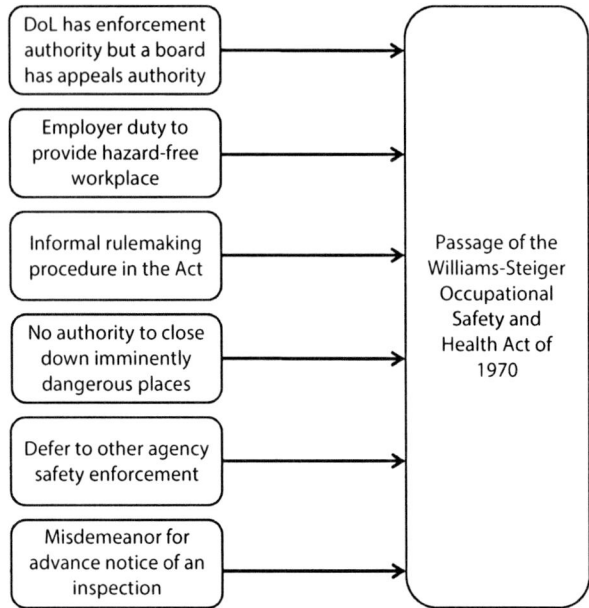

Figure 6-9. Diagram of the resolution of issues between the House and the Senate as an example of a complex parallel argument.

the bitter three-year legislative struggle on a note of harmony and bipartisanship.[29] Representative Leonor K. Sullivan expressed her support for the OSHAct, acknowledging its broader approach compared with her earlier proposals.[27]

6.4. THE PRECAUTIONARY PRINCIPLE AND ABDUCTIVE REASONING

What prompts a health worker, for example, to foresee a future epidemic in a presently healthy population is an act of creative thinking based on the best available information plus a trained capacity to look ahead for general trends of events or possible rearrangements of them.

—Martin Bloom[35]

Theofanis Christoforou wrote, "The precautionary principle is about scientific uncertainty. It permits and in some cases requires regulatory authorities to take action or adopt measures in order to avoid or reduce risk to health, safety, or the environment, if necessary by erring on the side of safety."[36] A decision-based precautionary principle has been advocated as a way to prevent crises in the future. Precaution goes beyond science-based results based on inductive arguments to hypotheses generating methods based on abductive reasoning as a practical method for anticipating plausible presumptions.[37] In a similar vein, intuition cannot be ignored in advocacy and critical thinking. Moreover, it is valued when creating hypotheses, especially in paradigm shifts. In the opening narrative, Wag Dodge used intuition in taking his action. These two forms of argument (inductive v abductive reasoning) are typically in conflict when minimizing false positives (critical in inductive reasoning) versus minimizing false negatives (critical in abductive reasoning).

6.4.1. Precautionary Principle

One established "precautionary" goal for U.S. society is "to assure so far as possible every working man and woman in the Nation safe and healthful working conditions," as stated in the OSHAct,[38] yet the public health professional is challenged as an advocate by the presence of uncertainty and with the burden of proof. Science-based policies to prevent damage to ecosystems and health depend upon foresight that involves long-term goals for the protection of health, such as smallpox eradication and smoking cessation. However, the scientific and public health communities need to define what precaution means in practice.

In the 1970s, concerns regarding the limitations of science and policy structures to address complexity and uncertainty in risks to health and the economy led to the precautionary principle. The essence of this principle is prevention of damage to health, founded upon the oath from the *Hippocratic Corpus,* "First do no harm." In 1998, the Wingspread Statement on the precautionary principle from a conference in Racine, Wisconsin, defined it as follows: "When an activity raises threats of harm to human health or the environment, precautionary measures should be taken even if some cause and effect relationships are not fully established scientifically." Central components of the principle follow:[39]

1. Take preventive action in the face of uncertainty.
2. Shift burdens onto proponents of potentially harmful activities.
3. Explore a wide range of alternatives to possible harmful actions.
4. Increase public participation in decision making.

6.4.2. Abductive Reasoning

Abductive reasoning is common in everyday thinking in a world of uncertainty and tentative reasoning. It is a conglomeration of best guesses and assumptions (presumptions). In this reasoning, the knowledge base as associated with previous propositions is used to gauge deviations toward a new proposition.[40]

Whereas inductive reasoning moves from premises to conclusions, abductive reasoning moves from conclusions (tentative propositions) to possible premises. It is also used in legal arguments and the generation of scientific hypotheses.[40] Abductive reasoning depends upon explanation and is educated guessing in which hypotheses are formed and evaluated. The hypotheses are generated as sufficient for further action but lacking in evidence to be accurate and are evaluated to determine if they are true.[9]

The process of abductive reasoning has three stages. First, it examines reports of known premises as associated with supporting evidence. Second, it searches for the various premises associated with the hypothetical evidence. Third, it selects the best explanation for an acceptable hypothesis.[40]

Abductive reasoning is also known as "inference to best explanation" (i.e., the most likely cause is the simplest),[40] resulting in the hypothesis being supported by the strongest inference as determined by six factors:[9]

1. Likelihood (the most important factor): the probability of the hypothesis given certain evidence or observations.
2. Explanatory power: based on the number of things a hypothesis explains, especially when compared with alternative hypotheses.
3. Simplicity: closely related to Occam's razor, used for making choices between competing explanations that involve uncertainty by choosing the option with the fewest assumptions.
4. Novelty: The hypothesis is inferred to be a discovery vehicle for seeking truth (some argue that this is an illegitimate factor, but public health surveillance follows this principle, e.g., sentinel events).
5. Appropriate explanatory content: There is a physical or natural basis rather than a moral or supernatural basis for the hypothesis.
6. Modesty of the conclusions relative to the premises: The more modest the proposed conclusions, the stronger the explanatory inference.

Watson is an IBM computer that competed on the game show *Jeopardy*. This is an artificial intelligence approach that attempts to imitate human reasoning, which holds promise in the future to gather evidence for legal cases or to reach a medical diagnosis given symptoms from a patient. It is an abductive reasoning technology that can be used to apply the precautionary principle. Watson receives a question; computes the similarity between things by examining thousands of examples from disparate sources, gathering evidence, getting matches for clues and phrases, and interpreting them in multiple ways; and comes up with hundreds of possible answers. Watson assumes that all answers might be right as competing hypotheses and retrieves evidence supportive of each answer, using statistics to determine the answer that is most likely to be correct. Watson uses probabilities to generate an evidence profile represented by a list and chooses the answer with the highest probability at the top of the list as an educated guess.[41]

Currently, onshore well drilling to recover natural gas using a technology called fracking has stimulated an advocacy movement to take precautions before environmental damage is done by the technology, especially the possibility of groundwater contamination and methane emissions into the air. Fracking is a combination of two technologies: directional drilling and hydraulic fracturing. As a precautionary tool, an artificial intelligence machine like Watson could be used to quickly generate hypotheses regarding releases from drilling emissions (e.g., radon gas).[42]

6.4.3. Errors of Our Ways

In addition, to reduce the potential for false positives, we may overlook their nemesis and key to precaution, minimizing false negatives. Scientists address two types of error. One is Type I error (false positive), which is the mistake of concluding that an association between cause and effect exists when, in truth, it does not. Scientists set the Type I error rate low at 5% (i.e., we are 95% confident that the true value of the parameter is in our confidence interval), for scientists do not want the stream of results to be founded upon a false positive finding. A finding with a 5% or less error rate is said to be significant. Type II error (false negative) is the failure to find an association when one actually exists.[5] This error rate is more lax at 20%—though this may vary because of the cost of reducing this rate with higher sample sizes. A disease in a person with this error rate could be missed 20% of the time. The way to minimize both types of error is to increase the sample size, which may not be feasible.

Inherent in this scientific approach is the bias toward less error regarding false positives rather than false negatives even though the potential victims of a malady may place a higher priority on less error regarding false negatives. Victims would not want to be told that they did not have a disease when they in truth actually did have the disease. The use of Bayesian methods offers one promise for decreasing the Type II error rate.[43]

6.4.4. The General Duty

The Wisconsin Industrial Commission Act of 1911 established the requirement of a safe workplace that expanded the duty of employers to go beyond proving safe apparatuses to making the whole of employment safe as a step toward precaution. Safety was redefined as freedom from danger, as reason would permit. The statute established a presumption of managerial responsibility and replaced factory laws with administrative rules for the implementation of safety standards.[44]

The OSHAct goes further, such that employers have a general duty to provide work and a workplace free from recognized hazards. As an attribute regarding the precautionary principle, the general duty clause shifts the burden to employers to provide a workplace free of recognized hazards, although the definition of a "recognized" hazard is in play as an issue, for its definition is a matter of policy and controversy. OSHA can issue citations for violations of standards or the general duty clause, even if no OSHA standard applies to the particular hazard. The OSHAct differs from environmental statutes by creating a general duty on both employers and employees to obey the law and to strive for safe and healthy workplaces. This general duty originally followed a doctrine under common law that there is a general duty to do no harm to others. Moreover, when the OSHAct was enacted in 1970, Congress identified a general duty in safety and health statutes in 36 states.[45]

6.5. AGENDA SETTING AND FRAMING

The Common Enemy: The common ground for discussing prevention is to define the problem as the disease or injury; For conversely, who would advocate for disease and injury!

—Melvin L. Myers (oral lecture, environmental health policy; Rollins School of Public Health, Emory University; January 13, 2014)

Occupational safety and health professionals within an organization are the advocates for workers' health, and framing the potential injury and illness problem is an important tool to use in their advocacy. Framing involves packaging facts to create a story.[8] Frames are mental structures of beliefs and assumptions that simplify people's understanding of the world around them, helping them to deal with complexity as they decide and act. How an issue is framed can affect the solution to a problem. One of the most influential frames is to anchor the argument to the problem: in this case, occupational injury or disease.

6.5.1. Agenda Setting

Evidence-based policy making is a complex process, but when the three stages of policy making are brought together, the likelihood of policy adoption is increased. The first stage is agenda setting, which establishes that a problem is worthy of governmental action. For example, miners trapped underground are of high salience regarding setting an agenda: this demands action by policy makers. The second stage is policy. In this stage, alternative policies are considered for action. The third stage is politics. In this stage, the policy needs to be technically sound, politically acceptable, and administratively feasible. Not considering politics can result in failure for an advocated policy.[24]

This process leads to building content for a policy, focusing on the aims of a policy that are likely to meet success.[24] The policy content is evaluated by following a logic diagram that tracks its context, inputs, process, and expected products (as shown in Table 6-3); it is known as the CIPP approach to evaluation.

Table 6-3. An Example of the Context, Inputs, Process, and Expected Products (CIPP) Evaluation Model, Applied to the Passage of the Occupational Safety and Health Act

Context →	Inputs →	Process →	Products
• Problem	• Moral high ground	• House bill	• Standards
• Alternative policies	• Presidential priority	• Senate bill	• Compliance
• Politics	• Agency backing	• Hearings	• Adjudication
	• Union support	• Argument	• Research findings
		• Resolution	• Reduced injuries and diseases

Source: Stufflebeam.[46]

Context evaluation identifies the strengths and weaknesses of pursuing and the knowledge status and deficiencies regarding each aim, remedies the deficiencies, and charts a path toward improvement. Input evaluation helps prescribe the partners and approaches through which changes can occur. Process evaluation is an ongoing review of the implementation of the planned schedule to achieve each aim and the efficient use of resources. Both quantitative and qualitative methods can be used. Product evaluation measures, interprets, and judges the attainment of the aims and can be extended to long-term outcomes.[46]

6.5.2. Threat and Opportunity Framing

A powerful framing technique is based on prospect theory, when one decides to frame an issue as a threat versus an opportunity. According to prospect theory, words matter a lot, and we act differently whether an issue is framed as a threat or loss versus an opportunity or gain. Framing as a threat causes us to take more risks, resulting in us committing more resources to protect against the loss. Conversely, framing as an opportunity can lead to using existing resources more effectively.[47] See Table 6-4 for a comparison of this binary approach to framing. Prospect theory is one technique developed under the new field of behavioral economics.

However, framing is not only a binary way of looking at the world. Everyone adopts mental models for understanding situations, but these models may be outdated. The world is continually changing regarding technology, demographics, the economy, and the environment. Governments and other

Table 6-4. Comparison of Framing Strategies to Influence More Effective Problem Solving Within an Organization

	Framing Option	
Factor	Threat (loss)	Opportunity (gain)
Resource allocation	Allocate more resources to the problem.	Use resources more effectively, but insufficiently.
Behavior	Act rigidly. May continue digging the hole that is the source of the problem.	Act creatively and adaptively.
Best approach	Initially assess the threat.	Reframe as an opportunity.

large organizations are slow to change in order to adapt to new situations and our updated mental models. Thus, reframing is critical to adapting to a changing world.[47]

6.5.3. Framing Steps

Sometimes a social justice advocate faces strong economic interests with a market justice ethic, and alas, different approaches to framing are necessary. While language is important, it is not the first and foremost concern. First is to articulate the change in concrete and specific terms (the issue), and second is to know how to make the change (the claim). Once the steps to a solution are articulated and the methods for their implementation are determined, language becomes important.[48,49]

Words or images can trigger frames for particular interpretations by an audience.[49] This author was once involved in a workshop with small-construction contractors. The words "sprains and strains" were valued terms for discussion because they are the vernacular in the workers' compensation realm, but as soon as the author used the term "ergonomics," a hot-button word, he lost respect in the group and was shunned. In the late 1990s, when this happened, an interest group had launched a widespread campaign against OSHA's proposed ergonomics standard, which will be discussed in more detail in Chapter 16. Another example is the word "government," which evokes the concepts of waste, inefficiency, and intrusion.

6.5.4. News Frames and Salience

News frames are another type of frame that bears on how to create messages for occupational safety and health. News-based frames organize messages into stories delineating what is important and not important. However, news stories rarely encourage audiences to understand the causes of the problem and policy solutions. The news focuses on episodes or individuals. While the science may be the foot in the door for a news story, the advocate needs to frame the story around individual-oriented stories as a "news-you-can-use piece."[49] Claims are remembered, so use of a memorable claim and repetition are important. If ambushed by a news team, one should immediately agree to an interview but arrange for some time to step aside and organize rational thoughts and claims.

6.6. FALLACIES AND ENEMIES OF PREVENTION

The assumption among Americans is, "If it's on the market, it's OK." Dream on. That fantasy is gone in Europe. We're asking the question: "Why should the government be in a position of proving that something is not safe?" But in the United States, there's still a level of confidence that if there is a problem, the government would do something about it, and the chemical wouldn't be there. That's the fallacy. That it's safe. I beg to differ."

—Robert Donkers[50]

In some cases, a salience threshold is reached that renders occupational safety and health policy effective, whereas in other cases, salience is lacking when other public policy goals counter occupational safety and health goals. Examination of these successes and failures offers a natural test bed for evaluating the salience of policy claims and the use of reason to effect policy or, conversely, fallacies that may have contributed to defeating policy claims.

Advocates need to be able to defend their claims with reasons against attacks or counterclaims. Advocates must recognize several pitfalls and defend their claims against counterclaims by recognizing their antagonist's pitfalls, which include hasty generalizations, unrepresentative samples, and fallacies. This section also describes the enemies of prevention that an advocate must overcome in argument and discusses examples of antiscience arguments that stand in the way of prevention. These arguments are a significant shift from attacks upon the rule making process to attacks on the underlying science behind regulation. Regulation is always seen as a constraint on the free market. The challenge is to overcome beliefs in individualism when shared responsibility is needed.[48]

6.6.1. Fallacies

An expert can appear befuddled if asked a complex question in which one question is embedded in another question. An advocate needs to be able to recognize this trick as well as fallacies in arguments. Fallacies include deficiencies of clarity that arise from inexact language, such as equivocation, in which the same word can convey different meanings, and this meaning can change during the argument (see Table 6-5). An example of equivocation is the use of the word "fairness," which can relate to equality of distribution but can also relate to getting what one deserves.[12]

Table 6-5. Panoply of Fallacies

Fallacy	Description
Ad hominem (kill the messenger)	The advocate is attacked personally instead of the argument. The opponent may dig up the person's past history in order to reduce the acceptance of his or her arguments by the public.
Begging the question (circular logic)	The conclusion is the same as the assertion—no argument is being made, only a statement.
Equivocation	Use of the same words in different senses in the same argument.
Non sequitur	Comments or claims that do not logically follow from what has gone before but are presented as if they do.
Only game in town	Accepted by default. Advocate must produce a more plausible explanation and if not, must accept the default explanation.
Poisoning the well	A form of ad hominem attack that occurs before an argument is complete, biasing the audience against the opponent's side before he or she can present the case.
Red herring	An irrelevant topic or premise brought into a discussion to divert attention from the topic at hand. It may appear relevant to those not paying close attention.
Scapegoating	Blaming a single person for a seemingly unsolvable problem.
Slippery slope	Assumes that a small effect will produce a much larger effect down the road without accurate causation.
Straw man (fallacy of relevance)	A method of creating a weaker form of an argument and then attacking that weaker position, which is a misrepresentation of an opponent's position. It is common because it is easy to misunderstand another person's position.

The problem of relevance has to do with a factor that has nothing to do with the relationship between the evidence and the claim. This problem includes an attack upon a person rather than against the argument (see Ad Hominem in Table 6-5), reference to someone without relevant expertise, appeals to popularity or tradition, or threats. An offshoot of this fallacy is a party bringing suit against a defendant when the party has no standing (e.g., the party is not affected or harmed by the defendant's actions).[12]

The name of the red herring fallacy came from animal rights activists dragging herring along a path away from a fox being chased by hounds in a foxhunt. The herring laid a scent that the hounds would follow rather than the scent of the fox. The advocate needs to be on guard against being led on a tangent away from the argument. The issue being discussed must remain germane and on agenda. Circular logic, as in begging the question, is present in almost all fiction, and fiction is used in many arguments. The fallacies discussed and listed in Table 6-5 are just a few for which the advocate needs to build an awareness.[51]

6.6.2. Enemies of Prevention

Advocates and leaders for occupational safety and health need to be aware of four great enemies of prevention: time, distance, greed, and ignorance.[52] An example of time as an enemy of prevention is the reversal of the elimination of silicosis in foundry work, when during World War II sand replaced steel shot as a blasting media for cleaning iron ingots. After the war, sand remained as the medium rather than returning to steel shot, as had been done during the 1930s to combat silicosis in the first place.

An example of distance as an enemy of prevention is the slow recognition of byssinosis in the United States. In the 1950s, the cotton textile industry claimed to have no problem with byssinosis, as their factories were so much cleaner than the older factories in Great Britain where byssinosis was a recognized disease related to exposure to cotton dust. Scientists from Great Britain traveled to the United States to discover how cotton dust was controlled, but instead they discovered that byssinosis was rampant among textile workers. This discovery broke the belief that what existed elsewhere was nonexistent in the United States.[53] Likewise, exporting hazardous work environments to foreign nations puts a distance between the United States and countries where occupational injuries and diseases are out of sight from the U.S. population that uses those imported products.[54] In addition, empathetic paternalism regarding care provided by the employer becomes more problematic when the employer moves to an adjacent (with fewer industry-related problems) neighborhood, as happened in Lawrence, Massachusetts, circa 1919.[55]

An example of greed as an enemy of prevention is the deliberate cover-up of health problems related to asbestos exposure. Companies around the world pursued the manufacture and use of asbestos products with knowledge of their latent effects upon workers and the public as a way to profit in the present and remain unconcerned with the future destruction of human health that it was known would occur.[56] As an example, for more than 30 years the Johns-Manville company manufactured and sold asbestos products and justified them as legal products as a foil against protective action despite knowledge of their danger as employees got sick and died; this is addressed further in Chapter 12.[57] Moreover, greed is endemic in "market justice," a method of operation based upon assumptions of rugged individualism, self-determination, strong individual control and responsibility, limited obligation to the collective good, and limited governmental involvement in social activity.[8,48]

Greed can also carry over to conspiracy for a cover-up of a danger in the workplace. In the early 1960s, industry discovered that vinyl chloride monomer (VCM) was the cause of a serious degenerative bone disease called acroosteolysis. A 1961 study found pathological changes in rabbit livers when exposed to VCM,[58] and in 1970, an Italian researcher reported tumors of the skin, lungs, and bones in rats when exposed to VCM gas.[59] Fearing liability, European and U.S. VCM producers conspired to keep secret studies indicating VCM carcinogenicity and evidence of angiosarcomas of the liver in VCM workers, a conspiracy that was effective when kept within the confines of a factory. The cover-up kept workers ignorant of the dangers that lay latent in their bodies from their work. In 1974, VCM exposures were conclusively linked to angiosarcomas of the liver in the deaths of four workers between 1968 and 1973, which was identical to earlier results of rat studies. In 1974, one company, B.F. Goodrich, broke ranks from the conspiracy to the dismay of the co-conspirators and reported the problem to NIOSH.[18] This conspiracy is discussed in more depth in Chapter 15.

The American adage "What you don't know won't hurt you" guides many policies to escape liability regarding the foreseeability of a hazard or the state-of-the-art technology that would eliminate or abate a hazard. Nonetheless, when it concerns hazards, they can hurt. This leads to the fourth enemy of prevention: ignorance. More specifically, ignorance is a reason for not taking preventive action rather than adopting policies of taking preventive action primarily because of uncertainty. Indeed, as Stuart Firestein described this pejorative side of ignorance,[60]

> One kind of ignorance is willful stupidity; worse than simple stupidity, it is a callous indifference to facts and logic. It shows itself as a stubborn devotion to uninformed opinions, ignoring contrary ideas, opinions, or data. The ignorant are unaware, unenlightened, uniformed, and surprisingly often occupy elected office. We can all agree that none of this is good.

However, moving from the pejorative side of ignorance to the provocative side of ignorance, a caveat is that ignorance is the driver for science, stimulating research to address the absence of the "fact, understanding, insight, or clarity" of a problem.[60]

THE MOUNTAIN DISEASE NARRATIVE

As far back as the 1500s, miners were employed to extract silver ore from mines in the Erz Mountains in Germany and in today's Czech Republic. Over the centuries, an illness known as *Bergkraukheit* or "mountain disease" struck these miners. Hundreds of miners died of this wasting disease within a year of starting their work in the mines. In the years just prior to 1900, miners were extracting uranium from these mines for use in dyes, and later for supplying radium for Pierre and Marie Curie's research. By the early 20th century, doctors suspected that the high mortality was caused by exposure to radiation and especially to radon gas. Detailed epidemiology records confirmed this suspicion.[61]

After World War II, the U.S. Atomic Energy Commission (AEC) launched an effort to purchase uranium for making bombs. A frenzy ensued in uranium mining in the West that included five states: Nevada, Utah, Colorado, Arizona, and New Mexico.[61] In 1948, Henry N. Doyle was sent to Salt Lake City, Utah, to set up a USPHS occupational health field station.[62] In 1949, the Colorado State Health Department contacted Doyle for assistance concerning the potential hazard of radiation exposure in uranium mines. Doyle had little to no knowledge about the measurement and effects of radiation exposure, but he knew whom to call: Duncan A. Holaday, a USPHS radiation industrial hygienist in Washington, DC. Holaday had been trained in radiation safety after the war and monitored radiation levels during nuclear bomb tests on Bikini Island. Moreover, he was familiar with the European literature regarding mountain disease and lung cancer. Duncan joined Doyle along with another four investigators and a secretary at the field station. Holaday gained access to the mines to study exposure levels but with the condition of not publishing the results and not warning workers lest they walk off the job. The radiation levels were a staggering 1,000 times what was considered safe. The USPHS launched a comprehensive uranium mining study in 1950. In the face of stupefying results of harm to the miners, the USPHS investigators were held to a "gag rule" ordered by the AEC and demanded by employers for national security reasons. Years passed with pleas for worker protection from Duncan and his colleagues, but to little avail.[61]

In 1959, Dr. Harold J. Magnuson, director of the Occupational Health Office at the USPHS, estimated that based upon the European experience, 1% of the uranium miners would die from lung cancer each year; more than 3,000 workers were mining uranium at that time.⁶¹ In that year, President Eisenhower established the Federal Radiation Council by executive order to address the health problems associated with radiation exposure.⁶³ A major study of lung disease among uranium miners was launched. The results of the study came in 1963 and got attention among government agencies. As the mines were under contract with the AEC, the DoL could use the Walsh-Healey Public Contracts Act to regulate exposure in the mines.⁶¹ In 1965, an article by USPHS investigators including Holaday as a co-author titled "Radiation as the Cause of Lung Cancer Among Uranium Miners" appeared in the *New England Journal of Medicine*.⁶⁴ As the media took notice of the problem, a *Washington Post* reporter published a 1967 article entitled "Hidden Casualties of Atom Age, Cancer: Uranium Mine Occupational Hazard."⁶⁵ On the same day, the reporter called Secretary of Labor Wirtz to ask about how the Walsh-Healy Act could be applied to protect these miners. Secretary Wirtz admitted little or no knowledge about the cancer problem or the act, whereupon the reporter published a story about Secretary Wirtz's ignorance. Secretary Wirtz was infuriated and embarrassed. He consulted Assistant Secretary of Labor Peterson and asked her to keep on top of the activities of the Federal Radiation Council. When the council became deadlocked on setting a protective standard for the miners, Secretary Wirtz was disenchanted with their callous disregard for worker health. As the council would not act, he would. He immediately invoked powers under the Walsh-Healey Public Contracts Act by setting a standard for exposure to radiation in mines.⁶¹ He had risen to be a strong advocate for occupational safety and health. Much wrangling ensued from this action, and struggles for payment of compensation for diseased miners and their survivors lasted for decades. However, this experience readied Secretary Wirtz, Assistant Secretary Peterson, and the DoL to actively engage in the creation of the OSHAct.⁶⁵

REFERENCES

1. Begley S. Critical thinking: part skill, part mindset and totally up to you. *Wall Street Journal*. October 20, 2006:B1.

2. Rothermel RC. *Mann Gulch Fire: A Race That Couldn't Be Won*. Ogden, UT: U.S. Department of Agriculture, Forest Service, Intermountain Research Station;1993. General Technical Report INT-299.

3. Turner D. The thirteenth fire. *Forest History Today*. 1999;Spring:26–28.

4. Matthews M. *A Great Day to Fight a Fire: Mann Gulch, 1949.* Norman, OK: University of Oklahoma Press;2006.

5. Hansson SO. *Setting the Limit: Occupational Health Standards and the Limits of Science.* New York, NY: Oxford University Press;1988.

6. Friedlaender E, Winston F. Evidence-based advocacy. *Inj Prev.* 2004;10:324–326.

7. Garvin DA, Roberto MA. Change through persuasion. *Harv Bus Rev.* 2005;83(2): 104–112.

8. Wallack L, Dorfman L, Jernigan D, Themba M. *Media Advocacy and Public Health: Power for Prevention.* London, UK: Sage Publications;1993.

9. Hendrickson N, St. Amant K, Hawk W, O'Meara W, Flage D. *The Rowman & Littlefield Handbook for Critical Thinking.* Lanham, MD: Rowman & Littlefield Publishers, Inc.;2008.

10. Verlinden J. *Critical Thinking and Everyday Argument.* Toronto, ON: Wadsworth, Inc.;2005:143.

11. Amidei N. *So You Want to Make a Difference: Advocacy Is the Key.* Washington, DC: OMB Watch;2002.

12. Zarefsky D. *Argumentation: The Study of Effective Reasoning.* Vol. 1, 2nd ed. Chantilly, VA: The Teaching Company;2005.

13. Domhoff GW. Alternative theoretical views. April 2005. Available at: http://sociology.ucsc.edu/whorulesamerica/theory/alternative_theories.html. Accessed August 15, 2012.

14. Meier KJ. *Regulation: Politics, Bureaucracy, and Economics.* New York, NY: St. Martin's Press, Inc.;1985.

15. Michaels D, Monforton C, Lurie P. Selected science: an industry campaign to undermine an OSHA hexavalent chromium standard. *Environmental Health: A Global Access Science Source.* 2006;5(5):8. doi:10.1186/1476-069X-5-5.

16. Michaels D. *Doubt Is Their Product: How Industry's Assault on Science Threatens Your Health.* New York, NY: Oxford University Press;2008.

17. Majone G. *Evidence, Argument, and the Policy Process.* New Haven, CT: Yale University Press;1989.

18. Markowitz G, Rosner D. *Deceit and Denial.* Berkeley, CA: University of California Press;2002.

19. Brownson RC, Baker EA, Leet TL, Gillespie KN. *Evidence-Based Public Health.* New York, NY: Oxford University Press;2003.

20. Moure-Eraso R. Statement from CSB Chairman Moure-Eraso on the four-year anniversary of the catastrophic Imperial Sugar explosion—chairman continues to encourage industry to support a combustible dust standard and applauds success of recommendations. U.S. Chemical Safety Board. February 2012. Available at: http://www.csb.gov/newsroom/detail.aspx?nid=399. Accessed October 24, 2012.

21. Occupational Safety and Health Act, 29 U.S.C. § 657 (1970).

22. Occupational Safety and Health Act, 29 U.S.C. § 654 (1970).

23. Perella J. *The Debate Method of Critical Thinking: An Introduction to Argumentation*. Dubuque, IA: Kendall Hunt Publishing Co.;1987.

24. Brownson RC, Chriqui JF, Stamatakis KA. Understanding evidence-based public health policy. *Am J Pub Health*. 2009;99(9):1576–1583.

25. Lindblom CE. The science of muddling through. *Pub Admin Rev*. 1959;19(2): 79–88.

26. Perrow C. *Normal Accidents*. Princeton, NJ: Princeton University Press;1999.

27. Hearing Before House Committee on Education and Labor, 2nd Sess, *Cong. Rec.* Vol. 166, H10688–H10690 (November 24, 1970) (testimony of Leonor K. Sullivan).

28. Department of Health, Education, and Welfare. *Protecting the Health of Eighty Million Americans: A National Goal for Occupational Health*. Special Report to the Surgeon General of the United States Public Health Service. Washington, DC: DHEW;1965. National Center for Urban and Industrial Health, Bureau of Disease Prevention and Environmental Health, Division of Occupational Health.

29. MacLaury J. The job safety law of 1970: its passage was perilous. *Monthly Labor Rev*. 1981;104:18–24.

30. Page JA, O'Brien M-W. *Bitter Wages*. New York, NY: Grossman Publishers;1973.

31. Mendeloff J. *Regulating Safety: An Economic and Political Analysis of Occupational Safety and Health Policy*. Cambridge, MA: MIT Press;1979.

32. Gromley WT. Regulatory networks in a federal system. *Polity*. 1986;18(4): 595–620.

33. Bokat SA, Thompson HA. *Occupational Safety and Health Law*. Washington, DC: Bureau of National Affairs;1988.

34. Rabinowitz RS. *Occupational Safety and Health Law*. 2nd ed. Washington, DC: Bureau of National Affairs;2002.

35. Bloom M. *Primary Prevention: The Possible Science.* Upper Saddle River, NJ: Prentice Hall;1981.

36. Christoforou T. The precautionary principle in European Community law and science. In: Tickner JA, ed. *Precaution Environmental Science and Preventive Public Policy.* Washington, DC: Island Press;2003:241–262.

37. Walton D. *Fundamentals of Critical Argumentation.* New York, NY: Cambridge University Press;2006.

38. Occupational Safety and Health Act, 29 U.S.C. § 651 (1970).

39. Tickner JA, Kriebel D, Wright S. A compass for health: rethinking precaution and its role in science and public health. *Int J Epidemiol.* 2003;32(4):489–492.

40. Walton DN. Abductive, presumptive, and plausible arguments. *Informal Logic.* 2001;21(2):141–169.

41. Ward J, Ferrucci D. How does the brain work [transcript]? *NOVA ScienceNow.* PBS. Available at: http://www.pbs.org/wgbh/nova/body/how-does-the-brain-work.html. Aired September 2001. Accessed October 27, 2012.

42. Nicoll G. Radiation sources in natural gas well activities. *Occup Health Saf.* 2012;81(10):22, 24, 26. Available at: http://ohsonline.com/Articles/2012/10/01/Radiation-Sources-in-Natural-Gas-Well-Activities.aspx?p=1. Accessed October 27, 2012.

43. Kriebel D, Tickner JA, Epstein P, et al. The precautionary principle in environmental science. *Environ Health Perspect.* 2001;109(9):871–876.

44. Rogers DW. *Making Capitalism Safe: Work Safety and Health Regulation in America, 1880–1940.* Urbana, IL: University of Illinois Press;2009.

45. Geiser K. Preface: Establishing a general duty of precaution in the environmental protection policies of the United States. In: Raffensberger C, Tickner JA, eds. *Protecting Public Health and the Environment: Implementing the Precautionary Principle.* Washington, DC: Island Press;1999:xxi–xxiv.

46. Stufflebeam DL. The CIPP model for evaluation. In: Stufflebeam DL, Madaus GF, Kellaghan T, eds. *Evaluation Models: Viewpoints on Educational and Human Services Evaluation.* 2nd ed. Boston, MA: Kluwer Academic Publishers;2000.

47. Roberto MA. *The Art of Critical Decision Making.* Chantilly, VA: The Teaching Company;2009. Course Guidebook.

48. Beauchamp DE. Public health as social justice. *Inquiry.* 1976;13(1):3–14.

49. Dorfman L, Wallack L, Woodruff K. More than a message: framing public health advocacy to change corporate practices. *Health Educ Behav.* 2005;32(3):320-336.
50. Schapiro M. Chemical revolution. In: *Exposed: The Toxic Chemistry of Everyday Products and What's at Stake for American Power.* White River Junction, VT: Chelsea Green Publishing;2007.
51. Tindale CW. *Fallacies and Argument Appraisal.* New York, NY: Cambridge University Press;2007.
52. Johnson BL. *Environmental Policy and Public Health.* Boca Raton, FL: CRC Press;2007.
53. Levenstein C, DeLaurier GF, Dunn ML. *Cotton Dust Papers: Science, Politics, and Power in the "Discovery" of Byssinosis in the U.S.* Amityville, NY: Baywood Publishing Company;2001.
54. Ives JH, ed. *The Export of Hazard: Transnational Corporations and Environmental Control Issues.* Boston, MA: Routledge & Kegan Paul;1985.
55. Cameron A. *Radicals of the Worst Sort: Laboring Women in Lawrence, Massachusetts, 1860-1912.* Urbana, IL: University of Illinois Press;1993.
56. Brodeur P. *Outrageous Misconduct: The Asbestos Industry on Trial.* New York, NY: Pantheon Books;1985.
57. Sells B. What asbestos taught me about managing risk. *Harv Bus Rev.* 1994;72(3):76-90.
58. Torkelson MS, Oyen F, Rowe VK. The toxicity of vinyl chloride as determined by repeated exposure of laboratory animals. *Am Ind Hyg Assoc J.* 1961;22:354-361.
59. Viola PL, Bigotti A, Caputo A. Oncogenic response of rat skin, lungs, and bones to vinyl chloride. *Cancer Res.* 1971;31:516-522.
60. Firestein S. *Ignorance: How It Drives Science.* New York, NY: Oxford University Press;2012.
61. Ringholz RC. *Uranium Frenzy: Saga of the Nuclear West.* Logan, UT: Utah State University Press;2002.
62. Doyle HN. The Federal Industrial Hygiene Agency: a history of the Division of Occupational Health, U.S. Public Health Service. Prepared for: History of Industrial Hygiene Committee; American Conference of Governmental Hygienists; 1974.
63. Fleming AS. The Federal Radiation Council. *Public Health Rep.* 1959;74(12):1107-1108.

64. Wagoner JK, Archer VE, Lundin FE, Holaday DA, Lloyd JW. Radiation as the cause of lung cancer among uranium miners. *N Engl J Med*. 1965;273(4):181–188.

65. MacLaury J. *Tragedy in the Uranium Mines: Catalyst for National Workers' Safety and Health Legislation*. Paper presented at: Symposium on Lyndon Baines Johnson's Legacy; April 27, 1998; Miami University, Oxford, OH. Available at: http://www.dol.gov/oasam/programs/history/lbjsym98.htm. Accessed December 16, 2013.

II. IMPLEMENTATION OF POLICY

In Part II, I cover Chapters 7 to 12. In Chapters 7, 8, and 9, I describe the complete Occupational Safety and Health Act (OSHAct; see Appendix), section by section. In Chapter 7, I address the first seven sections of the OSHAct, with an emphasis on standards. I also describe several court cases that shaped occupational safety and health policies regarding Occupational Safety and Health Administration (OSHA) rule making and standards. I describe the structure of OSHA and address the problem of overestimation of the cost of standards during rule making by both the affected industry and by OSHA.

In Chapter 8, I address Sections 8 through 19 of the OSHAct with an emphasis on enforcement policy. I describe the OSHA enforcement strategy and the state-based structure for enforcement. I discuss the role of the Occupational Safety and Health Review Commission. I describe the prosecution of occupational safety and health crimes beyond the OSHA jurisdiction, both by state and local governments and indirectly under environmental laws. I examine the fallacious claim that OSHA inspections are job killers.

In Chapter 9, I describe the last sections of the OSHAct (20–34). I highlight the research authorities of the National Institute for Occupational Safety and Health (NIOSH) and its structure. I describe the training and educational mandates for OSHA and NIOSH as well as the OSHA consultation program. I explain the role of the Bureau of Labor Statistics in compiling occupational safety and health statistics. I discuss the history of public health organizations that existed prior to and evolving into NIOSH and the policy roles of NIOSH directors over time, especially regarding science policy.

In Chapter 10, I describe the long history of catastrophic mine disasters along with how these drive a slow and incremental development of mine safety and health policy today. I describe the companion organization to OSHA, the

Mine Safety and Health Administration, as well as the rise of the Bureau of Mines and its eventual transfer of safety research functions to NIOSH in the last decade of the 20th century. I explain the delay in the recognition of silicosis as a disease followed by the delay of the recognition of coal workers' pneumoconiosis as an occupational disease. I describe the battle for black lung benefits and problems in the control of coal workers' pneumoconiosis. In Chapter 11, I address other statutes in the United States that provide for the protection of occupational safety and health and that can take precedence over OSHA's jurisdiction as established in the OSHAct. These statutes cover offshore drilling and fishing, operations of the Department of Energy, and transportation safety, and include some consumer, environmental, and labor protection laws. I look at other workers excluded from OSHA jurisdiction, including state and local government employees and self-employed workers.

In Chapter 12, I cover international policies regarding occupational safety and health. I address OSHA's involvement regarding international concerns and policies of the United Nations specialized agencies including the World Health Organization and the International Labor Organization. I also cover other international organizations such as the World Trade Organization, the European Community, and treaty-based organizations such as the Commission for Labor Cooperation arising from a side agreement to the North American Free Trade Agreement. In addition, I describe policies for international asbestos exposure elimination and control, as well as the recent problem of worker safety in textile factories in Bangladesh. I end the chapter with a description of the Bhopal disaster in India and of work-related human trafficking in nations of the world.

7

Standards and the Occupational Safety and Health Act

Fortunately, it [Occupational Safety and Health Act] *is an exceptionally well-crafted piece of legislation that is clearly organized, easily understood, and often eloquent.*

—Nicholas A. Ashford and Charles C. Caldart[1]

THE FORMALDEHYDE NARRATIVE

Eleven U.S. chemical companies created the Chemical Industry Institute of Toxicology (CIIT) in 1974 to address concerns about the effects of chemicals on environmental and human health. In a 1979 report to the U.S. Environmental Protection Agency (EPA), CIIT reported on the results of an animal study that suggested that formaldehyde was a carcinogen. The EPA participated in the Interagency Regulatory Liaison Group (see Chapter 3) in assessing the potential exposures to formaldehyde. As a result of toxicology studies and the exposure assessment, EPA's Office of Toxic Substances explored taking regulatory action under § 4(f) of the Toxic Substances Control Act (TSCA). In March 1981, EPA officials determined that there might be a reasonable basis to conclude that formaldehyde was a significant risk requiring action and prepared a draft notice. In May 1981, as President Ronald Reagan assumed office, the draft notice was also waiting for new EPA Administrator Anne Gorsuch and Deputy Administrator for Toxic Substances John Hernandez. In addition, a letter from the Formaldehyde Institute that disputed the draft notice awaited Gorsuch and Hernandez. After meeting with representatives of the Formaldehyde Institute,

Hernandez decided that further study was needed as the science was deemed insufficient for regulatory action.[2] The EPA's inaction led to a congressional hearing on the failure to regulate formaldehyde and to the Natural Resources Defense Council suing EPA for the same reason. The lawsuit was dropped following an EPA determination that two major groups were exposed: apparel industry workers and mobile home residents. As a result, EPA transferred the issue to the Occupational Safety and Health Administration (OSHA) in 1986, which promulgated a standard for formaldehyde in 1987.[1] Twenty-three years later, President Obama signed the Formaldehyde Standards for Composite Wood Products Act on July 7, 2010, as Title IV of the Toxic Substances Control Act, which directed EPA to promulgate final formaldehyde regulations by January 1, 2013.[3]

7.1. INTRODUCTION

[The Occupational Safety and Health Act is] *Probably one of the most important pieces of legislation from the standpoint of 55 million people ever passed by the United States Congress because it involves their lives.*

—President Richard Nixon[4]

After the passage of the Occupational Safety and Health Act (OSHAct; see Appendix), OSHA battled challenges to its standards in the courts and in Congress over employer duties to protect workers from occupational hazards. This chapter describes Sections 1 through 7 of the act; covers the purpose and findings of the act, definitions and their criticality to policy, and jurisdictional limitations under the act; and addresses safety and health standards and related court rulings. A full reading of the act appears at the end of this book.

Sections of legislation are numbered sequentially as in the act's sections, from 1 through 34. However, all federal statutes are codified by subject into the United States Code (U.S.C.). The U.S.C. consolidates all U.S. laws arranged according to subject matter under 50 titles and sets out the current status of the laws as amended.[5]

The OSHAct is placed under Chapter 15 of Title 29 of the U.S.C. The official citation of the statute is by title and section number, so the citation for the act is "29 U.S.C. § 650 et seq." with, for example, Section 2 of the act cited numerically as "29 U.S.C. § 651." Regulations are coded under the same title as the Code of

Federal Regulations (CFR), thus it is coded as "29 CFR." A standard is issued when it is submitted to the *Federal Register* and is promulgated when it is published in the *Federal Register*.

In writing standards, OSHA typically follows a hierarchy of controls based upon a precedence order of effectiveness in controlling the exposure to a hazard. The first line of defense is a physical change in the workplace with engineering controls that eliminate a hazard such as substituting a less hazardous substance, isolating the hazard, or ventilating the workspace. Protective safety devices that include interlocks, redundancy, fail-safe design, and fire suppression are a subset of engineering controls but are not as reliable as true engineering controls. The second line of defense is administrative controls that significantly limit daily exposure to hazards by control or manipulation of the work schedule or work habits (e.g., job rotation, training). This and the next level of control require the employer or worker to take protective action. The third line of defense is work practices that include hazard control programs such as compliance with OSHA requirements including hazard communication and process safety management standards as well as housekeeping and procedures for specific operations. Personal protective equipment (PPE) is the last line of defense and should only be used when all other hazard controls cannot be used (e.g., respirators when fighting fires) or in combination with other controls (e.g., gloves). This defense method requires the worker to wear protection.[6]

Employers must comply with two provisions of the OSH Act: (1) the general duty clause, and (2) interim, permanent, and emergency temporary standards. OSHA standards fall into four broad classifications: general industry, maritime, construction, and agriculture. General industry standards are broad, covering all workplaces for which OSHA has jurisdiction unless the standards exclude specific categories of workplaces. The other three classifications of workplaces address occupational safety and health in industries with unique working conditions and work practices.[7]

- General industry standards (29 § CFR 1910) may address either certain industry segments (vertical standards) such as logging or across all or many industry segments (horizontal standards) such as toxic substances (e.g., formaldehyde). As vertical standards, maritime, construction, and agricultural standards take precedence over general industry standards that cover similar hazards.

- Maritime standards (29 § CFR 1915–1919) address occupational hazards that involve waterborne commerce. These standards apply to work at shipyards, marine terminals, and longshoring activities such as shipbuilding, work at the docks, and loading vessels, respectively. These standards also apply to the safety certification of equipment in longshoring activities and accrediting responsible persons to insure that safety equipment is in working order. Under this classification, OSHA adopted previous standards established under the Longshore and Harbor Workers' Compensation Act of 1927 as interim standards.[8]
- Construction standards (29 § CFR 1926) cover work at construction sites, which presents a unique situation of multiple employers in flux with different trades moving onto and off of worksites continuously. Standards promulgated by the U.S. Department of Labor (DoL) under the Construction Safety Act of 1969,[9] which applied to work conducted under federal government contracts, were subsumed by OSHA as interim standards.
- Agriculture standards (29 § CFR 1928) are aimed at protecting employees on farms and other agricultural activities such as agricultural services. The agriculture classification addresses a range of unique working conditions that includes fishing and forestry with a typical feature of seasonal work in which much of it is affected by outdoor conditions, including field sanitation.

7.2. SECTIONS 1–7 OF THE OCCUPATIONAL SAFETY AND HEALTH ACT

To regulate Commerce with foreign Nations, and among the several States, and with the Indian Tribes.

—U.S. Constitution, Section 8, Clause 3

7.2.1. An Act (Section 1)

Congress enacted the act on December 29, 1970, to ensure safe and healthful working conditions for working men and women. The act authorizes the enforcement of standards developed under the act, encourages state efforts to assure safe and healthful working conditions, and provides for research, information, education, and training in the field of occupational safety and health.

7.2.2. Congressional Findings and Purpose (Section 2)

Congress stated in its findings that personal injuries and illnesses related to work pose a substantial burden on and hindrance to interstate commerce regarding lost production, wage loss, medical expenses, and disability compensation payments. The purpose of the act is "to assure so far as possible every working man and woman in the Nation safe and healthful working conditions."

The act's § 2(b)(12) provides "for appropriate reporting procedures with respect to occupational safety and health which procedures will help achieve the objectives of this Act and accurately describe the nature of the occupational safety and health problem." Based upon this authority, OSHA requires employers to maintain records of workplace injuries and illnesses that OSHA inspectors can access and heighten employer awareness of these problems. A recordable injury or illness involves medical treatment, loss of consciousness, restriction of work or motion, or transfer to another job.[1]

7.2.3. Definitions (Section 3)

Many definitions, which are easily passed over, are critical for establishing the authority of an agency. The definition of "commerce" restricts coverage by this act to the boundaries of states and territories and the outer continental shelf. The definition of "persons" includes not only people but also corporations and other legal entities. The act's definition of "employer" excludes the U.S. government, state governments, and their subdivisions (i.e., counties and cities). The definition of "occupational safety and health standard" was important in a later court case regarding a benzene standard with the ruling that a standard had to be "reasonably necessary or appropriate."

The definitions of "national consensus standard" and "established Federal standard" were important in establishing interim standards, which are addressed later regarding § 6(a). The OSHAct created both the Occupational Safety and Health Review Commission and the National Institute for Occupational Safety and Health (NIOSH), which are discussed in Chapters 8 and 9, respectively. While the act did not create OSHA by name, it provided for an Assistant Secretary of Labor for Occupational Safety and Health, and the U.S. Secretary of Labor established OSHA as the agency under the direction of the new Assistant Secretary.

Table 7-1. Section 4 of the Occupational Safety and Health Act

Section	Statement
§ 4(a)	This Act shall apply with respect to employment performed in a workplace in a State, the District of Columbia, the Commonwealth of Puerto Rico, the Virgin Islands, American Samoa, Guam, the Trust Territory of the Pacific Islands, Wake Island, Outer Continental Shelf Lands defined in the Outer Continental Shelf Lands Act,* Johnston Island, and the Canal Zone.
§ 4(b)(1)	Nothing in this Act shall apply to working conditions of employees with respect to which other Federal agencies . . . exercise statutory authority to prescribe or enforce standards or regulations affecting occupational safety or health.

*The Outer Continental Shelf Lands Act is addressed in Chapter 11.

7.2.4. Applicability of the Occupational Safety and Health Act (Section 4)

In the act, Section 4 specifies the geographical bounds for its coverage, as shown in Table 7-1. The act states that it does not apply to working conditions in which other federal agencies exercise their statutory authorities to enforce standards or regulations that affect occupational safety and health. As an example, the Mine Safety and Health Administration (MSHA) is responsible for protecting the occupational safety and health of miners.

In addition, other specific laws were subsumed by this act. These included the 1936 Walsh-Healey Public Contracts Act[10] and the 1965 McNamara-O'Hara Service Contract Act.[11] The OSHAct did not supersede or affect workers' compensation laws or common law or statutory rights and duties of employers and employees regarding work-related injuries or diseases.

The Supreme Court granted certiorari—a document that a losing party files with the Supreme Court asking for a review of a lower court's decision—to resolve a conflict among lower courts regarding the preemptive force of § 4(b)(1). On January 9, 2002, a unanimous court (Justice Antonin Scalia not participating) concluded that the U.S. Coast Guard had engaged in a limited exercise of its authority to regulate working conditions on uninspected vessels in the case, *Chao v. Mallard Bay Drilling, Inc.*[12] Therefore, OSHA's regulation of uninspected vessels had not been preempted, and OSHA properly exercised its jurisdiction over an uninspected drilling barge. The court noted that even though the Coast Guard regulates fire extinguishers, life preservers, and emergency floating equipment on uninspected vessels, these regulations fail to address overall safety and health. The court also found that the drilling barge was a "workplace" within the meaning of § 4(a) of the OSHAct because it was located within a geographic area of the state of Louisiana.[13]

7.2.5. Duties (Section 5)

The OSHAct establishes a duty for both employers and employees to protect employee safety and health. An important aspect of this act was the general duty clause, according to which it is the duty of each employer to provide its employees with a place of employment that is free from recognized occupational hazards. There is also a duty by both employer and employee, under the supervision of the employer, to comply with any standard established by this act. In the absence of a standard, the general duty clause can be invoked as long as the hazard has been recognized or should have been recognized by the employer (e.g., identified in the trade literature).

A "recognized hazard" carries a two-fold meaning. First, the employer or its industry must or should know of the hazard, including objective determinations (e.g., open and obvious). Second, the hazard must be preventable, insuring that the general duty is achievable. Expert consideration may render a method of hazard elimination unachievable if untested or unfeasible.[14]

Employees also have a duty to comply, but it is the employer's duty to enforce this compliance. OSHA enforces standards against only employers. Even though the 1977 Federal Mine Safety and Health Act[15] does not have a general duty clause, MSHA follows the same approach in holding employers responsible with one exception: MSHA can cite miners for carrying or smoking cigarettes or cigars in underground coal mines.

The general duty clause is important because it is the duty of the employer, not the government, to assure safe and healthful working conditions. The employer provides the safe working environment as a cost of doing business, following the environmental protection principle in which the "the polluter pays." The OSHAct provides for the promulgation of three types of standards: interim (§ 6[a]), permanent (§ 6[c]), and emergency temporary standards (§ 6[c]).

7.2.6. Interim Standards (Section 6[a])

In retrospect [OSHA] made a major mistake in 1971 when it hastily issued, en masse, a ramshackle collection of so-called national consensus standards ... this hodgepodge collection of standards and OSHA's early efforts to enforce them probably did more to damage the initial acceptance of the entire program than any other single action.

—Lane Kirkland[16]

The OSHAct gave the Secretary of Labor the authority to promulgate interim standards within two years of the passage of the act. Thus, the wholesale adoption of thousands of these standards resulted in many errors.[17] Nonetheless, Congress showed genius in establishing a panoply of start-up standards without going through rule making, for so much contention surrounded OSHA rule making in the years to come that the number of standards promulgated would have otherwise been small indeed. Moreover, nearly all of the safety standards remain current today.

The interim standards had to be based upon either a national consensus standard or an established federal standard, such as those promulgated for federal contractors—for example, the Threshold Limit Values (TLVs) established by the American Conference of Governmental Industrial Hygienists (ACGIH). A consensus standard was any standard established by a nationally recognized standards-producing organization in which opportunities for diverse views were considered. OSHA adopted many interim standards en masse using this authority during its first two years, except for standards that would not result in improved employee safety and health. OSHA was not required to adopt these standards verbatim as long as the change was not substantive.[18]

OSHA used consensus standards primarily from three organizations in setting interim standards: the American National Standards Institute (ANSI), the National Fire Protection Association, and the American Society for Testing and Materials. Other standards were adopted to a smaller degree by reference including a reference to the National Electrical Code.[18]

OSHA also adopted established federal standards. One set of standards was adopted in 1969 by the Secretary of Labor under the Walsh-Healey Public Contracts Act, based upon TLVs developed by ACGIH. Another set of standards was established in 1970 under the Construction Safety Act. In addition, OSHA adopted standards promulgated under the 1965 National Foundation on Arts and Humanities Act[19] and the Longshore and Harbor Workers' Compensation Act.[8,18]

Responding to criticisms of standards that were unnecessary or inappropriate, OSHA deleted 600 safety standards in 1978. The deletions of standards were based on the following criteria: they were either (1) obsolete, (2) directed at comfort rather than safety, (3) directed to public rather than private employees, (4) enforced by other agencies, (5) contingent upon manufacturer approval, (6) too detailed, or (7) covered by other standards.[16] An issue was raised following the adoption of these standards as to whether they were advisory (to be deleted) or mandatory (to remain as adopted). The words "should" or "shall" were used, respectively, to determine whether the standard was advisory or mandatory, and in 1984, OSHA revoked 153 interim standards adopted from ANSI that used the word "should."[18]

7.2.7. Permanent Standards (Section 6[b])

Permanent standards classified as safety standards include the logging operations standard and the crane and derricks standard that were established under the definition of standards in § 3(a). According to Stephen A. Bokat and Horace A. Thompson in 1988, virtually all permanent standards have been based upon language to promulgate "standards dealing with toxic materials or harmful physical agents" to protect employees from lifetime "material impairment of health or functional capacity."[16]

7.2.7.1. Rule Making. The Secretary of Labor may promulgate, modify, or revoke a standard by a rule-making process. Since this process is specified in the act, it supersedes the Administrative Procedures Act (APA) through a series of steps that lead to a final rule. These steps are as follows:

1. Determine that a rule should be promulgated based upon information provided to or by the Secretary.
2. The Secretary may establish an advisory committee.
3. The Secretary publishes a proposed rule in the *Federal Register* and provides an opportunity for public comment.
4. During this period, any person can request a public hearing on the proposed rule.
5. If a request is made, the Secretary must publish the details of the request and specify the time and place of a public hearing in the *Federal Register.*
6. Thereafter, the Secretary must either issue the rule or determine that the rule will not be issued.

However, OSHA follows a "hybrid" approach to rule making that complies with the six steps above and also complies with a substantial evidence test that was specified in the legislative conference report in deference to the bill (that became the OSHAct) presented by the House of Representatives. To comply with the substantial evidence test (a characteristic of formal rule making under APA), OSHA added to its rule-making procedure the following actions as described in the 1974 case, *Industrial Union Department, AFL-CIO v. Hodgson:*[20]

1. An oral hearing is held and presided over by a qualified hearing examiner.
2. Cross-examination is permitted.
3. A verbatim transcript is made.

7.2.7.2. Standard Promulgation. When the rule relates to toxic materials or harmful physical agents, the standard must be established under § 6(b)(5) to adequately assure, to the extent feasible and based upon the best available evidence, that no employee will "suffer material impairment of health or functional capacity" for his or her working lifetime. In the 1980 case of *Industrial Union Department v. American Petroleum Institute,*[21] the conflict between this definition of a standard and the earlier definition, "reasonably necessary or appropriate," was examined. The Supreme Court found that a significant risk must be shown to be potentially abated by the standard. A significant risk was defined as one case (of cancer) in 1,000, but the court defined an insignificant risk as one case in a billion.

The OSHAct conditions the protection of health on the feasibility to control hazards. The statute does not define the word "feasibility," but the legislative history allows that both technological and economic feasibility must be considered, thus delimiting health as the ultimate goal of the act.[1]

Over a period of 40 years after the passage of the OSHAct, OSHA had issued more than 80 safety and health standards. In some cases, OSHA uses the general duty clause to enforce against hazards where no standard exists or where a standard is not protective.[16] Table 7-2 lists the health standards that have been promulgated by OSHA.

Where appropriate, the standards must also include procedures for apprising workers of the hazards, the use of PPE, and medical examinations. Any employer may apply to OSHA for a variance with procedures to protect employees with a temporary procedure until technical or resource limitations can be overcome, and standards set by state programs may exceed the federal standards in protecting workers.

Table 7-2. Health Standards Promulgated by the Occupational Safety and Health Administration

1972–1983	1984–1992	1993–2006
Asbestos 1972	Ethylene oxide 1984	Lead (construction) 1993
14 carcinogens 1974	Asbestos**1986	Confined space entry† 1993
Vinyl chloride 1974	Field sanitation 1987	Asbestos* 1994
Coke oven emissions 1974	Formaldehyde 1987	1,3-butadiene 1996
Benzene 1978	Benzene** 1987	Methylene chloride 1997
DBCP 1978	Access to medical records** 1988	Respiratory protection 1998
Arsenic 1978	Air contaminants (vacated) 1989	Ergonomics 2000
Cotton dust 1978	Chemical exposure in laboratories 1990	Ergonomics (revoked) 2001
Acrylonitrile 1978	Bloodborne pathogens 1991	Bloodborne pathogens** 2001
Lead 1978	4,4'-methylenedianiline 1992	Hexavalent chromium* 2006
Cancer policy 1980	Cadmium 1992	
Access to medical records 1980	Asbestos* 1992	
Hearing conservation 1981	Formaldehyde* 1992	
Hazard communication 1983		

Note: DBCP = dibromochloropropane.
*Response to court remand.
**Modified or revised.
†Safety standard.

7.2.8. Temporary Standards (Section 6[c])

The OSHAct also provides for an emergency temporary standard, which takes effect upon publication in the *Federal Register*. This standard is based on employees exposed to "grave danger" from agents that are toxic or physically harmful or are a new hazard, making it necessary to protect the employees from the danger. The standard is effective for no more than six months but can be reissued in the *Federal Register*. The Secretary of Labor must issue a permanent standard while the temporary standard is in force. The temporary standard can be challenged in a court of appeals as provided for under § 6(f).

OSHA attempted to set a six-month emergency standard for workers' exposure to asbestos in the early 1980s. In staying the emergency standard in the 1984 case, *Asbestos Information Association v. OSHA*,[22] the Fifth Circuit Court (New Orleans) held that the urgency of the standard was not established because of the numerous uncertainties in the agency's risk assessment. Although "[t]he Agency need not support its conclusion with anything supporting scientific certainty" (citing the 1980 *Industrial Union Department v.*

American Petroleum Institute case[21]), the court rejected OSHA's risk assessment as too "speculative" because it attempted to make death predictions for only a six-month period, the term of an emergency temporary standard. The court's opinion stated, "Indeed, OSHA concedes some unreliability and uncertainty to be inherent in risk assessment generally. Applying the risk assessment process to a period of six months, one ninetieth of OSHA's estimated working lifetime, only magnifies those inherent uncertainties."[22]

The court also noted that contrary to OSHA's calculation that the six-month emergency standard might prevent 80 asbestos-related cancer deaths during that period, the agency's own data could be recalculated to predict that only about 14 deaths would be prevented during the six-month emergency period. The court held that the use of emergency temporary standards under § 6(c) was invalid because no emergency existed, the issue was not grave, and respirators could be used while permanent standards were promulgated.[1] Establishing a convincing significant risk of diseases of long latency for a six-month period curtailed the use of an emergency temporary standard as an instrument for OSHA action.

7.2.9. Variance, Publication, and Judicial Review (Section 6[d–g])

An employer may request a variance from a promulgated standard under § 6 with evidence that an alternative control is at least as effective. Employees are invited to the hearing regarding the employer's proposal. The Secretary of Labor can issue a rule for a variance. More broadly, the Secretary is required to publish any action related to a standard, including its enforcement, in the *Federal Register*.

Any person adversely affected by a standard can challenge the validity rule in a U.S. circuit court of appeals within 60 days after its promulgation, but the challenge does not stop the implementation of the standard unless the court later rules against it. The Secretary of Labor is also authorized to set priorities for the use of the agency's resources and to promulgate standards sequentially.

7.2.10. Advisory Committees (Section 7)

The OSHAct provides for two types of advisory committees. One type is the National Advisory Committee for Occupational Safety and Health (NACOSH). The act provides that NACOSH be composed of 12 persons. The Secretary of

Labor appoints these members and the committee's chair, but four of the 12 are designated by the Secretary of Health and Human Services, where NIOSH is based. NACOSH comprises representatives from management, labor, occupational safety and health professions (four from NIOSH), and the public (typically one of whom is named the chair). NACOSH advises on, consults with, and makes recommendations to the Secretary of Labor and the Secretary of Health and Human Services on the administration of the OSHAct.

The other type of advisory committee may be appointed to advise the Secretary of Labor on occupational safety and health standards promulgated under § 6(b) of the act. These committees typically comprise 15 members, but the representation on these committees must be balanced between representatives of employers and employees. However, OSHA has one standing committee under this authority, the Advisory Committee for Construction Safety and Health (ACCSH). This committee gained this status because of preexisting legislation, the 1969 Construction Safety Act, which was subsumed into the OSHAct. Any standard that is promulgated for the protection of construction workers must be brought before this committee before it is issued.

In 1972, the Secretary of Labor appointed members to the Standards Advisory Committee on Agriculture (SACA). The SACA convened a subgroup on rollover protective structures (ROPS) that year and based its advice on OSHA's proposed ROPS standard in 1974. OSHA published a final rule on ROPS in 1975, requiring employers to provide ROPS and safety belts on all agricultural tractors manufactured after October 25, 1976.[23]

With advice from SACA, OSHA published a reentry temporary emergency standard regarding pesticides in 1973. Courts overturned the emergency standard just one year later, deferring to EPA jurisdiction under the Federal Insecticide, Fungicide, and Rodenticide Act.[24]

This was when OSHA found itself the object of extreme criticism by Congress, influence by farmer special interests that despised federal intrusion into their operations. The nadir of this criticism was reached when Senator William Proxmire (R) of Wisconsin nominated the agency for one of his notorious "Golden Fleece" awards, mocking an OSHA contract to Purdue University for producing a brochure (among other publications) for low-literacy farm workers. The text of the brochure was written in simple, third-grade-level English in order to be more accessible to members of the target audience. Overlooking this important fact, Senator Proxmire gibbeted the brochure as an example of government waste, derisively reading the entire text into the *Congressional Record*.

The document quoted was one of many. House Representatives also made statements that ridiculed OSHA efforts, such as official safety precautions about "slippery manure." In effect, the ill-fated education effort for low-literacy farm workers led to OSHA disbanding the SACA in 1978. It also led to riders on the appropriations bill for OSHA that limited funding for the agency's enforcement at workplaces that exempted farms with 10 or fewer employees.[23]

In the final days of President Jimmy Carter's administration, OSHA promulgated a lead standard. This standard did not apply to the construction industry in part because the ACCSH was required by agency procedures to review any standard that applied to the construction industry prior to its promulgation, which time did not allow prior to the change in administrations.

OSHA must comply with the Federal Advisory Committee Act and the Negotiated Rulemaking Act (RegNeg), the latter of which Congress passed in 1990. In negotiated rule making, the agency is required to bring parties together in the early stages of the rule-making process to foster cooperation and solve regulatory problems.[25] As an example, OSHA established the Crane and Derrick Negotiated Rulemaking Committee in 2003 to develop a construction safety standard for cranes and derricks. The advisory committee consisted of 25 members chaired by a facilitator, and an OSHA representative was a member of the committee. OSHA issued the final rule in 2010.

7.3. SETTING PRECEDENCE

Courts make law by interpreting legislation when the laws omit agency direction or present ambiguity in meaning. This is true of the OSHAct. Many of these interpretations of important court cases that have affected the evolution of OSHA actions are shown in chronological order in Table 7-3. Earlier rulings guide later decisions and agency actions in this chronology.

During OSHA's first decade, court rulings strengthened its standard-setting process. In the 1974 asbestos case,[22] erring on the side of public health was affirmed, and regarding carcinogens in another 1974 case, the court recognized that for regulatory purposes an animal carcinogen can be a predictor of a human carcinogen. The vinyl chloride (VCM) case demonstrated the power of the emergency temporary standard to stop lethal exposures as permanent rule making takes place. It also affirmed control at the lowest detectable level for carcinogens and the hierarchy of controls in which engineering control technology is preferred over PPE. The 1978 coke oven case established no safe

Table 7-3. Precedent-Setting Judicial Interpretations of Standards Under the Occupational Safety and Health Act

Standard Promulgated	Case and Court	Interpretation
1972, Asbestos	1974, *Industrial Union Department, AFL-CIO v. Hodgson* (DC Cir.)	1. Affirmed OSHA substantial evidence review process 2. NIOSH recommendations were an aid to OSHA, not a requirement 3. OSHA could set a standard based on policy judgments on relative risks of underprotection compared with overprotection
1974, 14 Carcinogens	1974 *SOCMA v. Brennan*, 503 F.2d 1155 (3rd Cir.)	1. An animal carcinogen could be considered as a human carcinogen
1974, Vinyl chloride	1975, *Society of Plastics Industry, Inc. v. OSHA* (2nd Cir.)	1. Factual determinations were on "the frontiers of knowledge" 2. Favored positive over negative evidence in studies 3. Set policy of lowest detectible level for carcinogens 4. Engineering controls were more effective than PPE
1976, Coke oven emissions	1978, *American Iron and Steel Institute v. OSHA* (3rd Cir.)	1. Could require technology "looming on today's horizon" 2. Research and development provision was invalid and unenforceable 3. No absolutely safe level of exposure to a carcinogen
1978, 1987, Benzene	1980, *Industrial Union Department v. American Petroleum Institute* (U.S. Supreme Court)	1. OSHA had the burden of proof to show that an agent presented a significant risk of harm, but not with scientific certainty 2. One in a billion was an insignificant risk, whereas one in a thousand was a significant risk 3. OSHA could risk error on the side of overprotection rather than underprotection
1978, Lead	1980, *United Steelworkers of America, AFL-CIO-CLC v. Marshall and Bingham* (DC Cir.)	1. Clearly met significant risk test 2. Subclinical effects were "material impairment" in the continuum to overt lead disease 3. Both technologically and economically feasible 4. Affirmed medical removal protection
1978, Cotton dust	1981, *American Textile Manufacturers v. Donovan* (U.S. Supreme Court)	1. Rejected argument that Congress required cost-benefit analysis 2. Health standards subject to different criteria from safety standards 3. Financial cost of health and safety problem ≥ cost of eliminating the problem
1983, Asbestos	1984, *Asbestos Information Association v. OSHA*	1. Use of emergency temporary standard denied since the standard was not based on new information and consequences over six months would not be "grave"

(Continued)

Table 7-3. (Continued)

Standard Promulgated	Case and Court	Interpretation
1983, Hearing conservation	1985, *Forging Industry Association v. Secretary of Labor* (5th Cir.)	1. Standard did not seek to regulate nonoccupational exposures 2. Reasoning extended by example to air pollution exposures, which presented no reason to not regulate workplace lung exposures to fumes
1983, Hazard communication	1985, *United Steelworkers, AFL-CIO-CLC v. Auchter* (3rd Cir.)	1. Standard was a § 6(b) "standard," not a § 8 "regulation" 2. Thus, it could be used to preempt state laws 3. Include employees in all sectors, not just manufacturing
1984, Ethylene oxide	1986, *Public Citizen Health Research v. Brock* (DC Cir.)	1. Short-term exposure limit to be considered
1983, Hazard communication	1990, *Dole v. Steelworkers* (3rd Cir.)	1. OMB had no authority to interfere with OSHA substantive decision making under the Paperwork Reduction Act of 1980
1989, Air contaminants (not reissued)	1992, *AFL-CIO v. OSHA* (11th Cir.)	1. Supported "material impairment" determination 2. Substances posed a significant risk, but plaintiff failed to show exposure level of risk 3. Did not show how technology would meet the standard in different industries for each substance 4. No economic feasibility analysis for specific industries 5. Could rely on ACGIH recommendations for rule making 6. Mislabeled as generic standard

Note: OSHA = Occupational Safety and Health Administration; NIOSH = National Institute of Occupational Safety and Health; PPE = personal protective equipment; OMB = Office of Management and Budget; ACGIH = American Conference of Governmental Industrial Hygienists.

level of carcinogen exposure and specified that cutting-edge technology can be required but controls that are yet to be discovered and require research and development cannot be required.

While the 1980 benzene case affirmed again that OSHA standards can err on the side of public health, it dramatically changed the standard-setting process. The burden of proof was on OSHA to show quantitatively the risk reduction that occurs, corresponding with the increase in control of a substance. During that year, the lead case met this significant risk test and established that subclinical effects of an exposure qualify as material impairment and that medical removal from work is a valid control measure. In the following year, the cotton dust case resolved Congress's finding that the benefits of control (i.e., § 2(a), OSHAct) warrant the costs of the control. The 1985 noise control case determined that nonwork exposures do not lessen the need for reduced occupational exposures.

As for hazard communication, the 1985 case found that a standard cannot be limited to just one industrial sector when exposures occur in other sectors as well, and in the 1990 case, the court found that the Office of Management and Budget (OMB) lacks the authority to interfere with substantive rule making. The OSHA Hazard Communication Standard (HazCom Standard) is an example of a generic standard that addresses occupational hazards across multiple substances rather than a substance-by-substance approach for control. When OSHA attempted to update the interim permissible exposure limit (PEL) standards in 1989, the case that followed in 1992 found that the rule-making process for permanent standards was not met, thus rejecting this attempt at "generic" rule making. OSHA was required to address the significant risk and feasibility tests at the industry level for each substance.

While OSHA's first decade showed great promise for the OSHAct, in the second decade and since, court decisions, regulatory review procedures, and politics have stymied and slowed the standard-setting process. The exceptions include specific standards required by other statutes, such as for reduced lead exposure in the construction industry, or by court order, such as the health standard for hexavalent chromium.

Seven of the court cases are discussed in more detail below to contrast the empowering and delimiting effect of rulings: the VCM, asbestos, cotton dust, benzene, lead, hazard communication, and air contaminants standards. Also discussed is the OSHA "cancer policy" that has been shelved for nearly three decades because of the benzene case ruling. Furthermore, reviews of standards by the courts have not been the only challenge to OSHA; the "ergonomics standard was successfully invalidated by congressional action and is discussed as well.

7.4. CONGRESSIONAL INTENT AND THE VINYL CHLORIDE STANDARD

The structure of the standards promulgation process demonstrates how the OSHAct was designed to work. Prior to OSHA receiving new information on a possible workplace hazard, an ACGIH TLV standard would be adopted as an interim standard. So when NIOSH informed OSHA of the hazard of VCM exposure associated with a liver cancer, angiosarcoma, OSHA established an emergency temporary standard followed by a permanent standard to control VCM exposures. The standard was challenged in court in *Society of Plastics Industry, Inc., v. OSHA* (1975), but the court affirmed the standard.[26] The timeline for this process is shown below:

- January 1974: B.F. Goodrich notifies NIOSH.
- April 1974: OSHA issues emergency temporary standard.
- May 1974: OSHA proposes permanent standard.
- October 1974: OSHA issues final standard.
- November 1974: Society of Plastics Industry challenges standard.
- January 1975: Court of Appeals affirms standard.

The VCM case demonstrated the power of the standard-setting logic of the OSHAct. An interim standard had been set under § 6(a) of the act, § 6(c) was used to establish an emergency temporary standard, and OSHA concurrently promulgated a permanent standard under § 6(b). Based on health concerns that were published in 1970, OSHA promulgated regulations limiting occupational exposure to VCM on October 4, 1974. Under § 6(d) of the act, any person with standing (affected or harmed by) could challenge a rule by OSHA within 60 days after its promulgation. Various manufacturers of VCM and VCM products then challenged the OSHA regulation.[26]

In 1975, the decision of the 2nd Circuit Court (New York) denied the petition of the manufacturers and ruled that the Secretary of Labor's regulation prohibiting exposure (consistent with the NIOSH recommendation) to VCM concentrations in excess of one part per million (ppm) was warranted by the available scientific medical evidence where 13 workers had died from exposure and animal studies identified fatal liver angiosarcoma as an effect of the chemical; as such, the court denied the petitions for review. OSHA was allowed to force the development of technology beyond what was currently developed in order to meet the standard. In meeting this standard, respirators were allowed to be used while the technology was being developed.[27]

7.5. THE ASBESTOS STANDARD AT LAST

In the asbestos case, *Industrial Union Department, AFL-CIO v. Hodgson* (1974), the DC Circuit Court upheld an OSHA rule on an asbestos standard on the grounds that the policy "rests in the final analysis on a legislative policy judgment, rather than a factual determination, concerning the relative risks of under protection as compared to overprotection."[27] The American Federation of Labor-Congress of Industrial Organizations (AFL-CIO) challenged OSHA in this case over improper weighing of economic feasibility in the time frame allowed for compliance in this case. The court denied this challenge and supported the agency's discretion in allowing four years to comply. Nonetheless, the court made two important determinations in this case that were positive for protecting the health of workers. First, it affirmed the application of "no material impairment" as a result of exposure to workers. (In this case, OSHA was treating asbestos as a lung toxin rather than a carcinogen.) The court also established the definition of economic feasibility in that a standard may be feasible even if some employers were to go out of business as long as the whole industry was not disrupted.[27]

OSHA cannot ban a material, but EPA is authorized to ban a toxic material under the TSCA.[28] The EPA promulgated a rule to ban almost all asbestos products from commerce in the United States under this act, which would afford workers protection from exposure to asbestos fibers. However, in hearing the case *Corrosion Proof Fittings v. EPA*,[29] the 5th Circuit Court (New Orleans) vacated the standard and remanded the EPA rule because it failed to consider less burdensome alterative controls and failed to show that the benefits would exceed the costs of the regulation.[1]

7.6. EMPOWERING OSHA THROUGH THE COTTON DUST STANDARD

The OSHAct provides no guidance on how workplace hazards should be eliminated. OSHA has implemented a policy, consistent with the § 6(b)(5) statement to set a standard "which most adequately assures" that no employee will suffer material impairment, of using the hierarchy of controls with a precedence of environmental control prior to PPE.[17]

In May 1978, OSHA faced a major hurdle, overcoming advice in the White House from Charles Schultze, chairman of the Council of Economic Advisors, to relax the requirements under the cotton dust standard that was being developed. Secretary of Labor Ray Marshall was successful at convincing President Jimmy Carter to abide by the results of rule making for the standard and to

Table 7-4. Interpretation of Cost and Benefits

Section	Occupational Safety and Health Act
§ 2(a)	"The Congress finds that personal injuries and illnesses arising out of work situations impose a substantial burden upon, and are a hindrance to, interstate commerce in terms of lost production, wage loss, medical expenses, and disability compensation payments."
§ 6(b)(5)	"The Secretary, in promulgating standards dealing with toxic materials or harmful physical agents under this subsection, shall set the standard which most adequately assures, to the extent feasible, on the basis of the best available evidence, that no employee will suffer material impairment of health or functional capacity even if such employee has regular exposure to the hazard dealt with by such standard for the period of his working life."

protect workers from the occupational disease. The only condition placed on Secretary Marshall was to allow more time for implementation after promulgation of the standard.[30,31]

Cotton industry interests challenged OSHA's cotton dust standard in *American Textile Manufacturers v. Donovan* (1981),[30] contending that the OSHAct required OSHA to demonstrate a reasonable relationship between costs and benefits in promulgating a standard. In this case, the DoL contended that Congress had balanced the costs and benefits under § 2(a) of the OSHAct: "personal injuries and illnesses related to work pose a substantial burden on and hindrance of interstate commerce regarding lost production, wage loss, medical expenses, and disability compensation payments."

The Supreme Court ruled that a standard is economically feasible if industry can absorb or pass on the cost of compliance without threatening its long-term profitability or competitive structure. The court found that Congress had already weighed the benefits of the OSHAct in § 2(a) against the investment in occupational health under § 6(b), which is shown in Table 7-4. The court held that nothing in the act or its legislative history required OSHA to compare costs and benefits in promulgating a standard. Thus, OSHA was not required to conduct a cost-benefit analysis.[32]

7.7. THE BENZENE STANDARD AS A GAME CHANGER

In 1978, the Supreme Court emphasized the negative attributes of agency decision making and the potential abuse of discretion resulting from broad delegation in the benzene case, *Industrial Union Department v. American*

Table 7-5. A Comparison of the Two Sections of the Occupational Safety and Health Act at Issue in the Benzene Case

Industrial Union Department v. American Petroleum Institute (1978)

§ 6(b)(5)	§ 3(8)
"set the standard which most adequately assures, to the extent feasible, on the basis of the best available evidence, that no employee will suffer material impairment of health or functional capacity."	"occupational safety and health standard" is a standard that is "reasonably necessary or appropriate to provide safe or healthful employment."

Petroleum Institute (1978).[21] The OSHAct delegates broad authority to OSHA to promulgate standards to ensure safe and healthful working conditions for the nation's workers.

The argument in this case pitted § 3(8) against § 6(b)(5) of the OSHAct (see Table 7-5). When the toxic material or harmful physical agent to be regulated was a carcinogen, the Secretary of Labor would take the position that no safe exposure level could be determined, thus requiring an exposure limit at the lowest technologically feasible level that would not impair the viability of the industry.

After having determined that there was a causal connection between benzene and leukemia, the Secretary of Labor promulgated a standard reducing the PEL on airborne concentrations of benzene from the consensus standard of 10 parts benzene per million parts of air (10 ppm) to 1 ppm and prohibiting dermal contact with solutions containing benzene. On preenforcement review, the court of appeals held the standard invalid because it was based on findings unsupported by the administrative record. The court held that OSHA had exceeded its standard-setting authority because it had not shown that the 1 ppm exposure limit was "reasonably necessary or appropriate to provide safe and healthful employment" as required by § 3(8), and that OSHA had relied only on § 6(b)(5), which required a standard so "that no employee will suffer material impairment of health or functional capacity even if such employee has regular exposure to the hazard dealt with by such standard for the period of his working life." The court defined a range regarding the significance of occupational deaths from a one-in-a-billion chance of death as "insignificant" to a one-in-a-thousand chance of death as "significant." This ruling gave birth to the field of risk assessment.[1] The Supreme Court's 1980 decision on the benzene standard required OSHA to make a specific showing of significant risk, instead of assuming that workplace carcinogens always present a significant risk.[33]

The benzene case plurality aimed to resolve differences in § 3(8) and § 6(b)(5) language acting on the conjugation of the threshold requirement of "significant risk" under § 3(8) (the likelihood of harm) and conditions that result in "material impairment" under § 6(b)(5) (the severity of consequences). The ruling in this case was a split between four justices who invalidated the standard and four who dissented from the ruling of the plurality. The dissenters argued that even if § 3(8) constrained OSHA under § 6(b)(5), the plurality misread the section, which is written in the disjunctive, wherein a standard need only be "reasonably necessary *or* appropriate" (emphasis added). The dissenters claimed that the plurality read the phrase in the conjunctive, discarding whether the standard was "appropriate," defined as "especially suitable, compatible, or fitting."[17] Much rides on a conjunction.

The benzene standard was reissued in 1987 at 1 ppm, the same level as the 1978 standard. In a study of the human cost measured in disease for the 1978 to 1987 delay in promulgating the standard, workers exposed above the 1 ppm level experienced between 30 and 490 excess leukemia deaths. The authors of a study on the benzene standard warn against the health risk of regulatory delay.[34]

7.8. FACETS OF THE LEAD STANDARD

The DC Circuit Court found in the lead case, *United Steelworkers of America v. Marshall and Bingham* (1980),[25] that OSHA must act immediately to protect workers without waiting for scientific certainty. Furthermore, the court ruled that OSHA could use a phased approach in addressing feasibility in moving from a 100 µg/m^3 PEL for lead to a lower standard of 50 µg/m^3. This phased approach depended upon the use of respirators, the medical removal of exposed workers from the lead-contaminated environment, and no loss of wages as a result of that removal. The court found that OSHA met the threshold test of "significant" harm and also found that subclinical levels of lead in the blood above 50 µg/dl constituted "material" impairment.[1]

7.9. OFFICE OF MANAGEMENT AND BUDGET INTERFERENCE

In 1990, the Supreme Court held by a 7-2 majority that a lower court was correct in deciding that the Office of Management and Budget (OMB) had no authority under the Paperwork Reduction Act (PRA) to review regulations mandating disclosure by regulated entities directly to third parties (*Dole v. United Steelworkers of America*, 1990).[35] The 3rd Circuit Court of Appeals (Philadelphia) had ruled that OMB lacked authority under the PRA to consider the standard. The case arose out of OSHA's revised HazCom Standard that required employers to provide hazard information directly to employees. After OSHA submitted the standard to OMB for PRA review, OMB disapproved a provision for the maintenance and exchange of material safety data sheets on multiemployer worksites and two exemptions on the grounds that they were too narrow in scope. OSHA issued a new proposal inviting comment on a change to conform to OMB's objections.

The court ruled that under the PRA, OMB had impermissibly interfered with OSHA's substantive decision making. The Supreme Court affirmed the decision, holding that the language of the PRA applied only to information collections that a federal agency required for its own use or as an intermediary for dissemination to the public.[25]

7.10. UPDATING STANDARDS: THE AIR CONTAMINANTS STANDARD

Interim standards (i.e., PELs) for toxic substances were adopted in 1971 based on § 6(a) of the OSH Act from existing lists of federal and consensus standards, many of which were first published by the ACGIH. Those values were and are dated. Meanwhile, OSHA can only enforce the old values, notwithstanding more than four decades of evidence that these substances may be harmful.[33] In some cases, OSHA can use the general duty clause. The current ACGIH list contains different, and usually lower, values for many of the substances on the list, as well as a substantial number of additions. However, changing the PEL for any substance on the list requires extensive rule making.

OSHA had previously issued 24 PELs in about 17 years. The agency explained that it would take decades to review individual chemicals. In 1988, OSHA attempted to overcome this limitation by undertaking a large rule making for 428 substances. This was accomplished by "generic" rule making; substances were grouped into 18 categories by their primary health response.

Although OSHA applied case-by-case safety factors to determine the concentration level for each PEL, it never explained the method by which its safety factors were determined. The 11th Circuit (Atlanta) ruled in *AFL-CIO v. OSHA*

(1992)[36] that the PEL for each substance must stand independently, be supported by substantial evidence, and be accompanied by adequate explanation. The court found that the air contaminants rule was not truly a "generic" rule making, but a collection of 428 separate rules. The court vacated and remanded the rule for OSHA to make specific findings with respect to each substance. OSHA had based its rule on epidemiological or toxicological studies or, in their absence, simply adopted what it called "consensus levels" among scientists.

This case presents at least two implications for risk assessment: (1) regulation by classes of chemicals cannot be supported using a "generic" approach, and (2) the convention of using safety factors to superimpose conservative health risk policy on scientifically derived "lowest observable adverse effects levels" for noncarcinogens may not survive judicial review. The court also found that OSHA had not demonstrated that the PELs were economically feasible, which must be demonstrated industry by industry. OSHA had evaluated economic feasibility for broad industry sectors "without explaining why such a broad grouping was appropriate."[1]

7.11. THE DORMANT GENERIC CANCER STANDARD

We saw that with different chemicals and different situations, the agency had come to the same general policy conclusions. So we decided to try to answer the same general questions conclusively. It doesn't make sense to revisit—and re-litigate—the same general policy conclusions over and over again. It appeared there was an ultimate truth, that we could deal with some questions in a generic conceptual way.

—Grover C. Wrenn, OSHA[37]

In 1971, President Nixon announced that cancer would be cured by the year of the U.S. Bicentennial, 1976, but to no avail.[38] In 1976, CBS News aired a series of television programs that stimulated OSHA to take a preventive approach and develop a coherent cancer policy to combat environmental carcinogens in the workplace. The generic cancer standard, established in 1980, aimed to increase the speed and efficiency in protecting workers from exposures to carcinogens by resolving certain scientific issues as OSHA policy common to all rule making regarding carcinogens, as shown in Table 7-6.

This standard was extremely controversial, resulting in a quarter of a million written comments as well as numerous hearings during the 1977–1978

Table 7-6. Scientific Issues Resolved Through the Generic Cancer Standard

Issue	Resolution
Positive results from human epidemiological studies, or positive results from at least one animal bioassay meeting minimum standards of quality with supporting evidence	Sufficed to infer that a substance was a carcinogen.
Negative results in animal bioassays or human epidemiological studies	Not considered in deciding if a substance was a human carcinogen if positive results were found in either animal bioassay or epidemiological studies unless the negative studies were found to follow strict quality standards.
In animal bioassays, any malignant or benign tumor produced, or an increase of spontaneous tumors, or tumors that occur at the site of application of a substance by oral, inhalation, or dermal routes	Established the inference that the substance was a carcinogen.
Substance-induced tumors in animals at high doses	Evidence of carcinogenicity even at the maximum tolerated dose unless strong evidence showed that no carcinogenic metabolites are produced at a low dose.

rule-making period. In 1977, the Manufacturing Chemists Association established the American Industrial Health Council (AIHC), a task force to influence the standard. The council was made up of 120 U.S. producers of chemicals and other products and 60 trade associations.[39,40] Controversy arose because the standard would establish a presumption-rebuttal regulation as law, which stated premises and inference choices and allowed deviation from those choices only under specified conditions.[37] The standard followed three principles: (1) it was appropriate to extrapolate from animal bioassays, (2) positive results were generally superior to negative results, and (3) there was no evidence of the existence of a threshold.[37]

The standard classified substances as either Class I or Class II suspect carcinogens. Class I suspect carcinogens were substances that had been unequivocally shown to be carcinogenic through strong evidence such as data from human studies and positive results from one animal study and other supporting data. A standard that resulted from a Class I suspect carcinogen required the lowest level of exposure to the maximum extent feasible and no exposure if a less hazardous substance could be substituted. Class II suspect carcinogens were less conclusive, such as from one animal study, and any resulting standard would limit the exposure "as appropriate and consistent with statutory requirements."[1] Standards for Class II suspect carcinogens focused on control rather than elimination of exposure. The standard also required that OSHA publish two priority lists—about 10 each for Class I and Class II suspect carcinogens—every six months indicating those substances that OSHA might regulate in the future.[1]

Class III suspect carcinogens included substances suspected of carcinogenicity but for which evidence was lacking. Class IV suspect carcinogens covered chemicals not used in workplaces. Of 2,415 chemicals that were on the NIOSH list of suspect carcinogens, OSHA determined that 270 fell into the category of Class I suspect carcinogens, for which about 100 would ever require regulation. Further, OSHA determined that there about 196 and 300 of the chemicals on the NIOSH list were Class II and Class III suspect carcinogens, respectively. The burden of proof for investigating Class II chemicals fell upon the government.[39]

However, after the Supreme Court's ruling in the benzene case, OSHA could only promulgate a standard where the substance posed a "significant risk" of harm. In 1986, OSHA published its intent to revise its policy by January 1987, which has not occurred to this date. Even as it remains on the books the standard lies dormant, but it can reemerge. Nonetheless, OSHA would need to establish significant risk of harm and feasibility.[1]

7.12. THE ERGONOMICS STANDARD: THE HARD-WON FAILURE

In 1999, nearly 1 million people took time away from work to treat and recover from work-related musculoskeletal pain or impairment of function in the low back or upper extremities. Conservative estimates of the economic burden imposed, as measured by compensation costs, lost wages, and lost productivity, are between $45 and $54 billion annually.

—National Research Council and the
Institute of Medicine[41]

The separation of powers theory is at the heart of every administrative law, with a distinction that treats science, law, and politics as separate paradigms. If the agency rule in question mainly concerns scientific data (questions of fact), deference to agencies is greater than concerns of fairness (question of law) at stake. When a dispute is essentially over politics or congressional policy, the scope of review lies somewhere in between questions of fact and fairness.[42,43] The review of OSHA's action regarding the ergonomics standard is an example of politics as the paradigm of agency review.

NIOSH reported in 1983 that musculoskeletal injuries accounted for 580,000 (18%) of the estimated 3.2 million emergency-room-treated occupational injuries in the United States in 1982.[44] Physical demands of many jobs make the musculoskeletal system highly vulnerable to a variety of occupational disorders and injuries. Manual handling of materials and repetitive motions are especially important etiologic factors for these disorders.[44]

NIOSH found that approximately one-fourth of all workers' compensation indemnity expenditures in eight states were for back injuries.[44] Moreover, repetitive motion can cause cumulative trauma disorders, including carpal tunnel syndrome, tendinitis, ganglionitis, tenosynovitis, bursitis, and epicondylitis. Data from the Bureau of Labor Statistics indicated that in 1980, approximately 23,200 occupational injuries were associated with repetitive trauma.[44]

In the wake of a musculoskeletal disorders crisis in the meatpacking industry during George H.W. Bush's presidency, Secretary of Labor Elizabeth Dole announced in 1990 that OSHA would begin work on an ergonomics standard.[45] When President Bill Clinton's administration proposed new regulations to force employers to take steps to reduce the risk of musculoskeletal disorders on the job, business lobbies became fully mobilized to stop them once OSHA moved to issue ergonomics regulations. The National Coalition on Ergonomics (NCE) was formed with 300 members to coordinate the assault on OSHA, including both trade associations and individual corporations. Among the business associations, the National Association of Manufacturers and the U.S. Chamber of Commerce made the ergonomics regulations a major focus of their advocacy. A lobbyist for a trade group said, "Our main argument is that OSHA hadn't done its job in terms of science. They looked at the science, but they cherry-picked the things."[46] Business's main line of attack was that OSHA was exaggerating the problem.

A second line of attack was the cost of the regulations. OSHA estimated that the remedies required under the new ergonomic regulations would cost industry just $4.8 billion. Business groups ridiculed this estimate. For example, the United Parcel Service claimed that the new rules would cost it alone $20 billion initially and $5 billion annually. OSHA responded that business groups grossly exaggerated costs by basing their calculations on the most expensive solutions possible and then assuming that the agency would mandate the use of those solutions. At the same time, the proposed regulation did not specify the exact remedies to be used.[46,47]

Republicans in Congress sympathetic to the NCE were successful in attaching a rider to a series of appropriation bills to forbid OSHA from implementing the proposed rules. The Republicans asked for a study from the nonpartisan and highly respected National Academy of Sciences, mandating a moratorium on new ergonomic regulations pending completion of the research.[48] The following timeline shows the extent of public involvement in the rule making for the ergonomics standard:[49]

- Advanced notice of proposed rule making issued in 1992
- Stakeholder meetings held in 1994
- Draft rule distributed for comment in 1995
- Another series of stakeholder meetings held in 1998
- New draft standard released in February 1999
- Small Business Regulatory Enforcement Fairness Act panel review conducted from February to April 1999
- Proposed standard issued in November 1999, with a comment period of 100 days
- Nine weeks of public hearings from March 13 to July 7, 2000, at four locations around the country where more than 700 witnesses testified; hearings provided the opportunity to cross-examine other witnesses
- Forty-five-day period for post-hearing comments
- Additional 45-day period to submit post-hearing briefs

When the Republicans failed in their attempt to renew the moratorium in 1998, OSHA took the opportunity to prepare the final regulations and then issued them in late 2000, during the waning days of the Clinton administration. It was a significant victory for organized labor and a serious defeat for business lobbies.

The victory for labor was short-lived. Using a heretofore obscure law, the Congressional Review Act, Republicans in Congress were able to force a vote on the regulations in March 2001. Critically important was a provision in the law that prohibited a filibuster in the Senate, which kept the Democrats from stopping the vote. On a largely party-line vote, both the House and Senate voted to repeal the OSHA regulations.[46–49] President George W. Bush later signed the Joint Resolution of Disapproval of Ergonomics Regulation into law in 2001, shortly after taking office, and the OSHA ergonomic regulations were completely invalidated.[50]

7.13. THE OCCUPATIONAL SAFETY AND HEALTH ADMINISTRATION

Today, adequate protection does not exist. It is to the shame of a modern industrial Nation, which prides itself on the productivity of its workers, that each year: 14,500 workers are killed on the job, 2.2 million workers are injured.

—Lyndon B. Johnson[51]

Nearly 3,000 men worked at least part of the time inside the Hawks Nest Tunnel in West Virginia during its construction between 1930 and 1932. The tunnel was built to divert water through an electrical generating plant. In 1936, a news article reported the number of workers who had died from silicosis from dust exposure in the tunnel to be 476. A later epidemiological study placed that number at 764 dead.[52]

7.13.1. Precedents

As a result of publicity about and the enormity of the tragedy, Secretary of Labor Frances Perkins convened the National Conference on Silicosis in 1936. The conference pitted management against labor in describing the causes and solutions to the problem. The management perspective was that silicosis could be controlled through engineering and balancing the health of the workforce against the cost to industry, whereas labor argued that silicosis could be eliminated just like typhus was controlled by public health interventions and that protecting the health of the workforce was a public obligation.[53]

Following this exposé of the tragedy, attempts were made to enact federal legislation. In 1939, a Senate bill unsuccessfully proposed annual appropriations to the states for workers' compensation for silicosis and prevention plans based upon meeting standards to be approved by the Secretary of Labor.[53] Another attempt in 1940 was a bill to provide grants-in-aid to states so that they could set up industrial hygiene units in their labor department. In 1943, an attempt was made to fund state agencies responsible for administering state labor laws. Both bills failed as an intrusion on state rights. With a shift in focus from occupational diseases to injuries in 1951, Senator Hubert H. Humphrey (D) of Minnesota proposed an Accident Prevention Act to establish a bureau within the DoL to promulgate standards and an independent board to enforce them, but for naught. After 1962 House hearings, a committee reported about an Occupational Safety Act, which was blocked by the House Rules Committee.[54] Eventually, the executive branch took the leadership for new legislation for the Occupational Safety and Health Act. As discussed earlier, President Lyndon Johnson initiated the action, which made its way to Congress and President Richard Nixon finally signed in December 1970.

Along this path, the DoL gathered expertise that became useful for staffing OSHA upon its creation. President Franklin D. Roosevelt issued Executive Order No. 8071 in 1939 establishing a Federal Interdepartmental Safety Council, which was replaced by the Federal Safety Council by President Harry S. Truman in Executive Order No. 10194 issued in 1950 and later by President John F. Kennedy's Executive Order No. 10990 issued in 1962. The Employment Standards Administration (ESA) within the DoL was responsible for the promulgation and enforcing of safety and health standards regarding government contractors under the Walsh-Healey Public Contracts Act of 1936 prior to the passage of the OSHAct. Among other responsibilities, ESA enforces laws regarding child labor and administers laws governing workers' compensation for certain employees (including federal workers) injured on their jobs.

7.13.2. The Mandate and Mission

With the passage of the OSHAct on December 30, 1970, and its effective date on April 28, 1971, OSHA was established within the DoL. The mission of OSHA is to ensure the safety and health of America's workers by setting and enforcing standards; providing training, outreach, and education; establishing partnerships; and encouraging continual improvement in workplace safety and health. The agency established a training institute in the Chicago area in 1972 to instruct its inspectors and provide limited training to employers and employees. During the mid-1970s, OSHA expanded its expertise in occupational health through both increased training and hiring of industrial hygienists to address workplace health issues. In the mid-1990s, OSHA partnered with companies that wanted to improve their safety and health records, which was based upon the success of the Maine 200 pilot program. This program encouraged employers with many injuries at their sites to find and fix hazards and establish safety and health programs of their own. The employers were notified of enforcement targeted at them, but they could be placed on a secondary list for inspections if they submitted an abatement plan to be approved by OSHA. Of the 200 employers notified, 97.5% submitted plans to OSHA of which most were approved.[55] The impact of the agency on policy is shown in Table 7-7.

Table 7-7. Policies Under Each President and OSHA Administrator

President	OSHA Administrator	Policies
Nixon	George Guenther, 1971–1973	Organized OSHA; established interim standards and a permanent asbestos standard
	John H. Stender, 1973–1975	Set permanent standards for 14 carcinogens and coke oven emissions
Ford	Mort Corn, 1975–1977	Improved professionalism and technical expertise; improved communications with stakeholders, Congress, and NIOSH; launched generic cancer standard
Carter	Eula Bingham, 1977–1981	Focused on health hazards; issued 12 health standards (benzene, DBCP, arsenic, cotton dust, acrylonitrile, lead, cancer policy, access to medical records, hearing conservation); assisted small businesses; simplified safety rules; initiated New Directions Grants program to foster development of occupational safety and health training and education for workers
Reagan	Thorne G. Archter, 1981–1984	Minimized regulatory burdens on businesses; implemented lost workday rates inspection policy; promulgated hazard communication and noise standards
	Robert E. Roland, 1984–1985	Bhopal disaster prompted OSHA to increase inspections of chemical plants; promulgated ethylene oxide standard
	John A. Pendergrass, 1986–1989	Egregious penalty policy implemented; issued 11 safety and five health standards (revised asbestos and benzene, access to medical records, field sanitation, formaldehyde); oversaw air contamination standard rule making that was overturned in 1992
Bush, Sr.	Gerald Scannell, 1989–1992	Air contaminants standard vacated; promulgated chemical exposure in laboratories; bloodborne pathogens, 4,4′-methylenedianiline, and cadmium standards; on remand, issued asbestos and formaldehyde standards
Clinton	Joseph Dear, 1993–1997	OSHA reinvention (part of the Presidential Regulatory Reinvention Initiative, 1995–1997); site-specific targeting promulgated 1,3-butadiene and methylene chloride standards; asbestos standards on remand
	Charles Jeffress, 1997–2001	Substantive amendments to the OSHAct; promulgated respiratory protection, ergonomics, bloodborne diseases standards
Bush	John Henshaw, 2001–2004	9-11 response; ergonomics standard revoked; four-step ergonomics program; bloodborne pathogens standard revised*
	Ewin G. Foulke Jr., 2006–2008	Promulgated hexavalent chromium standard (court order); strong supporter of OSHA voluntary compliance efforts
Obama	David Michaels, 2008–	Updated PELs with reference to NIOSH recommended exposure limits; aligned HazCom Standard with Globally Harmonized System of Classification and Labeling of Chemicals; proposed silica exposure standard

Note: OSHA = Occupational Safety and Health Administration; NIOSH = National Institute for Occupational Safety and Health; DBCP = dibromochloropropane; OSHAct = Occupational Safety and Health Act; PELs = permissible emission limits; HazCom Standard = Hazard Communication Standard.
*Jonathan Snare acted as the agency's interim administrator from January 2005 until the appointment of Foulke as OSHA administrator.

OSHA and its state partners have approximately 2,100 (1,100 federal) inspectors, plus complaint discrimination investigators, engineers, physicians, educators, standards writers, and other technical and support personnel spread over more than 200 offices throughout the country. In 2005, OSHA's appropriation was $468 million, rising to $513 million in 2009. OSHA aims to ensure worker safety and health in the United States by engaging employers and employees to create better working environments. Since its inception in 1971, OSHA has helped cut workplace fatalities by more than 60% and occupational injury and illness rates by 40%. At the same time, U.S. employment has doubled from 58 million workers at 3.5 million worksites to more than 115 million workers at 7.2 million sites.[56] On August 27, 2002, OSHA announced an organizational restructuring as shown in Table 7-8. Table 7-9 lists the OSHA regional offices, which have responsibilities for both the OSHA area offices and the state plans within their jurisdiction.

During OSHA's first 20 years, the influx of the hundreds of interim standards it had set alarmed the business community. Concern was heightened as

Table 7-8. The Office of the Assistant Secretary for Occupational Safety and Health

Directorate of Administrative Programs provides administrative support to OSHA.

Directorate of Construction provides workplace safety standards and regulations to ensure safe working conditions for the nation's construction workers; coordinates with and provides assistance to other regulatory agencies on the implementation and enforcement of major construction laws and standards.

Directorate of Cooperative and State Programs (formerly Directorate of Federal-State Operations) coordinates OSHA's role in carrying out training and education for employers and employees, implementing consultation and cooperative programs, and coordinating the agency's compliance assistance and outreach activities as well as the agency's relations with state plans.

Directorate of Enforcement Programs (formerly Directorate of Compliance Programs) provides guidance (1) on how to comply with the requirements of OSHA standards, (2) in the form of directives and interpretations that detail or explain how compliance safety and health officers should enforce OSHA standards and how employers are expected to comply with OSHA standards, and (3) in the areas of general industry, maritime, whistle-blower investigations, and federal agencies and in health areas of construction.

Directorate for Evaluation and Analysis (formerly Directorate for Policy) focuses on performance measurement and program evaluations, including on-site audits of regional and area office operations.

Directorate of Information Technology manages OSHA's automated data processing resource requirements for planning, managing, tracking, and reporting on its programs, services, and assistance.

Directorate of Science, Technology, and Medicine (formerly Directorate of Technical Support) provides medical, toxicologic, and epidemiologic support to OSHA field offices and to the staff of the national office.

Directorate of Standards and Guidance (formerly Directorates of Health Standards Programs and of Safety Standards Programs) deals with both regulatory and nonregulatory approaches for safety and health standards and guidelines. A new function was added for planning, developing, and managing nonregulatory approaches to supplement the agency's rulemaking efforts.

Note: OSHA = Occupational Safety and Health Administration.

Table 7-9. Occupational Safety and Health Administration Regional Offices and Their Geographic Responsibilities

Federal Region	Regional Office	Geographical Coverage (area offices and state plans)
1.	Boston, MA	Connecticut, Massachusetts, Maine, New Hampshire, Rhode Island, Vermont
2.	New York, NY	New Jersey, New York, Puerto Rico, Virgin Islands
3.	Philadelphia, PA	District of Columbia, Delaware, Maryland, Pennsylvania, Virginia, West Virginia
4.	Atlanta, GA	Alabama, Florida, Georgia, Kentucky, Mississippi, North Carolina, South Carolina, Tennessee
5.	Chicago, IL	Illinois, Indiana, Michigan, Minnesota, Ohio, Wisconsin
6.	Dallas, TX	Arkansas, Louisiana, New Mexico, Oklahoma, Texas
7.	Kansas City, MO	Iowa, Kansas, Missouri, Nebraska
8.	Denver, CO	Colorado, Montana, North Dakota, South Dakota, Utah, Wyoming
9.	San Francisco, CA	Arizona, California, Guam, Hawaii, Nevada
10.	Seattle, WA	Alaska, Idaho, Oregon, Washington

OSHA promulgated a spate of health standards (and many more NIOSH-recommended standards held in reserve). The apex of OSHA achievement occurred with a move to generic rule making, specifically the cancer policy and the later HazCom Standard that was issued in the mid-1980s. But political reaction was mounting: Management fought vigorously against OSHA standards, challenging virtually every standard promulgated, and public interest organizations and unions contested standards regarding prevention issues as well. Nonetheless, as of 2013, of the more than 80 permanent standards issued by OSHA, just three have been overturned by the courts, one in 1980 and two in 1992: benzene (1978 standard, but reissued later), B 4,4-methylene bis (2-chloraniline), and air contaminants, respectively.[49]

In the early 1970s, it took six months to two years for OSHA to develop and issue major rules such as those on asbestos and VCM even though these rules were controversial and contentious. The preambles for the standards were only five to 10 pages, but the standards, evidence, and material were upheld by reviewing courts. In the mid- to late 1970s, the process was somewhat longer, taking three years for the promulgation of the lead standard and four years for standards on cotton dust and arsenic. During that time the agency developed and issued numerous other standards, including those for benzene, acrylonitrile, dibromochloropropane (DBCP), the cancer policy, access to exposure and medical records, hearing conservation, fire protection, and guarding roof perimeters.

7.13.3. The Great Slowdown

In the early 1980s, as a result of the antiregulatory philosophy of the Reagan administration, the time for standards development and issuance became even longer as action was taken only in response to congressional mandates or court orders. For example, it took six years and a lawsuit for OSHA to issue its formaldehyde standard and five years and a congressional mandate for the issuance of the bloodborne pathogens standard. Other standards initiated during the Reagan administration took much longer. Standards on 1,3 butadiene, methylene chloride, and respiratory protection each took 12 years from start to finish and were not completed until the Clinton administration.[57]

With the election of President Reagan, the pressure on employers was loosened. Agency appointees with management experience were appointed to bring with them business-friendly approaches for OSHA. Indeed, the HazCom Standard promulgated during President Reagan's term was sought by the chemical industry to standardize requirements being brought by the state and local governments.

Courts became more involved to force OSHA action, including broadening the HazCom Standard to all employees, requiring a short-term exposure limit for ethylene oxide exposures, lowering the exposure limits on the asbestos and the formaldehyde standards, and 20 years later requiring action on hexavalent chromium. In addition, congressional action has slowed the promulgation of and eventually stopped the ergonomics standard.[57]

The process has become more complex and burdensome as additional requirements have been imposed on the agency. The Paperwork Reduction Act, Regulatory Flexibility Act, Unfunded Mandates Reform Act, and Small Business Regulatory Enforcement Fairness Act have required additional analyses and reviews. Executive orders on regulatory reform and federalism impose further analytical and process requirements. These impediments to rule making slowed the process from six months to two years in the early 1970s, to three years at the end of the decade, five to six years in the 1980s, and one took 12 years into the 1990s before its promulgation. The ergonomics standard took nearly a decade to promulgate before it was terminated by Congress. Steel erection rule making took 15 years before its promulgation in 2001.

7.13.4. The Current Approach

OSHA places a priority on responding promptly to imminent danger situations; investigating fatalities, catastrophes, and worker complaints, and inspecting federal agencies to protect federal workers. The agency uses a targeted approach by directing inspections and outreach to work sites and industries with the highest injury and illness rates. In addition to workplace inspections, the agency employs a variety of compliance assistance and educational and outreach programs to improve employer health and safety management systems. The agency facilitates employers' readiness to respond to workplace emergencies such as natural disasters or terrorist attacks by focusing on emergency preparedness. It has been assigned the responsibility to enforce whistle-blower rights under another 23 statutes, perhaps diluting their work under the OSHAct. As OSHA faces many roadblocks for promulgating standards, it has shifted emphasis to enforcement, the subject of the next chapter.[56]

7.14. COST ESTIMATES

This regulation will put us out of business. . . . Our industry will not be able to compete.

—Ruth Ruttenberg[58]

When the OSHAct passed, opponents had substantially ignored the provisions regarding standards since they were based upon consensus standards that were industry-biased and "watered down" and were assumed to be guidelines rather than binding requirements. Moreover, the history of enforcement of federal standards up until that time was somewhat lax and thus did not "threaten" the regulated community. On a related note, since standards posed little threat to the status quo, alternatives such as economic incentives were ignored despite some economists' promotion and industry's general view of taxes as anathema. Thus, when OSHA promulgated consensus and previous federal standards en masse as interim standards, the industry was shocked. Furthermore, placing safety and health above all else further surprised the regulated community. In reaction, the regulated community mounted intense challenges to the standards,[58a] as has been noted. Indeed, cost-benefit analysis during President Reagan's administration was geared toward addressing the economic burden of the standards and not the disease burden to workers. The "Safety First" motto at many dangerous worksites has been subjugated by indifference when it comes to governmental intervention.

While scientific studies showed the dangers of exposure to VCM, for example, the industry fought OSHA during rule making, claiming that the 1974 VCM standard would lead to the demise of the industry and cost the national economy $65 to $90 billion based on the fewer products that would reach the market. No time frame was provided regarding this cost. Within months of the standard's promulgation, 90% of the producers were in compliance. In addition to protecting workers, the standard led to innovations that improved productivity: otherwise lost feedstock was captured by tightening piping and welding pipes together, a new reactor design increased efficiency and reduced exposures, a reclamation process led to reprocessing captured VCM, processes were merged to reduce exposure further, and computerization improved resin quality. Safety was improved by the standard, but it also forced innovation.[59] Congress's Office of Technology Assessment published a report in 1995 that found that actual costs to implement the VCM rule were at most $278 million, much lower than OSHA's $1 billion forecast.[60]

The 1972 asbestos standard led to the search for alternative materials, including new fire-retardant fibers and Nomex fiber as a substitute material with additional use beyond the utility of asbestos. These uses included fire-retardant clothing and Nomex paper insulation for motors.[59]

The textile industry also possessed a strong bias in overestimating the cost of compliance regarding the 1978 cotton dust standard. One estimate regarding the cost of compliance with the cotton dust standard was $171 million for ventilation and $428 million on new production equipment over the period required for full compliance. However, the standard was the tipping point for investing in better production equipment. For example, $353 million of the $428 million cost estimate was for increased productivity.[61] A side effect of the standard was reduced noise exposure from new equipment.

The exaggeration of the cost of compliance during rule making is aimed at stopping or limiting the rule in the economic interest of the industries that produce the hazard. It has nearly worked. In deliberations for the cotton dust standard, President Carter approved the worker protection rule in the face of strong advice from his economic councilors who argued against the standard. Regarding the estimates of the cost of standards, the Economic Policy Institute conducted a comparison in 1997 of the cost estimates prior to and after rule making for several OSHA and EPA standards. After a review of several

Table 7-10. The Pattern of Overestimating the Cost of OSHA Standards

Standard	Health Effect Prevented	Prerulemaking Estimate	Actual Cost or Revision
Asbestos, 1972	Asbestosis, mesothelioma, lung cancer	$150 million	$75 million
Vinyl chloride, 1974	Angiosarcoma	$109 million/year	$20 million/year
Coke oven emissions, 1976	Lung cancer	$200 million-$1 billion	$160 million
Cotton dust, 1978	Byssinosis	$700 million/year	$205 million/year

Source: Adapted from Hodges.[62]
Note: VCM = vinyl chloride monomer.

standards, the institute found that four OSHA standards had been analyzed before and after the promulgation of a standard. In these four, exaggeration of the cost prior to promulgation was identified in the study, as shown in Table 7-10.[62] The enforcement of standards is addressed in the next chapter.

THE LEAD STANDARD NARRATIVE

OSHA promulgated a permanent lead standard in 1978 with a PEL of 50 µg/m^3 under § 6(b) of the OSHAct, down from the interim standard of 200 µg/m^3 under § 6(a). An earlier court ruling had required that any standard that applied to construction workers be reviewed by ACCSH, which would slow down rule making for the general industry standard if a construction standard was issued as well. Moreover, exposures are different in construction since workers are involved in multiple worksites in contrast with general industry. In the interest of expediency, construction was excluded from the standard, for a permanent lead standard applied to construction could be promulgated later. The standard's exclusion was challenged, but nonetheless the court upheld the standard respecting OSHA's discretion. In the late 1980s, OSHA proposed a standard that updated all of the interim standards. The ACCSH recommended upgrading the lead standard as part of this proposal, but the courts overturned the final rule for this air contaminant standard. Construction workers were still protected at the old interim standard level until a young junior Senator Harry Reid (D) from Nevada proposed a bill, the Lead Exposure Reduction Act of 1991, with 16 cosponsors. Senator Reid held a concern for pregnant women and the potential exposure of fetuses to lead.

He proposed protection for construction workers under that bill as well. Congress passed the final bill, the Residential Lead-Based Paint Hazard Reduction Act of 1992 (§ 1031 and § 1032 of Title X of the Housing and Community Development Act of 1992), aimed at reducing exposures to children in home environments from lead, but the act also directed the Secretary of Labor to promulgate an interim final regulation followed by a permanent standard for the protection of construction workers from exposure to lead. OSHA promulgated a permanent lead standard with a PEL of 50 μg/m^3 for the construction industry in 1993 as authorized by Congress without the notice and comment procedure of the Act.[18]

REFERENCES

1. Ashford NA, Caldart CC. *Technology, Law, and the Working Environment.* Washington, DC; Island Press;1996.

2. Ashford NA, Ryan CW, Caldart CC. A hard look at Federal regulation of formaldehyde: A departure from reasoned decision-making. *Harv Environ Law Rev.* 1983; 7:297–370.

3. Formaldehyde Standards for Composite Wood Products Act, amendment to Toxic Substances Control Act, 15 U.S.C. 2697 (2010).

4. Nixon R. Remarks on signing the Occupational Safety and Health Act of 1970. December 29, 1970. In: Peters G, Woolley JT. The American presidency project. Available at: http://www.presidency.ucsb.edu/ws/?pid=2869. Accessed May 30, 2014.

5. Johnson CW. 2000. How our laws are made. January 2000. Available at: http://thomas.loc.gov/home/holam.txt. Accessed May 22, 2014.

6. Occupational Safety and Health Administration. OSHA's hierarchy of controls. Available at: https://www.osha.gov/dte/grant_materials/fy10/sh-20839-10/hierarchy_of_controls.pdf. Accessed June 6, 2014.

7. Blosser F. *Primer on Occupational Safety and Health.* Washington, DC: Bureau of National Affairs;1992.

8. Longshore and Harbor Workers' Compensation Act, 33 U.S.C. § 901 (1982).

9. Construction Safety Act, 40 U.S.C. § 327 (1976). Amendment to the Contract Work Hours Standards Act, Pub L. 91-54, August 9, 1969. Available at: http://www.gpo.gov/fdsys/pkg/STATUTE-83/pdf/STATUTE-83-Pg96.pdf. Accessed June 6, 2014.

10. Walsh-Healey Public Contracts Act, 41 U.S.C. § 35 (1982).

11. McNamara-O'Hara Service Contract Act, 40 U.S.C. § 327 (1982).

12. *Chao v. Mallard Bay Drilling, Inc.*, 534 U.S. 235 (2002). Available at: http://www.supremecourt.gov/oral_arguments/argument_transcripts/00-927.pdf. Accessed September 28, 2012.

13. Pawlenko KD. Recent developments: The Supreme Court finds room for OSHA to regulate working conditions of seamen aboard uninspected vessels: *Chao v. Mallard Bay Drilling, Inc. Tulane Law Rev.* 2002;76:1775–1784.

14. Kolesar DJ. Cumulative trauma disorders: OSHA's general duty clause and the need for an ergonomics standard. *Mich Law Rev.* 1992;90:2079–2112.

15. Federal Mine Safety and Health Act, 30 U.S.C. § 801 (1977).

16. Bokat SA, Thompson HA. *Occupational Safety and Health Law*. Washington, DC: Bureau of National Affairs;1988.

17. Mendeloff J. *Regulating Safety: An Economic and Political Analysis of Occupational Safety and Health Policy*. Cambridge, MA: MIT Press;1979.

18. Rothstein MA. *Occupational Safety and Health Law*. Eagan, MN: West;2009.

19. National Foundation on Arts and Humanities Act, 20 U.S.C. § 951 (1965).

20. *Industrial Union Department, AFL-CIO v. Hodgson*, 499 F2d 467 (DC Cir 1974). Available at: http://scholar.google.com/scholar_case?case=2499317818037189648&q=Industrial+Union+Department,+AFL-CIO+v.+Hodgson&hl=en&as_sdt=2,11&as_vis=1. Accessed September 28, 2012.

21. *Industrial Union Department, AFL-CIO v. American Petroleum Institute*, 448 U.S. 607 (1980).

22. *Asbestos Information Association/North America et al. v. OSHA*, 727 F2d 415 (5th Cir 1984).

23. McKnight RH, Myers ML. Agricultural safety and health in the U.S., 1900–1999. Paper presented at: Third International Conference on the History of Occupational and Environmental Health; sponsored by International Commission on Occupational Health (ICOH) and the Centre for the History of Medicine in the University of Birmingham School of Medicine; April 18–21, 2007; Dudley, West Midlands, United Kingdom.

24. Federal Insecticide, Fungicide, and Rodenticide Act, 7 U.S.C. § 136 et seq. (1980).

25. Rabinowitz RS. *Occupational Safety and Health Law.* 2nd ed. Washington, DC: Bureau of National Affairs;2002.

26. *Society of Plastics Industry, Inc. v. Occupational Safety and Health Administration,* 509 F2d 1301 (1975).

27. Ashford NA. Federal regulation of occupational health and safety in the workplace. In: Levy BS, Wingman DH, eds. *Occupational Health: Recognizing and Preventing Work-Related Disease.* Boston: Little, Brown and Co.;1983.

28. Toxic Substances Control Act, 15 U.S.C. § § 2601–2692 (1982).

29. *Corrosion Proof Fittings v. EPA,* 947 F2d 1201 (5th Cir. 1991).

30. *American Textile Manufacturers Institute, Inc., et al. v. Donovan, Secretary of Labor, et al.,* 452 U.S. 490 (1981).

31. *The Role of the Council on Competitiveness in Regulatory Review: Hearing before the Senate Committee on Governmental Affairs,* 102nd Cong, 1st Sess (October 21, 1991) (testimony of Robert V. Percival, assistant Professor of Law, director, environmental law program, University of Maryland School of Law).

32. Curran WJ, Boden LI. Occupational health values in the Supreme Court: cost-benefit analysis. *Am J Public Health.* 1981;71(11):1264–1265.

33. National Advisory Committee on Occupational Safety and Health. Report and recommendations related to OSHA's standards development process. 2000. Available at: http://www.osha.gov/dop/nacosh/nreport.html. Accessed November 2, 2006.

34. Nicholson WJ, Landrigan PJ. Quantitative assessment of lives lost due to delay in the regulation of occupational exposure to benzene. *Environ Health Perspect.* 1989;82(7):185–188.

35. *Dole, Secretary of Labor, et al. v. United Steelworkers of America, et al.,* 494 U.S. 26 (1990).

36. *American Federation of Labor and Congress of Industrial Organizations v. Occupational Safety and Health Administration,* 965 F2d 962 (1992).

37. Rushefsky ME. *Making Cancer Policy.* Albany, NY: State University of New York Press;1986.

38. Kolata G. Advances elusive in the drive to cure cancer. *New York Times.* April 24, 2009:A1. Available at: http://www.nytimes.com/2009/04/24/health/policy/24cancer.html?pagewanted=all&_r=0 Accessed May 31, 2014.

39. Epstein SS. *The Politics of Cancer Revisited*. Hankins, NY: East Ridge Press;1998:236.

40. Proctor RN. *Cancer Wars: How Politics Shapes What We Know and Don't Know About Cancer*. New York, NY: Basic Books;1995:123-125.

41. National Research Council and the Institute of Medicine. *Musculoskeletal Disorders and the Workplace: Low Back and Upper Extremities*. Washington, DC: National Academy Press, Panel on Musculoskeletal Disorders and the Workplace, Commission on Behavioral and Social Sciences and Education;2001:ES-1.

42. Edley CF. *Administrative Law: Rethinking Judicial Control of Bureaucracy*. New Haven, CT: Yale University Press;1990.

43. Harrington CB. *Review. The Law and Politics Book Rev*. 1991;1:90-92.

44. Centers for Disease Control and Prevention. Perspectives in disease prevention and health promotion leading work-related diseases and injuries—United States. *MMWR Weekly*. 1983;32(14):189-191.

45. *United Steelworkers of America v. Marshall and Bingham*, 647 F2d 1189 (DC Cir 1980).

46. Morgensen V. State or society? The rise and repeal of OSHA's ergonomics standard. In: Morgensen V, ed. *Worker Safety Under Siege: Labor, Capital, and the Politics of Workplace Safety in a Deregulated World*. Armonk, NY: M.E. Sharpe; 2006:108-142.

47. Baumgartner FR, Berry JM, Hojnacki ME, Kimball DC, et al. Advocacy and public policymaking: case overview, OSHA's proposed ergonomics standards. Available at: http://lobby.la.psu.edu/062_Ergonomics_Standards/frameset_ergonomics.html. Accessed April 20, 2012.

48. National Academy of Sciences. *Work-Related Musculoskeletal Disorders: A Review of the Evidence*. Washington, DC: National Academy Press;1998.

49. Hearings Before the House Committee on Employment and Education, Subcommittee on Workforce Protection on OSHA's Standard Setting Process, 107th Cong, 1st Sess (2001) [testimony of M. Seminario]. Available at: http://archives.republicans.edlabor.house.gov/archive/hearings/107th/wp/osha61401/seminario.htm. Accessed September 25, 2012.

50. Bush GW. Statement of administration policy: Joint Resolution of Disapproval of Ergonomics Regulation. March 6, 2001. In: Peters G, Woolley JT. American presidency project. Available at: http://www.presidency.ucsb.edu/ws/?pid=25633. Accessed May 31, 2014.

51. Johnson LB. President's message to Congress on manpower and occupational safety and health programs. *Weekly Compilation of Presidential Documents.* 1968;4(4):110–111.

52. Cherniak M. *The Hawk's Nest Incident: America's Worst Industrial Disaster.* New Haven, CT: Yale University Press;1986:17–21, 81, 104.

53. Rosner D, Markowitz G. *Deadly Dust: Silicosis and the Politics of Occupational Disease in Twentieth-Century America.* Princeton, NJ: Princeton University Press;1991.

54. Page JA, O'Brien M-W. *Bitter Wages.* New York, NY: Grossman Publishers;1973.

55. Fleming SH. OSHA at 30: Three decades of progress in occupational safety and health. *Job Safety & Health Quarterly.* 2001;12(3):23–32.

56. Occupational Safety and Health Administration. OSHAFacts. Available at: http://www.osha.gov/as/opa/oshafacts.html. Accessed June 15, 2010.

57. Robinson JC. *Toil and Toxics: Workplace Struggles and Political Strategies or Occupational Health.* Berkeley, CA: University of California Press;1991.

58. Ruttenberg R. Regulation is the mother of invention. *Working Papers of a New Society.* 1981;8:42–47.

58a. Ruth Ruttenberg and Associates, Inc. Why do regulatory agencies overestimate the compliance costs of their regulations? Prepared for Public Citizen Foundation. 2001. Available at: http://www.whitehouse.gov/sites/default/files/omb/assets/omb/inforeg/comments/comment72.pdf. Accessed January 30, 2015.

59. Ruttenberg R. *Not Too Costly, After All: An Examination of the Inflated Cost Estimates of Health, Safety and Environmental Protections.* Bethesda, MD: Ruth Ruttenberg and Associates, Inc.;2004.

60. Office of Technology Assessment. *Preventing Illness and Injury in the Workplace.* Washington, DC: U.S. Government Printing Office;1985. OTA-H-257.

61. Viscusi WK. Cotton dust regulation: An OSHA success story. *J Policy Anal Manage.* 1985;4(3):325–343.

62. Hodges H. *Falling Prices: Cost of Complying With Environmental Regulations Almost Always Less Than Advertised.* Washington, DC: Economic Policy Institute;1997. Briefing paper.

8

Enforcement and the Occupational Safety and Health Act

Trust, but verify.

—President Ronald Reagan[1]

THE CHILDBEARING CAPACITY NARRATIVE

In 1978, American Cyanamid Company officials informed 30 female workers in its Willow Island, West Virginia, plant of a fetal protection policy. Company managers met with and told the women that because hundreds of chemicals used at the plant were harmful to fetuses, the company had decided to exclude women of childbearing capacity from exposure to these chemicals. They said seven jobs could be filled by fertile women, and for the remaining jobs, women older than age 50 would be considered not of childbearing capacity. For the remaining women to keep their jobs, they would need to show proof of sterilization. The policy was soon narrowed to fetal protection from lead exposure in the plant's organic pigments department. Five women underwent sterilization, but two other women refused and were transferred to new jobs in a different department with lower pay. A worker complained to the Occupational Safety and Health Administration (OSHA) of the policy. As a result, OSHA inspected the plant and issued a citation to American Cyanamid under the general duty clause stating that the policy was a hazard to the reproductive health of the women. American Cyanamid appealed the citation to the Occupational Safety and Health Review Commission (OSHRC), which found that the legislative history for the general duty clause refers to materials and processes but not to policies. Thus, the OSHRC vacated the citation. As OSHA did not appeal this decision, the Oil, Chemical and Atomic International Union sought a reversal of the OSHRC decision in the DC Circuit Court.[2] The court concurred with the OSHRC decision: the American Cyanamid fetal protection policy did not constitute a hazard within the meaning of the Occupational Safety and Health Act (OSHAct; see Appendix) as a "hazard" of "employment" under the general duty clause.[3] In a later case under the Civil Rights Act, the Supreme Court reversed this policy in the Johnson Controls case, which is described in the narrative at the end of this chapter.

8.1. INTRODUCTION

With mounting obstacles for OSHA to promulgate standards, its strategy was directed at enforcement. The frontline for enforcement under the OSHAct falls upon the backs of OSHA compliance officers, and at the foundation of their enforcement actions is the general duty of employers to maintain their workplaces free of recognized hazards and to comply with standards promulgated under the OSHAct. Employees also have this responsibility as well but under the employer duty to supervise their safety. This chapter describes Sections 8–19 of the OSHAct. It explains the OSHA enforcement authorities and related court cases, the role of states in enforcement and consultation, and the responsibility of the OSHRC to adjudicate citations and penalties contested by employers. OSHA's strategic plan is examined, and the OSHRC and court rulings are reviewed, and the multi-employers doctrine (e.g., employees of an employer working on a site controlled by a different employer) and an employer's general duty when dated standards already exist are described. In addition, nonfederal prosecutions of workplace homicides are described. Penultimately, the U.S. Department of Justice's "worker endangerment initiative" is discussed, and finally, the issue of OSHA regulations and inspections as "job killers" is described.

8.2. SECTIONS 8–19 OF THE OCCUPATIONAL SAFETY AND HEALTH ACT

OSHA enforcement should send a clear message to companies and their subcontractors about their fundamental responsibility to provide a safe workplace.
—Senator Barack Obama. Senate Committee on Health, Education, Labor, and Pensions Hearing[4]

Section 6 of the OSHAct provides for the enforcement of the general duty clause and of standards. A flowchart of the process for standard setting and

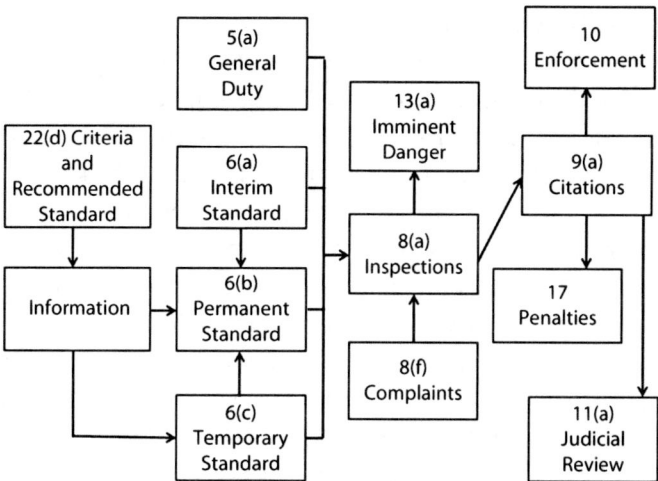

Figure 8-1. Flowchart of the Occupational Safety and Health Administration command-and-control process.

enforcement under the OSHAct is shown in Figure 8-1. As described in the previous chapter, OSHA can initiate rule making based on information, including a recommended standard from the National Institute for Occupational Safety and Health (NIOSH), as either a temporary standard that can lead to a permanent standard or directly to a permanent standard. Interim standards already in place can be updated through rule making. Under either the general duty clause or a standard, enforcement begins with inspections, which may be initiated by a worker's complaint. An inspection may find no violations, but if violations are found and there is an imminent hazard, a court-ordered injunction can be issued to stop exposures. Otherwise, violations can lead to OSHA issuing citations and proposed penalties from which an enforcement process with deadlines is initiated. Abatement conferences or adjudication can ensue through the OSHRC, and the courts can follow, leading to a final ruling.

8.2.1. Inspections, Investigations, and Recordkeeping (Section 8)

The OSHAct provides the authority for the government (both OSHA and NIOSH) to conduct inspections of places of employment and allows for access to records and entry without delay to inspect workplaces. The OSHAct also entitles an employee and an employer representative to accompany the OSHA compliance officer during the inspection. The act requires employers to maintain records that are necessary for OSHA enforcement and for developing information related to the causes and prevention of occupational injuries and illnesses so that researchers can determine the effectiveness of controls.[5]

An agency's action is unlawful when it is in conflict with the U.S. Constitution, even when the statute authorizes that action. Barlow's Inc. (*Marshall v. Barlow's Inc.*, 1978) brought action to obtain an injunction against a warrantless inspection of its business premises pursuant to § 8(a) of the OSHAct, which empowered agents of the Secretary of Labor to search the work area of any employment facility within OSHA's jurisdiction for safety hazards and violations of OSHA regulations.[6] The court ruled that the Fourth Amendment (Article IV) of the Constitution requires a warrant for the type of search involved and that the statutory authorization for warrantless inspections was unconstitutional.[7] The language involved in this case is shown in Table 8-1. The court held that the inspection without a warrant or its equivalent pursuant to § 8(a) of OSHA violated the Fourth Amendment of the Constitution.[3]

Under § 6(f) of the OSHAct, standards cannot be challenged after 60 days. When OSHA promulgated the Access to Employee Exposure and Medical Records rule, the 5th Circuit Court (New Orleans) determined that the rule was a regulation and not a standard (*Louisiana Chemical Association v. Bingham*, 1981).[8] This ruling against OSHA meant the 60-day limitation did not apply and the regulation could be brought to court beyond 60 days under

Table 8-1. Comparison of the Occupational Safety and Health Act § 8(a) and Article IV of the Constitution in Dispute in *Marshall v. Barlow's Inc.* (1978)

Marshall v. Barlow's Inc.

Occupational Safety and Health Act	Constitution
§ 8(a). In order to carry out the purposes of this Act, the Secretary, upon presenting appropriate credentials to the owner, operator, or agent in charge, is authorized (1) to enter without delay and at reasonable times any factory, plant, establishment, construction site, or other area, workplace or environment where work is performed by an employee of an employer (29 USC 657).	Article IV. The right of the people to be secure in their persons, houses, papers, and effects, against unreasonable searches and seizures, shall not be violated, and no Warrants shall issue, but upon probable cause, supported by Oath or affirmation, and particularly describing the place to be searched, and the persons or things to be seized.

the Administrative Procedures Act (APA). The court determined that while the salient issue regarding a standard is that it is to be used for "correcting and ameliorating a particular hazard," this rule was aimed at an enforcement action under § 8, so it was a regulation. The court also determined that this ruling would keep OSHA from bringing every recordkeeping regulation into the accelerated appeals process used for standards.[5,9]

8.2.2. Citations (Section 9)

An OSHA compliance officer can issue a citation, either immediately after an inspection or delivered later by mail, based upon the alleged violation of the OSHAct and its associated standards. The citation describes the violations observed during the inspection and sets reasonable deadlines for abating the violations, and OSHA must issue the citation within six months of the occurrence of the violation unless the OSHRC orders a stay for a longer period. Employers must post a copy of the citation at or near the locations where the violations occurred for a period of three days or until the violation is corrected, whichever is longer. If employers fail to post the citation, they can be fined and lose the right to contest the penalty. Citations can be grouped for multiple violations and are categorized by the degree of risk that they pose.[5] The categories of violations and associated degrees of risk are listed below:

- *De minimis*—conditions that violate a standard with no direct or immediate effect on safety and health,
- Other-than-serious—likely to not cause serious injury or illness,
- Serious—a substantial probability of serious harm,
- Repeat—conditions similar to earlier cited violations by the same employer,
- Willful—violations involving an intentional and knowing disregard of the OSHAct,
- Criminal/willful—a willful violation that resulted in the death of an employee.

8.2.3. Enforcement (Section 10)

As with anything else in law enforcement, if there's a law on the books and you don't enforce it, it becomes meaningless.

—Jane Barrett[10]

Following an inspection or failure to abate a violation, OSHA issues a citation followed by a notification of a proposed penalty to the employer by certified mail. The employer has 15 days to notify OSHA of its intent to contest the citation; otherwise, the citation and penalty are deemed final with no right of review. The employer can contest the time fixed in the citation as unreasonable, which will lead to a hearing before an administrative law judge of the OSHRC (see § 12 below). Affected employees can participate in the hearing. Based upon findings by the OSHRC, OSHA can modify the abatement period or the penalty or both.[3]

8.2.4. Judicial Review (Section 11)

Any person adversely affected or aggrieved by an order of the OSHRC issued under § 10(c) of the OSHAct may obtain a review of the order by filing a written petition in the court within 60 days following the issuance of an order. The petition can be filed in any U.S. court of appeals for the circuit in which the violation is alleged to have occurred or where the employer has its principal office, or in the DC Court of Appeals. The Secretary of Labor may also obtain a review of the enforcement of any final order of the OSHRC by filing a petition for relief in the court of appeals.

The OSHAct prohibits discrimination against employees for filing complaints with OSHA, and the courts have jurisdiction over alleged suits for discrimination. When the OSHAct was passed, Congress realized that OSHA inspectors would never be able to visit more than a small fraction of the nation's workplaces in any given year. Thus, the OSHAct relies heavily on workers to help identify hazards at their workplaces and to work with their employers to control those hazards. But Congress also understood that workers are not likely to participate in safety and health activities or report on hazardous conditions if they fear that they will lose their jobs or otherwise be retaliated against as a result of their activities. For this reason, § 11(c) protects employees from discrimination and retaliation when they report safety and health hazards or exercise other rights under the OSHAct—which was one of the first safety and health laws to contain a provision for protecting whistle-blowers.[11]

Early in 1980, the Supreme Court resolved a conflict among the circuits by upholding an OSHA regulation giving workers the right to refuse to perform hazardous jobs if they reasonably believed that there was no other way to avoid risk of serious injury or death, in *Whirlpool Corp. v. Marshall*.[3,12] Although the

OSHAct does not mention a right to refuse to work under unsafe conditions, Justice Potter Stewart's opinion for a unanimous court reasoned that the Secretary of Labor had the power to find an implied right in the law because Congress had intended to prevent injuries and to require employers to eliminate dangers in the workplace. However, the court made clear that employers have no obligation to pay workers for the time they have refused to work.[13]

The 5th Circuit Court (New Orleans) heard another case (*Donovan v. Square D. Company*, 1983) after an employee was allegedly fired in retaliation for safety-related activities.[14] The defense in this case was that a state-based two-year statute of limitations negated this action. The 5th Circuit Court judge found that the OSHAct superseded state law and that there was no statute of limitations on the OSHA action regarding discrimination in either the statute or in the policy.

8.2.5. Occupational Safety and Health Review Commission (Section 12)

The OSHRC rules on challenges by employers of citations or penalties from inspections conducted by OSHA. It functions as an administrative court, with established procedures for conducting hearings, receiving evidence, and rendering decisions. The mission of the OSHRC is to provide fair and timely adjudication of workplace safety and health disputes between OSHA and employers. It is an independent administrative law review board established at the creation of the OSHAct outside of the U.S. Department of Labor (DoL) through the influence of employers because business interest groups perceived the DoL as biased toward organized labor.

The OSHRC consists of three commissioners appointed by the president with six-year terms that are staggered with an appointment of one commissioner every two years. It functions as a two-tiered administrative court, with procedures for conducting hearings, receiving evidence, and rendering decisions by its administrative law judges as established by the APA. Five judges are located in Washington, DC; another three are in an Atlanta, Georgia, office; and four more are in Denver, Colorado. These judges interpret the statute and adjudicate disputes about whether OSHA has violated standards.[15] A panel of the commissioners provides discretionary review of these decisions. The petitioning party may request a review by an appropriate U.S. court of appeals within 60 days after the OSHRC's final decision is issued. Many other agencies establish administrative law judges as provided by the APA that are quasi-independent within the agency itself, such as in the U.S. Environmental Protection Agency (EPA).

8.2.6. Imminent Dangers (Section 13)

If OSHA finds that a work environment can cause imminent serious injury or death to a worker before normal enforcement procedures can abate the hazard, it can acquire a court injunction to close a workplace down. Moreover, in California, state law allows a "Cal/OSHA" compliance officer to immediately close a workplace if such conditions are found.[3]

8.2.7. Civil Litigation Representation (Section 14)

The U.S. Attorney General takes primacy in civil litigation before the Supreme Court. Although the Solicitor of Labor, who represents the Secretary of Labor, can represent the government before the Supreme Court, it must be under the direction and control of the Attorney General.

8.2.8. Trade Secrets (Section 15)

Whoever, being an officer or employee of the United States or of any department or agency thereof . . . publishes, divulges, discloses, or makes known . . . information [that] *concerns or relates to the trade secrets . . . shall be fined under this title, or imprisoned not more than one year, or both; and shall be removed from office or employment.*
 —18 USC § 1905: Disclosure of Confidential Information Generally[16]

The OSHAct provides procedures for maintaining the confidentiality of trade secrets obtained by inspecting officers. This section cross-references the 1948 Trade Secrets Act,[17] which provides that trade secret protection does not go beyond that afforded by state law. Trade secrecy is not a matter of federal constitutionality but is a matter of state-level legislation.

If a stated trade secret is readily discoverable through reverse engineering, then it is not protected as a trade secret. A trade secret exists only if its disclosure reveals a technological process or functional characteristic that is unknown to other companies. The secret must be a technology or technique that represents a clear advance in the field, must provide its owner with a competitive advantage, or not be available to a competitor through investigation or other fair means. When information is disclosed to the detriment of its owner, only then is trade secrecy violated.[18]

An employer can withhold information if it can support the assertion that it is a trade secret, release all information on the toxic properties and effects of the substance of the claimed trade secret, and inform the requesting party (e.g., OSHA, employee, employee representative) that it is a trade secret. Nonetheless, OSHA can require the employer to provide information claimed as a trade secret if a physician needs the information to treat an employee in an emergency situation, as long as the information is used for that treatment through a written confidentiality agreement as soon as circumstances permit. Similarly, OSHA can require disclosure of information to monitor worker exposures after a written confidentiality agreement is executed. OSHA can issue a citation if it determines that the information is not a trade secret or even if it is a trade secret and the requesting party has a legitimate need for the information, has executed a written confidentiality agreement, and has shown adequate means to comply with the agreement.[5] Chapter 14 will address further the veracity of trade secret claims.

8.2.9. Variations, Tolerances, and Exemptions (Section 16)

The OSHAct provides for variances, tolerances, or exemptions in compliance with standards for the national defense. However, these variances, tolerances, or exemptions cannot be in effect for more than six months without notifying the effected employees and affording them an opportunity for a hearing.

8.2.10. Civil Penalties (Section 17[a–d])

The penalties in the OSHA Act are inadequate to deal with people that don't take their safety responsibility seriously. The penalties were first established in 1970. They've only been increased one time since then and it's very low. A serious violation, something that might lead to someone's death, carries a maximum penalty of $7,000.

—Charles Jeffress[19]

The OSHAct authorizes OSHA to assign civil penalties for violations of the general duty clause or standards. The amounts of penalties depend on four factors: the gravity of the infraction, the size of the business, the employer's

Table 8-2. Maximum Civil Penalties Allowed by the Occupational Safety and Health Act and by a 1990 Amendment by the Omnibus Budget Reconciliation Act

Type of Violation	Original Act	1990 Amendment*
Serious and nonserious	$1,000	$7,000
Repeated and willful	$10,000	$70,000
Failure to abate violation	$1,000/day	$7,000/day

*Set a minimum penalty of $5,000 for a willful violation and a penalty of up to $7,000 per violation for failure to post a notification of citation.

good faith efforts to comply with the law during and after the inspection, and the employer's history of previous violations. In the late 1980s, critics claimed that the penalties were insignificant deterrents for violations; thus Congress increased the penalties sevenfold as shown in Table 8-2.[5]

An egregious-case policy for civil penalties grew out of an inspection policy established by President Ronald Reagan's administration in 1981. OSHA began exempting workplaces from comprehensive inspections if their records indicated that their injury rates were less than the national average,[5] which was known as the "records-check" policy.[20,21] After the catastrophic leak of the chemical methyl ethyl isocyanate at a Union Carbide Corporation plant in Bhopal, India, OSHA conducted inspections of two Union Carbide plants in West Virginia. The agency cited Union Carbide for alleged recordkeeping violations at these plants and, because of the seriousness of the hazard, moved toward a policy of large penalties. This egregious-case policy assesses a separate penalty for each instance of a violation rather than aggregating like violations with a single fine. When there is an egregious case, this policy can assign a violation to each source of a hazard and for each employee exposed. Thus, an aggregate $70,000 fine for a set of willful violations was changed to a $70,000 penalty for each individual violation or individual worker at risk. Indeed, $70,000 proposed penalties have been routinely issued for willful or repeat violations. This policy has led to several proposed fines that exceed $1 million. The violations are considered egregious in any of the following cases:[5]

- The employer knew of the violation when it occurred.
- The employer failed to act to correct the violation. The violation resulted in worker fatalities, a catastrophe, or several injuries or illnesses.
- The employer had a history of past violations.

- The employer intentionally disregarded its safety and health responsibilities.
- The employer clearly showed bad faith in compliance with standards.
- The employer committed multiple violations that rendered its safety and health program ineffective.

As examples, some recent egregious cases are described in Table 8-3.[21a]
Different penalties that may be proposed by type of violation follow:[22]

- Repeated violation—This violation occurs when a reinspection finds a substantially similar violation to an original citation that has become a final order. These violations can bring a fine of up to $70,000 for each violation over the previous three years.
- Failure-to-abate—Failure to correct a prior violation may bring a civil penalty of up to $7,000 for each day that the violation continues beyond the prescribed abatement date.
- Other-than-serious violation—This violation has a direct relationship to job safety and health but probably would not cause death or serious physical harm. OSHA may assess a penalty from $0 to $1,000 for each violation. The agency may adjust this penalty downward, depending on the employer's demonstrated efforts to comply with the OSH Act, history of previous violations, and size of business.
- Serious violation—This violation occurs where there is a substantial probability that death or serious physical harm could result. The agency assesses the penalty for this violation from $1,500 to $7,000 depending on the gravity of the violation and may adjust this penalty downward as well.
- Willful violation—A violation that the employer intentionally and knowingly commits. The employer is aware that a hazardous condition exists, knows that the condition violates a standard or other obligation of the OSH Act, and makes no reasonable effort to eliminate it. The penalty can range from $5,000 to $70,000 per violation.

8.2.11. Criminal Penalties (Section 17[e–l])

To willfully violate the law and kill someone is a misdemeanor.

—Charles Jeffress[19]

Violators are only open to criminal prosecution when a worker dies and the DoL reviews the case and refers it to the U.S. Department of Justice (DoJ).

Table 8-3. Recent Significant and Egregious Cases From Occupational Safety and Health Administration News Releases

Date and Place	Description
June 25, 2012, Jersey City, NJ	OSHA fined four contractors more than $460,000 for willful violations for exposing workers to falls and other safety hazards at a construction site.
June 18, 2012, Taunton, MA	OSHA proposed a fine of $702,300 for Tribe Mediterranean Foods following the death of a worker for the lack of employee training to prevent "needless and avoidable loss of life."
December 28, 2011, Houston, TX	OSHA proposed more than $1 million in fines to a piping technology and products employer for willful and serious violations and for misleading OSHA about an amputation hazard.
November 2, 2011, Alpha, IL	OSHA cited All-Feed Processing and Packaging Company for 23 health and safety violations with fines that exceeded $750,000 for failing to protect workers from dust and noise exposure.
April 19, 2011, Odell, IL	OSHA cited Wind Farm Servicing Company for six willful safety violations after a worker suffered burns in wind tower, with proposed fines of $378,000.
June 14, 2011, Phenix, AL	OSHA proposed more than $1.9 million in fines against Phenix Lumber Company for egregious and other safety violations.
June 10, 2011, Lewiston, ME	OSHA proposed more than $243,000 in fines against Lessard Brothers Construction for egregious fall hazards and other violations.
June 29, 2011, Colebrook, NH	OSHA cited Black Mag LLC for an explosion that killed two new workers and for 54 violations, fined the company $1.2 million, and permanently barred it from employing people to work with explosives.
June 30, 2011, Galva, IL	OSHA cited All-Feed Processing and Packaging for failing to provide respirator protection, with fines exceeding $167,000.
December 7, 2010, Coffeen, IL	OSHA fined U.S. Minerals $396,000 for 28 violations, including exposure to hazardous dust.
November 9, 2010, Pevely, MO	A judge upheld citations issued by OSHA for 19 violations to Thomas Industrial Coatings Inc. following an investigation of fatal 40-foot falls that killed two workers.
August 4, 2010, Burlington, WI	OSHA fined Cooperative Plus Inc. $721,000 after a worker was engulfed in frozen soybeans and rescued after four hours.
May 27, 2010, Aberdeen, SD	OSHA fined South Dakota Wheat Growers Association more than $1.6 million for grain-handling violations including a worker suffocation after being engulfed in grain.
May 27, 2010, Belvedere, IL	OSHA issued egregious willful and serious citations to NDK Crystals and fined $510,000 following an investigation into an explosion that killed a bystander.
March 8, 2010, Toledo, OH	OSHA proposed more than $3 million in fines to BP-Husky refinery for various alleged willful and serious violations that exposed workers to hazards that could cause serious injury or death.
February 12, 2010, Washington, PA	OSHA cited C.A. Franc $539,000 for willful fall hazard violations following a worker's death at the worksite, and the owner pleaded guilty to a related criminal charge.
July 7, 2012, Port Wentworth, GA	OSHA reached agreement with Imperial Sugar to pay more than $6 million and implement extensive safety and health abatement measures regarding the death of 14 workers in a sugar dust fire.
November 12, 2009, Cincinnati, OH	OSHA levied $321,000 in fines against Bridge and Tower Painter UCL Inc. for exposing workers to lead.

Table 8-3. (Continued)

Date and Place	Description
August 16, 2007, Tulsa, OK	OSHA fined industrial laundry giant Cintas $3 million in penalties for 42 willful violations found during an inspection after a worker fell into an operating dryer.
September 22, 2005, Texas City, TX	OSHA fined BP Products North America more than $21 million for 301 willful violations following the fatal explosion at its Texas City refinery complex that killed 15 workers and injured more than 170 other workers.

Note: OSHA = Occupational Safety and Health Administration.
Source: Multiple OSHA press releases.[21a]

If the DoJ chooses to prosecute under the OSHAct, the crime remains a misdemeanor with a possible jail sentence of not more than six months. The violation must be of a standard, so a violation under the general duty clause does not carry a criminal penalty. In such cases, OSHA turns that information over to the local U.S. attorney, and a local U.S. attorney can choose to bring criminal action or not. For the U.S. attorney, the matter is a priority of prosecuting felonies under other laws rather than expending resources on a misdemeanor violation. There is no criminal penalty under the OSHAct for endangerment for causing a serious bodily injury to an employee or exposing an employee to a risk of serious bodily injury. In addition, only employers can be prosecuted; thus supervisors are excluded.[23]

Interference with enforcement activities is a criminal act. A person knowingly making false statements may be liable for a fine of up to $10,000, a six-month imprisonment, or both.[3] For second convictions, the criminal penalties go up to $20,000, one year in prison, or both. Criminal penalties for giving advance notice of an inspection are no longer applied since an employer can request a warrant, thus eliminating the element of surprise.

During its first 32 years and more than 200,000 workplace-related deaths, OSHA referred only 151 cases to the DoJ for criminal prosecution. Federal prosecutors declined to pursue 79, or two-thirds, of these cases, and only eight of them resulted in prison sentences for company officials, which totaled 89 months of incarceration as shown in Table 8-4.[19,23] In many cases, penalties were increased because of attempts to bribe a government official or making false statements to a government investigator.

The Sentencing Reform Act of 1984 increased criminal penalties beyond those provided in the OSHAct. As a result, an employer and responsible management individuals convicted in a criminal proceeding of a willful violation

Table 8-4. Eight Cases of Felony Prosecutions Regarding the Occupational Safety and Health Act, 1988–2001

Year and Company	Description and Penalty
1988—Elliot Plumbing and Heating Co., South Dakota	Owner Howard Elliot pled guilty to criminal charges of willfully violating OSHA trenching safety standards after two of his employees were killed in a May 1988 trench collapse. He received a six-month sentence, suspended to 45 days, and three years of probation. Elliot also was ordered to pay restitution to the victims' families.
1994—Protech Construction Co., Illinois	Owner Kazimierz Chmielewski twice offered $1,000 cash bribes to OSHA officials to get out of a $35,000 willful violation charge for failure to install a protective guardrail on a scaffold. In 1998, he pled guilty to bribery and was sentenced to six months in jail and six months of home confinement.
1995—MIT Tank Wash, Georgia	Employees were required to clean fuel out of the tanks that included a hazardous fuel additive. In 1993, an employee entered a tank alone in violation of OSHA regulations and died from the toxic fumes. OSHA had warned owner Robert Swing to buy proper safety equipment, but he did not. Swing pled guilty to a willful violation and was sentenced to six months in jail, one year of probation, and a $190,000 fine.
1996—C&S Erectors, Pennsylvania	In 1996, employee Brian Smith fell 35 feet to his death while laying steel decking on the roof of a construction site. The company had a history of OSHA violations, and an investigation determined that the project's general contractor had previously warned C&S about its failure to provide fall protection. Owner Roy G. Stoops pled guilty to a willful violation and was sentenced to four months in prison and ordered to pay $6,000 in restitution to Smith's estate. The company was sentenced to one year of probation and held jointly liable for restitution.
1996— South East Towers, South Carolina	Employee John Christiansen was killed in 1995 when he fell 150 feet while retrieving equipment from a tower in Florida. According to OSHA, owners Theodore Smith and John Dennis tried to cover up that Christiansen was not wearing safety equipment when he fell. Smith and Dennis pled guilty to a willful violation, and each was sentenced to three months in prison and ordered to pay more than $7,300 restitution for Christiansen's funeral.
1997—LeMaster Steel Erectors, Ohio	In 1996, employee Jeffrey Highfill fell more than 25 feet from the roof of a construction site. The firm pled guilty to willfully violating fall protection regulations, and two of its officials—Michael Onyon and Jay Holloman—and foreman Ronald Lee Creighton pled guilty to making false statements to OSHA investigators. Hollomon and Onyon were sentenced to six months in prison, three years of probation, and fines of $2,000. Creighton was sentenced to four months in prison, three years of probation, and $1,000 in fines. LeMaster Steel was fined $300,000, ordered to pay $3,500 in burial expenses, and placed on five years of probation.
2000—Walter Marble, Illinois	A 1999 trench collapse killed employee Chad Sacker, who was buried under approximately eight feet of soil. Plumbing company owner Marble pled guilty to charges that he lied to investigators when he obstructed OSHA's investigation by creating fake documents to cover up the incident. He was sentenced to five months in prison, five months of home confinement, two years of supervised release following the home confinement, and a $3,000 fine.

Table 8-4. (Continued)

Year and Company	Description and Penalty
2001—Mordechai Rubbish, Inc., New York	An OSHA compliance officer had instructed the general contractor at a building demolition site not to begin work until an engineering survey was conducted to determine that the building could support the workers and their equipment. The general contractor advised demolition contractor Moshe Junger of this requirement, but he proceeded without the survey. Workers drove a 12-ton material handler onto the second floor of the building to remove several steel beams. The cement floor under the machine collapsed and worker Rogelio Villanueva-Daza was killed. Junger pled guilty and was sentenced to four months in prison and fined $100,000.

Note: OSHA = Occupational Safety and Health Administration.
Source: Public Broadcasting System.[19]

of a standard that has resulted in the death of an employee may be fined up to $250,000 for individuals or $500,000 for a corporation or imprisonment up to six months, or both.[5]

8.2.12. State Jurisdictions and Plans (Section 18)

OSHA organized its national network of inspectors in federal enforcement states by area offices. However, subject to OSHA certification, the OSHAct allows states to establish programs to issue and enforce standards. Wherever a state elects to not establish a program, OSHA retains authority. In order to be certified, a state submits a plan to OSHA describing the program, which is its proposal for developing and enforcing standards (at least as protective as federal standards), and its means for funding and staffing. A submitted plan approved by OSHA must be published in the *Federal Register* with an invitation for comments from the public. The state then has an opportunity to respond to challenges to the proposed plan. The agency may grant initial approval for the plan through a developmental period prior to certification. In 1972, OSHA approved the first state programs: South Carolina, Montana, and Oregon. The states with current certified plans are shown in Table 8-5.

Some states have withdrawn from agreements: Colorado, Connecticut (except public sector), Illinois, Montana, New Jersey (except public sector), New York (except public sector), and North Dakota. Any person can file a complaint to OSHA about a state program administration either orally or

Table 8-5. States and U.S. Territories With Approved State Plans, 2012

Alaska	Kentucky	New Mexico	Utah
Arizona	Maryland	New York*	Vermont
California	Michigan	North Carolina	Virgin Islands*
Connecticut*	Minnesota	Oregon	Virginia
Hawaii	Nevada	Puerto Rico	Washington
Indiana	New Jersey*	South Carolina	Wyoming
Iowa		Tennessee	

*The Connecticut, New Jersey, New York, and Virgin Islands plans cover public sector (state and local government) employment only.

in writing, which can lead to an OSHA investigation of the program. The agency may also act to withdraw its approval of a plan. A state can appeal such a decision to the U.S. Court of Appeals, and then to the Supreme Court.[5]

States may promulgate standards that are more restrictive than the corresponding federal standards. As an example, Oregon and Washington promulgated comprehensive standards for logging in the early 1970s, which preceded the federal standard for logging in 1996. Maryland promulgated a confined spaces standard in 1976 that preceded the federal standard of 1989. State-level standards for firefighting may also cover local government employees over whom OSHA lacks jurisdiction.

However, the OSHAct provides for a restriction on state standards if a rule affects interstate commerce unless justified by compelling local conditions. Industry groups in California brought such a challenge against a 1981 rule that was more stringent than the federal standard for the fumigant ethylene dibromide. The industry groups' claim was that the California rule would affect fumigant-treated produce exported beyond the state. OSHA sought public comment on the state rule and determined that the state standard was justified by local conditions.[5]

In addition to OSHA law, some 22 states, including California, Utah, Washington, and Michigan, have their own worker health and safety agencies with standards that meet or exceed the federal OSHA standards. As an example, Michigan promulgated safety standards for logging, firefighting, and automotive manufacturing that were more stringent than the federal standards. In fiscal year 2011, federal and § 18(b) state plan inspections totaled 40,648 and 52,056, respectively.

8.2.13. Federal Agency Programs (Section 19)

Even though the OSHAct specifically excludes federal agencies and employees from its jurisdiction under § 3, it requires the heads of each federal agency to establish and maintain an occupational safety and health program.[5] Following the passage of the OSHAct, President Richard Nixon issued Executive Order No. 11612 in 1971, which established the Federal Advisory Council on Occupational Safety and Health (FACOSH), and Executive Order No. 11807 in 1974, for occupational safety and health programs for federal employees, which affirmed a requirement that each agency assure protection for its employees consistent with OSHA standards. The advisory council consisted of 16 members appointed by the Secretary of Labor, of whom eight were representatives of federal agencies and eight represented labor organizations that stood for federal employees, and it advised the Secretary of Labor in carrying out responsibilities for federal employees under § 19 of the OSHAct.

In 1980, President Jimmy Carter issued Executive Order No. 12196 that provided for the application of OSHA standards and enforcement within federal agencies as well as the right of employees to request "health hazard evaluations" from NIOSH. Each federal agency was directed to name a person to be responsible for carrying out this order. In addition, FACOSH was continued in this capacity to advise the Secretary of Labor in carrying out responsibilities under the order.

8.3. OSHA STRATEGIC PLAN

OSHA's current strategic plan emphasizes enforcement, with a focus on increasing the number of inspections conducted in each year. The plan addresses the OSHA special emphasis programs, its Voluntary Protection Program (VPP), and its whistle-blower, ergonomic violations, and severe violators programs.[24,25]

8.3.1. Occupational Safety and Health Administration Emphasis Programs

National emphasis programs (NEPs) are intended to use enforcement resources more efficiently to help employers address hazards or industries that pose a particular risk to workers. These programs may be accompanied by outreach intended to inform affected employers of the program as well as the hazards that the programs are designed to reduce or eliminate. The agency targets facilities with a days-away-from-work, restricted work, or work transfer

(DART) rate of 10 or higher per 100 full-time workers. The current NEPs are listed and described in Table 8-6.[26]

Local Emphasis Programs (LEPs) are enforcement strategies designed and implemented at the regional OSHA office or area office levels to address hazards or industries that pose a particular risk to workers in the office's jurisdiction; at the regional level, the emphasis programs are applied to all of the area offices within the region. Outreach in the program may be in the form of informational

Table 8-6. Occupational Safety and Health Administration National Emphasis Programs, 2012

Date Established	Program	Policies and Procedures for Inspections
Reissued 03/11/2008	Combustible dust	Reduce the risk of deflagration, other fires, or explosion in workplaces that create or handle combustible dusts
12/23/2011	Federal agency targeting	Reduce the number of cases in specific federal agency service/operating locations with a high frequency of lost-time injuries or illnesses
10/30/2009	Flavoring chemicals/ diacetyl	Reduce exposure to diacetyl in facilities that manufacture food flavorings
10/27/2006	Amputations	Reduce workplace machinery and equipment hazards that cause or are likely to cause amputations
02/23/2010	Hexavalent chromium	Identify and reduce or eliminate health hazards associated with occupational exposure to hexavalent chromium and other toxic substances found in conjunction with hexavalent chromium
08/14/2008	Lead	Reduce occupational exposures to lead
04/05/2012	Nursing and residential care facilities	Address specific hazards including ergonomic stressors in patient lifting, bloodborne pathogens, tuberculosis, workplace violence, and slips, trips, and falls
05/19/2011	Primary metal industries	Identify and reduce or eliminate worker exposures to harmful chemical and physical health hazards in facilities
11/29/2011	Process safety management	Reduce or eliminate workplace hazards associated with catastrophic release of highly hazardous chemicals
09/28/2010	Injury and illness recordkeeping	Improve accuracy of occupational injury and illness recording and reporting requirements for establishments in selected industries
11/04/2010	Shipbreaking	Reduce and eliminate workplace hazards associated with shipbreaking operations
01/24/2008	Crystalline silica	Identify and reduce or eliminate health hazards associated with occupational exposure to crystalline silica
09/19/1985	Trenching and excavation	Eliminate or reduce incidence of trench/excavation collapses and accompanying loss of life

Source: Occupational Safety and Health Administration.[26]

Table 8-7. Occupational Safety and Health Administration Local Emphasis Programs

Region	States and Territories (postal abbreviations)	Example and Number of Programs
I	CT,** ME, MA, NH, RI, VT*	Fish processing industry ($n = 12$)
II	NJ,** NY,** Puerto Rico,* Virgin Islands**	Natural gas drilling operations ($n = 20$)
III	DE, DC, MD,* PA, VA,* WV	Healthcare industry ($n = 17$)
IV	AL, FL, GA, KY,* MS, NC,* SC,* TN	Powered industrial trucks ($n = 18$)
V	IL,** IN,* MI,* MN,* OH, WI	Dairy farm operations ($n = 7$)
VI	AR, LA, NM,* OK, TX	Marine operations ($n = 13$)
VII	IA,* KS, MO, NE	Grain handling industry ($n = 27$)
VIII	CO, MT, ND, SD, UT,* WY*	Roadway work zone activities ($n = 13$)
IX	AZ,* CA,* HI,* NV,* American Samoa, Guam, Northern Mariana Islands	Labor barracks ($n = 12$)
X	AK,* ID, OR,* WA*	Floating seafood processors ($n = 17$)

Source: Occupational Safety and Health Administration (OSHA).[27]
*These states and territories operate their own OSHA-approved job safety and health programs and cover state and local government workers as well as private sector workers.
**Plans cover public workers only.

mailings, training at local trade shows, or speeches at meetings of industry groups or labor organizations. Table 8-7 shows the 10-region structure of the LEPs, the states and territories covered by each region, and examples of LEPs within each region.[27]

8.3.2. Voluntary Protection Program

Whereas random, mandatory inspections are a worthwhile investment rather than voluntary compliance programs,[28] OSHA is shifting the VPP field inspection staff to enforcement activities. Moreover, OSHA is considering nongovernment funding to continue the VPP program with a fee-based system as an option, as suggested by the House Education and Labor Committee.[11]

VPP was launched in 1982 as a cooperative program between OSHA, management, and labor and recognizes employers and workers, in both private industry and the federal government, that have implemented safety and health management systems and maintained injury and illness rates below the national average for their industries. Participants at VPP worksites maintain comprehensive injury and illness prevention programs that share a number of important elements: (1) management commitment and worker involvement, (2) worksite analysis, (3) hazard prevention and control, and (4) training.

Employers who qualify for VPP view OSHA standards as establishing a minimum level of safety and health performance and go beyond OSHA requirements in protecting their workforce. As of May 31, 2012, there were 2,374 total active VPP sites (federal and state) protecting more than 911,000 workers. This figure has more than doubled since 2003.[11]

Applicants to the VPP must submit a written application and undergo a rigorous on-site evaluation by a team of safety and health professionals. In addition, union support is required for applicants represented by a bargaining unit. Program participants are exempt from OSHA-programmed inspections while they maintain their VPP status unless hospitalizations or fatalities occur. OSHA currently approves qualified employer VPP sites for participation in one of three VPP programs, described below.[11] The incentive to move from "Demonstration" to "Merit" to "Star" is decreased regulation but with OSHA oversight.

1. Star recognizes companies that demonstrate exemplary achievement in the prevention and control of occupational hazards and continuous improvement of their safety and health management system. Worksites in the Star program achieve injury/illness rates at or below the national average for their industries (approval is valid for 30–42 months).
2. Merit recognizes companies that develop and implement good safety and health management systems, but they need to take additional steps to achieve Star quality (approval is valid for 18–24 months).
3. Demonstration recognizes companies that show effective alternative methods of achieving safety and health management excellence (approval is valid for 12–24 months).

8.3.3. Whistle-Blower Program

Since the OSHAct was enacted in 1970, Congress has charged OSHA with enforcement responsibility for 22 additional whistle-blower antiretaliation statutes. Together, these laws protect employees who report violations of trucking, airline, nuclear power, pipeline, environmental, rail, mass transit, maritime safety, consumer product safety, and securities laws that are of fundamental importance in protecting the health, safety, and well-being of all Americans. Despite the increase in OSHA's statutory responsibilities, the staff charged with enforcing these laws did not grow significantly until fiscal year 2010, when 25 whistle-blower investigators were added to OSHA's ranks. Since

2010, however, four new whistle-blower laws have been added to OSHA's enforcement program. Even though these additional responsibilities dilute OSHA's attention to its responsibilities under the OSHAct, prompt responses of enforcement are vital for American workers to feel safe when reporting threats to their own safety and to public safety.[11]

8.3.4. Ergonomic Violations Program

In April 2002, OSHA developed a four-pronged ergonomics strategy designed to quickly and effectively address musculoskeletal disorders (MSDs) in the workplace with a combination of four elements: (1) industry-specific and task-specific guidelines, (2) outreach, (3) enforcement, and (4) research. OSHA's first ergonomic guidelines were released in 2003, for the nursing home industry; in 2004, for retail grocery stores and the poultry processing industry; and in 2008, for shipyards. Other industries developed voluntary ergonomics guidelines in cooperation with OSHA for the apparel and footwear industry and for jobs in the telecommunications industry.[29]

From 2002 through 2007, OSHA conducted 4,138 ergonomics inspections. As of September 2008, OSHA had 71 active strategic partnerships with an emphasis on ergonomics. In 2008, OSHA had 19 national alliances and 40 regional/area office alliances with a focus on ergonomics. Furthermore, OSHA has a 15-member National Advisory Committee on Ergonomics, with representatives from industry, academia, labor, and the legal and medical professions.[29]

The general duty clause is used to cite ergonomic violations. To document a general duty clause violation, OSHA demonstrates industry recognition and feasible ways to abate an ergonomics hazard. Agency field staff will increase their emphasis on recordkeeping logs, look for ergonomic hazards in their inspections, see if MSDs are accurately reported, and look for employer policies that discourage MSD reporting.[29] As of the publication of this book, no MSD column has been added to the OSHA log.

8.3.5. Severe Violator Enforcement Program

The Severe Violator Enforcement Program is aimed at employers that have demonstrated recalcitrance or indifference to their duties under the OSHAct by committing willful, repeated, or failure-to-abate violations. Enforcement actions include mandatory follow-up inspections, increased company/corporate awareness of

OSHA enforcement; corporate-wide agreements, where appropriate; enhanced settlement provisions; and federal court enforcement under § 11(b) of the OSHAct.[11] Moreover, the program provides nationwide referral procedures for criminal cases, which includes OSHA's state plan states. In addition, OSHA is reviewing and restructuring its penalties to ensure that they are consistent with the seriousness of the violation and serve as an effective deterrent.[30]

8.4. MULTI-EMPLOYER DOCTRINE

The term "occupational safety and health standard" means a standard which requires conditions, or the adoption or use of one or more practices, means, methods, operations, or processes, reasonably necessary or appropriate to provide safe or healthful employment and places of employment.

— § 3(8), Occupational Safety and Health Act of 1970

One of the most troubling areas for OSHA to address is the protection of all workers from workplace hazards at multiemployer worksites. To protect workers at these worksites, OSHA can cite more than one employer for the same violation. In a 1975 decision, the 2nd Court of Appeals (New York) ruled that the employers responsible for the creation or control of a hazard at multiemployer worksites are responsible for exposures to employees of other employers. There are two types of multiemployer situations. One type is joint employment, when equipment is leased along with an operator (e.g., a crane with a crane operator). The other type is when there is a prime contractor and a subcontractor (e.g., a general construction contractor and an electrical subcontractor).[31,32]

8.4.1. Joint Employers

Judicial review by the courts and the OSHRC has focused on business reality and the purposes of the OSHAct in joint employee situations. Factors considered in assessing liability for a violation include who has direct control of the loaned employees, who provides training and instruction for the loaned employees, and whom the loaned employees consider as their employer.[31]

8.4.2. Prime Contractors and Subcontractors

The most common prime contractor and subcontractor situations occur on construction sites but also include nonconstruction worksites. In this situation, an employee of one subcontractor may be exposed to a hazard caused by another subcontractor. Multiemployer problems can be described regarding two concepts: control and exposure.[31,33] The following employers normally can be cited, whether or not their own employees are exposed:

- The creating employer: creates the hazard.
- The controlling employer: responsible for safety and health conditions on the worksite by contract or through actual practice.
- The correcting employer: responsible for correcting the hazard.
- Exposure (the exposing employer): employees have access to a danger zone, and the employer normally shall be cited unless it (1) did not create the hazard, has the responsibility or the authority to have the hazard corrected, and has the ability to correct or remove the hazard; (2) can demonstrate that the creating, the controlling, and/or the correcting employers have been notified of the hazards to which its employees are exposed; (3) and has instructed its employees to recognize the hazard and, where necessary, informed them how to avoid the dangers associated with it.

8.5. GENERAL DUTY WHEN A STANDARD EXISTS

According to *International Union, United Automobile, Aerospace and Agricultural Implement Workers of America v. General Dynamics Land Systems Division* (1987),[34] OSHA had issued a citation under the general duty clause as a result of an employee being overcome by freon fumes. Other employees later were also affected by the fumes, and one died as a result. The OSHRC judge ruled that the employer had met the OSHA permissible exposure limit, which preempted a citation under the general duty clause. This ruling became a final order of the OSHRC. The U.S. Court of Appeals (DC Circuit) reversed this ruling by ruling that an existing standard does not absolve an employer from duties under the general duty clause. The Supreme Court denied certiorari in 1987, thus leaving the circuit decision in place.[3]

8.6. NONFEDERAL PROSECUTIONS

Nothing in this Act shall be construed to supersede or in any manner affect any workmen's compensation law or to enlarge or diminish or affect in any other manner the common law or statutory rights, duties, or liabilities of employers and employees under any law with respect to injuries, diseases, or death of employees arising out of, or in the course of, employment.

—§ 4(4), Occupational Safety and Health Act of 1970

8.6.1. Getting Away With Murder in the Workplace

There was, in effect, a culture of lawlessness.

—David Uhlmann[35]

Following hearings beginning at the first part of the year, on October 4, 1988, the House Committee on Government Operations submitted a report on a hearing entitled "Getting Away With Murder in the Workplace: OSHA's Non-use of Criminal Penalties for Safety Violations." The committee concluded that OSHA's record in referring cases for criminal action was "dismal." They observed that the statute precluded OSHA from seeking criminal sanctions where there was no fatality. They found an institutional reluctance by OSHA, the DoJ, and the U.S. Attorney's office to prosecute workplace safety cases. Indeed, the state plan states have also been reluctant to prosecute corporations or their officers, as shown in Table 8-8.[36]

The report noted that since the passage of the OSHAct 18 years earlier, OSHA had referred 42 cases to the DoJ for criminal prosecution, about one-third of which were prosecuted. They raised the concern that state and local criminal convictions were being overturned based upon preemption by the OSHAct and recommended that OSHA take an official position clarifying that the OSHAct does not preempt state and local criminal laws.

Table 8-8. State Plan Criminal Prosecutions or Referrals for Prosecutions, 1970–1988

>4	1–3	No prosecutions	No referrals
California	Maryland	Arizona	Alaska
	Michigan	Minnesota	Hawaii
	North Carolina	New Mexico	Indiana
	Utah	South Carolina	Iowa
	Washington	Vermont	Kentucky
	Wyoming		Nevada
			Oregon
			Tennessee

Source: Kinney.[36]

The U.S. Attorney's office found that there was no intent in the OSHAct or its legislative history that the act should preempt state criminal laws. With apparent anticipation of the upcoming Congressional report in October, in June 1988, OSHA Administrator, John A. Pendergrass signed a memorandum to regional administrators regarding cooperation with state or local criminal prosecutions. Pendergrass encouraged assisting states in prosecution efforts but declined to clarify the preemption issue, leaving resolution to the courts.

Nonetheless, several states have used their criminal statutes to prosecute employers for the death or serious injury of workers. These crimes have included murder, manslaughter, and criminal recklessness or negligence as defined below:[37]

- Murder—felonious homicide or the wrongful killing of a human being without justification or excuse.
- Manslaughter—reckless homicide or willful and wanton disregard of consequences that result in death; or the unlawful killing of another without malice, either expressed or implied.
- Criminal recklessness—awareness of the risk of harm and acting in disregard of that risk.
- Criminal negligence—failure to use the degree of care required to avoid criminal consequences.
- Criminal gross negligence—willful and wanton disregard for harm resulting from one's actions.

The states have prosecuted a number of employers for workplace crimes against the safety and health of workers. California leads other states in these prosecutions. In California, corporations are defined as a "person" in the criminal law; thus, they can be prosecuted for manslaughter. This is not uniform across states.[38] The following examples show the type of cases and issues involved in these prosecutions.

8.6.2. Illinois v. Chicago Magnet Wire Corp. (1985)

The Chicago Magnet Wire Corporation of Illinois was in the business of coating wire with various substances and chemicals. The case involved the exposure of 42 employees to toxic chemicals and overheated working conditions. In 1985, a Cook County grand jury delivered an indictment against Chicago Magnet Wire and five of its officials for multiple counts of aggravated battery and reckless misconduct and conspiracy. The Cook County court dismissed the charges, finding that the OSHAct preempted criminal prosecution. In an appeal, the state appellate court also ruled that the OSHAct preempted criminal prosecution. The state appealed the case to the Illinois Supreme Court, which ruled that the OSHAct does not preempt criminal prosecution.[37]

8.6.3. Illinois v. Film Recovery Systems Inc. et al. (1985)

Film Recovery Systems, Inc. engaged in the business of recovering silver from X-ray film acquired from hospitals and clinics. Workers would chop up the film and dump it into a vat of sodium cyanide to extract silver from the film. The silver adhered to electrodes from which workers scraped the silver. A Polish worker collapsed and died while convulsing of acute cyanide poisoning.[37]

Investigators found that the skull and crossbones labeling on the sodium cyanide drums had been scraped off, and the employer had instructed employees to refer to the drum's contents as "the chemical." Limited to civil penalties, OSHA fined Film Recovery Systems $2,000 for serious misconduct in this death.[39] OSHA had conducted an inspection at this site in 1982, but only conducted a records check based upon the policy of the Reagan administration.

The Cook County prosecutor in Illinois indicted the president of the company, the plant manager, and the plant foreman for murder and 20 counts of reckless conduct. The state also indicted the company and its parent company, Metallic Marketing, for involuntary manslaughter and reckless misconduct—Illinois law defines a corporation as a person that can be prosecuted for crimes.[37] The jury found the president, manager, and foreman guilty of murder and 14 counts of reckless misconduct and the company of involuntary manslaughter, but on appeal, the Illinois Supreme Court remanded the case for irregularities.[40]

8.6.4. People of the State of New York v. William Pymm, et al. (1987)

In January 1981, a worker at the Pymm Thermometer plant in New York wrote to OSHA, "Mercury is being used, gas and ovens. Please, we don't know how to describe any more violations, but we are sure there are more. Please send an inspector down to see for himself. We only make the minimum wage, so at least we will know our health is OK."[37] The agency inspected the plant in

March and found mercury on work surfaces including the lunch tables. It issued a citation with a $1,400 fine and a deadline of October 1 for compliance. However, OSHA extended the deadline. In 1984, a doctor reported elevated mercury levels in a Pymm worker. In 1985, a former Pymm worker informed OSHA of an unventilated and hidden cellar operated at the plant. An OSHA investigator found noxious vapors in the cellar operation and permanent brain damage in a worker named Vidal Rodriguez. Other workers were exposed as well.

Two months later, the Kings County district attorney, in cooperation with the New York State attorney general, charged owners and operators William and Edward Bynum with criminal assault and reckless endangerment for exposing workers to mercury, which they knew to be toxic. The Kings County jury convicted the defendants of assault with mercury; however, the judge set the verdict aside. The state appealed to the New York Supreme Court. In 1990, the New York Appellate Division reinstating the jury's guilty verdict against the defendants. However, on remand, the trial court changed the sentence to a misdemeanor with six months in jail and a fine of $10,000. The defendants served their sentences, but on appeal the case was dismissed because of a judge's error.[37]

8.6.5. *North Carolina v. Emmett Roe* (1992)

A September 1991 fire at the Imperial Food Products Inc. chicken-processing plant in Hamlet, North Carolina, killed 25 workers and injured another 56 workers. The fire began when oil from a conveyer belt leaked onto a gas-fired chicken fryer. Trying to escape, 100 employees found that many exit doors were barred. Emmett Roe, owner of the Atlanta-based company, had ordered that the doors be locked to prevent workers from stealing chicken parts and going outside for coffee breaks, and to keep insects from getting inside the plant.

In September 1992, Roe pled guilty in a plea bargain to 25 counts of involuntary manslaughter and was sentenced to 19 years in prison. The plea agreement dismissed charges brought against the plant's managers, James Hair and Roe's son Brad. Thus, there was no trial. Roe faced at least 19 lawsuits filed by the families of the victims. Dick Schultz, director of the North Carolina Occupational Safety and Health Project, said, "The penalty should have been more.... He'll be back on the streets in three years. The positive side is that

19 years is 19 years more than any other sentence for an employer in the state for workers' deaths."[41]

Assistant District Attorney David Graham said that the charges against Brad Roe and James Hair were dropped because the investigation found that the company was run "as a dictatorship." Graham said that Emmett Roe "personally formulated the locked door policy" and ensured that the policy was carried out by plant janitors. Under a state OSHA plan, North Carolina fined the plant $808,150—the largest fine in state history for workplace safety regulation violations. After the blaze, Roe declared bankruptcy and closed all of his operations.[41] Roe was paroled four and one-half years after his incarceration. This case harkens back to the Triangle Shirtwaist fire of 1912.[42]

8.6.6. *Contra Costa County v. KMGP Services Co.* (2012)

In November 2004, a high-pressure gasoline pipeline exploded when it was punctured by a backhoe in Walnut Creek, California, 20 miles east of San Francisco. The blast killed five workers and seriously injured four others. In October 2007, KMGP Services Co., a subsidiary of pipeline company Kinder Morgan, was convicted on six felony counts for violating worker-safety regulations. The company paid $15 million in criminal and civil penalties and more than $69 million in settlements to victims' families.[43]

8.6.7. *San Francisco City and County v. Digital Pre-Press International* (2012)

In December 2011, a California judge found sufficient evidence after three weeks of testimony at a preliminary hearing to the trial of the Digital Pre-Press International owner and foreman for the 2008 death of a pregnant worker. The decedent, 26-year-old Margarita Mojica, was an employee of the company, a printing plant in San Francisco. She was crushed to death on January 29, 2008, by a creasing and cutting machine while preparing the machine for a job. The machine suddenly activated as Mojica was reaching her upper body into the machine.

The District Attorney charged Sanjay Sakhuja (the company owner and CEO), Alick Yeung (the pressroom manager), and Pre-Press International, Inc. with felony involuntary manslaughter and felony violation of a California/OSHA regulation as a willful violation (causing death or permanent injury).

The "lockout" regulation, which the District Attorney claimed the company violated, means that power to a machine must be turned off and that the power switch must be locked in the off position. The penalty for involuntary manslaughter in California is two to four years in prison. By California law, California/OSHA fines for violations can add up to $250,000 per individual and $1.5 million for a applicable corporation.[44] In 2013, Sakhuja pleaded guilty to one count of involuntary manslaughter and five counts of labor code violations related to the death. Digital Pre-Press International previously settled with Mojica's family, including her surviving husband and daughter, for $6 million.[45] The OSHA fine for 14 violations was $62,000, reduced from $83,000, according to OSHA.[46]

8.7. WORKER ENDANGERMENT INITIATIVE

There's always companies that don't think it's important to comply with the law, and for those companies you need a strong enforcement scheme to bring them in line and to make sure that crime doesn't pay.

—David Uhlmann[35]

Criminal penalties under the OSHAct are weak in their application and consequence. They apply only to occupational deaths and not to endangerment of serious bodily harm or the risk of serious bodily harm. These penalties apply to the violation of a standard, not to a violation under the general duty clause, and only to employers, not to other culpable individuals. The criminal penalty for a willful violation of a standard that results in a death of a worker is six months' incarceration plus a fine, and the citation for a violation of a standard must be issued within six months of the incident. In contrast, penalties under a number of environmental laws apply to serious bodily harm or the risk thereof, and incarceration regarding a death or serious bodily harm can be up to 15 years incarceration, along with much larger fines. Thus, few cases under the OSHAct are prosecuted as a crime since resources in the DoJ can be more effectively used on prosecuting felonies rather than misdemeanors (i.e., incarceration for less than a year).

Because of the dissonance between possible criminal actions under the OSHAct and environmental laws, on March 17, 2005, the DoJ announced the Worker Endangerment Initiative, which rests on two principles: (1) environmental crimes lead to worker injuries, diseases, and deaths, and (2) employers who ignore worker safety laws in order to cut costs and maximize profits are almost certainly indifferent to environmental laws as well.[23] There is no system for tracking how this system affects prosecution rates. OSHA may have increased referrals to the DoJ, but prosecutors may use other statutes for criminal cases such as the crime of making false statements to federal investigators. Compliance officers for OSHA may also refer environmental crimes that originate from occupational safety and health investigations to the DoJ. Currently, the effectiveness of this program is unknown.

8.7.1. A Dangerous Business

This section discusses examples of the first principle of the Worker Endangerment Initiative. McWane Corporation is one of the nation's largest cast-iron pipe manufacturers, with various corporate entities located around the country. Between 1995 and 2003, there were 4,600 recorded injuries, nine deaths, and more than 400 violations of OSHA standards at McWane plants, which employed 5,000 workers.[47] In 2003, *Frontline,* the *New York Times,* and the Canadian Broadcasting Corporation joined forces to investigate the thousands of injuries and deaths at plants owned by the privately held McWane, Inc. Through interviews with current and former employees and executives, government officials, and environmental, health, and safety experts, McWane emerged as the most dangerous company in the United States in an inherently dangerous business.[19] The 2003 program drew the attention of the environmental crimes section of the DoJ.

Officials from the DoJ decided to reexamine the case from a criminal perspective. Investigators determined that one of nine deaths was in fact the result of the McWanes's willful disregard of safety rules at its New York plant. They described a corporate culture that put production and profits ahead of the well-being of its employees, who toiled in one of the nation's most dangerous industries.[35] But because of the weak criminal penalties for those violations, prosecutors looked to other laws under which to prosecute McWane and its Union Foundry. Their investigation revealed environmental crimes in addition to worker-safety violations. Occupational safety and health criminal law is weak, but environmental laws provide heightened penalties.[47]

The DoJ uses environmental laws to seek felony convictions when workers are seriously injured or killed on the job during the course of an environmental violation. The environmental laws include the Clean Air Act (CAA), the

Clean Water Act (CWA), and the Resource Conservation and Recovery Act (RCRA). Working with EPA's criminal investigators, OSHA's investigators, and the Federal Bureau of Investigation, these DoJ investigations led to the prosecution of McWane facilities in four federal jurisdictions.[48]

McWane and eight of its executives and managers were convicted of 125 environmental, health, and safety crimes, including lying to government officials and conspiracy. The nationwide investigation of McWane facilities focused on four states: Alabama, New Jersey, Texas, and Utah:[49]

- Alabama (Anniston)—In *United States v. Union Foundry* (N.D. Ala.), a McWane iron foundry division pled guilty in September 2005 to a willful violation of an OSHA standard. An employee had been caught in a conveyer belt pulley and crushed to death. In 2006, OSHA cited McWane Cast Iron Pipe for 38 safety and health hazards at the company's Birmingham plant and proposed civil penalties totaling $332,700.[50] This led to an EPA investigation of RCRA and CWA violations. The plant illegally treated baghouse dust contaminated with lead, a hazardous waste, and exposed workers to this waste. The company was ordered to pay a $3.5 million criminal fine and perform community service valued at $750,000, which included local lead and asbestos abatement.[49] In 2007, the 11th Circuit Court of Appeals (Atlanta) reversed the convictions of McWane and its managers in Alabama. The court ordered a new trial on charges related to the CWA (regarding discharges from the foundry onto wetlands, which were disputed), based on a recent Supreme Court decision interpreting part of that law regarding the definition of a navigable waterway (*Rapanos v. United States*, 2006).[51,52] The employee's widow filed a civil suit that resulted in a $2.27 million settlement with the company.[35]
- New Jersey (Phillipsburg)—The cast-iron pipe foundry had a long history of both environmental and worker safety violations. In 2002, OSHA proposed civil penalties of $130,000 to Atlantic States Cast Iron Pipe Company (a division of McWane) following an investigation of the amputation of a worker's fingers at the foundry that led to a citation for six repeat violations, three serious violations, and three other-than-serious violations.[53] In *United States v. Atlantic States Cast Iron Pipe Company* (D.N.J.), a seven-month trial lasting from mid-2005 to 2006—the longest environmental crimes trial ever—resulted in guilty verdicts

against Atlantic States and four manager defendants on 52 felony counts.[54] The primary means of tying together violations of the otherwise separate regulatory schemes was a conspiracy to defraud the United States by obstructing the lawful functions of OSHA and EPA in enforcing federal workplace safety and environmental laws. Evidence established a history of environmental violations, workplace injuries and fatalities, and activities intended to obstruct justice. The company was fined $8 million. The company and four current and former managers were found guilty of conspiracy to violate the CWA and CAA, and various substantive CWA, CAA, Comprehensive Environmental Response, Compensation, and Liability Act (CERCLA) violations, false statements, and obstruction charges. Individuals were sentenced to serve between six and 70 months in jail.[48]

- Texas (Tyler)—The Tyler Pipe division of McWane had a history of environmental and safety violations. In 2000, the company pled guilty to a willful violation of OSHA standards that resulted in the death of an employee. Earlier that year, OSHA issued multiple civil citations under its egregious penalty policy in the death of maintenance mechanic Rolan Hoskin at the Tyler Pipe plant. There, citing 17 willful safety and health violations, OSHA levied a cumulative fine of $1 million, in addition to a $250,000 criminal penalty.[49] In 2003, OSHA issued citations to Tyler Pipe for violations of health and safety requirements that put its employees in danger and imposed penalties of $196,000 for 13 serious violations and four repeat violations. The citations resulted from an inspection because of a serious occupational injury at the facility.[55] In addition, when Tyler Pipe replaced a large furnace, known as a cupola, it falsely claimed that the cupola was not new, in an attempt to avoid equipping it with updated "best available control technology," as required by the CAA; the company was charged by the DoJ with a felony. In this case (*United States v. Tyler Pipe Company*, 2005), the charge was for a false statement concerning a permit application and to a knowing violation of the CAA for illegally operating its facility without notifying authorities of a major modification. The company was sentenced to pay a fine of $4.5 million and ordered to replace and upgrade structures at its iron foundry facility at a cost of about $20 million.[48]

- Utah—A Utah division of McWane was convicted of making false statements and sentenced to pay a $3 million fine (*United States v. Pacific

States Cast Iron Pipe Company, 2006). The company's vice president and general manager was sentenced to serve 12 months' incarceration for violating the CAA.[48]

8.7.2. Environmental Alliance

The Worker Endangerment Initiative also addresses a moral deficiency in employers who are willing to ignore worker safety laws in their efforts to maximize production and cut costs, and ignore environmental laws as well. Accordingly, the DoJ and EPA have provided OSHA compliance officers with criminal investigative and environmental training so that serious environmental crimes can be identified. More than 1,000 OSHA inspectors, managers, and DoL solicitors have received training. In the pilot case for joint enforcement actions under the OSHAct and environmental statutes, *United States v. Atlantic States Cast Iron Pipe Co., et al.* (D.N.J.), as discussed above, a McWane pipe foundry and four of its managers were convicted of numerous environmental and worker safety violations committed over the course of an eight-year period.[48]

Joint enforcement actions under the OSHAct and the environmental laws present a problem. Under the OSHAct, the citations need to be issued within six months, which can lead to discovery by the defendant before the investigation is complete under the environmental laws. Attorneys for joint prosecutions need to plan for receiving a stay for a longer period of time from an OSHRC administrative law judge.[23]

8.7.3. Endangerment Crimes

The DoJ training of OSHA compliance officers included an understanding of the endangerment laws under the CAA, CWA, and RCRA. Unlike the OSHAct, these environmental endangerment statutes carry felony penalties of up to 15 years in prison and a $1 million fine for organizations. Endangerment prosecutions can be brought for causing a death or serious bodily injury, or the imminent danger of a risk of death or serious bodily injury. The CAA also has a negligence provision that carries a penalty of up to one year in jail. A limitation in the CAA is its application to emissions into the ambient air outside of an enclosed building; thus, a release into the air inside of a building is beyond the scope of this law. The CWA is limited to any release into the water that endangers the health of a person, including workers. RCRA can apply to workers when they are exposed to hazardous wastes.[23]

Worker endangerment has a history prior to the Worker Endangerment Initiative regarding prosecutions under environmental laws. As an early example (*United States v. Company B and Two Individuals*, 1987), Company B, a corporation in Colorado, was the first prosecution for violating the knowing endangerment provision of an environmental statute, specifically RCRA, and was convicted of multiple RCRA, CWA, and false statement counts. Evidence showed that three employees at the facility were exposed to toxic chemicals while working in the drum-cleaning area without respirators, protective clothing, or adequate ventilation. After a three-week jury trial in 1987, Company B was sentenced to pay a $7.5 million fine, although all but $440,000 of the fine was suspended on the condition that the company pay $950,000 restitution to the three workers for neurological damages and other health effects and for site cleanup at an estimated at a cost of $2.4 million.[56]

Another early endangerment prosecution (*United States v. Elias,* 2001) convicted a company owner under RCRA to 17 years in prison and ordered the company to pay $6.3 million in restitution and $400,000 in cleanup costs. In this case, the owner of a fertilizer company in Soda Springs, Idaho, ordered his employees to clean out a 25,000-gallon tank that contained more than a foot of hardened cyanide-laced sludge in 1999. During a second entry into the tank, a 20-year-old employee collapsed. The owner insisted to emergency responders that only water and mud were in the tank, but by the time a cyanide antidote was finally administered, the employee had suffered irreversible brain damage. The owner was tried for knowing endangerment for his conduct toward the employee, illegal disposal of hazardous waste (which occurred after the incident), and a false statement for creating a confined-space permit after the fact and presenting it to OSHA.[57]

The first case under the Worker Endangerment Initiative (*United States v. Motiva Enterprises,* 2003) was the result of the 2001 explosion of a 415,000-gallon tank for sulfuric acid that killed one worker, injured eight others, and spilled 99,000 gallons of acid into the Delaware River. The tank belonged to an oil refining business named Motiva, which was owned by Shell Oil Company and Saudi Refining, Inc. The tank that exploded had a history of significant corrosion and leaks. Moreover, Motiva had improperly converted the tank from fresh acid service to spent acid service. In 2005, Motiva pled guilty to negligent endangerment and to two CWA violations and was guilty of negligently releasing sulfuric acid into the air in violation of the CAA. As part of a plea bargain, Motiva was sentenced to pay a $10 million dollar criminal fine and serve three years of probation. It was also required to pay a $12 million civil penalty and spend at least $3.96 million on environmental projects. The new owner of the refinery agreed to implement a series of enhanced safety procedures at an estimated cost of $7.5 million.[58] The OSHA penalty totaled $175,000, which was a civil and not a criminal fine.

8.7.4. Unanticipated Releases

The worst industrial disaster in history took place in Bhopal, India, in December 1984. Gaseous methyl isocyanate leaked from an insecticide-manufacturing plant owned by a subsidiary of Union Carbide Corporation and killed and injured thousands of people. In response to the Bhopal disaster, Congress passed § 112(r) of the CAA, authorizing the United States to sue industries that fail to design and maintain safe facilities. Under this section, the DoJ brings civil actions against those responsible for unsafe industrial practices that threaten the public health and the environment.[58]

In the Motiva release, as described above, the United States and the State of Delaware sued Motiva Enterprises under § 112(r) of the CAA and the CWA (*U.S. v. Motiva Enterprises LLC, et al.*, 2003). The governments alleged that the tank's explosion-prevention system was badly designed, that Motiva failed to inspect the tank thoroughly, and that Motiva continued to use the tank after corrosion created holes in the tank. The settlement of that action was valued at more than $23 million, which included a $12 million civil penalty, $7.5 million in injunctive relief, cash expenditures of nearly $4.0 million on environmental projects, and placing 285 acres under a conservation easement.[58]

Another prosecution (*United States v. BP Products North America*, 2007) was in response to an explosion at BP's Texas City Refinery that killed 15 employees and injured more than 170 other workers. This 2005 explosion resulted in the release of thousands of gallons of explosive hydrocarbons from a "blowdown stack" during the start-up of an unleaded gasoline refining unit. The vapor ignited when it reached an idling truck. BP pleaded guilty to violating § 112(r)(7) of the CAA and agreed to pay a $50.6 million fine. The conditions of a three-year probation included compliance with the requirements set out in civil agreements between BP and OSHA and BP and the Texas Commission on Environmental Quality to implement safety and environmental improvements at the refinery.[23]

Earlier in 2005, OSHA had assigned $21,361,500 in penalties to BP regarding the explosion in Texas City. When BP failed to comply with the 2005 citations, OSHA proposed penalties of $87,430,000 to BP for the company's failure to correct potential hazards faced by employees. The DoJ agreements resolved OSHA's failure-to-abate citations issued after the 2009 follow-up investigation with a penalty of $50.7 million, and BP agreed to take immediate steps to protect workers with improvements at the refinery by allocating a minimum of $500 million to that effort.[59–61]

8.7.5. National Emission Standards for Hazardous Pollutants

The CAA's National Emission Standards for Hazardous Air Pollutants (NESHAP) provide for work practice standards regarding asbestos abatement and lead abatement as well as hazardous waste cleanup under the Resource Conservation and Recovery Act of 1976 when workers are exposed to a hazard because of a violation of either a work standard or an emissions limit. The Justice Department has successfully prosecuted a large number of CAA cases involving the unlawful removal of regulated asbestos-containing materials from buildings and other structures in connection with renovations and demolitions. Three illustrative examples follow:[23]

- Buddy Frazier and his associates, Chance Gaines and James Bragg, exploited homeless and itinerant workers for illegal asbestos work. Frazier, Gaines, and Bragg recruited homeless men in Tennessee, obtained fraudulent asbestos training identification cards for these workers, and directed them to strip asbestos pipe insulation without first wetting the material, exposing them to airborne asbestos. After an indictment for conspiracy in 1998, Frazier, Gaines, and Bragg were prosecuted for multiple CAA asbestos work practice and worker identification violations at an asbestos-abatement project that preceded a demolition of a manufacturing building in Marshfield, Wisconsin (*United States v. Buddy Frazier*, 2010). They were sentenced to prison for 30, 33, and 24 months, respectively.[62]
- Alex and Raul Salvagno caused more than 500 employees to violate the work practice standards set out in the CAA's asbestos NESHAP, and expert testimony concluded that these workers' exposure would lead to them contracting asbestosis, mesothelioma, and lung cancer. The Salvagnos

were convicted in New York of conspiracy and violations of the CAA, the Toxic Substances Control Act, and the Racketeer Influenced and Corrupt Organizations Act for illegal asbestos abatements that spanned nearly a decade (*United States v. Salvagno*, 2004). Alex and Raul Salvagno were sentenced to 25 and 19 years in prison, respectively; to forfeit $3.7 million; and to pay $23 million in restitution for the victims. On appeal, the sentences were affirmed by the court in 2009.[63]

- A jury found guilty verdicts against two defendants for knowingly violating regulations controlling asbestos removal during demolition of housing in a low-income neighborhood in 2002 (*United States v. Cleve Allan George*, 2007). The defendants knowingly allowed friable asbestos to be removed improperly and filed false air monitoring documents. Cleve Allan George and Dylan C. Starnes were employees of the Environmental Contracting Company in Atlanta, and both were sentenced to 33 months in prison and three years of probation plus a special assessment of $1,600 each for improperly removing asbestos from a low-income public housing project on St. Thomas, in the Virgin Islands. In addition to the jail sentence, they were also required to pay for the cost of medical surveillance required for any people who were exposed to the asbestos. Starnes was sentenced on July 27, 2007, and George was sentenced on February 28, 2008.[64,65]

8.8. JOB KILLERS?

It is a truth universally acknowledged that OSHA workplace regulations are unduly burdensome, negatively impacting an employer's competitiveness and destroying jobs for workers.

—Robin E. Kobayashi[66]

OSHA is one of the most controversial regulatory agencies in the United States. A debate has raged for years over whether workplace safety regulations and inspections correlate with a decline in injury rates and with lower productivity. However, a recent study makes clear that OSHA inspections save money for the firm and for society, and jobs are not lost.[28]

In the 1990s, the California OSHA office began a program of inspections selected at random—not just at workplaces with recent complaints or incidents. This approach to inspections provided a natural field experiment that uses the powerful method of randomization, similar to a medical clinical trial. Researchers included 818 companies with more than 10 employees in a study that included the 409 companies that were randomly selected for inspections compared with 409 other similar companies that qualified for inspection but were not inspected. The study was informed by other data sources. This sample allowed the researchers to assess the actual impact of inspections on operating costs, credit rating, job retention, company survival, and sales.[28]

The study reported that companies subject to random inspections by the California OSHA office showed a 9.4% decline in injury rates compared with uninspected firms in the four years following the inspection, which led to a 26% decrease in workers' compensation costs. There was no evidence of a negative impact on employment or profitability of the inspected firms. Indeed, the results showed slight gains in firm survival, payroll, creditworthiness, sales, and employment in the inspected cohort. An average of $355,000 over five years was saved in worker injury claims and compensation per firm, with savings observed among both small and large employers. The savings were about 14% of the average annual payroll of these companies. When extrapolated nationally, OSHA inspections would save about $6 billion annually nationwide.[28]

THE PREGNANCY DISCRIMINATION NARRATIVE

Between 1979 and 1983, seven women working at Johnson Controls, Inc. became pregnant and exceeded the critical level for blood lead levels in excess of 30 µg/dL as mandated by OSHA for a worker who expected to have a family. In 1982, Johnson Controls implemented a policy of excluding women capable of childbearing from jobs that exposed them to lead. Exclusion did not apply to women whose inability to bear children was medically documented. Mary Craig chose sterilization in order to keep her job; 50-year-old divorcee Elsi Nason had her compensation reduced when she was transferred from lead work; Donald Penny, with plans to be a father, was denied a request for a leave of absence so as to lower his blood lead level. They sued the company in a U.S. district court in Wisconsin, which certified it as a class action that represented other employees as well. The suit was brought under the Civil Rights Act of 1964 as amended by the 1978 Pregnancy Discrimination Act (i.e., Title VII). The district court found for Johnson Controls on the weight of evidence for the protection of the fetus, which was affirmed at the 7th Circuit Court of Appeals (Chicago). In the ruling for Johnson Controls, the court held that the defense met the test of business necessity: (1) there is a substantial health risk to the fetus, (2) transmission of the risk occurs only through women, and (3) and there is a less discriminatory alternative equally capable of preventing the health hazard to the fetus. Johnson Controls brought an additional defense for a safety exception provided by the "bona fide occupational qualification reasonably necessary to the normal operation of that particular business" under Title VII. By 1991, the case wound its way to the Supreme Court, which reversed the previous rulings, finding that the Johnson Controls defense met neither the business necessity nor the occupational qualification tests. Regarding the former test, the court found that the policy was discriminatory against women since the lead exposure also affects men's reproductive abilities. As for the second test, the court's strict interpretation of the law concluded that the job qualification exception was by no means central to the mission of battery making. Moreover, within the legislative history, the congressional standard had been to protect female workers.[3,67,68]

In this case, the controversy was framed as a conflict between fetal and women's rights, hinging on the implicit view of patriarchy that privileges the interests of men over women. While Johnson Controls advocated the policy as altruistic, with the protection of future generations of the unborn at stake, economic factors could not go unnoticed: (1) traditionally women's role in the U.S. economy is to forgo employment to produce babies, (2) a woman's job may be the only way to escape poverty, (3) women can be replaced in jobs by men, (4) companies fear postnatal liability for birth defects, and (5) companies say that they can move the jobs offshore to avoid liability (counter to altruism). In patriarchy, the male is the norm and women are different from the norm, which nonetheless was the essence of the court's ruling in the Johnson Controls case. The approach was different when dibromochloropropane exposure was found to sterilize men and the EPA banned the use of the pesticide. A reframing of the issue would consider the pregnant worker as normal and to be protected and not make the argument about women versus fetuses.[69]

REFERENCES

1. Watson WD. Trust, but verify: Reagan, Gorbachev, and the INF Treaty. *Hilltop Rev.* 2011;5(1):22–39.

2. *Oil, Chemical and Atomic Workers v. American Cyanamid Co.*, No. 81-1687 (D.C. Cir. 1984).

3. Ashford NA, Caldart CC. *Technology, Law, and the Working Environment.* Washington, DC: Island Press;1996.

4. Obama B. When a worker is killed: Do OSHA penalties enhance workplace safety? A statement from Barack Obama on OSHA violations. Senate Committee on Health, Education, Labor, and Pensions Hearing. April 29, 2008. Available at: http://www.boilermakers.org/resources/news/Obama_issues_statement_on_Senate_OSHA_report. Accessed May 30, 2014.

5. Blosser F. *Primer on Occupational Safety and Health.* Washington, DC: Bureau of National Affairs;1992.

6. *Marshall v. Barlow's Inc.*, 436 U.S. 307 (1978).

7. U.S. Const. amend. IV.

8. *Louisiana Chemical Association v. Bingham*, 657 F.2nd 777 Supp. 1188 (5th Cir. 1981).

9. Bokat SA, Thompson HA. *Occupational Safety and Health Law.* Washington, DC: Bureau of National Affairs;1988.

10. Heath B. Justice Department is prosecuting fewer cases of benefits fraud. *USA Today.* June 20, 2011:1A.

11. *Hearings Before the House Subcommittee on Workforce Protections, Committee on Education and the Workforce* (June 28, 2012) (statement of Jordan Barab, Deputy Assistant Secretary for Occupational Safety and Health, U.S. Department of Labor).

12. *Whirlpool Corp. v. Marshall*, 445 U.S. 1 (1980).

13. Mounts GJ. Labor and the Supreme Court, 1979–80. *Monthly Labor Rev.* 1981;104(4):12–22.

14. *Donovan v. Square, D Co.* 709 F.2nd 335 (5th Cir. 1983).

15. Gostin LO. *Public Health Law: Power, Duty, Restraint.* New York, NY: Milbank Memorial Fund;2000.

16. Disclosure of Confidential Information Generally, 18 USC § 1905 (2000). Available at: http://www.gpo.gov/fdsys/pkg/USCODE-2011-title18/pdf/USCODE-2011-title18-partI-chap93-sec1905.pdf. Accessed May 30, 2014.

17. Cohen J. Federal issues in trade secret law. *J High Tech Law.* 2003;2(1):1–26. Available at: http://www.suffolk.edu/documents/jhtl_publications/JCOHENV2N1LA.pdf. Accessed May 30, 2014.

18. Ashford NA, Caldart CC. The right to know: toxics information transfer in the workplace. *Annu Rev Public Health.* 1985;6:383–401.

19. A dangerous business: Criminal prosecutions of workplace fatalities. *Frontline.* Public Broadcasting System. 2003. Available at: http://www.pbs.org/wgbh/pages/frontline/shows/workplace/osha/referrals.html. Accessed November 21, 2012.

20. Ruser JW, Smith RS. The effect of OSHA records check inspections on reported occupational injuries in manufacturing establishments. *J Risk Uncertain.* 1988;1(4):415–435.

21. Gray WB, Mendeloff JM. *The Declining Effects of OSHA Inspections on Manufacturing Injuries: 1979 to 1998.* Cambridge, MA: National Bureau of Economic Research;2002. Working Paper 9119.

21a. Occupational Safety and Health Administration. OSHA press releases. Available at: https://www.osha.gov/dep/index.html. Accessed November 20, 2012.

22. Occupational Safety and Health Administration. Employer rights and responsibilities following an OSHA inspection. 2003. Available at: http://www.osha.gov/Publications/osha3000.html. Accessed November 22, 2012.

23. Harris DL. Achieving worker safety through environmental crimes prosecutions. *US Attorneys' Bull.* 2011;59(4):58–64.

24. Occupational Safety and Health Administration. Draft strategic plan FY 2010-2016. Stakeholder consultation. February 22, 2010. Available at: http://www.dol.gov/_sec/stratplan/2010/osha. Accessed November 22, 2012.

25. Enforcement a key issue in OSHA strategic plan. Safety/OSHA. April 21, 2010. Available at: http://hr.cch.com/news/safety/042110a.asp. Accessed November 22, 2012.

26. Occupational Safety and Health Administration. OSHA's active national and special emphasis program index, 1985–2012. Available at: http://www.osha.gov/dep/neps/nep-programs.html. Accessed November 22, 2012.

27. Occupational Safety and Health Administration. Local emphasis programs. Available at: http://www.osha.gov/dep/leps/leps.html. Accessed November 22, 2012.

28. Levine DI, Toffel MW, Johnson MS. Randomized government safety inspections reduce worker injuries with no detectable job loss. *Science.* 2012;336(6083):907–911.

29. Occupational Safety and Health Administration. Four-pronged, comprehensive approach. Available at: http://www.osha.gov/SLTC/ergonomics/four-pronged_factsheet.html. Accessed November 22, 2012.

30. Occupational Safety and Health Administration. Severe violator enforcement program (SVEP). OSHA instruction. Available at: http://www.osha.gov/dep/svep-directive.pdf. Accessed November 22, 2012.
31. Rothstein MA. *Occupational Safety and Health Law.* Eagan, MN: West;2009.
32. Mintz BW. *OSHA: History, Law, and Policy.* Washington, DC: Bureau of National Affairs;1984.
33. Occupational Safety and Health Administration. Multiemployer worksites. construction safety and health outreach program. December 10, 1999. Available at: http://www.osha.gov/doc/outreachtraining/htmlfiles/multi.html. Accessed October 4, 2012.
34. *International Union, United Automobile, Aerospace and Agricultural Implement Workers of America v. General Dynamics Land Systems Division.* 815 F.2d 1570 (D.C. Cir. 1987).
35. Barstow D. Iron pipe maker is fined $8 million for violations. *New York Times.* April 24, 2009. Available at: http://www.nytimes.com/2009/04/25/nyregion/25pipe.html?_r=2&scp=1&sq=mcwane&st=cse&. Accessed November 22, 2012.
36. Kinney JA. Criminal job safety prosecutions: lessons learned, prospects for the future: Chicago, IL: National Safe Workplace Institute;1990.
37. Bingham E, Reddick E, Meader W, Rankin L. Public health aspects of criminal prosecution of workplace-related deaths, injury, and disease. *Int J Occup Med Tox.* 1994;3(4, special issue):34–55.
38. Bixby MB. Workplace homicide: Trends, issues, and policy. *Oregon Law Rev.* 1991;70(2):333–379.
39. Bureau of National Affairs. *Occupational Safety and Health: 7 Critical Issues for the 1990s.* Washington, DC: Bureau of National Affairs;1989.
40. Cranor CF. Editorial. *Int. J Occup Environ Health.* 2006;12(2):177–179.
41. Govekar PL, Govekar MA. A tale of two fires: igniting social expectations for managers' responsibility. *J Manage Hist.* 2006;12:90–99. Available at: http://www.essential.org/monitor/hyper/issues/1992/11/mm1192_12.html. Accessed October 24, 2012.
42. Von Drehle D. *Triangle: The Fire that Changed America.* New York, NY: Grove Press;2003.

43. Lee HK. Energy firm convicted in Walnut Creek pipeline blast that killed 5. *San Francisco Chronicle*. September 21, 2007. Available at: http://www.sfgate.com/bayarea/article/Energy-firm-convicted-in-Walnut-Creek-pipeline-2539356.php#ixzz2CVd0B4Dz. Accessed November 21, 2012.

44. Stillman SO. Judge finds sufficient evidence to order printing company, owner and foreman to trial in 2008 death of pregnant worker [press release]. December 28, 2011. Available at: http://www.sfdistrictattorney.com/index.aspx?page=155. Accessed September 17, 2012.

45. Richardson K. Digital Pre-Press International owner pleads guilty in death of pregnant employee. *Promo Marketing Magazine*. April 18, 2013. Available at: http://magazine.promomarketing.com/article/digital-pre-press-international-owner-pleads-guilty-death-employee/1#. Accessed May 30, 2014.

46. Occupational Safety and Health Administration. Inspection data. Available at: https://www.osha.gov/pls/imis/establishment.inspection_detail?id=307399246. Accessed May 30, 2014.

47. Barstow D, Bergman L. At a Texas foundry, an indifference to life. *New York Times*. January 8, 2003. Available at: http://www.nytimes.com/2003/01/08/us/at-a-texas-foundry-an-indifference-to-life.html?pagewanted=all&src=pm. Accessed November 22, 2012.

48. U.S. Department of Justice. Worker endangerment. October 2010. Available at: http://www.justice.gov/enrd/3391.htm. Accessed November 22, 2012.

49. U.S. Department of Justice. *United States v. McWane Corporation (New Jersey, Texas, Utah, Alabama)* [press release]. November 2010. Available at: http://www.justice.gov/enrd/3409.htm. Accessed November 22, 2012.

50. Occupational Safety and Health Administration. OSHA proposes more than $332,000 in penalties for workplace hazards at Birmingham foundry [news release]. February 16, 2006. Available at: http://www.osha.gov/pls/oshaweb/owadisp.show_document?p_table=NEWS_RELEASES&p_id=12008. Accessed November 22, 2012.

51. Bowling T. Eleventh Circuit uses "significant nexus" test. *United States v. Robison*, U.S. App. LEXIS 24825 (11th Cir. 2007). *SandBar*. 2008;6(4). Available at: http://nsglc.olemiss.edu/SandBar/SandBar6/6.4nexus.htm. Accessed November 22, 2012.

52. *Rapanos v. United States*. U.S. No. 04-1034, 376 F. 3d 629, and No. 04-1384, 391 F. 3d 704, vacated and remanded (2006). Available at: http://www.law.cornell.edu/supct/html/04-1034.ZS.html. Accessed July 24, 2014.

53. Occupational Safety and Health Administration. Accident, safety and health violations bring OSHA citations, $130,000 penalty to McWane facility in New Jersey [news release]. June 4, 2003. Available at: http://www.osha.gov/pls/oshaweb/owadisp.show_document?p_table=NEWS_RELEASES&p_id=10238. Accessed November 22, 2012.

54. *United States v. Atlantic States Cast Iron Pipe Company.* No. 3:03-CR-00852 (D.N.J. 2006).

55. Occupational Safety and Health Administration. OSHA fines Tyler Pipe Co. of Tyler, Texas, $196,000 for safety and health hazards [news release]. April 14, 2003. Available at: https://www.osha.gov/pls/oshaweb/owadisp.show_document?p_table=NEWS_RELEASES&p_id=10169. Accessed November 22, 2012.

56. U.S. Department of Justice. *United States v. Company B and Two Individuals* (D. Colo.). October 2010. Available at: http://www.justice.gov/enrd/3438.htm. Accessed November 22, 2012.

57. U.S. Department of Justice. Idaho man given longest-ever sentence for environmental crime. *United States v. Elias* (D. Idaho) [news release]. April 27, 2000. Available at: http://www.justice.gov/opa/pr/2000/April/239enrd.htm. Accessed November 24, 2012.

58. U.S. Department of Justice. *U.S. v. Motiva Enterprises LLC, et al.* (D. Del.). November 2010. Available at: http://www.justice.gov/enrd/4463.htm. Accessed November 22, 2012.

59. Occupational Safety and Health Administration. OSHA fines BP Products North America more than $21 million following Texas City explosion company agrees to make extensive plant-wide improvements [news release]. September 22, 2005. Available at: http://www.osha.gov/pls/oshaweb/owadisp.show_document?p_table=NEWS_RELEASES&p_id=11589. Accessed November 24, 2012.

60. Occupational Safety and Health Administration. BP to pay $50.6 million to resolve U.S. Labor Department litigation: penalty stems from 2005 explosion at Texas City, Texas, refinery [news release]. August 12, 2010. Available at: http://www.osha.gov/pls/oshaweb/owadisp.show_document?p_table=NEWS_RELEASES&p_id=18156. Accessed November 24, 2012.

61. Occupational Safety and Health Administration. U.S. Department of Labor's OSHA issues record-breaking fines to BP [news release]. October 30, 2009. Available at: http://www.osha.gov/pls/oshaweb/owadisp.show_document?p_table=NEWS_RELEASES&p_id=16674. Accessed November 24, 2012.

62. U.S. Department of Justice. *United States v. Buddy Frazier* (W.D. Wisc.) November 2010. Available at: http://www.justice.gov/enrd/3517.htm. Accessed November 22, 2012.

63. U.S. Department of Justice. Two men sentenced for criminal violations relating to illegal asbestos removal activities throughout New York state: jail sentences imposed are the longest ever for environmental crime. December 23, 2004. Available at: http://www.justice.gov/opa/pr/2004/December/04_enrd_803.htm. Accessed November 24, 2012.

64. U.S. Department of Justice. Summary of litigation accomplishments fiscal year 2005. Environment and Natural Resources Division. Available at: http://www.justice.gov/enrd/ENRD_Assets/ENRD_2005_Accomplishments_Report.pdf. Accessed November 22, 2012.

65. U.S. Court of Appeals for the 3rd Circuit. No. 07-3341. U.S.A. v. Dylan C. Starnes, Appellant. No. 08-1691. U.S.A. v Cleve-Allan George, Appellant. On Appeal from the District Court of the Virgin Islands. Argued December 11, 2008. Available at: http://federalevidence.com/pdf/2009/09-Sept/US_v._Starnes.pdf. Accessed June 7, 2014.

66. Kobayashi RE. The OSHA regulatory burden: new study debunks job killer, anti-competitive theories. May 20, 2012. Available at: http://www.lexisnexis.com/community/workerscompensationlaw/blogs/reformlegislation/archive/2012/10/24/the-osha-regulatory-burden-new-study-debunks-job-killer-anti-competitive-theories.aspx. Accessed November 21, 2012.

67. Scannell TM. Fetal protection no longer bona fide occupational qualification success. International Union, UAW v Johnson Controls, 11 S Ct. 1196 (1991). *Marquette Law Rev.* 1992;75(2):489–507.

68. *International Union, United Automobile, Aerospace & Agricultural Implement Workers of America, UAW, et al. v. Johnson Controls, Inc.*, 499 U.S. 187 (1991). Available at: http://www.law.cornell.edu/supremecourt/text/499/187. Accessed September 17, 2012.

69. Keehner M. Arguing about fetal "versus" women's rights: An ideological evaluation. In: Schiappa E, ed. *Warranting Assent: Case Studies in Argument Evaluation.* Albany, NY: State University of New York Press;1995:193–210.

9

Research and the Occupational Safety and Health Act

Two general rules have been formulated as complementary expressions of beneficent actions: first, do no harm; and second, maximize possible benefits and minimize risks.

—Cynthia McGuire Dunn and Gary Chadwick[1]

THE RIGHT-OF-ENTRY NARRATIVE

H. Montague Murray, a British physician, diagnosed asbestosis for the first time in 1900. In 1931, Dr. Anthony J. Lanza of the Metropolitan Life Insurance Company, at the request of Johns-Manville (a manufacturer of asbestos-containing products) and a brake lining firm, completed a health hazard evaluation of the asbestos industry. The U.S. Public Health Service (USPHS) published the results in 1935, but a Johns-Manville lawyer intervened in the message published in the report. Lanza complied with the industry request stating that asbestosis is milder than silicosis, emphasizing favorable aspects of the survey, and toning down "undesirable" results of the survey.[2] This industry influence extended into governmental surveys as well, where the USPHS Division of Occupational Health had to sign a pledge of confidentiality before being granted access to factories. This was the case in a 1967 investigation of possible hazards of industrial exposure to asbestos at a factory in Tyler, Texas. The results of the investigation informed the company (Pittsburgh Corning) that the asbestos fiber counts were considered high in more than half of the samples. The company's medical director warned the factory manager that the results constituted a "significant health hazard." The USPHS division, renamed the Bureau for Occupational and Safety Health (BOSH), conducted additional surveys at the Tyler plant in 1969 and 1970. However, since the government had no legal authority to enter and inspect factories, and to do so, they succumbed to a pledge of confidentiality, the workers were not informed of the hazardous exposure to asbestos.[3] In December 1970, the president signed the Occupational Safety and Health Act (OSHAct; see Appendix), and four months later BOSH became the National Institute for Occupational Safety and Health (NIOSH), which was now empowered with the right-of-entry into workplaces and to access workers' records. Almost overnight, the investigators moved from apologists for industry to advocates for workers' health, issuing their first recommended standard to the Occupational Safety and Health Administration (OSHA) in 1972: the control of occupational exposure to asbestos.[4]

9.1. INTRODUCTION

Policy makers often have to act, even though we may not fully understand the full range of possible outcomes, let alone each possible outcome's likelihood. As a result, risk management often involves significant judgment as we evaluate the risks of different events and that our actions will alter those risks.

—Alan Greenspan[5]

This chapter describes the remainder of the OSHAct: § 20–34. It addresses NIOSH and its creation and role under the OSHAct and the role of the Bureau of Labor Statistics (BLS) and OSHA in collecting statistics. Training and education are discussed, which involve both OSHA and NIOSH. The National Workman's Commission on State Compensation Laws is described but is examined in more detail in Chapter 13. NIOSH is located within the Centers for Disease Control and Prevention (CDC) and therefore within the Department of Health and Human Services (DHHS). The origins of NIOSH—important regarding its public health legacy—and its uneasy relationship within the CDC are described. An important feature of this legacy is the continuing power of field investigations over a century that informs both science and policy of the hazards associated with work in the United States. The legacy also gives NIOSH broad authority that goes beyond the OSHAct under the Public Health Service Act of 1912 to those not covered by OSHA,[6] such as self-employed farmers, local government employees (e.g., firefighters), and exposed family members as bystanders to work-related hazards (e.g., contaminated take-home clothing). Finally, court rulings regarding NIOSH are described.

9.2. SECTIONS 20–34 OF THE OCCUPATIONAL SAFETY AND HEALTH ACT

The following congressional verbatim statements of purpose and policy under § 2 of the OSHAct are addressed in this section:

§ 2(1): encourage employers and employees in their efforts to reduce the number of occupational safety and health hazards at their places of employment, and to stimulate employers and employees to institute new and to perfect existing programs for providing safe and healthful working conditions

§ 2(5): provide for research in the field of occupational safety and health, including the psychological factors involved, and by developing innovative methods, techniques, and approaches for dealing with occupational safety and health problems

§ 2(6): explore ways to discover latent diseases, establishing causal connections between diseases and work in environmental conditions, and conducting other research relating to health problems, in recognition of the fact that occupational health standards present problems often different from those involved in occupational safety

§ 2(7): provide medical criteria which will assure insofar as practicable that no employee will suffer diminished health, functional capacity, or life expectancy as a result of his work experience

§ 2(8): provide for training programs to increase the number and competence of personnel engaged in the field of occupational safety and health;

§ 2(12): provide for appropriate reporting procedures with respect to occupational safety and health which procedures will help achieve the objectives of this Act and accurately describe the nature of the occupational safety and health problem.

9.2.1. Research (Section 20)

The Secretary of Health and Human Services (HHS) is authorized (through NIOSH) to conduct research on new safety and health problems and develop information on safe levels of exposure to toxic materials and harmful physical agents and substances. The first four paragraphs of this section authorizes research, experiments, and demonstrations relating to innovative methods and techniques in dealing with occupational safety and health problems, to new problems (e.g., created by new technology) and ameliorative actions beyond what was anticipated within the OSHAct, and to criteria for recommended safety and health standards that describe workplace exposure levels to toxic or physical agents so no worker will suffer impaired health, functional capacities, or diminished life.

This section also authorizes NIOSH to require employers to measure, record, and make reports on the exposure of employees to substances or physical agents, but this authority has never been used, for NIOSH would be required—at the request of the employers—to reimburse the affected employers for any expenses incurred as a result of this requirement.

The Secretary of HHS is required (through NIOSH) to publish a list of known toxic substances and concentrations at which these substance cause toxic effects. This list has been published several times as the Registry of Toxic Effects and Chemical Substances (RTECS). This section also provides for the conduct of on-site investigations called Health Hazard Evaluations (HHEs) at the request of an employee or employer to determine the toxicity of materials used in workplaces and industry-wide studies, which focus on agents to develop criteria for recommending standards to OSHA. Through § 8 of the OSHAct, NIOSH is provided with access to records and worksites for research purposes.

9.2.2. Training and Education (Section 21)

The Secretary of HHS is required (through NIOSH) to promote the training of an adequate supply of professionals in occupational safety and health. In addition, the Secretary of Labor is required to provide training for employers and employees in the nation's workplaces. Moreover, OSHA has established a free consultation program for small businesses.

In 1977, NIOSH funded the first nine academic education and research centers (ERCs) to provide "an adequate supply of qualified personnel to carry out the purposes" of the OSHAct by offering education for occupational health and safety professionals: Harvard University, University of Cincinnati, Johns Hopkins University, University of Texas-Houston, University of Minnesota, University of North Carolina, University of Washington-Seattle, University of Illinois-Chicago, and University of Arizona. As of 2012, NIOSH had established 17 ERCs. The core areas of programming are industrial hygiene, occupational health nursing, occupational medicine, and occupational safety. NIOSH also funds individual academic training programs (project grants) that support undergraduate and graduate training in single disciplines (e.g., toxicology). In addition, NIOSH funds a special category of project grants to provide firefighters, paramedics, and other emergency responders with knowledge and skills in handling hazardous substances.

In 1972, OSHA established its training institute to instruct OSHA inspectors and the public regarding rights and duties under the OSHAct. The agency created training institute education centers in 1992 to make its training courses more widely available to employers, workers, and the public. The initial 12 centers grew to 20 centers and trains more than 300,000 students each year.

In 1978, OSHA launched the New Directions Grants program to promote occupational safety and health training and education for employers and workers. This program was renamed the Susan Harwood Training Grants program after the death of 17-year OSHA veteran Harwood in 1996. The focus of the program is to provide training and education for workers and employers on the recognition, avoidance, and prevention of safety and health hazards in their workplaces, and to inform workers of their rights and employers of their responsibilities under the OSHAct. Target audiences include underserved and low-literacy workers, and workers in high-hazard industries. Since 1978, more than 1.8 million workers have been trained through this program. In 2012, OSHA awarded grants to 72 nonprofit organizations.[7]

In 1975, OSHA created a free consultation service in which more than 500,000 businesses participated during its first 30 years. In fiscal year 2010, the agency's on-site consultation program conducted more than 30,000 visits to worksites covering more than 1.5 million workers nationwide, with priority given to high-hazard worksites. This service is available in each state and assists employers with the identification, evaluation, and recommendations for control of potential worksite hazards. The service is delivered by state governments, which may be provided by state agencies or sometimes through state universities, and is separate from the OSHA enforcement effort. In addition, no citations are issued or penalties proposed, and a consultation qualifies the employer for a one-year exemption from routine OSHA inspections.

The on-site consultation program's Safety and Health Recognition and Achievement Program (SHARP) recognizes small employers who operate exemplary injury and illness prevention programs and serves as a model for workplace safety and health. Upon receiving SHARP recognition, OSHA exempts a worksite from programmed inspections during the period that the SHARP certification is valid.[8,9]

9.2.3. National Institute for Occupational Safety and Health (Section 22)

Congress created NIOSH by raising the status of an existing organization—BOSH—to research institute status in the DHHS, which was placed within the CDC in 1974. The NIOSH Director is appointed by the Secretary of HHS for a term of six years. The institute is responsible for recommending standards to OSHA with supporting criteria and fulfilling the mandates authorized in § 20 and part of § 21. Table 9-1 lists the criteria documents with recommended standards that NIOSH has submitted to the Secretary of Labor since the early 1970s. This section of the OSHAct also authorizes the funding of research in other agencies or private organizations through grants, contracts, and other arrangements. Under the Federal Mine Safety and Health Act of 1977 (Mine Act), NIOSH has similar responsibilities.

9.2.4. Grants (Section 23)

Under § 23, the OSHAct provides an incentive through grants for states to establish programs under § 18 by authorizing the Secretary of Labor to award grants for approved programs. In the first two years of the OSHAct, OSHA awarded up to 90% of costs to individual states for program development in the two years following the passage of the OSHAct. Currently, OSHA funds 50% of the cost of administering and enforcing the state programs. These limits on OSHA funding support are specified in § 23.

This matching funds approach has been problematic for some state programs that are subject to the whim of state budget cutters. As an example, the California program was eliminated in July 1987, which led to the layoff of state employees and a massive influx of federal OSHA employees tapped from across the nation to fill the void. However, the California program was restored in November 1988, when organized labor was successful in marshaling public support for a ballot initiative that called for reinstating the program. For a short period of time, the Michigan governor in 1991 targeted the state

Table 9-1. National Institute of Occupational Safety and Health Criteria Documents/ Special Hazard Reviews Submitted to the Occupational Safety and Health Administration and the Mine Safety and Health Administration

Year	Document	Year	Document
1972	Asbestos*	1976	Methyl Alcohol
1972	Beryllium	1976	Oxides of Nitrogen
1972	Hot Environments	1976	Chlorine
1972	Carbon Monoxide	1976	Parathion
1972	Noise*	1976	Malathion
1972	Ultraviolet Radiation	1976	1,1,1-Trichloroethane
1972	Inorganic Lead*	1976	Tetrachloroethylene
1973	Coke Oven Emissions*	1976	Logging From Felling to First Haul*
1973	Chromic Acid	1976	Acetylene
1973	Toluene Diisocyanate	1976	Phenol
1973	Toluene	1976	Benzene‡
1973	Inorganic Mercury	1976	Cadmium*
1973	Trichloroethylene	1976	Carbon Dioxide
1974	Inorganic Arsenic*	1976	Allyl Chloride
1974	Sulfur Dioxide	1976	Epichlorohydrin
1974	Sulfuric Acid	1976	Methyl Parathion
1974	Ammonia	1976	1,1,2,2-Tetrachloroethane
1974	Chloroform	1976	Hydrogen Cyanide and Cyanide Salts
1974	Cotton Dust*	1976	Acrylamide
1974	Crystalline Silica	1976	Organotin Compounds
1974	An Identification System for Occupationally Hazardous Materials*	1976	Carbaryl
		1976	Boron Trifluoride
1974	Vinyl Chloride*	1976	Formaldehyde*
1974	Benzene*	1976	Asbestos‡*
1975	Inorganic Arsenic‡	1977	Nickel Carbonyl
1975	Xylene	1977	Waste Anesthetic Gases and Vapors*
1975	Inorganic Fluoride	1977	Alkanes (C5-C8)
1975	Zinc Oxide	1977	Fibrous Glass
1975	Sodium Hydroxide	1977	Sulfur Dioxide‡
1975	Emergency Egress From Elevated Workstations	1977	Carbon Disulfide
		1977	Hydrogen Sulfide
1975	Carbon Tetrachloride	1977	Use of Ethylene Oxide as a Sterilant in Medical Facilities*
1976	Chromium (VI)*‡		
1976	Phosgene	1977	Benzoyl Peroxide
1976	Kepone (1976)	1977	Refined Petroleum Solvents
1976	Ethylene Dichloride	1977	Beryllium‡
1976	Methyl Chloride	1977	Inorganic Nickel
1976	Nitric Acid	1977	Chloroprene
1976	Isopropyl Alcohol	1977	Ethylene Dibromide
1976	Hydrogen Fluoride	1977	Vanadium

(Continued)

Table 9-1. (Continued)

Year	Document	Year	Document
1977	Tungsten and Cemented Tungsten Carbide	1979	Vinyl Halides
1977	Decomposition Products of Fluorocarbon Polymers	1979	Confined Spaces*
		1980	Benzidine-Based Dyes
		1981	Coal Liquefaction, Vol. 1
1977	Asphalt Fumes	1981	Coal Liquefaction, Vol. 2
1977	Dioxane	1981	Cobalt
1977	Polychlorinated Biphenyls (PCBs)	1981	Controlling Animal Rendering Processes
1977	Coal Tar Products		
1978	Dibromochloropropane (DBCP)*	1983	Alternatives to Di-2-Ethylhexyl Phthalate (DOP) in Respirator Quantitative Fit Testing
1978	Acrylonitrile*		
1978	Trichloroethylene		
1978	Dinitro-Ortho-Cresol	1983	Construction Safety Standards for Excavations, Vol. 1*
1978	Cresol		
1978	Hydroquinone	1983	Construction Safety Standards for Excavations, Vol. 2*
1978	Nitroglycerine and Ethylene Glycol Dinitrate		
		1983	Styrene
1978	Chrysene	1983	Controlling Hazardous Energy During Maintenance and Servicing*
1978	Glycidyl Ethers		
1978	Manufacture and Formulation of Pesticides	1983	Occupational Safety in Grain Elevators and Feed Mills*
1978	Hydrazines	1983	Land-Based Oil and Gas Well Drilling
1978	4,4'-Methylenebis (2-Chloraniline)*	1984	Precast Concrete Products Industry
1978	Inorganic Lead*‡	1984	Manufacture of Paint and Allied Coating Products
1978	o-Tolidine		
1978	Benzyl Chloride	1985	Foundries
1978	Ketones	1986	Hot Environments‡
1978	Coal Gasification Plants	1987	Radon Progeny in Underground Mines**
1978	DDT		
1978	Aldrin/Dieldrin	1988	Welding, Brazing, and Thermal Cutting
1978	Carbon Black	1988	Grain Dust, Health Hazards of Storing, Handling, and Shipping Grain
1978	Vinyl Acetate		
1978	Ethylene Dichloride (1,2-Dichloroethane)‡	1989	Hand-Arm Vibration
		1989	Di (2-Ethylhexyl) Phthalate
1978	N-Alkane Mono Thiols, Cyclohexanethiol, and Benzenethiol	1990	Propylene Glycol Ethers and Their Acetates
1978	Nitriles	1990	Ethylene Glycol Monobutyl Ether and Ethylene Glycol Monobutyl Ether Acetate
1978	Diisocyanates		
1978	Antimony		
1978	Ethylene Thiourea	1991	Acrylamide
1978	Carbon Tetrachloride‡	1991	Ethylene Glycol Monomethyl Ether, Ethylene Glycol Monoethyl Ether and Their Acetates
1979	Chloroform‡		
1979	Furfuryl Alcohol		

Table 9-1. (Continued)

Year	Document	Year	Document
1993	Chlorobenzene	1996	2-Diethylaminoethanol
1993	Ethyl Ether	1998	Metalworking Fluids
1994	2-Ethyl-2-Hydroxymethyl-1,3-Propanediol*	1998	Occupational Noise Exposure
1995	Respirable Coal Mine Dust**	2006	Refractory Ceramic Fibers

*OSHA Standard Promulgated.
**Recommendation to the Mine Safety and Health Administration.
‡Revised recommendation.

OSHA program for elimination, but the state Department of Labor was able to adjust internal funds to maintain the program.[10]

9.2.5. Statistics (Section 24)

At the beginning of the 20th century, the BLS conducted its first full-scale survey of safety and health conditions in American workplaces with a 1912 study of industrial injuries in the iron and steel industry. The bureau also sponsored industrial hygiene investigations, such as Dr. Alice Hamilton's early 20th-century research on work-related lead poisoning, and initiated studies of nationwide work injury data in the late 1930's. However, the work injury data were compiled only from employers who volunteered to record and report that information, and only disabling injuries defined in the American National Standards Institute's American Standard Method of Measuring and Recording Work Injury Experience Z16.1 were counted. Numerous work injuries that required medical treatment but did not result in a full day away from work were excluded from survey estimates, as were, with few exceptions, occupational illnesses.[11]

The OSHAct addressed these and other limitations. The act directed the Secretary of Labor to compile accurate statistics on occupational injuries and illnesses and to make periodic reports on such occurrences. The Secretary of Labor delegated responsibility to the BLS to

> compile accurate statistics on work injuries and illnesses which shall include all disabling, serious or significant injuries and illnesses, whether or not involving loss of time from work other than minor injuries requiring

only first aid treatment and which do not involve medical treatment, loss of consciousness, restriction of work or motion, or transfer to another job.[12]

Employers are required to participate in this data collection as authorized under OSHAct § 8.

Each year OSHA collects work-related injury and illness data from employers within specific industry and employment size specifications. This data collection is called the OSHA Data Initiative. The agency uses the data to calculate injury and illness incidence rates for specific establishments. This searchable database contains a table with the name, address, industry, and associated total case rate; days away, restricted, and transfer case rate; and the days away from work case rate for establishments since 1996. In 1999, OSHA established the Site-Specific Targeting Program to focus resources on individual worksites with the highest injury and illness rates.

9.2.6. Audits and Annual Report (Sections 25–26)

The OSHAct prescribes procedures for grantees to maintain financial records of grant funds awarded by NIOSH and the right of access to these records for audits to be conducted by the DHHS. The act also requires the submission of an annual report to the president for submission to Congress. The Secretaries of Labor and of HHS must report on progress toward achieving the purpose of the OSHAct and needs in the field of occupational safety and health. In the first report submitted to Congress, OSHA and NIOSH bound the report into a single volume. Thereafter, each agency submitted their reports bound separately. Over time, the annual report was discontinued through a combination of a lack of oversight by Congress and a broad attempt by the government to reduce costly reporting requirements embedded in a multitude of national statutes.

9.2.7. National Commission on State Workmen's Compensation Laws (Section 27)

The OSHAct established the National Commission on State Workmen's Compensation Laws to "undertake a comprehensive study and evaluation of State workmen's compensation laws in order to determine if such laws provide an adequate, prompt, and equitable system of compensation." President Richard Nixon appointed the members of the commission in 1971.

The *Report of the National Commission on Workmen's Compensation* was submitted in July 1972 to the president and Congress as specified in the 1970 legislation, then later in summer 1972, the commission released two additional publications: *Supplemental Studies of National Commission on Workmen's Compensation Laws* and *Compendium on Workmen's Compensation Laws*. The commission concluded that state laws were not achieving their potential. They made 84 recommendations, 19 considered essential, for improving the system although the focus was on coverage and benefits and not on prevention. The report included extensive testimony by workers' compensation experts. The use of the term "workmen's" was abandoned in favor of "workers" in later references to workers' compensation. The commission stated that a workers' compensation system should (1) provide broad coverage of employees and work-related injuries and diseases, (2) provide substantial protection against the interruption of income, (3) provide sufficient medical care and rehabilitation services, (4) encourage workplace safety, and (5) deliver benefits in an efficient and effective manner.[13,14] Many states modified their workers' compensation statutes based upon these recommendations, which dealt primarily with insurance fairness and consistency across states.

In January 1976, members of the Interagency Workers' Compensation Task Force, composed of federal government departments and agencies, reported on needs to reform the state-based workers' compensation systems. Their report warned that without reform, the system would become more expensive, less equitable, and less effective. To date, federal bills brought in Congress to establish a federal workers' compensation law to supplant state laws have not passed.[15]

9.2.8. Small Business (Section 28)

The OSHAct amended the Small Business Act of 1958 to provide financial assistance to small businesses to comply with the act. This assistance includes support for altering equipment, methods of operation, or facilities. When OSHA recognizes substantial economic injury, loans are available to these businesses.[16]

9.2.9. Occupational Safety and Health Administration (Sections 29–30)

When the OSHAct was promulgated, the Secretary of Labor was authorized to establish a position for an Assistant Secretary of Labor for Occupational Safety and Health plus additional executive positions with responsibilities for carrying out the purposes of the act. The Secretary of Labor created OSHA with the new assistant secretary as its administrator. In addition, positions were authorized to staff the Occupational Safety and Health Review Commission (OSHRC).

9.2.10. Emergency Locator Beacons, Separability, Appropriations, and Effective Date (Sections 31–34)

Section 31 added a section regarding emergency locator beacons to another law. It appears odd that a section on emergency locator beacons appears in the OSHAct, but § 31 represents a common practice in legislation in which a "rider" is attached to active legislation so as to amend another piece of existing legislation. This rider amended the Federal Aviation Act of 1958, with no direct relevance to the OSHAct save this section.

Section 32 provides that if any part of the act is held to be invalid—such as inspections absent a warrant—that such findings are to be separate from and not invalidate the rest of the act.

The penultimate section of the act, § 33, provides that funds be approved annually for the implementation of the act. The appropriations process has led to directives to OSHA and NIOSH—a common practice by appropriations committees—to emphasize areas of concern or to restrict expenditures for certain actions. For example, through this process, Congress has exempted certain industry components from OSHA inspections through language that accompanies the annual appropriations, such as the following regarding small businesses:[9]

- Work activities involving hunting, shooting, and fishing,
- Employees having 10 or fewer employees, in industry categories having a lost-workday occupational injury rate lower than the most recently published national average rate,
- Farming operations that do not maintain temporary labor camps and that employ 10 or fewer employees (i.e., family farms).

The final section, § 34, establishes the effective date of the OSHAct as 120 days after its enactment. The OSHAct was approved on December 29, 1970, and became effective on April 28, 1971, when OSHA, NIOSH, and the OSHRC were created.

9.3. EARLY PUBLIC HEALTH AGENCIES FOR OCCUPATIONAL SAFETY AND HEALTH

In the century preceding the OSHAct, the USPHS was limited in scope to the authorities given to the federal government, which included foreign and interstate commerce, federal territory (e.g., not yet a state, Hawaii was the first to provide workers' compensation for occupational diseases), federal administrative affairs (e.g., the Walsh-Healey Public Contracts Act of 1936), and the customary sovereign power of investigation and research.[17] In addition, the taxing power of the federal government was used to control the disease of phosphorous necrosis (phossy jaw) with the enactment of the White Phosphorus Matches Prohibition Act of 1912.[18] Other than USPHS investigations of match factories prior to passage of the OSHAct, USPHS investigators lacked the legal authority to enter and inspect workplaces and had to pledge confidentiality if they did so.

Congressional interest in occupational health protection in the 1910-1914 period was centered in the mining and steel industries. In 1910, Dr. Anthony J. Lanza was assigned to the Bureau of Mines (BoM) in the Department of Interior (DoI) to investigate consumption (silicosis) among miners in Missouri and Montana. In 1913, while on assignment from the USPHS to the BoM, Dr. James A. Watkins began a series of studies of working conditions in the U.S. Steel Corporation's Homestead and Duquesne plants in the Pittsburgh, Pennsylvania area.[19]

9.3.1. The Public Health Service Act

Congress passed the Public Health Service Act in 1912, which placed the USPHS in the U.S. Treasury Department. The types of diseases addressed shortly after the passage of this act were listed in a model law for morbidity reports from the states that were occupational in nature: poisoning by arsenic, brass, carbon monoxide, lead, mercury, natural gas, phosphorus, wood alcohol, naphtha, bisulfide of carbon, and dinitrobenzene; caisson disease; and other work-related disabilities.[17] These diseases were acute, and this model law survives today as a list of notifiable diseases as reported in the *Morbidity and Mortality Weekly Report* (*MMWR*), which no longer includes occupational diseases. The last work-related national notifiable disease was silicotuberculosis, which remained on the list into the 1970s. This checkered history of acceptance of occupational health as part of public health stemmed from the

USPHS's avoidance of controversy (e.g., labor versus business) and commitment to state health departments, the general public's concern and fear regarding "communicable" diseases (e.g., a general threat versus a threat to subpopulations such as workers), and the shift of public health protection to other agencies as described in Chapter 3.

The increased number and frequency of studies related to occupational health protection led to the creation of the USPHS's Office of Industrial Hygiene and Sanitation (the predecessor agency to BOSH and then NIOSH) in 1914. Dr. Joseph W. Schereschewsky was the first chief of the office, which was stationed at Pittsburgh's Marine Hospital in close proximity to the BoM so as to better investigate injuries and illnesses in mining. While resuming silicosis studies in Pueblo, Colorado, in conjunction with the BoM, Schereschewsky broadened investigations into women's occupational health, child labor problems, eyestrain and shop lighting, and hazards in the chemical and textile industries. In addition, the office conducted investigations of the New York garment industry, the steel industry, and diverse companies in the Cincinnati, Ohio, area.[19,20]

Schereschewsky served as chief of the office until 1918, when he became director of the new Division of Scientific Research within the USPHS. In 1922, he implemented a cancer research program at the USPHS Marine Hospital in Boston, Massachusetts, which grew into the National Cancer Institute.[19]

9.3.2. World War I

The United States declared war on Germany in 1917. The U.S. Army placed a half million men in 32 training camps called cantonments. Four million men eventually moved through these camps. The Office of Industrial Hygiene and Sanitation was assigned two roles in the war effort: (1) the control of disease around the cantonments, including water safety, mosquito control, and venereal disease control; and (2) occupational disease investigations and prevention in the war industries and related construction activities, particularly munitions production.[19,21]

Upon Schereschewsky's promotion in 1918, Lanza was named the new chief of the office. In that year, office personnel were detailed to the DoL as part of the Working Conditions Services (WCS). This group was then renamed as the Division of Industrial Hygiene and Medicine (DIHM) and was transferred to Washington, DC. Based upon British experience, the DIHM's initial focus was on health protection and control of work hours. Six offices were set up nationwide, and hygiene codes were established for munitions work. Medical care services were investigated in the manufacture of trinitrotoluene (TNT) and picric acid, loaded shells and hand grenades, poisonous gases, airplanes, and military balloon fabrics.[19]

A particular concern was the occupational hazard associated with TNT poisoning. Deaths from TNT poisoning exceeded the battlefield death rate among soldiers. In one plant, 17,000 cases of poisoning resulted in 475 deaths. Another plant reported 7,000 cases and 105 deaths. The DIHM investigated the absorption of TNT and the detection and prevention of TNT poisoning. It conducted animal studies, developed diagnostic criteria for early recognition of poisoning, and developed methods for detecting airborne TNT.[22,23]

After the signing of the armistice, the DIHM supervised plants under the U.S. Employees' Compensation Commission until the WCS ceased to exist; with the lack of appropriated funds, the regional offices were closed. The commission had the responsibility for compensating all federal employees (or their survivors) who were injured or killed in the line of duty.[24] In 1921, Lanza resigned, and the DIHM was returned to the authority of the USPHS and renamed as the Office of Industrial Hygiene and Sanitation once again.[19]

9.3.3. Between the Wars

Dr. Lewis R. Thompson became chief of the office and began to recruit engineers. The office and the BoM collaborated on a number of projects. Since the office had no laboratory facilities, Thompson assigned investigators to universities where laboratories were available. One result of this work was the Greenburg-Smith impinger that was used for dust sampling for many years. The "dusty trades" became a focus of investigations, including Vermont granite and anthracite coal studies. In 1923, investigators studied radium exposures of employees at the Bureau of Standards.[19]

In 1925, news emerged about 139 cases of lead poisoning and 13 deaths associated with the manufacture of tetraethyl lead, a new product used as an antiknock compound in gasoline. As a result, Surgeon General Hugh S. Cumming called for a conference to address the prevention of tetraethyl lead poisoning. In 1926, agreement was reached at a follow-up conference for the industry to regulate the use and handling of the additive to be administered by Thompson's office. Several states made lead poisoning a reportable disease up until

World War II. This conference became a model for other conferences. In 1928, the Surgeon General convened a conference to control exposures to radium during the painting of luminous-dial watches from which several deaths from poisoning among women had occurred. Similar conferences were convened that addressed methanol, volatile chlorinated liquid hydrocarbons including carbon tetrachloride, carbon tetrachloride fire extinguishers, aniline oil, carbon disulfide, benzol, and occupational cancer. Another was convened in 1941 to address mercurial poisoning in the hat making industry.[25] Modeled after these early conferences, Surgeon General Antonia C. Novello convened the Surgeon General's Conference on Agricultural Safety and Health in 1991.[26]

Thompson served as chief of the Office of Industrial Hygiene and Sanitation until 1930, when Dr. James P. Leake became chief. In that same year, a sister organization to the office was established: the Office of Dermatoses Investigations. Its chief, Dr. Louis Schwartz, studied industrial dermatoses in a series of investigations in 1931. During the Depression years of 1930 to 1937, USPHS policy focused on sanitation and communicable disease control, leaving industrial hygiene as a minor priority. Fieldwork for industrial hygiene was halted for lack of funds. The perception of the times at the USPHS was that industrial diseases were limited to silicosis and to lead and mercury poisoning. Skin diseases were of a low priority since they rarely resulted in disability. The only occupational cancer concern was exposure to coal tar derivatives. During this hiatus, office staff wrote reports and articles documenting their findings from previous years. Industrial management did not support cooperation in studies, organized labor was struggling for national recognition and was suspicious of government objectives, and workers were more interested in jobs than industrial disease.[17] Nonetheless, more than 500 poisonous materials and hazardous conditions were identified that could be detrimental to worker health.[27]

Title VI of the Social Security Act of 1935 provided funds for the USPHS to conduct research and provide grants-in-aid to the states, which included industrial hygiene. In 1937, the Office of Industrial Hygiene and Sanitation combined with the Office of Dermatoses Investigations as the Division of Industrial Hygiene, headed by Dr. Royd R. Sayers. The division was placed within the new National Institutes of Health (NIH), located on a campus in Bethesda, Maryland. NIH was directed by former office chief Thompson. In 1938, a meeting of state directors of newly funded industrial hygiene programs established the National Conference of Industrial Hygienists, which was soon renamed as the American Conference of Governmental Industrial Hygienists.[19]

9.3.4. World War II

With the advent of World War II, Dr. James E. Townsend was appointed as chief of the Division of Industrial Hygiene.[19] Emerging health and sanitation appropriations included industrial hygiene to convert state industrial hygiene programs from peacetime to the war effort. The division assumed national leadership for industrial health and medicine. In this effort, it led:[28]

- The evaluation and control of health hazards in the war industries (e.g., exposure to dusts, fumes, gases, and vapors, and to other materials and conditions),
- Advice to industry regarding the construction and renovations of plants,
- The promotion of physical examinations and medical services for workers, and
- The control of communicable diseases among workers in cooperation with local health departments.

Representative Frances Payne Bolton (R) of Ohio proposed a bill to fill a critical shortage of occupational nurses. Her bill passed without a dissenting vote in 1943. Furthermore, the division assisted the War and Navy Departments in the inspection of industrial military establishments.[28]

The division worked with the Army Ordnance Department to prevent mortality from TNT poisoning. The division also provided direct medical and industrial hygiene services to 90 government-owned, contractor-operated arsenals with more than 140 investigations. The services were applied to plants that manufactured TNT, Royal Demolition Explosive, tetryl, and smokeless powder as well as shell loading plants. Lanza, the former chief of the Office of Industrial Hygiene and Sanitation (a.k.a. DIHM) during World War I, returned from employment at the Metropolitan Life Insurance Company to public service as the chief medical officer for the Army Ordnance Department. Even though the United States was producing ordnance for all of the Allies, the prevention of mortality from TNT poisoning was significantly down from the tragic World War I numbers to 22 deaths during World War II.

One member of the Division of Industrial Hygiene was killed in an explosion at a shell loading plant in Indiana.[19,29] The Division also conducted investigations of shipyards operated by the U.S. Maritime Commission that included research of the effects of exposure to welding fumes.[28]

Another major division service during World War II was providing grants and personnel assignments to the states for industrial hygiene work, because all U.S. industry was on a war footing. By 1944, 360 personnel were assigned to 47 units in 38 states. This service was continued into the post–World War II period. Furthermore, a mimeographed quarterly newsletter, *Industrial Hygiene*, was begun in 1941, becoming the *Industrial Hygiene Newsletter* in 1944.[19,28]

The division also engaged in confidential industrial research from which more than 100 reports were submitted to the armed services. These investigations covered evaluations of physiology regarding oxygen breathing devices, a variety of clothing and equipment, and the potential dangers of exposure to metals, explosives, and solvents. A related investigation by the NIH that concerned the toxicology of a new explosive, pentaerythritol tetranitrate (PETN), was conducted before production was undertaken.[28]

9.3.5. The Postwar Years

After the war, the division's focus concentrated on state programs supported by field investigations, and as a result, it was transferred from NIH to the Bureau of State Services. Much of the division's research staff transferred to other NIH programs in 1946. The division established consultants at USPHS regional offices to support state programs and administer division programs in the region. In 1948, USPHS policies modified this approach by staffing the regional offices with general consultants rather than program (i.e., industrial hygiene) consultants. One result was the establishment of a field station in Salt Lake City, Utah, to provide technical assistance to the western states. The field station began an investigation of the uranium mining industry in 1950, which soon consumed its attention. In addition, the division established a field station in Cincinnati that returned the division to a research role, especially regarding toxicology and engineering. Rather than distributing mimeographed copies, the division started printing its *Industrial Hygiene Newsletter* in a magazine format monthly in 1947.[19]

During this period after the war, both management and organized labor were more interested in occupational safety and health issues. For management, the war had brought industrial hygiene into the staffing and conscience of companies, and for organized labor, an interest in occupational diseases had emerged. This dual interest led to requests to the division for field investigations. In 1946, the United Steelworkers of America requested division assistance to determine the health effects of exposure to fluorides. In 1947, because of the incidence of bronchogenic carcinoma among workers in chromate production, the industry requested help in determining the relationship of exposures in the industry and the incidences of cancer. The result was the identification of a rate of 1,115 cases per 100,000 workers compared with a control group of 20.8 cases per 100,000 subjects.[19] The industry requested assistance for medical and engineering controls. A union request for an investigation of the health effects of tungsten carbide was stymied because of the lack of cooperation by management. Other requests included one in 1952, by the United Gas, Coke, and Chemical Workers of America, to investigate the health effects of exposures to diatomite mining and processing, which was linked to a request by the State of California to determine the health effects (pneumoconiosis) associated with diatomite mining and processing.[19]

Townsend chaired the Medical Advisory Committee on Beryllium to industry regarding the metal's use as a phosphor in fluorescent lights. Beryllium disease resulted from dust inhalation from broken lights, and cuts from contaminated broken glass resulted in poor wound healing, particularly among children. Following a meeting between Townsend and industry representatives, Surgeon General Leonard A. Scheele announced that companies would stop using beryllium in the manufacture of fluorescent lamps after June 30, 1949. However, the industry did not agree to destroy the inventory of unsold lamps.[30]

The division was assigned to investigate an air pollution episode in Donora, Pennsylvania, in 1948. It sought additional funding for more air pollution research, but neither the USPHS nor Congress supported the request. Later, the division was asked to provide technical assistance to Mexico for an air pollution study at Tampico and to the U.S. Department of State for a joint U.S.-Canada air pollution study in the Detroit (Michigan) and Windsor (Ontario) areas.[19]

In 1951, having served previously with the Communicable Disease Center in Atlanta, Georgia, and now "moved to a higher position,"[31] Dr. Seward E. Miller was named chief of the division. He increased its breadth to include occupational medicine and psychiatry. Since funds were lacking, he relinquished air pollution studies. However, soon thereafter, congressional interest in air pollution emerged, resulting in a significant USPHS program that was destined to grow over time into a major federal program.

Miller established a rapport with the DoL's Bureau of Labor Standards by supporting a proposed grant-in-aid program to strengthen occupational safety and health at state labor departments, which was against the traditional turf interests of the USPHS. Even though funding was denied for this proposal, the effort led to a more unified interest in protecting workers' safety and health. Miller also proposed a National Institute of Occupational Health, which was bureaucratically buried. The proposal was unearthed later in the debate for the creation of NIOSH.[18]

Reduced funding in 1953 saw the demise of several projects, including Miller's program for occupational psychiatry. By 1954, the Bureau of State Services consolidated into two divisions. Miller was named director of the new Division of Special Health Services (the other was the Division of Sanitary Engineering), within which the Division of Industrial Hygiene became the Occupational Health Program with Henry N. Doyle as its chief. Without significant funding, the program denied several requests for studying the problem of coal workers' pneumoconiosis, and the production of the *Industrial Hygiene Newsletter* ceased. (A complete set is available in the DoL library.) However, in 1955, as a result of a study by the new program, congressional interest reemerged in silicosis, which led to the funding of a larger study in the metal mining industry. Training was emphasized and, in 1958, the program published the first edition of *The Industrial Environment—Its Evaluation and Control*. For a time, the program developed radiological health expertise, which was shunted to the new and separate Radiological Health Program.[17]

In 1957, Dr. Harold J. Magnuson became chief of the Occupational Health Program. He focused on major field investigations: silicosis in metal mines, lung cancer among uranium miners, and hearing loss among U.S. prison workers. Magnuson moved away from a drift toward secondary prevention in providing care to workers (under Miller) back toward primary prevention through environmental controls (e.g., a shift from studying microbiology to studying microchemical risk factors) and from promotion of personal health services to protection through environmental controls. In 1959, the Division of Special Health Services was abolished and the Occupational Health Program was reconstituted as the Division of Occupational Health. By 1962, this division received appropriations for a study of coal workers' pneumoconiosis.[19]

Magnuson accepted another position in 1963, and Dr. Murray C. Brown became chief after some intermittent leaders. Results of the study of lung disease among uranium miners gained visibility and led the DoL to set standards under the Walsh-Healey Public Contracts Act and the BoM for the protection of uranium miners. Over time, increased funding led to the establishment of the Appalachian Laboratory for Occupational Respiratory Diseases in Morgantown, West Virginia, in 1967. The 1967 results of the coal miners' pneumoconiosis study had an important role in the passage of the Federal Coal Mine Health and Safety Act of 1969; more description of this act appears in the next chapter.

The division had no specific authority in law, which Brown aimed to change. To initiate this change, Brown called on Dr. William W. Frye in 1965, chancellor of the medical center at Louisiana State University, to assist in developing a report regarding the occupational health needs of the country. John (Jack) F. Hardesty was among the division staff members working on the report; his brother was President Lyndon Johnson's speechwriter described earlier in Chapter 5. The "Frye report" included 17 recommendations supported by 29 position papers; all 17 recommendations later found their way into the OSHAct in some form.[17] The goals in the report were based on two principles, which in addition are paraphrased parenthetically from the OSHAct:

1. The elimination of any factor that makes the worker pay with his or her health for the privilege of having a job (i.e., § 2[b], "to assure so far as possible every working man and woman in the Nation safe and healthful working conditions").
2. The active promotion of the nation's economy (a $10 billion annual gain in 1965 dollars) through the reduction of sick absence and lower productivity because of correctable health factors associated with the workplace (i.e., § 2[b], "to preserve our human resources"; § 2[a], "[so as not to] impose a substantial burden upon, and [...] a hindrance to, interstate commerce in terms of lost production, wage loss, medical expenses, and disability compensation payments").

Chaired by Dr. Norton Nelson of the New York University Medical Center and with George Taylor of the American Federation of Labor-Congress of Industrial Organizations (AFL-CIO) participating, the National Advisory Environmental Health Committee prepared a 1965 report entitled *Protecting the Health of Eighty Million Americans—A National Goal for Occupational Health.* Nelson was helped by the staff of the Division of Occupational Health, and he consulted with Frye in writing the report. The division submitted a report to Surgeon General William H. Stewart in 1965, from which President Johnson often quoted as he promoted the OSHAct. By 1967, the DoL took the lead in preparing proposed legislation. In that same year, the division was elevated in status and renamed as BOSH. Brown retired in 1969, and Dr. Marcus M. Key was appointed director of the new bureau.[19]

In 1970, Congress passed the OSHAct, which created NIOSH at USPHS but placed responsibility for standard setting and enforcement within the DoL. BOSH became NIOSH and was given authority like OSHA to enter and inspect factories, but for research purposes only. This authority changed the attitude of NIOSH investigators—instead of gaining access through cooperation, they could now enter sites by the force of law.[19]

9.4. THE NATIONAL INSTITUTE FOR OCCUPATIONAL SAFETY AND HEALTH

The research and recommendations of the institute will be of critical importance in continually improving occupational health and safety standards promulgated under the act.

—Senator Jacob Javits[32]

The National Institute for Occupational Safety and Health—created by § 22 of the OSHAct—is the federal agency responsible for conducting research and making recommendations for the prevention of work-related injury and illness. Its parent agency, the CDC, is charged with tracking and investigating public health trends. CDC's stated mission is "To promote health and quality of life by preventing and controlling disease, injury, and disability." As stated earlier, the CDC is an agency within DHHS.

While OSHA is responsible for developing and enforcing workplace safety and health regulations, NIOSH was established to provide research, information, education, and training in the field of occupational safety and health. The institute is authorized to develop recommendations for occupational safety and health standards and perform all functions of the Secretary of HHS under § 20 (research) and part of § 21 (training and education) of the OSHAct.

The Mine Act delegated additional authority to NIOSH for mine health research. The act authorized NIOSH, as under the OSHAct, to develop recommendations for mine health standards for the Mine Safety and Health Administration (MSHA) and conduct on-site investigations in mines. In addition, NIOSH was mandated to administer a medical surveillance program for miners, including chest X-rays to detect coal workers' pneumoconiosis and to test and certify personal protective equipment (PPE) and hazard-measurement instruments. The U.S. Department of the Interior (DoI) abolished the BoM on March 30, 1996, but two laboratories of the bureau—one in Pittsburgh, Pennsylvania, and another in Spokane, Washington—were transferred to NIOSH. Thus, NIOSH not only addresses "health" problems pursuit to the Mine Act, but it now addresses "safety" research as well—the former province of BoM. More is described about BoM in the next chapter.

The institute is headquartered in Washington, DC, with research laboratories and offices, as shown in Table 9-2. It is a professionally diverse organization with a staff of more than 1,400 people representing a wide range of disciplines including epidemiology, medicine, industrial hygiene, safety, psychology, engineering, chemistry, and statistics. Institute scientists work in multidisciplinary teams and carry out intramural and extramural research focused on preventing or reducing work-related injury and illness. The OSHAct directs the Secretary of the Department Health, Education, and Welfare—DHEW, which was later named the DHHS—to appoint a director of NIOSH for a six-year term.

9.4.1. The Formative Years (Marcus Key, 1971–1974)

Elliot Richardson, the Secretary of DHEW, appointed Dr. Marcus Key as the first NIOSH director. Key was an occupational dermatologist and the director of the NIOSH predecessor agency, BOSH. He joined the USPHS in the Division of Occupational Health in 1956. Key had worked closely with George H.R. Taylor, the director of occupational safety and health for the AFL-CIO, and Jack Sheehan, legislative director of the United Steelworkers, in writing and promoting the OSHAct. Thus, Key's hand had been active in the OSHAct sections that related to NIOSH: (1) a broad range of discretionary research authorities, (2) RTECS, (3) right-of-entry and access to records, (4) HHEs, (5) industry-wide studies, and (6) training. A NIOSH mandate was spelled out in

Table 9-2. National Institute for Occupational Health and Safety Research Laboratories, Offices, and Locations

- Office of the Director (Washington, DC)
- Office of Extramural Programs facilitates and oversees extramural research and training grants and cooperative agreements. (Atlanta, GA)
- Alaska Pacific Office (Anchorage, AK)
- Western States Office (Denver, CO)
- Education and Information Division develops and transfers information and provides recommendations to foster the prevention of occupational injuries and diseases. (Cincinnati, OH)
- Division of Surveillance, Hazard Evaluations, and Field Studies conducts surveillance of the nation's workforce and workplaces to assess job-related illnesses, exposures, and hazardous agents, and researches the causes of diseases in the working population and their offspring. (Cincinnati, OH)
- Division of Applied Research and Technology provides national and international leadership in applied research focused on the prevention of occupational illness and injury and on intervention effectiveness. (Cincinnati, OH)
- Office of Compensation Analysis and Support conducts activities to assist claimants and support the role of the Secretary of HHS under the Energy Employees Occupational Illness Compensation Program Act of 2000. (Cincinnati, OH)
- Health Effects Laboratory Division conducts laboratory research, develops intervention programs, and designs, tests, and implements effective methods of health communications for controlling and preventing workplace safety and health problems. (Morgantown, WV)
- Division of Safety Research serves as the focal point for the institute's traumatic occupational injury research program focused on injury prevention. (Morgantown, WV)
- Division of Respiratory Disease Studies provides national and international leadership toward the identification, evaluation, and prevention of occupational respiratory disease, such as asthma, chronic obstructive pulmonary disease, and pneumoconiosis. (Morgantown, WV)
- National Personal Protective Technology Laboratory, established in 1999, focuses expertise from many scientific disciplines to advance federal research on respirators and other personal protective technologies for workers. (Pittsburgh, PA)
- Pittsburgh Research Laboratory occupies 180 acres of experimental property and conducts research on the safety and health hazards of mining and on mining disaster prevention. (Pittsburgh, PA)
- Spokane Research Laboratory conducts research on metal and nonmetal mining safety. (Spokane, WA)

Note: HHS = Health and Human Services.

OSHAct § 22, which created NIOSH: to recommend standards to the DoL with supporting criteria.[33] It is noteworthy that the preposition used in the institute's name is "for" rather than "of" as is used in the names of other health institutes, indicating the advocacy stance envisioned for NIOSH. Many organizational changes at CDC eventually adopted the word "for" as well (e.g., "Communicable Disease Center" to "Center for Disease Control").

While OSHA's immediate focus was on safety, Key placed a focus on the health aspects of the OSHAct. He emphasized HHEs; producing criteria documents; research into the chemical and biological precursors to occupational diseases, especially cancer; and epidemiological studies across entire industries.[34] By 1972, NIOSH had launched 22 industry-wide epidemiological studies across several hundred thousand workers, including printing press operators, foundry workers, construction machinery operators and stationary engineers, cotton textile workers, asbestos workers, uranium miners and millers, and dentists.[35] In addition, Key began a two-tier peer review process with NIH for extramural research grants.[36] Key's hallmark contribution was advocating the lowest detectable level as a policy in recommending standards for carcinogenic agents, since there is no known threshold level for carcinogens.[36a]

In the 1970s, NIOSH conducted a wide range of research projects in-house or through grants concerning the effects of exposure to toxic substances and harmful physical agents and to combinations of exposures. Instruments were developed to monitor levels of environmental hazards in workplaces, and personal monitoring devices were designed for use by individual workers. A two-year National Occupational Hazard Survey got under way to assess potential health hazards in a sample of 8,000 representative workplaces for a national estimate of industrial health hazards, as did educating a cadre of occupational safety and health professionals.[37,38]

Criteria documents and recommended standards to OSHA were a priority.[39] This priority focused on toxic substances and physical agents guided by five indexes: (1) number of workers exposed, (2) expert opinion on relative toxicity, (3) incidence of disease, (4) amount of agent produced, and (5) trend of usage.[40] In 1974, NIOSH and OSHA jointly initiated the development of OSHAct § 6(b) occupational health standards based on existing § 6(a) permissible exposure limits. This joint effort was called the Standards Completion Program (SCP) and involved the cooperative efforts of personnel from various divisions within NIOSH and OSHA and several of their contractors. The SCP developed 387 substance-specific draft standards with supporting documentation that contained technical information and recommendations needed for the promulgation of new occupational health standards. In addition, the SCP was the basis for establishing "immediately dangerous to life and health" values and the *Pocket Guide to Chemical Hazards* for industrial hygienists.

Following the wholesale loss of environmental programs to EPA in 1970, the USPHS assembled several programs, including NIOSH and CDC, into the Health Service and Mental Health Administration (HSMHA). Assistant Secretary for Health Charles Edwards assigned CDC Director David Sensor to temporarily direct and ultimately dissolve HSMHA. Sensor elevated the CDC to the agency level equivalent with NIH and FDA, sent the National Institute of Mental Health to NIH, and brought some organizational remnants into the CDC, including NIOSH. An alternative for NIOSH was considered in which it would be elevated as an agency and located in Research Triangle Park, NC. Industry input was sought regarding this proposal, which led to a DuPont Company representative examining the possibility, who was "horrified" at the possibility, and as result the idea "fizzled."[31] On July 1, 1973, NIOSH was transferred to the CDC.[41]

While the CDC and NIOSH shared common public health principles, their traditional constituencies were different.[31] Consistent with USPHS tradition, the CDC worked closely with state health departments, but NIOSH stakeholders included the unions, enlightened companies that took occupational safety and health seriously, OSHA, and the changing mine safety agencies that were morphing toward becoming the MSHA; all were headquartered in Washington, DC. Moreover, by naming NIOSH as an "institute," the OSHAct originally envisioned it as part of NIH. As one author put it, this organizational "miscarriage" has been at the root of NIOSH's problems since its birth.[42] Another viewpoint has been that NIOSH should be at an organizational level more equivalent to OSHA, in the DoL, rather than "tucked" under the CDC.[34]

Key resigned on September 1, 1974.[43] Deputy Director Edward J. Baier served as acting director following Key's resignation, and many within the institute expected Baier to be appointed as the new director.

9.4.2. Following the Letter of the Law (John Finklea, 1975–1978)

The CDC was looking for a replacement to fill Key's vacancy. A CDC search committee recommended Dr. John Finklea as a candidate, and he and CDC Director Sensor met. Sensor agreed with the choice and submitted Finklea's name up the line to the Secretary of HHS's office to make the appointment.[31]

In April 1975, DHEW Secretary Caspar Weinberger named Finklea director of NIOSH in the midst of congressional complaints that NIOSH was too soft on industry, industry claims of sloppy research, and organized labor accusations of delays in sharing health information. Finklea was an epidemiologist and formerly served as the director of EPA's National Environmental Research Center at Research Triangle Park in North Carolina, where he advocated the need to control sulfates emitted into the ambient air. Strong reaction from the utility industry preceded his removal from that post.

One condition struck between Finklea and Sensor was that Sensor would protect Finklea from political backlash as he mounted a major effort at producing criteria documents and recommended standards. With NIOSH's limited resources, Finklea chose to direct the researchers under him toward the completion of criteria documents. Emboldened by Sensor's reputation as a tough bureaucratic survivor and by his pact to foil attacks counter to the protection of workers' health, Finklea took an aggressive stance for the protection of workers, making enemies along the way. Following are examples of his experience:

- He pushed the NIOSH staff hard to inform and generate criteria documents, leading to internal resentment.[31]
- He closed the Salt Lake City field station, transferring the program to Morgantown, West Virginia, to consolidate mining research, causing added resentment.
- He suggested that medical malpractice existed among company medical directors in their use of prophylactic chelation therapy for lead-exposed workers.[44]
- He wrote "Dear Colleague" letters to company medical directors alerting them to NIOSH *Current Intelligence Bulletins* and thereby establishing hazards as recognized under the general duty clause of § 5(a) of the OSH Act.
- He suggested that diesel exhaust in underground coal mines may be complicit in causing lung cancer,[45] exciting mine operators to throw expletives his way.

Finklea worked to accelerate health hazard research, especially in the chemical industry. Within months of his appointment, Finklea had NIOSH issuing a steady stream of *Current Intelligence Bulletins* on toxic substances. He encouraged cooperation between NIOSH and OSHA, and in 1978, NIOSH and OSHA jointly published the *Pocket Guide to Chemical Hazards,* developed from the SCP. Courts affirmed NIOSH's authority to enter workplaces, examine medical records, and disseminate research findings. Under Finklea's leadership, NIOSH issued a register of 100 chemical compounds considered potential carcinogens. He increased awareness for birth defects, miscarriages, and other reproduction-related problems stemming from chemical and radiological exposure. In addition, Finklea called on Congress to adopt toxic substances legislation related to carcinogenic pesticides and Kepone when the Toxic Substances Control Act of 1976 was being debated.[46] Over Finklea's tenure, NIOSH identified 65 potentially dangerous substances found at job sites compared with 23 such warnings issued during the first four years of NIOSH's existence. Finklea announced the creation of ERCs in 1977.

In January 1977, President Jimmy Carter named Joseph A. Califano Jr. as Secretary of HHS. Two weeks later, Secretary Califano fired Sensor in the aftermath of a controversy surrounding the swine flu campaign. But more than that, Secretary Califano believed in "out with the old and in with the new" and replaced all of the directors of USPHS agencies except for the NIH director. Serving at the pleasure of the Secretary of HHS, Finklea was vulnerable now that his pact of protection with Sensor was void. Two months after Sensor was fired, Secretary Califano named Dr. William Foege as the new CDC director.[31]

In 1972, before Finklea became NIOSH director, NIOSH had published a criteria document with a recommendation to control exposure to prevent acute and chronic beryllium disease,[47] recommending an interim standard of 2 µg/m^3. Beryllium was used in making atomic weapons. Much happened in 1975, when OSHA asked NIOSH to review the evidence of beryllium as a potential carcinogen, and in September, NIOSH concluded that it was a potential carcinogen.[48] Animal studies had indicated the carcinogenic potential of beryllium, and by 1975, three NIOSH field studies indicated that beryllium was associated with lung cancer. As a result, OSHA issued a proposed standard for beryllium in 1975 at 1 µg/m^3. In December 1975, Finklea wrote a letter to OSHA Administrator Morton Corn amending the recommended standard for beryllium as a carcinogen at a level of 0.5 µg/m^3.[49] The agency held a hearing for the beryllium standard in 1977,[48] at which Finklea's deputy, Edward Baier, testified on the carcinogenic potential of beryllium.[50] He related that the 1972 criteria document did not recommend a standard based upon carcinogenicity since the evidence available at that time was that it was an animal carcinogen. Finklea and Baier updated their recommendation that beryllium be controlled as a carcinogen now that human carcinogenicity had been associated with beryllium exposure. A December 2, 1977, issue of *Science* reported on a battle between Finklea and two beryllium industry companies over several months. The NIOSH position was that beryllium was a human carcinogen, and the industry position was that it was not. Fearing failure in the rule-making process regarding feasibility, the industry challenged the science, calling NIOSH studies "shoddy." Investigators for NIOSH openly acknowledged weaknesses in their three studies, some emanating from the lack of industry cooperation. Over the telephone, Finklea challenged the veracity of industry expert claims, and the industry claimed that he made "naked threats" to their witnesses prior to the earlier OSHA hearing.[51]

In short order, Secretary Califano decided to remove Finklea as NIOSH director. After several meetings between Foege and Finklea, on January 6, 1978, Finklea resigned.[52] Foege named Dr. J. Donald Millar as interim NIOSH director. Millar had served on Sensor's 1975 search committee that had recommended Finklea as director. Under Finklea's three-year directorship, 55% of all NIOSH criteria documents with recommended standards were issued, as shown in Figure 9-1 along with the number of criteria documents and recommended standards produced

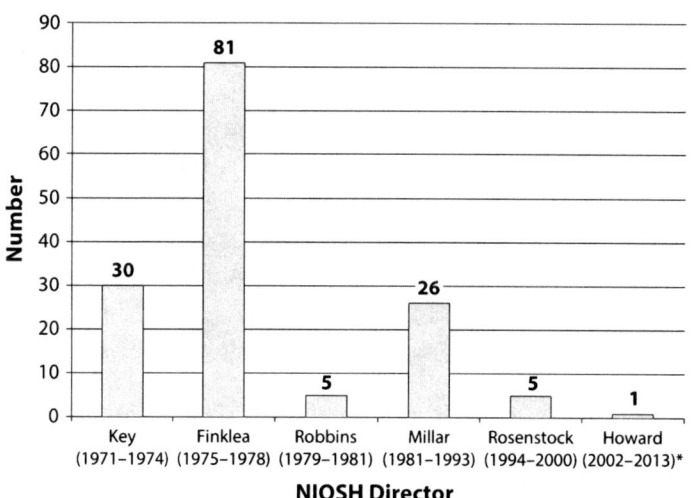

Note: NIOSH = National Institute for Occupational Safety and Health.
*Howard's first term ended in 2008; he was reappointed later in 2009.

Figure 9-1. Number of recommended standards and criteria issued by the National Institute for Occupational Safety and Health (NIOSH) to the Secretary of Labor by each NIOSH director.

under other NIOSH directors. In 1977, the Government Accountability Office concluded that at the rate that NIOSH and OSHA were issuing standards, it would "take more than a century to establish needed standards for substances already identified as hazards."[53]

The beryllium industry continued to frame beryllium as a benign cancer-causing agent. Through its public relations company, an expert panel called the Beryllium Industry Scientific Advisory Committee was convened that challenged the quality and credibility of NIOSH studies. One month after Finklea's resignation, this panel of eight consultants charged NIOSH investigators with prejudice and incompetence in a letter addressed to Secretary Califano and Secretary of Labor Ray Marshall.[54] Two weeks later, the dominant company in the two-company industry sent a copy of the letter to the Office of Management and Budget (OMB). At about the same time, OSHA received letters from prominent congressional representatives and senators demanding a "truly independent review" of the science behind OSHA's proposed rule.[55,56] The CDC convened a seven-member "blue ribbon panel" to examine the science. Foege charged the panel to answer three questions (verbatim), which the panel answered (paraphrased), as follows:[57]

1. Question: Are the animal studies credible in showing beryllium carcinogenicity in at least two studies? Answer: Yes, with some qualifications.
2. Question: Is beryllium copper alloy a carcinogen? Answer: Insufficient data are available to answer this question. A very low dose in a small number of animals has been examined, but studies of human populations are needed, and the alloy needs to be tested for carcinogenicity.
3. Question: Is there evidence indicating that beryllium is a carcinogen in man? Answer: The epidemiologic evidence suggests that beryllium is a carcinogen in humans. Beryllium should be considered as a carcinogen for exposed workers.

The attacking-the-science card had been played, but the industry had another card up its sleeve. Because of national defense, the Secretaries of Defense and Energy convinced Secretary Marshall in 1979 to place the beryllium rule making on hold. Outside of rulemaking, the issue of national security was used to pressure Secretary Marshall to drop the promulgation of an occupational standard for beryllium. The industry had trumped the science and the regulators; OSHA Administrator Dr. Eula Bingham expressed her disappointment with the decision.[56]

9.4.3. Strong Advocacy (Anthony Robbins, 1979–1981)

Secretary Califano named Dr. Anthony Robbins NIOSH director in 1979. In the years 1979 to 1981, Robbins moved the NIOSH focus from generating criteria documents and recommending standards to a broader agenda. This agenda followed three principles:[58]

1. A focus on control technology and substitution for hazardous agents was to be pursued until workers were safe.
2. Worker right-to-know was emphasized by reporting research results broadly to the affected workers and through public media, and assisting anyone capable of improving worker safety and health.
3. Traditional public health through field investigations was increased along with a three-pronged approach to epidemiology: micro-epidemiology by investigating individual cases, meso-epidemiology by conducting industry-wide studies, and macro-epidemiology by collecting and analyzing nationwide data regarding hazards and health effects.

Robbins also collaborated closely with OSHA Administrator Bingham, and John Froines moved from OSHA to NIOSH as deputy director. Robbins worked with Bingham and Dr. David P. Rall, the director of the National Institute of the Environmental Health Sciences (NIEHS), in the creation of the National Toxicology Program at NIEHS. Regarding field investigations, Robbins recruited a substantial number of CDC Epidemic Intelligence Officers to NIOSH to conduct HHEs.[59] In 1980, NIOSH funded its first state-based occupational health cooperative agreements.

In 1979, Senator Richard Schweiker (R) of Pennsylvania sought to exempt from safety inspections all employers, large or small, regardless of industry, who had good safety records. They would still have to conform to OSHA regulations and be subject to health inspections. Schweiker was an original supporter of the OSHAct, but he believed that Congress had mistakenly cast the DoL as a "policeman" for all the nation's workplaces. He hoped to focus enforcement on the smaller number of workplaces in a policy of "worst first" and stimulate cooperation and voluntary compliance in the rest. Organized labor campaigned strongly against the Schweiker amendment to the OSH Act, claiming that his proposal would dilute enforcement, and Robbins joined in the campaign. The amendment was defeated in 1980.[60]

When Ronald Reagan took office as president in 1981, he named Senator Schweiker as Secretary of HHS, home of the CDC, the parent agency for NIOSH. Schweiker recalled Robbins's strong advocacy against his amendment and removed him as director of NIOSH. Moreover, Schweiker thought NIOSH a rogue organization and considered its abolition. To gain control over the "politicization" of NIOSH, he decided to move its headquarters from Rockville, Maryland, which is close to Washington, DC, to its parent organization's headquarters in Atlanta.

9.4.4. Leading Work-Related Diseases and Injuries (J. Donald Millar, 1981–1993)

In 1981, Secretary of HHS Schweiker named Donald Millar, a CDC veteran and interim NIOSH director after Finklea had been forced out, as director of NIOSH. He served two six-year terms as director, whereas former director Key resigned after three years, and both Finklea and Robbins were fired.[32] Millar was expected to bring NIOSH into the mainstream of public health prevention efforts and practice—and enhance and maintain NIOSH's scientific credibility. Moreover, he was to move the NIOSH headquarters from Rockville to Atlanta where CDC was headquartered. Millar named veteran NIOSH toxicologist, Elliott Harris, as his deputy and strengthened peer review requirements at NIOSH and established the Board of Scientific Councilors (BSC) to review and recommend improvements to NIOSH programs. The first meeting of the BSC occurred in 1984. The national cadre of industrial hygienists increased from about 5,000 in the 1970s to 12,000 by the end of the 1980s.[61]

Millar strengthened the safety research program, emphasizing the epidemiology of injuries.[61] In the early 1980s, he established the Fatal Accident Circumstances and Epidemiology program to conduct field investigations of occupational fatalities, and the National Traumatic Occupational Fatality system that used death certificates to include self-employed worker deaths, which was a forerunner to the BLS Census of Fatal Occupational Injuries system. In 1987, the Sentinel Event Notification System for Occupational Risk program was established and landmark studies of the hazards of vermiculite from Libby, Montana, were published. In 1990, NIOSH established the Centers for Agricultural Disease and Injury Research, Education, and Prevention and funded a construction safety and health research center at the Center to Protect Workers' Rights, (i.e., the Center for Construction Research and Training). The CDC's *MMWR* was used routinely to inform the public of occupational hazards and their control.

Under Millar, NIOSH suggested a list of 10 leading work-related diseases and injuries in 1983 as a basis for forming research strategies for improving national occupational health and safety.[62,63] The problems on the list were selected based on three criteria: (1) the frequency of the condition, (2) the severity of the condition in the individual case, and (3) the preventability of the condition. The list is shown below:[64]

- Occupational lung diseases—asbestosis, byssinosis, silicosis, and coal worker's pneumoconiosis, lung cancer, occupational asthma[65]
- Musculoskeletal injuries and disorders—disorders of the back, trunk, upper extremity, neck, lower extremity; traumatically induced Raynaud's phenomenon[66]
- Occupational cancers—leukemia, mesothelioma, cancers of the bladder, nose, and liver[67]
- Severe occupational traumatic injuries—amputations, fractures, eye loss, lacerations, and traumatic deaths[68]
- Cardiovascular diseases—hypertension, coronary artery disease, acute myocardial infarction[69]
- Disorders of reproduction—infertility, spontaneous abortion, teratogenesis[70]
- Neurotoxic disorders—peripheral neuropathy, toxic encephalitis, psychoses, extreme personality changes (exposure-related)[71]
- Noise-induced loss of hearing—a discovery arising from this priority was exposures to ototoxic chemicals[72]
- Dermatologic conditions—dermatoses, thermal burns, chemical burns, contusions[73]
- Psychological disorders—neuroses, personality disorders, alcoholism, drug dependency[74]

At the end of Millar's second term in 1993, Richard Lemen became the acting director. Lemen convened a 1994 NIOSH conference, "Silent Epidemics in the Workplace," regarding workplace violence, asbestos-related disease, noise-induced hearing loss, and musculoskeletal disorders.

9.4.5. National Occupational Research Agenda
(Linda Rosenstock, 1994–2000)

Secretary of HHS Donna Shalala named Dr. Linda Rosenstock as NIOSH director on April 11, 1994. Rosenstock moved from her position at the University of Washington in Seattle, where she was the director of the Occupational and Environmental Medicine Program. Her appointment by Secretary Shalala came with a promise of a return of the NIOSH headquarters back to Washington, with offices in the DHHS Humphrey Building. Rosenstock said the relocation of headquarters would enhance the visibility of NIOSH with an advantage of educating people there of the importance of occupational safety and health. The move would mean co-location with sister federal agencies OSHA, MSHA, EPA, and NIH. Moreover, her credibility had been secured with OSHA Administrator Joe Dear, since she had formerly worked with him in Washington State. She had also developed a relationship with the U.S. Department of Energy (DoE) and its worker protection program. Her priorities included delivering timely information of current workplace concerns, focusing on emerging technologies, and expanding extramural programs. A NIOSH presence remained in Atlanta under Deputy Director Lemen.[75]

In 1997, mine safety research authority under the Mine Act was transferred to NIOSH following the elimination of the BoM in the DoI. This transfer added laboratories to NIOSH in Pittsburgh and Spokane with a substantial increase in safety research and engineering personnel.

In 1996, NIOSH issued recommendations for preventing workplace homicides and assaults, and in 1999, it issued recommendations for preventing work-related needlestick injuries. Recognizing that the research effort was much broader than its programs, NIOSH launched the National Occupational Research Agenda (NORA) as a stakeholder partnership to stimulate innovative research and improved safe workplaces. Unveiled in 1996, NORA became a research framework for NIOSH and the nation. Diverse parties collaborated to identify the most critical issues in workplace safety and health based upon relevant information: (1) the number of workers at risk for a particular injury or illness, (2) the seriousness of the hazard or issue, and (3) the probability that new information and approaches would make a difference. Participants in NORA included stakeholders from universities, large and small businesses, professional societies, government agencies, and worker organizations. The collaboration resulted in 21 research priorities grouped into three categories, as shown in Table 9-3.[76]

Table 9-3. National Occupational Research Agenda Priorities by Category

Disease and Injury	Work Environment and Workforce	Research Tools and Approaches
Allergic and irritant dermatitis	Emerging technologies	Cancer research methods
Asthma and chronic obstructive pulmonary disease	Indoor environment	Control technology and personal protective equipment
	Mixed exposures	
	Organization of work	Exposure assessment methods
Fertility and pregnancy abnormalities	Special populations at risk	Health services research
		Intervention effectiveness research
Hearing loss		Risk assessment methods
Infectious diseases		Social and economic consequences of workplace injury and illness
Low-back disorders		
Musculoskeletal disorders of the upper extremities		Surveillance research methods
Traumatic injuries		

The priorities addressed both current and emerging problems, and partnerships were struck in implementing research toward these priority areas. Some partnerships were with labor and management, others were in the development of safer technologies, and others involved joint funding of research grants with institutes from within NIH. At the end of Rosenstock's six-year term in 2000, NIOSH's Dr. Kathleen M. Rest was named acting director.

9.4.6. National Academy Review (John Howard, 2002–2008, 2009)

Secretary of HHS Tommy G. Thompson selected Dr. John Howard as the new director of NIOSH on July 15, 2002. From 1991 to 2002, Howard had been the director of the Division of Occupational Safety and Health in California.[77]

Under Howard, NIOSH shifted its research efforts to emerging technologies and practical applications for new research findings. This included an initiative called "research-to-practice" (r2p) to ensure that NIOSH's findings would turn into practices and products that would ultimately benefit workers. He emphasized research on mining, nanotechnology, job stress, and ergonomics. After the 9/11 terrorist attacks, Howard oversaw federally funded health care programs for responders, including many laborers who became ill as a result of their work at the stricken Twin Towers in New York City. In 2005, NIOSH provided technical and humanitarian assistance after Hurricane Katrina.

Howard used the NORA priorities to conduct program reviews required by OMB. The Government Performance and Results Act of 1993 requires federal agencies to provide strategic and performance plans and reports. The President's Management Council released the Program Assessment Rating Tool (PART) as developed by OMB in 2002, which provided a method to assess the performance of program activities. The purpose of PART was to require federal agencies to evaluate their programs' overall effectiveness in four areas: (1) program purpose and design, (2) strategic planning, (3) program management, and (4) program results and accountability.[78]

To pursue this requirement, NIOSH enlisted the National Academy of Sciences to review eight NIOSH programs from 2005 to 2008. The purpose of the reviews was to assess the impact on policy or outcomes and relevance regarding worker protection in each program and to identify emerging issues. The National Academy and its National Research Council and Institute of Medicine provided independent expert reviews of the relevance and impact of the eight NORA programs. Relevance addressed the NIOSH mission in the

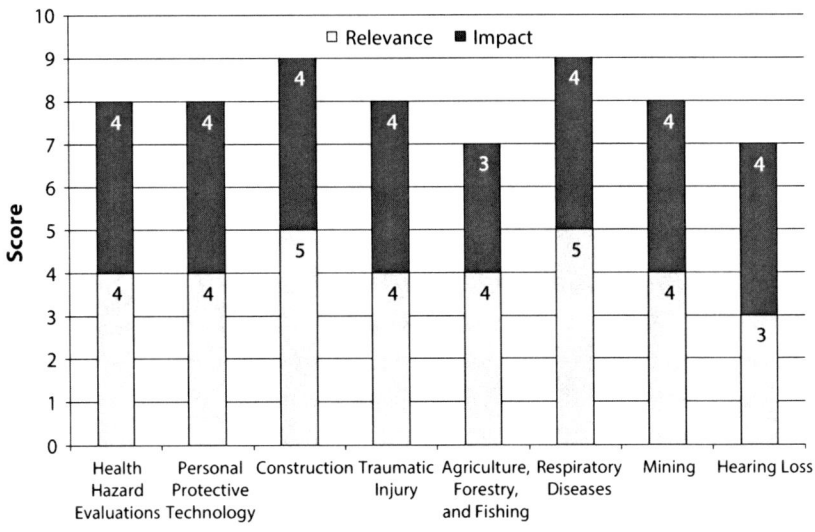

Note: NIOSH = National Institute for Occupational Safety and Health. 5 is the highest score.

Figure 9-2. Scores for relevance and impact by the National Academy of Sciences for National Institute for Occupational Safety and Health programs.

targeting of new and significant emerging research areas that appeared especially important, and impact addressed progress in reducing workplace illness and injuries through research. The scoring from these reviews is shown in Figure 9-2, and the programs are described below:

1. HHE Program: The HHE program responded to requests from employers, labor unions, and federal and state agencies to investigate previously unknown potential occupational health hazards or known health hazards found in new occupational settings. The academy found that the program had a positive impact on workforce conditions, responded well during public health emergencies, and offered exemplars in training programs for occupational health professionals.[79]
2. Personal Protective Technology (PPT) Program: Created when the National Personal Protective Technology Laboratory was established in 1999, the program consolidated the congressionally mandated respirator certification program under the Mine Act with research and standards development activities in advancing the state of knowledge and application of PPT. The academy found that the program made meaningful contributions to improving workers' safety and health.[80]
3. Construction Research Program: In 1990, Congress directed NIOSH to develop a comprehensive prevention program directed at safety and health problems affecting construction workers by expanding existing NIOSH activities in areas of surveillance, research, and intervention. The academy found that the program made meaningful contributions to improving construction worker safety and health and was significantly engaged in appropriate transfer activities for program results.[81]
4. Traumatic Injury Research Program: NIOSH is tasked with conducting research and making recommendations for the prevention of occupational injuries. The academy concluded that the research addressed priority areas and led to demonstrated effects on some end intermediate (research-to-practice) or end (reduced injuries and diseases) outcomes. It also concluded that the program's strategic goals were focused on major contributors to occupational injuries and deaths and to populations and groups at disproportionate risk.[82]
5. Agriculture, Forestry, and Fishing Research Program: In 1989, Congress directed NIOSH to develop a comprehensive prevention program directed at safety and health problems affecting agriculture, forestry, and fishing

sector workers in areas of surveillance, research, and intervention. The academy found that the program made meaningful contributions regarding knowledge to improve worker safety and health in the sector. However, research varied in relevance among its elements, and knowledge transfer activities were moderate, owing mainly to populations of self-employed workers and their resistance to interventions from the government, particularly regarding improvements to agricultural safety and health. There was little evidence that research activities contributed to reducing workplace injury and illness.[83]

6. Respiratory Diseases Research Program: The National Institute for Occupational Safety and Health had a range of research activities in this program with a focus on work-related airway diseases, interstitial lung diseases, respiratory infectious diseases, and respiratory cancers. The academy concluded that most elements of the program made major contributions to worker safety and health outcomes.[84]

7. Mining Research Program: This program was authorized by the Mine Act, which is the subject of the next chapter. The academy considered that contributions to workplace improvements were major in respiratory disease and traumatic injury prevention, moderate in hearing loss and ground failure prevention, and likely in disaster and musculoskeletal injury prevention. Moreover, it found that program outputs were incorporated into stakeholder operations and training.[85]

8. Hearing Loss Research Program: This program conducted research to contribute to effective hearing loss prevention, reduce hearing loss through the use of PPE; develop engineering controls to reduce noise exposures; and improve understanding of occupational hearing loss including exposure to ototoxic chemicals. The academy found that over the past decade, the program made meaningful contributions to improving worker safety and health and moderate contribution to improvements used by stakeholders.[86]

9.4.7. The Research Councils

In 2006, the NORA emphasis changed toward a sector-based structure, which was in accord with the OSHAct § 20 authorization for industry-wide studies.

The approach was made to better move r2p within workplaces, which was evidenced by the programs in the Construction Research Program; the Agriculture, Forestry, and Fishing Research Program; and the Mining Research Program. The national agenda was developed and implemented through 10 NORA Sector Councils, as described in Table 9-4,[87-96] to improve occupational safety and health through research and partnerships. The NORA Sector Council membership built broad and diverse participation with organizational members (e.g., trade associations, labor groups, governmental agencies,

Table 9-4. National Occupational Research Agenda Councils

Sector	Target Population*
Agriculture, forestry, and fishing	More than a million paid workers in 2005 (and many more self-employed workers) faced risks that included animal handling, falls, infectious diseases, overexertion, tractor overturns, chemicals, and machinery.[87]
Construction	An estimated nine million public and private sector workers in 2011 faced risks that included motor vehicles, falls, overexertion, and chemicals.[88]
Health care and social assistance	An estimated 19 million paid workers in 2010 faced risks that included infectious diseases, workplace violence, overexertion, chemicals, shift work, and psychosocial stressors.[89]
Manufacturing	An estimated 14 million paid workers in 2011 faced risks that included machinery, repetitive motion, overexertion, chemicals, and shift work.[90]
Mining (not counting the oil and gas extraction subsector)	More than 300,000 paid workers in 2005 faced risks that included falling materials, explosions, fires, powered haulage, overexertion, electrical equipment, and exposure to particulates and dusts including diesel emissions, coal dust, and silica dust.[91]
Oil and gas extraction	More than 400,000 paid workers in 2010 faced risks such as motor vehicle crashes, contact with tools and equipment, fire and explosions, exposure to chemicals, and shift work.[92]
Public safety	About 1.8 million paid workers and 800,000 volunteer firefighters in 2005 faced risks that include infectious diseases, workplace violence, overexertion, chemicals, shift work, and psychosocial stressors.[93]
Services	Nearly 65 million paid workers in 2011 faced risks that included workplace violence, overexertion, shift work, and psychosocial stressors.[94]
Transportation, warehousing, and utilities	An estimated six million paid workers in 2005 faced risks that included motor vehicle crashes, workplace violence, overexertion, shift work, and psychosocial stressors.[95]
Wholesale and retail trade	Nearly 20 million paid workers (including many young workers) in 2011 faced risks that included workplace violence, overexertion, machinery, chemicals, shift work, and psychosocial stressors.[96]

*Self-employed workers add to the magnitude of these populations.

and professional organizations) and individual members (e.g., researchers and safety and health professionals).[97]

9.4.8. The Argument About Reducing NIOSH Status

In April 2005, CDC Director Dr. Julie Gerberding announced a reorganization of the CDC to "cope with the challenges of 21st-century health threats."[98] In a reversal of President Bill Clinton's "reinventing government" position to reduce layers of government, the reorganization established coordinating centers with the stated purpose to "help CDC's scientists combine their expertise to solve public health problems, streamline the flow of information for leadership decision making, and better leverage the expertise of CDC partners."[97] The reorganization put NIOSH into a Coordinating Center for Environmental Health, Injury Prevention, and Occupational Health along with the Agency for Toxic Substances and Disease Registry, the National Center for Environmental Health, and National Center for Injury Control and Prevention.

The four living former heads of NIOSH—Key, Robbins, Millar, and Rosenstock—collaborated in writing a letter to the editor of *Science* critical of the reorganization and its adverse effect on NIOSH.[99] They were concerned that the reorganization would reduce NIOSH one more layer lower, having to report through the Coordinating Center director to the CDC director. This would diminish NIOSH visibility and lower its status further relative to its partners at the Assistant Secretary level in the DoL: OSHA and MSHA. The four former NIOSH directors also sent a letter to Secretary of HHS Thompson expressing "great concern" regarding the reorganization.[100] Arguably, this also would be an additional layer of management that would tap overhead funds from the NIOSH appropriated budget and might diffuse appropriated NIOSH funds into other CDC priorities. Suspicion arose that one of Gerberding's primary advisors on the reorganization was the chairman of the CDC Foundation board of directors and former chair and CEO of UPS, the company that had led the campaign against the OSHA ergonomics standard.[42]

The CDC announcement created a broad opposition from both NIOSH advocates and partners against the reorganization. Secretary Thompson also received a letter from former OSHA administrators Dr. Eula Bingham, Gerald Scannell, and Joe Dear, as well as former MSHA Administrator J. Davitt McAteer and former Assistant Secretary of Energy for Environment, Safety, and Health Dr. David Michaels. Scannell served under President George H.W. Bush and Bingham under President Carter. The others served in the Clinton administration. They asked Secretary Thompson to suspend the reorganization, arguing that moving NIOSH lower in the departmental structure would obscure its distinct identity and special role and would diminish its effectiveness in helping OSHA and MSHA to bring science-based considerations to the rule-making process. The congressional intent was not for the head of OSHA to communicate with someone five levels down in the bureaucracy. Other letters came to Secretary Thompson from the AFL-CIO, the American College of Occupational and Environmental Medicine, the American Association of Occupational Health Nurses, the American Society of Safety Engineers (ASSE), and the American Industrial Hygiene Association (AIHA).[100]

Despite opposition from a broad array of forces, the CDC moved ahead to relocate NIOSH within the Coordinating Center, to take effect on October 1, 2005. However, Congress intervened. The Senate Appropriations Committee, reviewing the fiscal year 2005 DHHS budget passed by the House, added language directing the CDC to make no changes in NIOSH's operating procedure or organizational structure and to ensure that no funds or personnel were transferred from NIOSH to other components of the CDC. Until reconciled with the Senate, the CDC-NIOSH structure remained static under a temporary, continuing resolution until a regular appropriations bill was adopted.[101] The CDC's reorganization went ahead but without moving NIOSH to a lower level in the organization.

As Howard's six-year term approached its end, the Laborers' Health and Safety Fund of North America was among the many organizations that pushed for his reappointment. Ignoring such endorsements, the CDC announced on July 3, 2008, that Gerberding met with Howard to inform him that the agency would begin a search for a new NIOSH director. Howard's term ended a week and half later, with Christine M. Blanche named as acting director of NIOSH.[102]

Sharp criticisms pummeled Gerberding from labor unions, members of the House and Senate, the U.S. Chamber of Commerce, the AFL-CIO, ASSE, AIHA, both of New York's senators, and New York Governor David Paterson (D). New York Democratic Representatives Carolyn Maloney and Jerrold Nadler protested Howard's dismissal alongside 9/11 responders at Ground Zero on July 8. Representative Maloney said,

> Only the [George W.] Bush administration would fire a respected public servant who has received near-universal praise for doing a good job.

Dr. Howard is out of a job because he wanted to help the heroes of 9/11 and his superiors didn't. We demand that the administration take back this outrageous slap at sick 9/11 responders and reappoint Dr. Howard to a well-deserved second term.[102]

Some members of Congress believed that the Bush administration wanted Howard out because he was pushing for costly 9/11 health programs, since he had coordinated and championed health programs over the previous two years, including screening, monitoring, and treatment, for workers who were sickened at Ground Zero.[103] Others believed that it came from running afoul of Gerberding in the failed reorganization plan four years earlier.[102] Another explanation of the "icy" relationship between Howard and Gerberding was when Howard, as the California OSHA Office director, had cited Gerberding for refusing to buy safer needles when she ran the HIV prevention program at the San Francisco General Hospital.[104]

With the change of administration to President Barack Obama, Secretary of HHS Kathleen Sebelius named Howard to reassume the dual role of NIOSH director and the World Trade Center Programs Coordinator for HHS on September 8, 2009.[105] Howard continued to address the NIOSH challenge of shifting from agents with a widespread risk associated with chemical or physical agents like asbestos and radiation to current hazards requiring different design strategies for eliminating risks, such as musculoskeletal disorders and work-related stress. Thus, NIOSH shifted from a traditional and specific focus on health protection and initiated a Total Worker Health program that integrates health protection and promotion. This initiative brings together the two-part purpose of the OSHAct: (1) "to assure so far as possible every working man and woman in the Nation safe and healthful working conditions," and (2) "to preserve our human resources."

The Total Worker Health program seeks to promote workplace programs, policies, and practices that result in healthier and more productive employees through a simultaneous focus on disease prevention, health promotion, and accommodations to age, family, and life stage. The initiative incorporates NIOSH's foundational commitment to workplaces free of recognized hazards into a broader consideration of the factors that affect worker health and well-being. The goal is to integrate state-of-the-art occupational health, health promotion, and chronic disease research findings to benefit working-age populations, regardless of workplace size, work sector, or region of the country.[106] Other NIOSH programs outside of the OSHAct are addressed in later chapters.

9.5. NIOSH AT COURT

The Secretary of Health and Human Services is authorized to make inspections and question employers and employees as provided in section 8 of this Act in order to carry out his functions and responsibilities under this section.
—§ 20(b). Occupational Safety and Health Act of 1970

Two legal issues have brought NIOSH to court. One issue is its subpoena power for access to records, and the other issue concerns its power of right-of-entry. Additional legal issues concern its involvement in standards setting and its authority under the Mine Act for certifying respirators.[107]

9.5.1. Access to Records

NIOSH exercises its authority for access to records under § 8(b) of the OSHAct. With clear judicial backing, NIOSH has the power of subpoena to access records from employers or from third parties (i.e., insurance companies). The authority is the same as that used by OSHA. An employer's lack of compliance with a subpoena can result in a contempt citation from the court against the employer.[107]

An issue brought by companies regarding NIOSH access to records is employee privacy. For the most part, courts have concurred with plaintiffs that privacy must be protected, and NIOSH must assure the confidentiality of employee records. In this regard, a claim was made against NIOSH that the employers release the records with personal identifiers marked out. NIOSH needs the personal identifiers to conduct epidemiology studies to associate causal factors of a health effect with the health effect. The courts sided with NIOSH on this issue, stating that the benefit to society outweighed the interest for privacy.[107] Employee consent arose as an issue with a ruling that employees should be notified of a NIOSH request for access to records; a nonresponse would imply consent and that a company must release the records.

Plaintiffs in a case must have standing, meaning that they are or potentially can be injured in the legal sense by the action of a defendant. The issue of standing by a company to resist disclosure of employee records to NIOSH when the affected party is the employee has been addressed by the courts in two ways. One way is when companies have possession of the records and thus have standing. The other way is when employers or insurance companies may be affected by a liability claim because of the possession of records.[107]

Another objection to NIOSH access to records is the protection of medical records based upon physician-patient privilege found in state law. This argument has failed since there is no federal law that protects this privilege. Another defense arose against NIOSH in California with the claim that access to records subverts the California OSHA office's authority. The court stated, "It was the intent of Congress to grant the Secretary [of HHS] the widest possible powers to engage in research and study of industrial problems."[107]

9.5.2. Right-of-Entry

Under the OSHAct and the Mine Act, NIOSH has the right to enter private workplaces to carry out its investigations and inspections. All court cases brought on this issue have been brought under the OSHAct. Cases that apply to OSHA can also apply to NIOSH regarding right-of-entry (e.g., *Marshall v. Barlow's, Inc.*, 1978). The difference lies with a criterion of "reasonable legislative or administrative standards" in which OSHA has enforcement authority but NIOSH does not. However, NIOSH has research authority that warrants its right-of-entry. The most contentious issue arises when an employee or an employee representative (i.e., a union) requests an HHE from NIOSH. The institute has this authority, as documented in its regulation regarding procedures for entry; NIOSH authority for entry has been upheld when it is based on a research protocol or for technical assistance to OSHA.

The scope of a warrant has also been raised as an issue. The courts have found that NIOSH investigations are limited only by the OSHAct language of reasonable limits and manner under § 8(a) and the warrant clause of the U.S. Constitution. Reasonable limits include obtaining employee consent for physical examinations, investigations at NIOSH's expense, and avoiding unreasonable disruption of employer operations. In one case regarding an HHE in which the NIOSH regulation requires the employer provide space for a physical examination, an employer argued that NIOSH must provide compensation for the "taking of property." The court sided with NIOSH as a reasonable authority given to NIOSH under the congressional purpose of promoting health.[107]

BUREAU OF MINES CLOSURE NARRATIVE

In response to a spate of mine explosions and the need to understand their prevention, Congress passed the Organic Act (Public Law 61-179) on May 16, 1910, establishing the BoM. Indeed, its initial mission was to provide the mining industry with information on blasting materials and techniques that could be used safely in the presence of flammable mine gases and dust. One of the first actions of the new BoM was to request and accept details of USPHS medical officers for assignment to mine rescue cars (railroad) placed around the country. During the early 20th century, USPHS predecessor agencies to NIOSH had worked closely with the BoM, including conducting toxicology studies in the 1920s. Except for a short stint under the authority of the Secretary of Commerce and future President Herbert C. Hoover, the BoM was part of the DoI. Over the years into the 1990s, BoM had made considerable progress in improving the health and safety of miners by providing much of the breakthrough technology that reduced fatal and nonfatal injuries and occupational diseases in the mining industry. After 85 years of existence, in the summer of 1995, the House proposed the abolition of the BoM. In September 1995, the Conference Committee of Congress recommended the closure of BoM within an unprecedented 90 days. Congress also directed that the BoM health and safety research programs in Pittsburgh and Spokane be assigned on an interim basis to the DoE. Then in October 1996, these programs were permanently transferred to NIOSH. The transfers included 413 positions, with 336 in Pittsburgh and 77 in Spokane. NIOSH named an Associate Director for Mining in charge of these programs and established the Pittsburgh Research Laboratory and the Spokane Research Laboratory.[108]

REFERENCES

1. Dunn CM, Chadwick G. *Protecting Study Volunteers in Research: A Manual for Investigative Sites*. Boston, MA: CenterWatch, Inc.;1999.
2. Kotelchuck D. Asbestos: "The funeral dress of kings"—and others. In Rosner D, Markowitz G, eds., *Dying for Work*. Bloomington, IN: Indiana University Press;1987:192–207.

3. Brodeur P. *Outrageous Misconduct: The Asbestos Industry on Trial*. New York, NY: Pantheon Books;1985.

4. National Institute for Occupational Safety and Health. Criteria for a recommended standard: occupational exposure to asbestos. HSM 72-10267. 1972. Available at: http://www.cdc.gov/niosh/docs/72-10267/pdfs/7210267.pdf. Accessed September 22, 2012.

5. Greenspan A. Remarks by Chairman Alan Greenspan (Federal Reserve Board) at: Meetings of the American Economic Association; January 3, 2004; San Diego, CA.

6. Public Health Service Act, 42 U.S.C. 241, Ch. 6A, Subch. XXXI. Public Health Service. § 241 Research and investigations generally (1912).

7. Occupational Safety and Health Administration. Susan Harwood training grants program. Available at: http://www.osha.gov/dte/sharwood/index.html. Accessed November 28, 2012.

8. Barab J. *Hearing before the House Subcommittee on Workforce Protections Committee on Education and the Workforce*, 112th Cong, 2nd Sess (June 28, 2012) (statement of Jordan Barab, Deputy Assistant Secretary for Occupational Safety and Health, U.S. Department of Labor).

9. Occupational Safety and Health Administration. OSHA fact sheet: the OSHA consultation program. Available at: http://www.osha.gov/OshDoc/data_General_Facts/factsheet-consultations.pdf. Accessed November 28, 2012.

10. Blosser F. *Primer on Occupational Safety and Health*. Washington, DC: Bureau of National Affairs;1992.

11. Bureau of Labor Statistics. History of BLS safety and health statistical programs. October 10, 2012. Available at: http://www.bls.gov/iif/oshhist.htm. Accessed November 27, 2012.

12. Statistics, 29 U.S.C. § 673 (2003).

13. Little JW, Eaton TA, Smith GR. *Cases and Materials on Workers' Compensation*. 3rd ed. St. Paul, MN: West Publishing Co.;1993.

14. National Commission on State Workmen's Compensation Laws. *Report of the National Commission on State Workmen's Compensation Laws*. Washington, DC: U.S. Government Printing Office;1972.

15. U.S. Chamber of Commerce. *2004 Analysis of Workers' Compensation Laws*. Washington, DC: U.S. Chamber of Commerce;2004.

16. Ashford NA Caldart CC. *Technology, Law, and the Working Environment.* Washington, DC: Island Press;1996.

17. Kerr JW. Relation of the Public Health Service to problems of industrial hygiene. *Am J Pub Health.* 1917;7:776–782.

18. Myers ML, McGlothlin JD. Matchmakers' "Phossy Jaw" eradicated. *AIHA Journal.* April 1996; 57:330-332.

19. Doyle HN. The Federal Industrial Hygiene Agency: A History of the Division of Occupational Health, U.S. Public Health Service. Prepared for the History of Industrial Hygiene Committee, American Conference of Governmental Hygienists. 1974.

20. Mock HE. Industrial medicine and surgery—a resume of its development and scope. *J Ind Hyg.* 1919; 1(1):1-8.

21. Trask JW. The work of the United States Public Health Service in relation to the present war. *Am J Public Health.* 1917;7(12):987–994.

22. Schereschewsky JW. Trinitrotoluol: practical points in its safe handling. *Public Health Rep.* 1917;32(46):1919–1926.

23. Goodwin JW. Twenty years handling TNT in a shell loading plant. *Am Ind Hyg Assoc. J.* 1972;33(1):41–44.

24. Nordlund WJ. Federal Employees' Compensation Act. *Monthly Labor Rev.* 1991;114(9):3-14.

25. Guinan M. The Surgeon General's conferences on occupational health. *Dateline: CDC.* 1989;22(9):12.

26. Myers ML, Herrick RF, Olenchock SA, et al., eds. *Papers and Proceedings of the Surgeon General's Conference on Agricultural Safety and Health.* Cincinnati, OH: National Institute for Occupational Safety and Health;1992. DHHS (NIOSH) Publication Number 92-105.

27. Sayers RR, Bloomfield JJ. Industrial hygiene activities in the United States. *Am J Public Health.* 1936; 26(11):1087–1096.

28. Parran T. The United States Public Health Service in the war. In: Fishbein M, ed. *Doctors at War.* New York, NY: E.P. Dutton & Company, Inc.;1945:247–274.

29. McConnell WJ, Flinn RH. Summary of twenty-two trinitrotoluene fatalities in World War II. *J Ind Hyg Toxicol.* 1946;28:76-86.

30. Anonymous. Beryllium phosphor to be discontinued by major manufacturers of fluorescent lights. *Am Ind Hyg Assoc Q.* 1949;10(1):16.

31. Etheridge EW. *Sentinel for Health: A History of the Centers for Disease Control.* Berkeley, CA: University of California Press;1992.

32. Sun M. Reagan reforms create upheaval at NIOSH. *Science.* October 9, 1981;214:166–168.

33. Seagle EF. The Occupational Safety and Health Act of 1970 and the Department of Health, Education, and Welfare. *Am J Public Health.* 1972;62(3):11–13.

34. Tabershaw IR. NIOSH has lost its Key. *J Occup Med.* 1974;16(10):678–679.

35. Key MM. New horizons in industrial health. *Health Serv Rep.* 1973;88(3): 195–200.

36. Key MM. Letter to Gershon Fishbein. Houston, TX: The University of Texas, School of Public Health, Southeast Center for Occupational and Environmental Health; September 23, 1992.

36a. Gelman JL. Vinyl chloride conspiracy documents: part 4 (Jun 1974–Dec 1974). May 18, 2003. Available at: http://www.johngelman.com/ReadingRoom/tabid/65/ctl/ArticleView/mid/372/articleId/357/Vinyl-Chloride-Conspiracy-Documents-Part-4-Jun-1974--Dec-1974.aspx. Accessed January 30, 2015.

37. *Hearing Before Subcommittee on Environmental Problems Affecting Small Business* (June 22, 1972) (testimony of MM Key, National Institute for Occupational Health and Safety). Abstract available at: http://www2a.cdc.gov/nioshtic-2/BuildQyr.asp?s1=testimony+1972&f1=%2A&Startyear=&Adv=0&terms=1&whichdate=DP&D1=10&Limit=500&Sort=DP+DESC&EndYear=&PageNo=2&RecNo=12&View=f&. Accessed December 1, 2012.

38. *Hearing Before Subcommittee on Labor* (September 27, 1972) (testimony of MM Key, National Institute for Occupational Safety and Health). Available at: http://www2a.cdc.gov/nioshtic-2/BuildQyr.asp?s1=testimony+1972&f1=%2A&Startyear=&Adv=0&terms=1&whichdate=DP&D1=10&Limit=500&Sort=DP+DESC&EndYear=&PageNo=2&RecNo=11&View=f&. Accessed December 1, 2012.

39. Key MM. Health standards and standard setting in the United States. *Ann N Y Acad Sci.* 1972;200(1):707–711.

40. Ashford NA. *Crisis in the Workplace: Occupational Disease and Injury, A Report to the Ford Foundation.* Cambridge, MA: MIT Press;1976.

41. Office of Technology Assessment. *Preventing Illness and Injury in the Workplace.* Washington, DC: U.S. Government Printing Office. OTA-H-256.

42. Barab J. NIOSH reorganization: good, bad or ugly? *Confined Space: News and Commentary on Workplace Health and Safety, Labor and Politics.* Blog dated

May 24, 2004. Available at: http://spewingforth.blogspot.com/2004/05/niosh-reorganization-good-bad-or-ugly.html. Accessed December 1, 2012.

43. Page JA, Munsing PN. Occupational health and the federal government: the wages are still bitter. *Law Contemp Probl.* 1974;38(4):651–668.

44. Finklea JF. Prophylactic chelation therapy for lead exposure. *JAMA.* 1976;235(15):1553.

45. Mastromatteo E. Occupational health: Current priorities. Proceedings: Seminar on Pollution Control and Environmental Health. Pollution Control Association of Ontario, Ontario Ministry of the Environment; May 17, 1979; Toronto, ON: 3–24. Available at: https://archive.org/stream/proceedingsofsem00onta/PROCEEDINGSOFTHE_00_SNSN_02443_djvu.txt. Accessed June 24, 2014.

46. *Hearing Before House Subcommittee on Manpower, Compensation, and Health and Safety, Committee on Education and Labor,* 94th Cong, 1st Sess (May 11, 1976) (testimony of JF Finklea, National Institute for Occupational Safety and Health). Available at: http://www2a.cdc.gov/nioshtic-2/BuildQyr.asp?s1=finklea+legislation&f1=%2A&Startyear=&Adv=0&terms=1&D1=10&EndYear=&Limit=10000&sort=&PageNo=1&RecNo=1&View=f&. Accessed December 5, 2012.

47. National Institute for Occupational Safety and Health. *Criteria for a Recommended Standard: Occupational Exposure to Beryllium.* Cincinnati, OH: NIOSH; 1972. NIOSH 72-10268.

48. Government Accountability Office [author]. Delays in Setting Workplace Standards for Cancer-Causing and Other Dangerous Agents, HR Doc. No. 77-71 (1977).

49. Finklea JF. Letter to Assistant Secretary of Occupational Safety and Health, U.S. Department of Labor, "Update of NIOSH Criteria Document on Beryllium." Washington, DC; December 10, 1975.

50. Public Hearing on the Occupational Standard for Beryllium, Occupational Safety and Health Administration (OSHA), U.S. Department of Labor (August 19, 1977) (testimony of EJ Baier, OSHA). Available at: http://www.cdc.gov/niosh/pdfs/77-bery.pdf. Accessed December 2, 2012.

51. Shapley D. Occupational cancer: Government challenged in beryllium proceeding. *Science.* 1977;198(4320):898–899, 901.

52. Shapley D. Finklea quits as chief of occupational health institute. *Science.* 1978;199(4327):408.

53. Magnuson HJ. Ten years' progress—real or imagined? *J Occup Med.* 1978;20(4):247–250.

54. Eisenbud M, Goldwater LJ, Higgens I, et al. Letter to Joseph A. Califano, Secretary of Health, Education and Welfare, and Ray Marshall, Secretary of Labor. February 10, 1978.

55. McGarity TO. Resisting regulation with blue ribbon panels. *Fordham Urban Law J.* 2005;33(4):100–139.

56. Roe S. Industry, defense establishment twist a proposal to protect beryllium workers into a secret deal protecting their own interests. *ToledoBlade.com*. September 29, 2000. Available at: http://www.toledoblade.com/frontpage/1999/03/29/Industry-defense-establishment-twist-a-proposal-to-protect-beryllium-workers-into-a-secret-deal-protecting-their-own-interests.html. Accessed December 10, 2012.

57. Discher DP. Letter to William H. Foege. Atlanta, GA: Centers for Disease Control and Prevention; October 13, 1978.

58. Robbins A, Froines JR. On the mission of NIOSH. *Am J Public Health.* 1979;69(9):957.

59. Robbins A. Letter to Gershon Fishbein. Morelos, Mexico: Instituto Nacional de Salud Publica; January 2, 1993.

60. Occupational Safety and Health Administration. Reflections on OSHA's history. 2009. Available at: http://www.osha.gov/history/OSHA_HISTORY_3360s.pdf. Accessed November 29, 2012.

61. Millar JD. 10% inspiration. *Appl Occup Environ Hyg.* 1991;6(9):742–746.

62. Millar JD. Summary of proposed national strategies for the prevention of leading work-related diseases and injuries, Part 1. *Am J Ind Med.* 1988;13(2):223–240.

63. Millar JD. The NIOSH-suggested list of the ten leading work-related diseases and injuries. *J Occup Med.* 1984;26(5):340–341.

64. Millar JD, Myers ML. Occupational safety and health: Progress toward the 1990 objectives for the nation. *Public Health Rep.* 1983;98(4):324–335.

65. Centers for Disease Control and Prevention. Leading work-related diseases and injuries—United States (Occupational Lung Diseases). *MMWR Morb Mortal Wkly Rep.* 1983;32(2):24–26, 32.

66. Centers for Disease Control and Prevention. Leading work-related diseases and injuries—United States (Musculoskeletal Disorders). *MMWR Morb Mortal Wkly Rep.* 1983;32(14):189–191.

67. Centers for Disease Control and Prevention. Leading work-related diseases and injuries—United States (Occupational Cancers). *MMWR Morb Mortal Wkly Rep.* 1984;33(9):125–128.

68. Centers for Disease Control and Prevention. Leading work-related diseases and injuries—United States (Severe Occupational Traumatic Injuries). *MMWR Morb Mortal Wkly Rep.* 1984;33(16):213–215.

69. Centers for Disease Control and Prevention. Leading work-related diseases and injuries—United States (Occupational Cardiovascular Diseases). *MMWR Morb Mortal Wkly Rep.* 1985;34:219–222, 227.

70. Centers for Disease Control and Prevention. Leading work-related diseases and injuries—United States (disorders of reproduction). *MMWR Morb Mortal Wkly Rep.* 1985;34(35):537–540.

71. Centers for Disease Control and Prevention. Leading work-related diseases and injuries—United States (neurotoxic disorders). *MMWR Morb Mortal Wkly Rep.* 1986;35(16):113–116, 121–123.

72. Centers for Disease Control and Prevention. Leading work-related diseases and injuries—United States (noise-induced loss of hearing). *MMWR Morb Mortal Wkly Rep.* 1986;35(12):185–188.

73. Centers for Disease Control and Prevention. Leading work-related diseases and injuries (dermatologic conditions). *MMWR Morb Mortal Wkly Rep.* 1986;35(35):561–563.

74. Centers for Disease Control and Prevention. Leading work-related diseases and injuries—United States (psychological disorders). *MMWR Morb Mortal Wkly Rep.* 1986;35(39):613–614, 619–621.

75. Cockrill L. Rosenstock named director of NIOSH. *Dateline: CDC.* 1994;27(2):1, 5.

76. Rosenstock L, Olenec C, Gregory R, et al. The national occupational research agenda: A model of broad stakeholder input into priority setting. *Am J Public Health.* 1998;88(3):353–356.

77. Thompson TG. Secretary Thompson announces new director of CDC's National Institute for Occupational Safety and Health [press release]. June 21, 2002. Available at: http://archive.hhs.gov/news/press/2002pres/20020621c.html. Accessed December 4, 2012.

78. Stalebrink OJ. National performance mandates and intergovernmental collaboration: an examination of the Program Assessment Rating Tool (PART). *Am Rev Public Admin.* 2009;39(6):619–639.

79. National Research Council. *The Health Hazard Evaluation Program at NIOSH.* Washington, DC: The National Academies Press;2008. Committee to Review the NIOSH Health Hazard Evaluation Program. Report No. 7, Reviews of Research Programs of the National Institute for Occupational Safety and Health.

80. Institute of Medicine and National Research Council. *The Personal Protective Technology Program at NIOSH.* Washington, DC: The National Academies Press;2008. Committee to Review the NIOSH Personal Protective Technology Program. Report No. 5, Reviews of Research Programs of the National Institute for Occupational Safety and Health.

81. National Research Council and Institute of Medicine. *Construction Research at NIOSH.* Washington, DC: The National Academies Press;2009. Committee to Review the NIOSH Construction Research Program. Report No. 8, Reviews of Research Programs of the National Institute for Occupational Safety and Health.

82. Institute of Medicine and National Research Council. *Traumatic Injury Research at NIOSH.* Washington, DC: The National Academies Press;2009. Committee to Review the NIOSH Traumatic Injury Research Program. Report No. 6, Reviews of Research Programs of the National Institute for Occupational Safety and Health.

83. National Research Council and Institute of Medicine. *Agriculture, Forestry, and Fishing Research at NIOSH.* Washington, DC: The National Academies Press;2008. Committee to Review the NIOSH Agriculture, Forestry, and Fishing Research Program. Report No. 3, Reviews of Research Programs of the National Institute for Occupational Safety and Health.

84. National Research Council and Institute of Medicine. *Respiratory Diseases Research at NIOSH.* Washington, DC: The National Academies Press;2008. Committee to Review the NIOSH Respiratory Diseases Research Program. Report No. 4, Reviews of Research Programs of the National Institute for Occupational Safety and Health.

85. National Research Council and Institute of Medicine. *Mining Safety and Health Research at NIOSH.* Washington, DC: The National Academies Press;2007. Committee to Review the NIOSH Mining Safety and Health Research Program. Report No. 2, Reviews of Research Programs of the National Institute for Occupational Safety and Health.

86. Institute of Medicine and National Research Council. *Hearing Loss Research at NIOSH.* Washington, DC: The National Academies Press;2006. Committee to Review the NIOSH Hearing Loss Research Program. Report No. 1, Reviews of Research Programs of the National Institute for Occupational Safety and Health.

87. National Occupational Research Agenda (NORA) Agriculture, Forestry, and Fishing Sector Council. *National Agriculture, Forestry, and Fishing Agenda.* Washington, DC: NIOSH;2008. Available at: http://www.cdc.gov/niosh/nora/comment/agendas/AgForFish/pdfs/AgForFishDec2008.pdf. Accessed June 12, 2014.

88. NORA Construction Sector Council. *National Construction Agenda.* Washington, DC: NIOSH;2008. Available at: http://www.cdc.gov/niosh/nora/comment/agendas/construction/pdfs/ConstOct2008.pdf. Accessed June 12, 2014.
89. NORA Health Care and Social Assistance Sector Council. *National Health Care and Social Assistance Agenda.* Washington, DC: NIOSH;2013. Available at: http://www.cdc.gov/niosh/nora/comment/agendas/hlthcaresocassist/pdfs/HlthcareSocAssistFeb2013.pdf. Accessed June 12, 2014.
90. NORA Manufacturing Sector Council. *National Manufacturing Agenda.* Washington, DC: NIOSH;2010. Available at: http://www.cdc.gov/niosh/nora/comment/agendas/manuf/pdfs/ManufJune2010.pdf. Accessed June 12, 2014.
91. NORA Mining Sector Council. *National Mining Agenda.* Washington, DC: NIOSH;2013. Available at: http://www.cdc.gov/niosh/nora/comment/agendas/mining/pdfs/MiningApr2013.pdf. Accessed June 12, 2014.
92. NORA Oil and Gas Extraction Sector Council. *National Oil and Gas Extraction Sector Agenda.* Washington, DC: NIOSH; 2011. Available at: http://www.cdc.gov/niosh/nora/comment/agendas/oilgas. Accessed June 13, 2014.
93. NORA Public Safety Sector Council. National public safety sector agenda. 2013. Available at: http://www.cdc.gov/niosh/nora/comment/agendas/pubsafsub/pdfs/PubSafOct2013.pdf. Accessed June 13, 2014.
94. NORA Services Sector Council. National services sector agenda. 2013. Available at: http://www.cdc.gov/niosh/nora/sectors/serv/pdfs/ServAug2013.pdf. Accessed June 12, 2014.
95. NORA Transportation, warehousing, and utilities Sector Council. National services sector agenda. 2013. Available at: http://www.cdc.gov/niosh/nora/sectors/twu/. Accessed June 12, 2014.
96. NORA Wholesale and Retail Trade Sector Council. National wholesale and retail trade sector agenda. 2009. Available at: http://www.cdc.gov/niosh/nora/comment/agendas/wholrettrade/pdfs/WholRetTradeOct2009.pdf. Accessed June 12, 2014.
97. National Institute for Occupational Safety and Health. The National Occupational Research Agenda (NORA): Sector programs. Available at: http://www.cdc.gov/niosh/nora/sectorprograms.html. Accessed December 9, 2012.
98. Centers for Disease Control and Prevention. Notice to readers: CDC announces landmark reorganization. *MMWR Morb Mortal Wkly Rep.* 2005;54(15):387. Available at: http://www.cdc.gov/mmwr/preview/mmwrhtml/mm5415a8.htm. Accessed June 4, 2014.

99. Key MM, Robbins A, Millar DJ, et al. NIOSH and the CDC reorganization. *Science.* 2004;305(5684):607.

100. Barab J. Opposition to NIOSH reorganization growing. *Confined Space: News and Commentary on Workplace Health and Safety, Labor and Politics.* Blog dated July 27, 2004. Available at: http://spewingforth.blogspot.com/2004/07/opposition-to-niosh-reorganization.html. Accessed December 1, 2012.

101. Anonymous. Critics object to NIOSH reorganization. *Life Lines.* 2004;1(5). Available at: http://www.lhsfna.org/index.cfm?objectid=468EB25F-D56F-E6FA-9046C03073411551. Accessed December 1,2012.

102. Jones JE. CDC faces backlash after ousting NIOSH Director. *Life Lines.* 2008;5(3). Available at: http://www.lhsfna.org/index.cfm?objectID=6F1D6829-D56F-E6FA-96973B26575DEF63. Accessed December 1, 2012.

103. Editorial. A pointless departure. *New York Times.* July 11, 2008. Available at: http://www.nytimes.com/2008/07/11/opinion/11fri3.html?ref=julielgerberding. Accessed December 1, 2012.

104. Borwegen B. Nominees for the 2007 Alice Hamilton Award. 2007. Available at: http://www.google.com/#hl=en&sugexp=les%3B&gs_nf=3&gs_rn=0&gs_ri=serp&gs_mss=Dr.%20julie%20Gerberding&pq=dr.%20gerberding&cp=29&gs_id=1s&xhr=t&q=Dr.%20julie%20Gerberding%20cal%2Fosha&pf=p&tbo=d&rlz=1W1ADRA_enUS445&sclient=psy-ab&oq=Dr.+julie+Gerberding+cal/osha&gs_l=&pbx=1&bav=on.2,or.r_gc.r_pw.r_qf.&fp=76f70bb515aa5578&bpcl=39650382&biw=1366&bih=584. Accessed December 10, 2012.

105. American Society of Safety Engineers. ASSE applauds appointment of Dr. John Howard as NIOSH leader (9/9). *Today's News.* September 9, 2009. Available at: p://www.ishn.com/articles/asse-applauds-appointment-of-dr-john-howard-as-niosh-leader-9-9. Accessed November 30, 2012.

106. Cherniack M, Henning R, Merchant JA, et al. Statement on national worklife priorities. *Am J Ind Med.* 2011;54(1):10–20.

107. Rabinowitz RS. *Occupational Safety and Health Law.* Washington, DC: Bureau of National Affairs;2002.

108. National Institute for Occupational Safety and Health. NIOSH mining program briefing book. 2005. Available at: http://www.cdc.gov/niosh/nas/mining/pdfs/whatis-history.pdf. Accessed September 23, 2012.

10

The Mine Safety and Health Act

Death in the mines can be as sudden as an explosion or a collapse of roof and ribs, or it comes insidiously from "black lung" disease. . . . The time has come to replace this fatalism with hope by substituting action for words. Catastrophes in the coal mines are not inevitable. They can be prevented and they must be prevented.

—President Richard Nixon[1]

THE MINE GAS NARRATIVE

On May Day 1900, miners began work in the coal mines near Scofield, Utah. At mid-morning, mineshaft No. 4 unexpectedly exploded. John Wilson, a miner who had been standing at the mine entrance at the time of the blast, was blown 820 feet away and against a tree. The relief crew was horrified by the scene as they approached the mine. It took nearly 20 minutes to clear debris away from the entrance to get to the trapped miners. When they cleared it, the crew entered the mine and found that some men were still alive but quickly suffocating from the deadly gases left by the explosion; gases known at that time were called firedamp, blackdamp, afterdamp, and more (see Table 10-1). Miners in an adjoining mining shaft were also dying from the toxic gases. The blast took the lives of 200 miners that day. It was the worst mine disaster in the United States up to that time.[2]

Tragedy returned to Utah in 1984. An overheated compressor ignited a fire at the Wilberg Mine, filling the two designated escapeways with fire, heat, and smoke. There were three other escapeways. One was called a dogleg (abrupt, angular change in direction) entry that was unrestricted and was open. The only miner to escape took this route, feeling his way in the dark and opening a

Table 10-1. Early Names of Coal Mine Gases Called Damps*

Damp	Description	Example
Firedamp	Flammable gases in coal mines	Methane
Blackdamp	Other lethal gases	Carbon dioxide
Stinkdamp	Poisonous, explosive gas with rotten egg odor; also creates oxygen-deficient environment (heavier than air)	Hydrogen sulfide
Afterdamp	Lethal gases from firedamp or coal dust explosions	Carbon monoxide
Whitedamp	Noxious gases from coal combustion (also afterdamp)	Carbon monoxide
Chokedamp	Lack of oxygen after an explosion (also blackdamp)	Oxygen deficiency

From the German Dampf.

"man door" to escape the smoke. Several corpses were later found in the dogleg escapeway. A second escapeway was blocked by a roof fall and was impassable. Another escapeway, named the bleeder entry, was restricted but passable. One miner made it past an obstruction there but died before he reached the opening to ambient air. He held an unused self-contained self-rescue (SCSR) device in his hand. The lone survivor used two SCSRs over about four hours to find his way out. This was a survivable fire except for the lack of proper training in the use of SCSRs. An SCSR properly placed into a person's mouth generates oxygen for the miner to breathe.[3] The Mine Safety and Health Administration (MSHA) called off the rescue attempts after 17 hours and sealed off the mine to extinguish the fire. This fire resulted in 27 dead, ranging in ages from 22 to 37 years; there were 26 men and one woman; and 18 were miners and nine were mine company officials. The oversized crew and nine officials were present to break a 24-hour world record for coal extraction using a highly mechanized longwall machine. All of the bodies were located and recovered over the next year.[4] Death was from carbon dioxide poisoning, which SCSRs are designed to counter, and the dead—miners and officials—failed to activate their SCSRs.[5] This failure led to research in training for emergency decision making and the use of SCSRs. The key finding was that most underground coal miners never actually donned the SCSR. Instead, procedures for donning the unit were covered in annual refresher classes and were typically explained by a trainer who stood before the class, demonstrating the steps involved. Since donning an SCSR is a motor task in harsh and dark conditions, the only way to learn is by doing, so the training had to be repeated often. A simple 3+3 linear procedure was developed and became effective as a training tool to save lives.[6,7]

10.1. INTRODUCTION

This chapter describes the history of mining hazards and their implications for formulating occupational safety and health policies. The problem is international, with working conditions in developing countries reflective of those in the United States more than a century ago. Moreover, the United States provides a rich history of mine safety and health policy evolution. This history is instructive in several ways. First, it shows how disasters lead to governmental intervention, which has been recognized as "disaster→law," even though other factors affect the enactment of protective legislation, including low unemployment when labor stability is important.[8] Second, it shows the cumulative steps over time toward more intense governmental intervention (i.e., incrementalism). Third, it shows how the acute problem of literally thousands of worker deaths overshadows the incidence of chronic occupational disease. Moreover, it is a story about reactionary policies of secondary and tertiary prevention (e.g., mine rescue and workers' compensation, respectively) that precede progressive policies for primary prevention such as dust control. Fourth, it shows that individual workers need training to avoid and escape disaster. Fifth, it demonstrates that governmental intervention can save lives despite mine owner and at times union obstructions. Finally, sordid in its details, the story for the control of and compensation for coal workers' pneumoconiosis (black lung disease, or CWP) is a natural experiment in advocacy. This evolution informed the later Occupational Safety and Health Act (OSHAct; see Appendix).

In the 1800s, miners' unions became active in representing miners' safety, and in the early 1900s, mine disasters raised the salience of the miners' plight as victims in mines who were clearly not to blame for their deaths. In response to this attention, the U.S. government created the Bureau of Mines (BoM), which enlisted the U.S. Public Health Service (USPHS) to help in disaster responses from mine safety cars and investigate the problem of silicosis. While the Organic Act of 1910 created the BoM, this congressional action was an inchoate march toward improved miner protection, for the BoM was not yet authorized to establish or enforce standards. Slowly, through the 20th century, policies developed to protect miners with a significant impact on reduced fatalities.[8]

This chapter reviews the evolution over a century of how mine disasters led to the Federal Coal Mine Health and Safety Act of 1969 (Coal Act), the

Federal Mine Safety and Health Act of 1977 (Mine Act), and most recently the Mine Improvement and New Emergency Response Act of 2006. It describes the organizations created by the Mine Act: the MSHA and the Federal Mine Safety and Health Review Commission—and the history of another organization linked to the Mine Act, the BoM. It discusses the protection of both miners' safety and health and the issue of CWP. It reviews the denial of the existence of CWP over decades and the battle to recognize it as an occupational disease. Finally, the chapter describes the issue of tampering with coal mine dust samplers.

10.2. EARLY MINE SAFETY AND HEALTH STATUTES

Coal is already saturated with the blood of too many men and drenched with the tears of too many surviving widows and orphans.

—John L. Lewis[9]

Prior to the current Mine Act, a series of governmental laws grew stronger incrementally over time. Moreover, each law was typically preceded by disaster, raising public angst and salience for action. Indeed, in a five-year period from 1906 to 1911, 13,228 miners were killed in U.S. coal mines. Table 10-2 shows the impact of disasters on governmental intervention and the incremental approach of these actions to increase the effectiveness of the interventions, and Figure 10-1 is a flowchart showing the progression of these disasters and resulting statutes.

10.2.1. An Act for the Protection of Lives of Miners in the Territories

In 1865, a bill was introduced in Congress to create a federal mining bureau, but the bill failed to pass.[10] Then in 1891, Congress passed the first federal statute governing mine safety, An Act for the Protection of Lives of Miners in the Territories, marking the beginning of an extended evolution of increasingly comprehensive federal legislation regulating mining activities. The 1891 law was limited to underground coal mines in U.S. territories. It established minimum ventilation requirements in the mines, the construction of escape shafts, and prohibitions from employing children younger than age 12. Failure to abate a violation could lead to a fine as high as $500, and courts could order injunctions to restrain mining operations.[11-13] Ironically, between 67 and more than 100 miners were killed and another 200 injured in an Oklahoma

Table 10-2. A Chronology of Congressional Prevention Statutes Preceded by Mine Disasters

Year	Tipping Point for Action	Intervention, *Public Law*
1910	In 1907, Monongah, WV, 362 men and boys were killed by explosions and gas.	Organic Act, *PL 61-179*
1941	Several 1940 explosions, including Willow Grove Mine, OH, and Pond Creek Mine, WV, killed 72 and 91 miners, respectively.	Coal Mine Inspection and Investigation Act, *PL 77-49*
1947	A 1947 Centralia, IL, explosion killed 111; eight more were rescued and 24 escaped.	Coal Mine Act, *PL 80-326*
1952	A 1951 West Frankfort, IL, explosion killed 119 of 256 miners.	Federal Coal Mine Safety Act, *PL 82-552*
1966	Explosions in small mines killed all miners including in two Tennessee mines where all five in one mine and all nine employees in the other mine were killed in 1965.	Federal Coal Mine Safety Act, *PL 89-376*
1969	In a 1968 Farmington, WV, mine, 78 of 99 miners were killed in 15 separate explosions.	Federal Coal Mine Health and Safety Act, *PL 91-173*
1977	In the Sunshine Mine, Kellogg, ID, 91 miners died from carbon monoxide poisoning in 1972, and the 1976 Scotia Mine explosion in Overnfork, KY, killed 26 miners.	Federal Mine Safety and Health Act, *PL 95-164*
2006	The 2006 Sago Mine, WV, and Darby Mine, KY, explosions killed 12 and five miners, respectively, and two miners died in an Alma No. 1, WV, fire from carbon monoxide exposure.	Mine Improvement and New Emergency Response Act, *PL 109-236*

Territory coal mine explosion in 1892; many may have been children. The federal rules were not implemented until 1893, according to when the Federal Mine Inspector records were available to the public.[14]

10.2.2. Organic Act of 1910 (Public Law 61-179) and Organic Act Amendments of 1913 (Public Law 62-386)

On December 6, 1907, explosions occurred at the No. 6 and No. 8 mines at Monongah, West Virginia, killing 362 miners. The explosions ripped through the mines, shaking the earth as far as eight miles away, shattering buildings and pavement, hurling people and horses violently to the ground, and knocking streetcars off their rails. Rescue workers cleared away the wreckage at the entrance and tried to force their way into the mine. The rescuers soon began to succumb to the toxic mine air and had to be rescued themselves.[15] The public was outraged with the incessant loss of life from these tragedies. An estimated 30,000 miners had been killed in the three decades before 1910,[16] and the

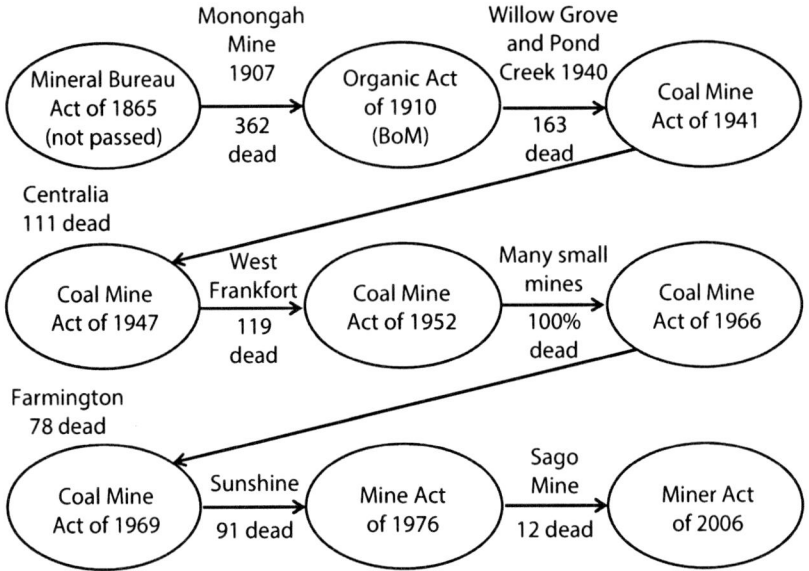

Note: BoM = Bureau of Mines.

Figure 10-1. A flowchart of disasters leading to a series of federal statutes.

period 1900 through 1909 was the deadliest decade in U.S. underground coal mining. These events, including five disasters in December 1907, caused citizens and lawmakers to focus on coal mining and the dangers it presented to workers.

Congress passed the Organic Act of 1910, which created the BoM from the U.S. Geologic Survey (USGS) within the U.S. Department of the Interior (DoI), with the aim to apply research to the mitigation of underground coal mine disasters.[17] In fact, the act specifically denied the BoM "any right or authority in connection with the inspection or supervision of mines or metallurgical plants."[18] The 1913 Organic Act amendments expanded the BoM research authority into improved mining technology.

10.2.3. The Coal Mine Inspection and Investigation Act of 1941 (Public Law 77-49)

After the establishment of the BoM, coal mine disasters continued to occur. Two explosions in 1940 raised public outrage again: Willow Grove Mine, at

St. Clairsville, OH, and Pond Creek Mine, Bartley, WV, killed 72 and 91 miners, respectively. These and earlier disasters, coupled with the overall high death rate among underground coal miners, revealed the widespread failures of state-level protections. Compensation for CWP was also an unresolved issue. Thus, the United Mine Workers of America (UMWA) and New Deal advocates joined in giving the BoM authority to improve coal miner safety and health. The Neely-Keller bill was introduced in Congress in 1939 to prevent mine explosions and work-related disease.[19]

Against strong industry objections, Congress passed the Coal Mine Inspection and Investigation Act in 1941, which later became known as Title I of the 1969 Coal Act.[19] This law gave BoM mine inspectors the right of entry to carry out annual "investigations in coal mines for the purpose of obtaining information relating to health and safety conditions, accidents, and occupational diseases." The act left all enforcement up to the states. The BoM was authorized to use its investigations as "the basis for the preparation and dissemination of reports, studies, statistics, and other educational materials pertaining to the protection and advancement of health and safety in coal mines." While the law did not authorize standard setting, the BoM developed tentative standards as benchmarks for its inspections. The BoM implemented the law regarding explosion prevention but lacked the capacity for disease investigation, which resided in the USPHS.[19,20]

10.2.4. Coal Mine Act of 1947 (Public Law 80-326)

In the interest of national defense and the economy, President Harry S. Truman seized control of the coal mines to stop a long strike over a labor contract in 1946. Secretary of the Interior Julius Albert Krug was named the administrator of the mines and signed an agreement with UMWA President John L. Lewis that covered the terms and conditions of work. Regarding these conditions, the BoM promulgated the Federal Mine Safety Code, which it enforced until the mines were returned to the mine owners in 1947.[12]

A March 1947 explosion in the Centralia No. 5 mine in Illinois killed 111 miners. Another eight miners were rescued, and 24 managed to escape after the explosion.[21] The Centralia mine explosion led Congress to enact the Coal Mine Act of 1947. This new law, which expired one year after its enactment because of a "sunset" provision in the legislation, authorized the crafting of a code of federal regulations for bituminous and lignite coal mine safety.

However, there were no provisions in the law for enforcement of the regulations. Investigators from the BoM were authorized to notify the mine operator and state mine agency of violations of the code.[7,20]

10.2.5. Federal Coal Mine Safety Act of 1952 (Public Law 82-552)

An explosion in December 1951 at the Orient mine at West Frankfort, Illinois, killed 119 of the 256 miners working underground, again inflaming public outrage.[21,22] This explosion, along with a lack of government intervention beyond a year in response to the earlier 1947 Centralia explosion, prompted Congress to enact the Federal Coal Mine Safety Act of 1952 (known as the Coal Act of 1952). The law emphasized the prevention of major mine explosions and provided that mandatory safety standards for underground coal mines be set. More stringent standards were mandated for "gassy" mines. It required annual mine inspections and provided the BoM with the power to issue violation notices and imminent danger withdrawal orders with fines of up to $2,000 (see 10.2.8). The BoM was empowered to issue civil penalties against mine operators for refusing inspectors access to mine property with fines of up to $500. However, no monetary penalties were authorized for noncompliance with the safety standards. While the focus of the act was on eliminating fatalities caused by disasters such as explosions and fires, states retained the authority to prevent the other 90% of the deaths that were associated with normal operating hazards, such as working at cutting and loading the coal at the face of extraction. Surface mines, anthracite coal mines, and mines employing fewer than 15 workers were exempt from the law. States were allowed to enforce federal standards under a state plan system. In 1953, the act was extended to cover anthracite mines.[7,12]

The Coal Act of 1952 established the three-member Federal Coal Mine Safety Board of Review as a quasi-judicial body to decide coal operators' appeals of actions of federal mine inspectors or of the BoM pursuant to the act. The board was deactivated in 1970, pursuant to the Coal Act of 1969.[23]

10.2.6. Metal and Nonmetallic Mines Act of 1961 (Public Law 87-300)

After years of contending with inadequate workers' compensation for work-related diseases, the International Union of Mine, Mill, and Smelter Workers (Mine-Mill) threatened federal legislation, with few results. As it became clear that workers' compensation and state-level regulations were insufficient incentives in noncoal mines for preventing work-related disorders and, more specifically, silicosis, the union agitated for federal legislation.[24] In 1961, federal legislation came with the Metal and Nonmetallic Mines Act, which authorized the Secretary of the Interior to conduct a study of the causes and prevention of injuries, health hazards, and other health and safety conditions in metal and nonmetal mines.[7] Federal officials were given right of entry to collect information. This act resulted in the Mine Safety Board Report in 1963 after an 18-month study issued by DoI in 1963.[21]

10.2.7. Federal Metal and Nonmetallic Mine Safety Act of 1966 (Public Law 89-577)

With persistent agitation by Mine-Mill and based upon the 1963 Mine Safety Board Report, the first federal statute directly regulating noncoal mines was enacted in 1966 as the Federal Metal and Nonmetallic Mine Safety Act. The act provided procedures for developing and promulgating standards (many of which were advisory) for both underground and open-pit mines and for inspections and investigations. One annual inspection was required for underground mines. Federal inspectors were authorized to issue violation notices and withdrawal orders. State inspectors were allowed to enforce federal standards under a state plan system, and education and training programs were expanded. Mine-Mill merged with the United Steelworkers of America in 1967.[24]

10.2.8. Federal Coal Mine Safety Act of 1966 (Public Law 89-376)

Mine operators avoided inspections under the 1952 law by opening a series of small mines with fewer than 15 employed miners. The growth of small mines led to an increase in fatalities in small mines. In 1965, explosions in two Tennessee mines caught the public's attention, where all five in one mine and all nine employees in the other mine died.[9] Moreover, 23 coal mine disasters killed 299 persons from 1952 to 1966, including those in Tennessee. The Federal Coal Mine Safety Act of 1966 extended provisions of the 1952 act to all underground coal mines. The new law permitted mine inspectors to issue withdrawal orders in the event of an unwarranted failure on the part of a mine operator to comply with the standards. Withdrawal orders required operators to move all workers from the affected area until the hazard had been mitigated.[7]

10.2.9. Federal Coal Mine Health and Safety Act of 1969 (Public Law 91-173)

Like almost all legislation on this subject, the bill before us was triggered by a coal mine disaster—one in which 78 men lost their lives. Every significant advance in federal coal mine safety law has required that men die—that they die dramatically and in substantial numbers—before the Congress would undertake to afford them a greater measure of protection.

—Representative Carl Perkins[25]

The frequency and severity of underground coal mine disasters continued to decline in the 1950s and 1960s. Then in November 1968, an enormous explosion occurred in a mine in Farmington, West Virginia, during which 15 major and four minor explosions ignited. After 10 days, the mine was sealed.[15] This disaster shocked many mine safety practitioners, who believed the day of major disasters had ended with the provisions of the 1952 act, strengthened in 1966. When the mine was unsealed, the bodies of 59 victims were removed between September 1969 and April 1978. The mine was permanently sealed in November 1978, leaving 19 victims entombed. The cause of the explosion was never determined, but it had a far-reaching effect that shaped U.S. mine safety and health policy.

This disaster led to the passage of the Federal Coal Mine Health and Safety Act of 1969 (Coal Act). This new law was the most sweeping and comprehensive mine safety legislation ever in the United States and forever changed the face of coal mine health and safety.

After Sections 101 through 104, Title I of the Coal Act covered the major provisions of the act. Title II and Title III of the act established interim health and safety standards, respectively. Title IV provided for benefits of coal miners who developed CWP. Longer statutes such as the Coal Act are divided into titles, with a sequential numbering of sections within each title.[12]

The BoM had primary authority under the Coal Act, but the USPHS had research authority regarding miner health standards and the U.S. Department of Labor (DoL) had the responsibility for CWP benefits after 1972, which were initially administered by the Social Security Administration. The Coal Act covered both surface and underground coal mines, mandated two annual inspections at surface mines, and required four inspections per year for underground mines. Enforcement powers were increased, safety standards for all coal mines were strengthened, many safety standards were specified, and new health standards were adopted. The law established fines for violations, criminal penalties for willful violations of the law, and basic safety and health training requirements. In addition, a training grant program was instituted.[7]

Miners could request a federal inspection, and state enforcement plans were discontinued. The Coal Act provided compensation (black lung benefits) for miners who were disabled by the progressive respiratory disease caused by the inhalation of coal mine dust that resulted in CWP.

In 1973, the Secretary of the Interior, through administrative action, created the Mining Enforcement and Safety Administration (MESA) as a new departmental agency separate from BoM. MESA assumed the safety and health enforcement functions formerly carried out by BoM to discourage any appearance of a conflict of interest between the enforcement of mine safety and health standards and the BoM's other responsibilities for mineral resource development.

10.3. FEDERAL MINE SAFETY AND HEALTH ACT OF 1977 (PUBLIC LAW 95-164)

In 1972, an underground fire at the Sunshine silver mine in Kellogg, ID, caused the death of 91 miners from carbon monoxide exposure and suffocation, while another 80 miners escaped and two more were rescued.[26] In March 1976, two explosions occurred within days of each other at the Scotia Mine in Kentucky. The explosions killed 26 people, three of whom were MESA inspectors who were investigating the first of the two explosions.[12] After the 1976 Scotia Mine disaster, Congress enacted the Federal Mine Safety and Health Amendments Act of 1977 (Mine Act). The Mine Act amended the 1969 Coal Act and incorporated metal and nonmetal mining within the law, and thereby repealed the much weaker Federal Metal and Nonmetallic Mine Safety Act of 1966.[27] Except for the BoM and the National Mine Health and Safety Academy, the functions and resources of the Secretary of the Interior under the Coal Act of 1969 and the Federal Metal and Nonmetallic Mine Safety Act were transferred to the Secretary of Labor. The Mine Act applies to all mines, but it excludes liquid mining (e.g., oil) unless it is conducted with workers located underground.

Section 2(g) of the Mine Act states its purpose:

(1) to establish interim mandatory health and safety standards and to direct the HHS Secretary and the Secretary of Labor to develop and promulgate

improved mandatory health or safety standards to protect the health and safety of the Nation's coal or other miners; (2) to require that each operator of a coal or other mine and every miner in such mine comply with such standards; (3) to cooperate with and provide assistance to the States in the development and enforcement of effective State coal or other mine health and safety programs; and (4) to improve and expand, in cooperation with the States and the coal or other mining industry, research and development and training programs aimed at preventing coal or other mine accidents and occupationally caused diseases in the industry.

Separate safety and health standards for coal and for metal and nonmetal mines were retained. As in the Coal Act, the Mine Act requires four annual inspections at all underground mines and two at all surface mines. Advisory standards for metal and nonmetal mines were eliminated, and state enforcement plans in metal and nonmetal sectors were discontinued.

While the Mine Act set up different research authorities for the National Institute for Occupational Safety and Health (NIOSH) regarding health standards in the U.S. Department of Health and Human Services (DHHS) and BoM for safety standards in the DoI, Congress abolished the BoM in 1995 as described in Chapter 9. The abolition was followed by the transfer of two BoM laboratories to NIOSH in 1996. Thus, NIOSH became responsible for research regarding both health and safety standards.[28] The Mine Act is organized into five titles, as shown in Table 10-3. The strategy for preventing occupational disease and injury in the coal mining industry employs several elements. Standards are set and enforced; technical assistance, research, and development are provided; and surveillance is conducted. Compensation for CWP is a vivid reminder of the consequences of failure to prevent disease.

However, there are significant problems in each of these elements. Regulatory reform threatens to weaken many standards, there is a decline in government research budgets, surveillance is not well monitored, and compensation for CWP is significantly more difficult to obtain now than in the past. Moreover, recent conservative governments are not friendly toward unions.[29]

10.3.1. Title I—General

The Mine Act amended the 1969 Coal Act to include metal and nonmetal mines by adding the words "and other" to read "coal and other mines." The

Table 10-3. Titles and Sections of the Mine Act

Title I: General	Title II: Interim Mandatory Health Standards	Title III: Interim Mandatory Safety Standards for Underground Coal Mines	Title IV: Black Lung Benefits	Title V: Administration
• Mandatory standards • Advisory committees • Inspections, investigations, and recordkeeping • Citations and orders • Procedures for enforcement • Judicial review • Procedures to counteract dangerous conditions • Injunctions and posting • Penalties • Entitlements • Administration • Review commission • Appropriations • Mandatory training	• Coverage • Dust standard and respiratory equipment • Medical examinations • Dust from drilling rock • Dust standard when quartz is present • Noise standard	• Coverage • MSHA created • Roof support and ventilation • Combustible materials and rock dusting • Electrical equipment • Trailing cables • Grounding • Underground high and low voltage distribution • Trolley and feeder wires • Fire protection • Maps • Blasting and explosives • Hoisting and mantrips (miners' trips into and out of mines on trolleys) • Emergency shelters • Communications • Special report	• Part A—General • Part B—Claims for benefits filed on or before December 31, 1973 • Part C—Claims for benefits after December 31, 1973 (in the original Coal Act of 1969)	• Research, training, and education • State assistance • Economic assistance to small business • Inspectors • State laws in effect • Administrative procedures • Regulations • Operative date and repeal • Separability, reports • Special report

Mine Act gives MSHA jurisdiction over lands, structures, facilities, equipment, and other property used in, to be used in, or resulting from mineral extraction and mineral milling, including regulation of mine construction.

The Mine Act holds mine operators responsible for the safety and health of miners, provides for the setting of mandatory safety and health standards, mandates miners' training requirements, prescribes penalties for violations, and enables inspectors to close dangerous mines. The safety and health standards address numerous hazards including roof falls, flammable and explosive gases, fire, electricity, equipment overturns and maintenance, airborne contaminants, noise, and respirable dust. The MSHA enforces safety and health requirements at more than 13,000 mines, investigates mine injuries, and offers mine operators training, technical, and compliance assistance. Mine rescue teams are required for all underground mines.

The authorities under the Mine Act are similar to those under the OSHAct, as shown in Figure 10-2. However, NIOSH-recommended standards under the Mine Act require MSHA to take action, where under the OSHAct no action is required as a result of a recommended standard from NIOSH. If rule making is

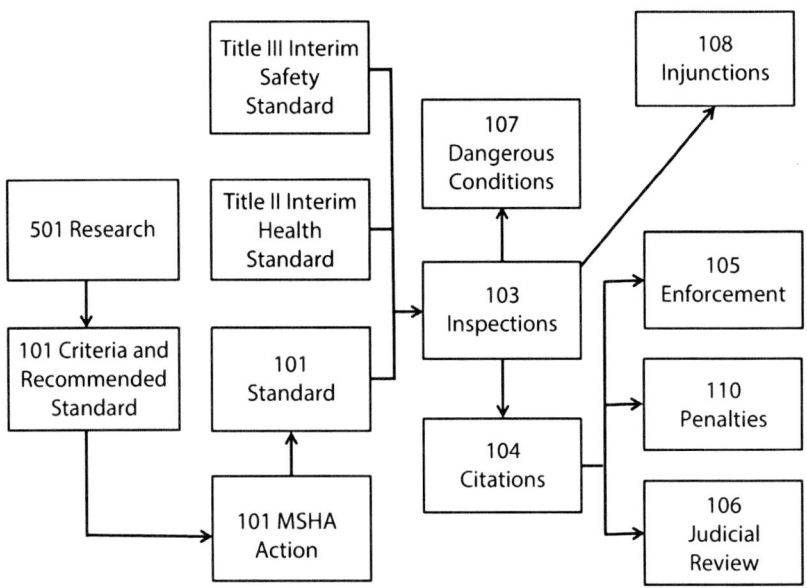

Note: MSHA = Mine Safety and Health Administration.

Figure 10-2. Flowchart of the standard-setting and enforcement steps in the 1977 Mine Act.

initiated, then a standard may result, joining other standards specified within the Mine Act. Next, MSHA proceeds to the enforcement of the standards through inspections and issuing citations and orders as appropriate. Employers may appeal citations to the Mine Safety and Health Review Commission (MSHRC). They may request variances from standards and can receive technical assistance from MSHA or NIOSH. Miners can request inspections and have protections against discrimination. However, different from the Occupational Safety and Health Administration (OSHA), as authorized under the Coal Act, MSHA must inspect all mines: surface mines semiannually and underground mines quarterly. Inspectors can and have closed mines when an imminent danger is observed. Miners are required to undergo extensive training prior to working in a mine and annually thereafter. The Mine Act does not have a general duty clause as in the OSHAct.[20] During a closure order, the operator is still liable for providing full-time pay to the miners.

Mandatory safety and health standards under MSHA can be either an emergency temporary or permanent standard. An emergency temporary standard stays in force until superseded by a permanent standard. The Mine Act requires the Secretary of the Interior to establish an advisory committee on safety research and the Secretary of HHS to establish an advisory committee on mine health research. However, with the abolition of the BoM in the DoI, the DHHS committee combines safety and health research into its advisory committee, the Mine Safety and Health Research Advisory Committee.

When an inspector finds a violation, the mine operator gives a date by which to abate the cited hazard and is assessed a penalty. If the violation is not corrected, then the inspector can issue a closure order, which directs the operator to remove all miners from the affected area of the mine. A closure order can also be issued to protect miners from imminent danger to life or limb.[30] The Mine Act also established the MSHRC, similar to the Occupational Safety and Health Review Commission (OSHRC).

While the penalty structure stated in the Mine Act is similar to the penalties found in the OSHAct, the maximum criminal fine exposure is significantly greater than stated in that act because of the "alternative sentence" provisions, which assess fines for an individual found guilty. The fines are doubled for organizations. Misdemeanors are subject to maximum imprisonment of six months to a year, and a felony has a maximum term of imprisonment of more than one year.

- A felony or any misdemeanor resulting in death may receive a criminal fine as follows:
  - For an individual, up to $250,000
  - For an organization, up to $500,000
- A misdemeanor not resulting in death is subject to a fine as follows:
  - For an individual, up to $100,000
  - For an organization, up to $200,000

10.3.2. Title II—Interim Mandatory Health Standards

The health standards set forth in this section are considered as interim, which can be replaced with permanent standards. The Coal Act, followed by the Mine Act, established measures to control CWP, commonly called "black lung." These measures include the setting of a mandatory coal mine dust exposure limit and requires mine operators to provide miners with X-rays at regular intervals. If an X-ray shows disease, the miner can be transferred to a less dusty work environment.[31]

To allow time for compliance pursuant to the 1969 Coal Act, the mandatory dust standard was established at 3.0 μg/m^3 in 1970 before it was reduced to 2.0 μg/m^3 in 1972. The 2.0 μg/m^3 standard was consistent with the results of British research that indicated that coal mine dust exposure at or less than 2.0 μg/m^3 protected miners from Category II (respiratory impairment from 55% to 80%, which is more impairment than Category I but less than Category III) or more of pneumoconiosis during a working lifetime of 35 years.[32]

Under this title, NIOSH is responsible for research and for certifying X-ray readers, respirators, and dust monitors. Dust exposure monitoring is also covered for silica in both surface and underground mines. This title also provides for a dust standard when quartz is present and a noise standard. NIOSH also provides for autopsies for coal miner decedents to determine whether they have CWP.[20]

10.3.3. Title III—Interim Mandatory Safety Standards for Underground Coal Mines

This title created MSHA as part of the DoL to protect miners' safety and health and uniquely specifies standards typically left to the experts in the regulatory agency. Nonetheless, the intent of Congress cannot be questioned when the law specifies the standard. This title specifies standards for roof support, electrical equipment and grounding, underground electrical distribution and circuits, trolley wires, maps, blasting and explosives, hoisting and mantrips (miners' trips into and out of mines on trolleys), emergency shelters, and communications.

10.3.4. Title IV—Black Lung Benefits

This part of the Mine Act is discussed in a later chapter regarding compensation. In 1972, the Coal Act was amended with the Black Lung Benefits Act, which liberalized benefits given for compensation. Corresponding to the passage of the Mine Act, the Black Lung Benefits Reform Act of 1977 provided for an excise tax on the sale of coal to pay black lung benefits. This act also improved and defined provisions for awarding black lung benefits, and required that DoL and NIOSH conduct a detailed study of lung disease. The Black Lung Benefits Act of 1981 was enacted to increase revenue for the Black Lung Disability Fund with a new tax on coal production.[10]

10.3.5. Title V—Administration

This title specifies that research regarding health will be conducted within DHHS (by NIOSH) and regarding safety within the DoI (by BoM). The DoI abolished the BoM in 1996, but the safety research components of that bureau were transferred to NIOSH, where complete research authority currently lies. This title also provides for the National Mine Health and Safety Academy for the training of mine operators and miners and, like the OSHAct, for assistance to states as well as for small business.

This title provides broad authority for NIOSH to conduct studies, research, experiments, and demonstrations to improve working conditions and practices in coal or other mines, and to prevent injuries and occupational diseases originating in the coal or other mining industry.

It also provides for the training and education of mine operators and miners by MSHA and by the DoI through the National Mine Health and Safety Academy. By the Supplemental Appropriations Act of 1979 (Public Law 96-38), the activities and functions of the National Mine Health and Safety Academy were transferred from the DoI to the DoL. The Mine Safety and Health Administration (MSHA) provides grants to states to assist in complying with the Mine

Act and has improved workers' compensation for miners. The Mine Act also provides for MSHA appointment of qualified employees for the inspection of mines and the training of these employees.

As in the OSHAct, economic assistance is provided through the Small Business Act for mine companies to comply with the Mine Act, and a "separability" clause is included so that no one part of the law found to be invalid will invalidate the rest of the law in whole or in part. No state law should be held in conflict with the Mine Act. The Secretary of Labor is required to submit an annual report on the progress in fulfilling the purpose of the Mine Act, and the Secretary of HHS must submit an annual report on the health of miners through the president to Congress.

10.4. MINE IMPROVEMENT AND NEW EMERGENCY RESPONSE ACT OF 2006 (PUBLIC LAW 109-236)

Mine safety and health gained public salience again when in the first five months of 2006, the Sago (West Virginia) and Darby (Kentucky) mine explosions and the Alma No. 1 (West Virginia) fire all occurred. Following these disasters, Congress passed the Mine Improvement and New Emergency Response Act of 2006 (Miner Act). It requires U.S. mine operators to develop and maintain emergency preparedness and response plans to reduce delay and improve response quality, requiring that every mine have at least two rescue teams located so as to be able to travel to the mine within one hour. It requires new regulations regarding mine rescue teams, sealing of abandoned areas, and prompt notification of mine incidents. The act also requires mine operators to provide additional SCSRs, escapeway lifelines, wireless two-way communication and tracking, and refuge alternatives, and mandates care for the families of trapped miners.[7]

In addition, the act calls for several studies into ways to enhance mine safety and the establishment of a new office within NIOSH devoted to improving mine safety. It also creates a scholarship program to mitigate an anticipated shortage of trained and experienced miners and MSHA enforcement personnel, and it established the Brookwood-Sago Mine Safety Grants program to better identify, avoid, and prevent unsafe working conditions in and around mines.

The Miner Act gives MSHA the ability to temporarily close a mine that fails to pay the penalties or fines. The legislation raises the criminal penalty cap to $250,000 for first offenses and $500,000 for second offenses, as well as establishing a maximum civil penalty of $220,000 for flagrant violations.

10.5. THE MINE SAFETY AND HEALTH ADMINISTRATION

The Mine Safety and Health Administration (MSHA) was created in 1978 under Title III of the 1977 Mine Act with the transfer of the federal mine safety program from MESA in the DoI to the DoL. The Mine Act instructs MSHA to help reduce deaths, injuries, and illnesses in all U.S. mines by developing and enforcing safety and health standards, assisting mine operators to comply with the standards, and providing technical, educational, and other assistance. Headed by an Assistant Secretary of Labor, MSHA's authority applies to all U.S. mining and mineral milling operations, regardless of size, number of employees, or method of extraction. Its authority ranges from two-person sand and gravel pits to large underground coal mines. The agency cooperates with industry, labor, and other federal and state agencies to improve safety and health for all miners. It issues regulations covering health and safety in the nation's mines, and its inspectors enforce these regulations by issuing citations and orders to mine operators.

Inspectors are trained to investigate areas or activities that place miners at most risk. Strong enforcement is augmented by assisting mine operators to understand the law and compliance requirements. Enforcement of safety and health standards is carried out by two activities. First, the "Coal Mine Safety and Health" activity conducts mine inspections, investigations, and trainings through 11 district offices and a system of subordinate offices. Second, the "Metal and Nonmetal Mine Safety and Health" activity administers its programs for all noncoal mines through six district offices. Other MSHA operations include the following:

- The Office of Standards, Regulations, and Variances coordinates the development and issuance of safety and health rules and the revision of existing rules.
- The Office of Assessments administers civil penalties against mine operators for failing to comply with health or safety requirements.
- The Directorate of Technical Support applies scientific and engineering solutions to mitigate hazards (with facilities in Pennsylvania and West Virginia).

- The Directorate of Educational Policy and Development administers training programs at the National Mine Health and Safety Academy and through the Educational Field Services Division, extending training to mine operators and miners throughout the country.
- The Directorate of Program Evaluation and Information Resources reviews and evaluates the effectiveness of agency programs; compiles and analyzes national mine injury and illness data at the Office of Injury and Employment Information located in Denver, Colorado; and publishes data on the prevalence of work-related injuries and illnesses.
- The Directorate of Administration and Management plans and directs all MSHA administrative and management services.

10.6. FEDERAL MINE SAFETY AND HEALTH REVIEW COMMISSION

Patterned after the OSHRC, the Federal Mine Safety and Health Review Commission was created through Title I of the Mine Act. The five-member commission is an independent adjudicative agency that provides administrative trial and appellate review of legal disputes arising under the Mine Act, including the determination of appropriate penalties. The president appoints and the Senate confirms the commissioners.

Most cases deal with civil penalties assessed against mine operators and address whether the alleged safety and health violations occurred as well as the amount of the proposed penalties. Other types of cases include orders to close a mine, miners' charges of safety-related discrimination, and miners' compensation when a mine is idled by a closure order.

The commission's administrative law judges (ALJs) decide cases at the trial level, while the commission provides appellate review. A vote by two commissioners can lead to a review of an ALJ decision at the request of an adversely affected party or based on the commission's own direction for review. An ALJ decision that is not accepted for review is a final order of the commission, which can be appealed by a party to the U.S. Court of Appeals. The commission's headquarters and the ALJ office are co-located in Washington, DC, with additional ALJ offices located in Denver, Colorado, and in Pittsburgh, Pennsylvania.

10.7. MINE SAFETY AND HEALTH ADMINISTRATION AND OCCUPATIONAL SAFETY AND HEALTH ADMINISTRATION MEMORANDUM OF UNDERSTANDING

Section 4(b)(1): Nothing in this Act shall apply to working conditions of employees with respect to which other Federal agencies (that) . . . exercise statutory authority to prescribe or enforce standards or regulations affecting occupational safety or health.

—Occupational Safety and Health Act of 1970

In 1979, MSHA and OSHA entered into an agreement to clarify areas of authority and jurisdiction, improve administration, and coordinate in areas of mutual interest.[32] Generally the Secretary of Labor applies the Mine Act and its standards to eliminate unsafe and unhealthful working conditions on mine sites and in milling operations. Congress's intent was that doubts be resolved in favor of inclusion of a facility (e.g., a mill) within the coverage of the Mine Act. However, the OSHAct is applied to those working conditions if the following applies:

1. The Mine Act does not apply to occupational safety and health hazards on mine or mill sites (e.g., hospitals on mine sites).
2. No MSHA standards apply to particular working conditions on the sites.
3. An employer is neither a mine operator nor an independent contractor but has direct control of the working conditions at the mine site or mill.

The jurisdiction of MSHA includes salt processing facilities on mine property, electrolytic plants where the plants are an integral part of milling operations, stone cutting and stone sawing operations on mine property where such operations do not occur in a stone polishing or finishing plant, and alumina and cement plants. The jurisdiction of OSHA includes brick, clay pipe, and refractory plants; ceramic plants; fertilizer product operations; concrete batch, asphalt batch, and not-mix plants; and smelters and refineries. The agency's jurisdiction also includes salt and cement distribution terminals not located on mine property and milling operations associated with gypsum board plants not located on mine property.

When either agency receives information concerning unsafe or unhealthful working conditions under the jurisdiction of the other agency, it forwards that information to the other agency for appropriate action. When MSHA receives information regarding a possible unsafe or unhealthful condition in an area for which MSHA has authority and determines that none of the Mine Act's provisions with respect to imminent danger authority or enforceable standards provide an appropriate remedy, then MSHA refers the matter to OSHA.

10.8. BUREAU OF MINES (1910–1996)

For a generation or so machinery has had to wait its turn in the mine, it is simply because for a time men were cheaper than machinery. In Northumberland and Durham, in the early days of coal mining, they were so cheaply esteemed that it was unusual to hold inquests on the bodies of men killed in mine disasters. Trade Unionism was needed to alter that state of affairs.

—H.G. Wells[33]

In November 1906, UMWA President Francis Feehan forwarded a miner's complaint about the constant danger of an explosion in the Naomi mine near Pittsburgh to mine inspector Henry Louttit. He inspected the mine three times in 1907, warning the mine foreman that the mine was gassy and poorly ventilated. The foreman said, "The law is being complied with." A year after the miner's warning, an explosion in the mine killed all 35 miners at work that day. On a typical workday, 350 miners would have been in the mine. The explosion occurred on a Sunday. Pennsylvania's chief mine inspector James Roderick wrote to a fellow inspector of his dread of the conditions in the mines but was frustrated with having no authority to intervene to remedy the conditions.[34]

10.8.1. The Technologic Branch

In 1899, the USGS director had recommended establishing a Division of Mines and Mining, and Congress appropriated funds in 1904 for analyzing and testing coal. As a result, the USGS formed the Technologic Branch, headed by Dr. Joseph A. Holmes, a former North Carolina State University geologist and professor. Under Holmes, the branch also investigated mine explosions.[28] Over time, it sought out the mysteries of death caused by the many gases associated with the explosions (see Table 10-1).

In 1910, the Technologic Branch was determining whether the miners killed in an Alabama mine explosion died from either injury or from suffocation.[35]

Holmes asked Surgeon General Walter Wyman of the Public Health and Marine-Hospital Service (which became the USPHS in 1912) to analyze blood samples from the dead miners to determine if the cause of death was blackdamp (carbon dioxide) or whitedamp (carbon monoxide). Dr. John F. Anderson, the director of the Service's Hygienic Laboratory, reported the results of the analyses to the Technologic Branch. The determination was that in at least six of seven cases, the cause of death was suffocation and that each of the six miners had inhaled the toxic gas carbon monoxide before dying.[36]

Holmes became an influential advocate for the creation of a BoM separate from the USGS. In 1907, President Theodore Roosevelt recommended the establishment of the BoM in a year when coal mine disasters took more than 3,000 lives and during a decade when coal mine fatalities exceeded 2,000 annually. Although much controversy surrounded the creation of the BoM,[37] an aroused public moved Congress to act on President Roosevelt's recommendation by establishing the BoM in 1910.[18,28,38]

10.8.2. Bureau of Mines Created

The Technologic Branch was elevated into the new BoM on July 1, 1910, but it took three months for President William Howard Taft to be convinced to appoint Holmes as its director. The USGS director and Holmes's boss, George Otis Smith, was his major antagonist in his bid to be appointed as BoM director. Smith claimed that Holmes showed only perfunctory allegiance to the USGS. Even though Holmes was a Democrat and had been named as Technologic Branch chief by Theodore Roosevelt, Taft could not ignore Holmes's popularity and his superior qualifications and experience. Thus, with Holmes's assurances of his loyalty, Taft named him BoM director.[37] Holmes served until his death in 1915.

While he was Technologic Branch chief, Holmes outfitted six mine rescue cars (railroad), which were the most visible presence of the new BoM to the country. These cars were placed in major U.S. coal fields as a mobile resource to assist in coal mine safety. The mine rescue car operators' task was to investigate mining conditions, train mine rescue squads, train miners in first aid, and investigate sanitary conditions. In a mining emergency, the cars were immediately dispatched to the scene of the incident.[28]

Based upon a 1910 request by Holmes to the Surgeon General, Assistant Surgeon W. Colby Rucker accompanied personnel on a mine rescue car in West

Virginia in January 1911 to investigate sanitary conditions in mines.[39] Later in 1911, Dr. Samuel C. Hotchkiss from the Public Health and Marine-Hospital Service was assigned to a BoM mine rescue car; his task was to investigate silicosis in Joplin, Missouri, while other physicians were detailed to serve in other cars.[40] This activity led to the creation, within the USPHS, of an industrial hygiene activity in 1912 that conducted studies of working conditions in factories and the Office of Industrial Hygiene and Sanitation in 1914.[41]

Because of continued concern for the survival and rescue of miners in the event of a disaster, Congress mandated the BoM "to make diligent investigation of the methods of mining, especially in relation to the safety of miners, the use of explosives, [and] the prevention of accidents." Research addressed safer blasting materials for underground coal mines and the prevention of underground mine gas and dust explosions based on the identification of chemical and physical characteristics of explosives that could perform usefully without causing disastrous fires and explosions.[28]

10.8.3. Pittsburgh Mining Experiment Station

From its Pittsburgh Mining Experiment Station,[38] the BoM tested explosives and demonstrated coal dust explosions in a mine in Bruceton, Pennsylvania, about 13 miles south of Pittsburgh. At this experimental mine, demonstrations showed that coal mine dust by itself was capable of propagating an explosion even in the absence of any methane gas, which was contrary to the widely held belief that coal mine dust could not explode without gas. These early experiments proved that the widespread practice of using loose coal dust in mines to pack explosives in boreholes was dangerous, had cost thousands of lives, and had to be stopped. Research determined that weak methane explosions could initiate violent coal dust explosions, and experiments demonstrated how rock dust, water, and other quenching agents could be applied to arrest these explosions.[28]

There were neither permissible types of safe explosives nor certified permissible equipment for use in U.S. coal mines. The Experiment Station tested and approved explosives with detonation products that had temperatures low enough and flames short enough in duration to be considered safe in flammable mine atmospheres. To be classified as permissible for use in underground coal mines, explosives now had to pass a series of safety and performance tests.[28]

Upon its creation, the BoM also conducted research on safety requirements for electrical equipment, safety lamps, and electrical types of methane indicators; the occurrence of methane gas in coal mines and the adequacy of ventilation to prevent the accumulation of dangerous concentrations of the gas; and the flammability of coal mine dust and quenching of flames by using rock dust. In 1917, the BoM received an appropriation for a detail of three officers (Drs. J.F. Worley, R.R. Sayers, and R.C. Williams)—in addition to Lanza—from the USPHS, which was continued until World War I, when only Dr. Sayers continued on detail with the BoM, where he remained for 17 years.[42]

10.8.4. World War I

When the United States entered World War I in April 1917, disinterest in coal mine safety accelerated as the BoM was pressed into other activities. While the coal mine safety budget remained fixed, it was hampered by an engineer shortage as other war-related programs grew. The BoM was involved in nitrate and new alloy production, fuel conservation, and domestic production of metals (e.g., nickel, manganese). Explosives research focused on war applications rather than mine safety. It also engaged heavily in chemical warfare research.[37]

Regarding gas warfare, and because of the BoM's investigation into poisonous and asphyxiating gases in mines, the bureau had offered its services to the Military Committee of the National Research Council (NRC) on February 8, 1917, before the United States declared war on Germany on April 2. The BoM's Van H. Manning, BoM director from 1915 to 1920, directed the chemical warfare research program. On April 3, the Military Committee formed the Subcommittee on Noxious Gases, composed of U.S. Army and Navy officers and members of the committee, chaired by Manning.[28, 43]

In May 1917, the BoM was authorized to accept help from laboratories at 21 universities, three companies, and three government agencies. The need for more chemists quickly arose, and in cooperation with the American Chemical Society and the NRC, it started recruiting. By July, 15,000 chemists responded to a recruitment survey, and lacking the authority to pay civilian employees, the bureau granted the chemists military commissions. Furthermore, a central laboratory was established that month at American University in Washington, DC. It was called the American University Experimental Station, and its mission was weapons development and testing. By September, the BoM enlisted additional laboratories into the war effort. At the beginning of the war,

American University graduated its first class with one building on the campus, but by the end of the war that number had expanded to a 509-acre campus with 153 office buildings, laboratories, and test facilities.[43,44]

In September 1917, the War Department began suggesting that the American University Experimental Station be militarized, and 10 months later, in June 1918, President Woodrow Wilson agreed, transferring the extensive work at American University to a newly formed army subdivision, the Chemical Warfare Service. Eventually, more than 10% of all the chemists in the United States became directly involved with chemical warfare research during the war.[44]

In addition, the Army assigned the BoM responsibility for military research on and production of respirators, and George A. Burrell of the BoM directed research on a suitable gas mask for American soldiers, which resulted in an assortment of gas masks.[43,45] The BoM established the War Gas Investigations program at American University and produced the first 25,000 gas masks for Army soldiers during the war.[46] Despite the uncomfortable mouthpiece and nose clip of the British Small Box Respirator, the Army decided that this type of mask provided the best protection. In June 1917, the BoM completed an initial attempt to copy the mask, but without success. The next attempt was the training mask in July 1917. More than 600,000 of the masks were manufactured and used for training in the United States.[46] By 1918, the Gas Defense Service of the Army Medical Department produced 3 million of an improved mask, the Richardson-Flory-Kops mask.[47] The war ended on November 11, 1918.

10.8.5. The Department of Commerce

In 1921, President Warren G. Harding named future President Herbert Hoover as Secretary of Commerce. Hoover had sought this role to make the Department of Commerce (DoC) a powerful service organization and to forge cooperative voluntary partnerships between government and business out of a philosophy of "associationalism," which meant crossing class lines to bring together people from diverse identities and conditions.[48] Hoover was a successful mining engineer and in 1912, he and his wife, Lou Henry Hoover, had published Georgius Agricola's 1556 Latin edition of the *De Re Metallica* ("About Metal Things") in English in *The Mining Magazine*.[49] With his interest in mining, Secretary Hoover may have encouraged President Calvin

Coolidge to transfer the BoM and its employees (except those involved in oil leasing work) into the DoC in 1925. The stated purpose of the transfer was to permit a closer coordination of BoM activities with other activities in the department. When President Coolidge decided not to run for office for a second term, Hoover resigned as Secretary of Commerce to successfully run for president.[28]

In 1926, the BoM conducted a study to ascertain the diseases and types of injury incidents most prevalent among miners. It also conducted physical examinations and X-ray studies of miners and a study of the value of the helium-oxygen atmosphere in diving and caisson operations.[28] It was during this period that the BoM cooperated with the USPHS in conducting investigations for the Surgeon General's conferences, which were described in Chapter 9. The first of these conferences, in 1925, regarded tetra-ethyl lead. Instrumental in that study was the BoM's Frank A. Patty, whom General Motors employed after the study. In 1948 he wrote a detailed handbook for the industrial hygiene profession, *Patty's Industrial Hygiene and Toxicology,* that continues in updated editions to this day.[49a]

10.8.6. The Depression Years

In 1928, the Pittsburgh Mining Experiment Station was engaged in the (1) control of mine gases and dusts, (2) disposal of mine wastewaters, (3) mine sealing against acid mine drainage, (4) catalytic treatment of automobile exhaust; and (5) research regarding explosives, injury hazards, mine ventilation, and falls of roof and coal sections. The BoM was returned to the umbrella of the DoI in 1934.[23] By 1936, its research emphasis narrowed to explosives, explosions, and combustion but expanded to include fundamental research into the structure of flames, explosions, and detonations by 1946.[28]

Over the years, the BoM sought to reduce the use of unsuitable explosives and specifically black powder the cause of many underground disasters. It required 30 years of education and demonstration to overcome the use of black powder as an explosive used in coal mines.

In 1940, after UMWA President Lewis recommended his long-term neighbor Sayers as the BoM director, Congress stipulated in appropriations language that Sayers should direct the BoM while maintaining his commission in the USPHS. After his confirmation by the Senate that year, he held the post of BoM director until 1947.[40,49]

10.8.7. Inspection Authority and Closure

The Coal Mine Act of 1952 provided for annual inspections in underground bituminous coal mines with more than 15 employees and gave the BoM authority to issue violation notices and withdrawal orders for imminent dangers. The 1952 act also authorized civil penalties for noncompliance with withdrawal orders or for mine operators refusing inspectors access to mine property. However, no provision was made for monetary penalties for safety violations. In 1966, Congress extended the 1952 Coal Act to all underground coal mines.

Also in 1966, Congress enacted the Federal Metal and Nonmetallic Mine Safety Act, which regulated noncoal mines and provided for the promulgation of standards and for inspections and investigations. However, its enforcement authority was minimal, with many advisory standards. The BoM gained much stronger enforcement authority with the passage of the Coal Act of 1969, but the Secretary of the Interior created MESA in 1973 and transferred standard-setting and enforcement responsibilities to MESA from the BoM. However, safety research responsibilities remained at the BoM. The administrative change was made to avoid the perceived conflict of interest regarding BoM responsibilities for research into technologies for mineral exploitation.

In September 1982, the BoM coal mining technology program was assigned to the Department of Energy (DoE),[38] then in 1995, Congress closed the BoM completely. The health and safety research program at the BoM Pittsburgh (Pennsylvania) and Spokane (Washington) research centers (see Chapter 9) was assigned on an interim basis to DoE, and in 1997, the program was permanently transferred to NIOSH.

10.9. A SORDID CONSPIRACY OF IGNORANCE AND GREED

The majority of coal miners killed on the job, however, do not lose their lives in dramatic disasters. They die by ones and twos in accidents that do not generate national headlines. And more, many more, are killed not on the job but by the job, victims of the insidious "black lung" disease that results from the daily breathing of coal dust.

—Representative Carl Perkins[25]

In 1831, Dr. J.C. Gregory reported a *Case of Peculiar Black Infiltration of the Whole Lungs, Resembling Melanosis*. He had conducted an autopsy on a British miner who had worked in the coal mines for at least 12 years and found that both lungs of the decedent presented a uniform black color throughout the lungs. Gregory determined that the black pigment was likely coal, the consequence of the inhalation of coal mine dust. Separately in that year, the term "black lung" described the lungs of a Scottish coal miner.[50]

This section tells an insidious story of scientific confirmation bias with an inability to break out of an existing paradigm. Two paradigms are described that acted as foils against the identification and prevention of two occupational lung diseases. One paradigm is the germ theory, which helped control infectious diseases but obscured the identification and prevention of silicosis, and once overcome as a public health scourge, the new silicosis paradigm was held as "the" only dust-related lung disease, becoming an intellectual foil against recognizing and preventing another scourge, CWP. Relatedly, this section discusses how greed by mine operators and union higher-ups alike used these and other foils to obscure the disease and avoid remedial and preventive costs associated with CWP.

10.9.1. Silicosis

During most of the 1800s, doctors and workers accepted dust as a source of phthisis (to waste away) that was associated with coughing, wheezing, spitting blood, and becoming weak. With the discovery of the tuberculosis bacillus and the development of germ theory in the 1880s, the cause of phthisis, sometimes called consumption, was believed to be caused by infection. Thus, silicosis was identified as consumption (i.e., tuberculosis), and the strategy for dealing with consumption was finding treatments (i.e., the panacea bias). While silicosis may have been the killer of workers in the grinding trades for centuries, the germ theory was a foil against its prevention until studies confirmed that it was not the result of infection.

Such a study came in 1900—of gold miners in South Africa—concluding that silica was the cause of a fibroid form of phthisis. This led to a British commission investigating lung disease among miners there that found in 1902 that the disease resulted from irritation by dust and not tubercle. The Miner's Phthisis Commission, appointed by the Union of South Africa, concluded in 1912 that silicosis was the primary cause of all cases of gold miners' phthisis.[51]

Meanwhile, in the United States, Frederick L. Hoffman, a statistician with Prudential Life Insurance Company, "unmasked" silicosis as a distinct disease of the dusty trades. He contended that dust-laden air and not the paucity of bacteria in the dusty air was the cause of workers' consumption. By 1908, he was able to demonstrate his claim with a statistical analysis of death rates of workers in the "dusty trades" compared with the death rates from lung diseases in the general population.[51]

The USPHS officer Lanza mounted a tristate (Missouri, Kansas, and Oklahoma) study of miners' consumption in zinc and lead mines while on detail to the BoM in 1914. He showed a high incidence of nontubercular lung disease with injury resulting from exposure to rock dust. He also found that tuberculosis accelerated workers' deaths from miners' consumption—a condition later named silicotuberculosis. Lanza determined that of 9,000 miners, one-third had some stage of silicosis. Moreover, Lanza had identified something different from germ theory: the existence of a chronic form of a disease (silicosis can be acute or chronic, e.g., causing death in two years or 15 years, respectively). While confirmation bias driven by the germ theory dominated scientists' belief that all disease could be diagnosed in the laboratory as either a germ or a poison, by 1915, USPHS officers were struck by the importance of consumption and other diseases that were associated with workplace exposures. Follow-up studies by the USPHS and BoM across the nation and in other industries including foundries discovered that silicosis was a tragic public health epidemic. The term "silicosis," and not "consumption," became widely used in the United States by 1917.[51]

Silicosis became a new paradigm, the "King of Occupational Diseases," and later the "Depression disease." The USPHS conducted studies of coal miners' health three times between 1924 and 1945. The first survey found excessive pulmonary fibrosis in X-rays of miners but concluded that it was not work-related (the X-ray films were inconsistent with silicosis). Later studies in the 1930s led to the conclusion that the fibrosis among anthracite miners was silicosis.[52]

During the Great Depression, silicosis killed more than 700 workers when they drilled through high-quartz rock to form a tunnel at Gauley Bridge, West Virginia.[53] The spoils from the drilling were mined as a byproduct and sold for their high quartz content.[53] Because of the deaths from this incident, a joint resolution of Congress mandated that the DoL call a National Conference on Silicosis in 1936, and a second conference was called in 1937.[54] The conferences resulted in a USPHS voluntary standard of 10 million particles per cubic foot of air, which even the USPHS admitted was an inadequate preventive measure against silicosis and, more particularly, silicotuberculosis.[51] Silicosis had become an economic "hazard" to some industries, which led to naming silicosis as a condition under state workers' compensation laws, thus limiting liability.[54]

In December 1956, the House Committee on Education and Labor held hearings on mine safety. As a result of those hearings, the USPHS and BoM conducted a four-year study on the prevalence of silicosis among metal miners. An examination of nearly 15,000 metal miners concluded that there had been an "extraordinary" reduction in the silicosis prevalence rate when compared with the 1930s and that control measures "can eradicate silicosis."[55] Further study was mandated when Congress enacted the Metal and Nonmetallic Mines Act in 1961.

10.9.2. Miners' Asthma

The miners' asthma is caused by the miners inhaling the dust. I was laid up last week with asthma . . . though I have not worked in the mines since 1898.
—William B. Wilson[19]

In 1822, the term "miners' asthma" was first used to describe a lung disease among coal miners who had symptoms that included spitting, coughing, and breathlessness. Coal miners' asthma was generally attributed to inhalation of coal dust.[54]

During the 1860s and 1870s, European medical studies confirmed that inhalation of coal mine dust caused miners' asthma, but after 1870, many physicians did not understand the pathology of this lung disease and rather believed that coal mine dust protected against tuberculosis. Some U.S. physicians associated sunlight deprivation with miners' ill health. This misinformation continued for the lack of investigation and statistical analysis. Few physicians or state mine inspectors held a concern about miners' asthma, even though manual labor shifted to coal cutting machines that increased dust exposures in the coal mines.[56]

In the United States, miners' asthma became an issue of economic conflict when the 1902 UMWA anthracite strike lasted for five months with 150,000 strikers off the job. To resolve the conflict, UMWA President John Mitchell met with President Theodore Roosevelt. The president suggested a resolution and established the U.S. Anthracite Coal Strike Commission of 1902–1903. The union used the commission hearings to draw public attention to miners' asthma,[57] and Mitchell testified for an 8-hour workday to reduce the exposure to the dust at the commission's public hearing in Pennsylvania. Clarence Darrow, representing the union, spoke of the unhealthy working conditions in underground mines and argued for increased compensation to offset the disease of miners' asthma: "If he [the miner] escapes death or injury by falls of rock or coal, he cannot escape attacks of miners' asthma, a disease peculiar to those who mine anthracite coal."[57] Many miners and physicians testified to the problem of miners' asthma.

The industry countered with how the coal mine dust instilled immunity to infections such as tuberculosis, and the autopsies proved nothing more than a benign discoloration of the lungs. They looked to British data that indicated that miners did not die from miners' asthma, which Darrow countered by arguing that the data did not include those who had left the mine but had fallen ill (today, known as the healthy worker effect).[57]

Mining company physicians testified to the rarity of seeing patients with miners' asthma, and mine superintendents and foremen also testified to this rarity and that any miners' asthma was caused by previous exposures before the advent of modern ventilation methods. To resolve the strike, the commission faced more than 10,000 pages of testimony but had to act quickly. It submitting a report to the president recommending that wages be increased because of the hazard of employment, but with no mention of the respiratory hazard. Nonetheless, the testimony built a growing awareness among miners of the respiratory hazard.[57]

In 1915, the UMWA agitated for workers' compensation benefits for victims of miners' asthma that continued for a number of years. At the request of Governor Gifford Pinchot (R) of Pennsylvania in 1933, the USPHS conducted a study of miners' asthma. Nearly one-fourth of the miners examined were found to suffer from this disease. The study was conducted in cooperation with the state departments of labor and industry and of health, the anthracite coal operators, and the UMWA.[40] The 1935 report, *Anthraco-Silicosis among Hard Coal Miners*, resulted; thus, silicosis remained as the principal recognized cause of occupational lung disease.

10.9.3. United Mine Workers of America Welfare and Retirement Fund

Now it feels like I've got a heavy wet sack on each lung.

—Mark McCowan[58]

When President Truman seized the mines in 1946 to end a strike, Secretary of the Interior Krug and UMWA President Lewis signed an agreement that created the United Mine Workers Welfare and Retirement Fund. The fund was supported through coal royalty payments intended for health and pension benefits. The agreement provided for a national survey of health conditions in the mining industry, which was headed by Rear Admiral Joel T. Boone of the U.S. Navy Medical Corps. The "Boone report" was issued in 1947. As a result, Lewis was moved to learn more about CWP.[59]

Lewis named Sayers as the fund's first chief medical officer. As the BoM director, Sayers got at cross-purposes with the Truman administration and was dismissed earlier in 1946, ostensibly because Sayers had tried to help Lewis force a renegotiation of a contract several weeks after it was signed. Sayers lasted only a year as the fund's first chief medical officer. He remained fixed in the belief that silicosis was the only occupational lung disease, denying that CWP was a disease. However, his downfall occurred when he came up against Josephine Roche, who had worked under the Franklin D. Roosevelt administration advocating for her national health insurance plan from the U.S. Department of the Treasury (DoT). The USPHS was located in the DoT, so she was aware of Sayers's work in the USPHS and his detail to head the BoM. The Sayers proposal for the fund was patterned after an American Medical Association (AMA) proposal to decentralize the program at the district level for setting prices and standards, monitoring professional conduct, and billing the fund for payment. This decentralization was anathema to Roche's way of thinking. She convinced Lewis that the Sayers plan was too expensive, at a cost of $60 million per year, and Sayers left his post after a year.[49]

Lewis then named Dr. Warren F. Draper as chief medical officer in 1948, following his retirement from the USPHS as Assistant Surgeon General. He remained in this position until 1969. Since Sayers's initial approach of fee-for-services led to costly and poor care, an advisory committee that included AMA representatives concluded that direct care in fund-owned hospitals was the answer. As a result, by 1956, the fund had built 10 hospitals with 1,000 beds in three states: Kentucky (seven), West Virginia (two), and Virginia (one). Full-time medical care personnel were hired, and they were bound together in their care and expertise through a regional hospital system. By 1962, the system had reached into all 25 of the coal mining states.

Miners' asthma became a "new" occupational disease reported by British investigators in 1942 as CWP, which was defined as a chronic lung disease caused by inhalation of coal mine dust. Throughout the 1950s and 1960s, the fund disseminated information on advances in understanding chronic pulmonary diseases of mining. In particular, the fund promoted the British conceptualization of a distinctive CWP.[57]

Dr. Lorin E. Kerr came to work at the fund's office in Morgantown, West Virginia, in 1948. To better understand CWP, he read the British research papers on CWP and recognized that some fund patients exhibited the symptoms of the disease. In 1951, he was transferred to Washington, DC, as an assistant to Draper.[60,61] Draper asked Kerr to become versed in dust-related disease, persuade the scientific community that CWP was a disabling disease caused by inhaling coal mine dust, and challenge the denial of the disease.[25] Kerr was on his way to breaking the silicosis paradigm and for the recognition of CWP as a disease.[60]

Kerr wrote his first scholarly article on the subject in a 1956 edition of the *Industrial Medicine and Surgery* journal entitled "Coal Workers' Pneumoconiosis."[60] Within the UMWA, the persistent efforts of physicians associated with the fund, especially Kerr, created awareness of CWP among coal miners exposed to excess dust.[62] In 1952, Alabama became the first state to provide compensation for CWP.[54]

10.9.4. Black Lung Advocacy

Y'all got black lung, and y'all gonna die!"

—Isadore E. Buff[62]

In the 1960s, discontent smoldered among coal miners, and much of it against their own union. The source of this discontent traced back to two policies established by UMWA President Lewis 25 years earlier. One was political, in which Lewis grabbed control of naming the presidents of 19 of 23 mining districts and the subsequent loss of local autonomy rather than depending on local elections. The other was economic. Coal prices were going down because of shifts to diesel fuel by the railroads and oil for household heating. In Lewis's vision, the mines had to become more mechanized to reduce the cost of production. This would mean fewer miners, but those remaining could be paid more. Ancillary to this policy was ridding competition from small mines and negotiating with the Bituminous Coal Operators Association (BCOA), in which the chronic disease problem among the coal miners was ignored.[63]

Advocacy was primed first by Dr. Isadore E. Buff, who charged that companies should pay the cost resulting from CWP, but he also criticized the union leadership, naming them culpable along with the mining companies for ignoring the disease. Shortly after the Farmington (West Virginia) tragedy in November 1968, he enlisted the help of two other physicians, Donald L. Rasmussen and Hawey Wells, to form the Physicians' Committee for Miners Health and Safety. Together they organized a "traveling medicine show," which visited many communities in the West Virginia coal fields to educate miners about black lung and to argue forcefully for a compensation system that, they hoped, would force companies to reduce the dust hazard. Wells, a pathologist in the USPHS, was working in Johnstown, Pennsylvania, and Rasmussen had come to work as a physician with the fund in 1962, where he developed an expertise on CWP. He supervised a USPHS study of CWP in West Virginia that was completed in 1965 before he returned to care for sick miners.[19,62]

What really galled the miners was UMWA President W.A. (Tony) Boyle—who had taken over the presidency from Lewis—when he rushed to the Consolidation Coal's mine explosion site in Farmington where 78 miners were killed. Boyle was dressed impeccably, avoided the victims' families, and attempted to defend Consolidation Coal as "one of the best companies to work with as far as cooperation and safety are concerned." This was in sharp contrast to former UMWA President Lewis, who donned a miner's helmet at the 1951 West Frankfort (Kentucky) disaster and went underground. He emerged with blackened cheeks and was visibly stricken with grief, which was captured by news report pictures. From these pictures, miners took pride in Lewis's concern for the dead miners.[63,64]

The miners had accepted the fate of generations—to work and then to die—but now earned benefits were being taken away as the fund started denying benefits with increasing frequency. Declining union membership meant that the cost of maintaining the fund-based infrastructure was spread among fewer miners, and Boyle had built stronger ties with the mining companies at the expense of benefits for the miners. The most severely affected were widows, the disabled, and the old.

The plight of the sick and the widows kindled flames of discontent. In 1964, coal miners started rebelling against mine operators and their union because nothing was done to stop or compensate for CWP. A decline in the mining population led to the sale of the 10 fund hospitals to the Appalachian Regional Hospitals, Inc., which was funded by a federal grant.[59] Moreover, a 1964 union contract negotiated by Boyle with the BCOA only provided a "measly" raise in pay, no sick pay provision, and seniority loopholes that would not protect the employment of older (and diseased) workers.[63]

Advocates for the miners and their families came from a program in President Lyndon Johnson's War on Poverty, Volunteers in Service to America (VISTA). VISTA volunteers worked closely with the Association of Disabled Miners and Widows in 1966 to qualify its members for union benefits, including displaced and disenfranchised miners who were denied UMWA benefits that were either illegally or improperly withheld. In addition, they helped formulate a state workers' compensation bill with a West Virginia legislator.[19,62]

A young lawyer from West Virginia named J. Davitt McAteer (later named assistant secretary of the MSHA under the Clinton administration) was on the staff of consumer advocate Ralph Nader in 1966. McAteer convinced Nader of the cozy relationship of the BoM and the UMWA with the coal operators, and the problem of dust disease among the miners.[63] As Nader learned more about the issue, he became outraged and acted by working with VISTA and physician advocates, leading to a national agenda of protective legislation through another of his public interest attorneys, Gary Sellers.[19]

Kerr spoke on CWP at the UMWA annual convention in fall 1968, lighting the spark to organize for changes in the workers' compensation laws for CWP. Kerr's strong presentation on black lung led to a resolution obligating the union to lobby in all coal mining states to secure the recognition of CWP as an occupational disease compensable under state workers' compensation programs.[62] Boyle stopped any such resolution at the national level. Returning from the convention, West Virginia miners started to press for a workers' compensation law for black lung. They modeled their advocacy on a 1965 Pennsylvania law that resulted from the work of a UMWA district president, Joseph A. (Jock) Yablonski, that was extended to cover bituminous as well as anthracite coal miners.[63]

As knowledge of the scourge of black lung fueled the miners' discontent, Rasmussen, Buff, and Wells approached UMWA district officials in West Virginia to advocate to change the law to make CWP compensable. The officials were not interested, but encouraged by the three doctors, a dozen rank-and-file miners on a street corner formed the Black Lung Association (BLA) late in 1968, bent on workers' compensation reform. The BLA hired an attorney and lobbied in the state capitol. In February 1969, 2,000 miners marched on the West Virginia legislature. Some miners had lung tissue from Kerr that they carried around in a coffin at the statehouse with a sign saying, "Black Lung Kills." Big rallies were held across the state. While the UMWA had authorized no strikes since 1952, wildcat strikes emerged against the UMWA, the fund, and lawmakers for the lack of workers' compensation for disease, and against their traditional target, the mine operators. In a spontaneous reaction mine-by-mine, within a week one-third of the miners in the state had walked out.[52,62]

Even though many in the West Virginia legislature had close ties to the mine operators, they agreed to consider the provisions that the BLA wanted. Hearings were held with testimonies favoring the BLA proposal, but after the hearings, the legislature claimed the transcript had been lost and came out with a new proposal that was worse than what existed previously. In reaction, 42,000 of 44,000 miners statewide went on strike and shut down every coal mine in the state.[52,62]

As the legislature reconsidered the bill, hundreds of miners watched from the legislative galleries. They understood little about the making of laws, but they were informed by janitors at the statehouse. The janitors, many of whom were disabled miners, could explain the legislative process, and moreover, they had access to the legislators' wastebaskets and thus could determine friend and foe to the miners' cause. The legislature approved a bill in the closing minutes of the 1969 session. Its most significant provision was the Presumption Clause, which said that if someone had worked 10 years or more in the mines subjected to dust exposure, an X-ray was unneeded, and many miners benefited from the provision. Nonetheless, the law was full of loopholes and special conditions that could deny benefits to many other miners. Moreover, nothing was done to control coal mine dust exposure. When Governor Arch A. Moore Jr. (R) signed the bill, the miners went back to work after 23 days of strident advocacy.[52,62]

10.9.5. Federal Action

On September 11, 1968, President Johnson proposed new health and safety legislation that essentially would have extended existing regulations, provided for penalties for violations, and set limits for exposure to coal mine dust. Representative Ken Heckler (D) of West Virginia was a quiet and modest man hidden behind stacks of paper at his desk, but he cosponsored President Johnson's proposed bill with two Pennsylvania representatives. However, in the waning days of the Johnson administration, Congress took no action on the bill.[63]

Three issues soon gained salience in Congress: (1) the 1968 explosion at the Farmington mine, (2) the publicity of the West Virginia strike, and (3) the ineffective state response to the BLA proposal. Representative Heckler became galvanized to do more following the 1968 explosion. In January 1969, the BLA invited Heckler to speak at a rally in Charleston, West Virginia. He appeared in front of 3,000 miners in a packed civic center and became a champion. He challenged Boyle as an unworthy leader, to the cheers of the miners. As their cheers subsided, Heckler spoke again and unveiled a sign that read, "Black Lung is Good for You," and he lifted a 12-lb. piece of baloney into the air to a crescendo of wild applause from the miners, as he thrust the baloney higher, saying, "This is what the UMWA thinks of coal mine safety and health." Two weeks after his speech in Charleston, Heckler redrafted President Johnson's coal mine safety bill that incorporated both safety and health measures against a strategy by the industry and the UMWA to separate the two issues and let black lung agitation dissipate with the passage of a safety bill.[63]

Then on March 3, 1969, President Richard Nixon submitted coal mine health and safety proposals that he said were "essential to meet our obligation to the nation's coal miners." Those miners, he said in his message to Congress, "had too long endured the constant threat and often sudden reality of disaster, disease, and death. The time has come to replace this fatalism with hope by substituting action for words. Catastrophes in the coal mines are not inevitable."[65]

Along with consideration of the president's proposals, congressional committees were reworking versions of the original proposals submitted by President Johnson. In opening the hearings for these legislative proposals before the Senate Labor and Public Welfare Committee, Chairman Harrison Williams (D) of New Jersey said that mechanization in the mines had increased the miners' chances of contracting disease. He added that the search for legislative solutions should not be impeded by "industry assertions that it was unable to bear the financial burden of complying with the new requirements" and cited several reports indicating that the coal industry was in an economic resurgence. Testimony was provided by coal company representatives as well as by Buff, Rasmussen, and Wells. Kerr testified, discounted the ability of masks or respirators to aid in reducing coal mine dust inhalation, and backed the inclusion of black lung in workers' compensation coverage. Others also testified against respirators as a "crutch" and added that Great Britain had effectively controlled black lung through dust limits.[65a]

The bill was finally passed in the House on December 17, 1969, and a day later in the Senate, followed by a conference committee to iron out differences in the two versions of the bill. Congress passed the bill, the Federal Coal Mine Health and Safety Act,[19] on December 18, 1969, but the battle was not over. President Nixon, whose original proposal excluded provisions for black lung compensation, was incensed by the congressional action to provide compensation. He threatened to veto the bill because of the cost of compensation, estimated at $150 to $300 million a year. Miners' fury followed the president's threat. About 1,200 miners at four West Virginia mines went on strike in protest. On December 29, several widows of miners killed in the Farmington explosion arrived at the White House to see the president and demand approval of the bill. To avoid an unpleasant meeting with the seven widows and faced with the possibility of a nationwide strike, President Nixon sent word to the widows that he would sign the bill. The next day, he signed the Federal Coal Mine Health and Safety Act into law, the striking miners went back to work, and the seven women were given a tour of the White House, including the empty Oval Office where they were given pens that President Nixon had used to sign the bill.[19]

The law excluded a tort provision that was introduced by Representative Margaret M. Heckler (R) of Massachusetts whereby a miner or miner's survivors could sue for damages against the coal mine operator and the mine equipment manufacturer as compensation for injury. Nevertheless, the legislation resulted in both remedial and preventive outcomes with the following provisions:[8,66]

1. An interim dust standard for all U.S. coal mines,
2. Promulgation of standards by the Surgeon General and the Secretary of the Interior,
3. Civil penalties of up to $25,000 per violation,
4. Compensation for totally disabled miners from CWP,
5. Appropriations for health and safety research.

As a postscript, with the encouragement of Nader, Jock Yablonski challenged Tony Boyle for the UMWA presidency. Yablonski lost but was contesting the election when he, his wife, and their daughter were murdered on December 31, 1969, as they slept in their Pennsylvania farmhouse. Boyle denied any connection to the five thugs charged with the murders. Then in March 1971, Boyle canceled a trip to Charleston when he was indicted for embezzling union funds and making illegal political contributions. He was convicted on those charges. Boyle was also charged with paying the assassins $20,000 to execute Yablonski, and he tried to kill himself. Eventually, Boyle was convicted and sentenced to three life sentences.[62,63]

10.10. COAL MINE DUST SAMPLER TAMPERING SCANDALS

You see, an explosion can ruin a district manager's career. People dying of black lung 20 years later can't do that.
—Bill Sutherland[67]

The 1969 Mine Act set the legal limit for exposure to coal mine dust at 2.0 μg/m^3 so as to eliminate permanent disability from CWP. Diagnoses of CWP plunged 90% after the passage of the Mine Act, but by the mid-1990s, CWP diagnoses began to increase in younger miners with rapid progression to severe stages of CWP. These observations were most acute in eastern Kentucky, southern West Virginia, and southwestern Virginia. Thousands of coal miners continued to suffer and die from black lung during the 40-plus years since the new limits to coal mine dust exposure were supposed to provide protection. In the decade ending in 2012, NIOSH reported that the number of CWP cases had doubled.[68] Thus, either the standard is not stringent enough or the standard lacks compliance.

When the 1969 law first took effect, Richard Allen, a federal underground coal mine inspector, was party to the discovery of suspicious small blue fibers in each mine dust sample from a mine. The investigators compared the fibers in these samples to the blue carpet fibers in the coal mine manager's office and found that the samples came from the office and not from deep inside the mine. The mine manager was later convicted of defrauding BoM and served time in prison.[68]

This foreshadowed events to come. Noncompliance has been found to be at the core of this public health failure. Mining companies have exploited loopholes and defrauded government regulators, and regulators have placed a prevention priority on acute situations of disasters and fatalities from injury rather than the chronic condition of CWP. Since 1970, the United States has witnessed the CWP-related deaths of more than 70,000 miners, with a cost to the government and industry of more than $45 billion in compensation for CWP victims and their families. After the Massey Energy (West Virginia) mine explosion in 2010, miners told investigators they were ordered to manipulate mine dust sampling. Autopsies of the explosion's 29 victims showed a CWP rate 10 times the average for southern West Virginia.[68]

10.10.1. An Addiction to Cheat

In 2003, James Weeks wrote an article with the title, "The Fox Guarding the Chicken Coop."[69] He addressed the problem of the mine operators' role of taking samples in their own mines to determine compliance with the exposure limit to coal mine dust.[69] MSHA's respirable coal dust control program requires mine operators to collect periodic coal dust samples from the mines. To collect samples, miners wear personal sampling devices while performing specific tasks in each section of the mine. These devices consist of a pump that collects respirable dust from the air in sealed, preweighed filter cassettes. Mine operators subsequently submit the cassettes to MSHA for analysis. The dust collected on the filters shows if an operator is complying with MSHA'S respirable dust standard.[70] Reasons for monitoring the workplace are:

- To eliminate CWP disability by controlling exposure,
- To measure the dust level to which workers are exposed,
- To determine the effectiveness of dust control measures.

A scandal involving tampering with coal dust samples occurred in the mid-1970s, but court actions resulted in no convictions. Between January 1980 and January 1991, eight operators of coal companies were convicted for tampering with coal dust samples or related violations. In April 1991, the DoL announced that MSHA had issued 4,710 citations to more than 500 companies for tampering with respirable coal mine dust samples at nearly 850 coal mines. Proposed civil penalties against mine operators totaled $6.5 million. The violations occurred as a result of the operators' removal of coal mine dust from the cassette filters to decrease the weight of the samples in order to comply with MSHA's standards.[70,71]

Six years after the creation of the 1969 Coal Act, the Government Accountability Office (GAO) conducted an audit of the coal mine dust sampling program and reported to Congress and MESA evidence of cheating everywhere it looked. In 1975, the GAO reported that 18% of the air samples submitted by operators from the dirtiest areas of mines had 0.1 µg/m^3 of coal mine dust in the air, but just days after samples were submitted, federal inspectors were finding the legal limit of 2.0 µg/m^3. The GAO investigators tested whether these very low readings were possible by measuring dust levels inside and outside of coal mines. Measurements taken in mine offices had more than 0.2 μg/m³, and measurements taken entirely outdoors had 0.1 μg/m³.[72]

In 1978, University of Kentucky graduate student Gerald Sharp wrote to an MSHA training center in Lexington, Kentucky, that he had witnessed that almost everyone taking coal dust samples in mines had cheated, often flagrantly. At the mines he visited, Sharp found up to two-thirds of measurements taken had 0.2 μg/m³ of dust or less, which he concluded were impossibly low. Operators had little to lose from cheating, Sharp wrote, "because [MSHA] never refuses a sample for being suspiciously low." Moreover, since the mine owners control the sampling within their own mines, and with a penalty of noncompliance that could result in closing the mine, they err toward lower dust level submissions. In addition, MSHA laboratory technicians recorded the results of these tests with samples nearly free of dust, which experts said must be fraudulent. Sharp said in an interview, "There was this whole charade of empty samples being sent to [the MSHA lab in] Pittsburgh, and they'd say they were fine. I was amazed that there were millions of dollars being spent for absolutely nothing."[53,67,73]

Mine operators found ways to game the system or cheat when taking dust samples. Some of these methods exploited loopholes, and other methods were illegal.[69] When dust samples were taken, operators would:

- Reduce production, increase ventilation, and assign miners who wore "samplers" to less dusty jobs.
- Place samplers in clean areas of the mine.
- Turn the samplers off before the shift was over.
- Take samples outside the mine.
- Discard filter cassettes (the part of the sampler on which respirable dust is collected) that looked too dirty.
- Intentionally void samples.

Prior to 1984, employees of three large mining companies were accused of willfully submitting incorrect sampling data. In that year, Leslie I. Boden, a professor at Harvard University's School of Public Health, published a study that concluded that most of the 0.1 μg/m³ and 0.2 μg/m³ dust readings submitted by operators were likely inaccurate. Ten consecutive dust measurements at 2.1 μg/m³ or more will result in MSHA issuing a citation, and with noncompliance, MSHA may close a hazardous section of the mine. Thus, there is an inherent incentive to lower the risk of penalties by submitting inaccurate data.[74]

Boden and Gold[73] demonstrated that low weight samples (less than 0.3 μg/m³) were significantly and consistently more frequent in operator measurements than they were in MSHA measurements in 1984. Similarly, Seixas et al.[75] also reported a disproportionate number of low weight samples in operator measurements in 1990, which can result in a systematic bias from operators when they improperly take samples in places or at times where and when dust concentration is low. These places and times include outside a mine, in intake airways, in idle areas of a mine, or when production is low.[28]

A yearlong investigation reported in 1998 by the Louisville, Kentucky, *Courier-Journal* found that cheating remained widespread and efforts to stop it have been ineffective. In fact, 15% of air samples—up from 10% four years earlier—taken by operators in 1997 had so little dust that experts claimed they were inaccurate. In Kentucky, for example, the percentage of tests with 0.1 μg/m³ increased from 12% in 1993 to 20% in 1997. As a result, MSHA Administrator McAteer, under President Bill Clinton, directed mine inspectors to conduct monthly spot checks of mines where 0.1 μg/m³ samples were common.[67]

10.10.2. MSHA's Blind Spots

I won't say the agency was as attentive as it should have been. They just had a blind spot.

—Thomas A. Mascolino[67]

The federal enforcement system has focused on preventing the immediate acute conditions of explosions and miner fatalities rather than the chronic conditions of delayed death from CWP. Moreover, blinded to the billions of dollars in future compensation costs for CWP, in the short run, requiring operators to collect the samples has been less expensive than hiring more inspectors to supervise the tests. Furthermore, why not focus on those mines where the legal limit is exceeded and not on those mines that are in compliance (even when compliance is in doubt)?[67]

When the GAO audit uncovered the problem of biased samples in 1975, Congress authorized MSHA to hire 100 more inspectors to conduct dust tests. However, rather than conducting these tests, MSHA officials assigned the new inspectors to spend most of their time making safety inspections. Jim Day,

MESA director from 1973 to 1975, said years later that he believed cheating by operators was common, but when he tried to prosecute a few operators, most of the cases were thrown out of court on technicalities.[67]

Robert Barrett, the next MESA director from 1975 to 1978 (MESA became MSHA in 1977), years later acknowledged that cheating was going on and assigned more inspectors to collect dust samples underground. Barrett increased the percentage of at least one dust test supervised by an MSHA inspector annually from 44% in 1975 to 67% in 1978.[67]

To address concerns documented in Sharp's 1978 report and the 1975 GAO report, MSHA proposed regulations in 1978 to improve the dust-monitoring program. In addition, the BoM was developing tamper-resistant instruments to be mounted on a mining machine. These instruments would display dust concentrations in real time. However, Ronald Reagan became president in 1981, and was intent on curtailing regulations, which included MSHA's power. Development of the machine-mounted dust monitor stopped in the election year of 1980, and virtually all of the MSHA reforms came to a halt by 1985.[69]

President Reagan appointed Ford B. Ford as MSHA director. In his confirmation hearings, Ford vowed to make the agency more cooperative with industry, saying that enforcement was "by no means the only or even necessarily the overriding tool." He reduced fines to $20 for most citations, and during his two years at MSHA, penalty collections plummeted by more than 70%. The average number of mines assigned to each inspector rose from six to eight. In 1985, 21% of the samples submitted by operators had 0.1 µg/m^3 of coal mine dust, a level never proven to exist that low in underground coal mines.[67]

Joseph A. LaMonica was chief of MSHA's Division of Health in 1978. LaMonica's first priority was reducing fatalities, and regarding the dust standard, he instructed his inspectors to spend their time in mines where air samples exceeded the legal dust limit and not waste time on mines that complied with the 2.0 µg/m^3 dust standard. In 1980, 407 underground coal mines (nearly 20% of the U.S. total) submitted at least half of their samples with a measurement of 0.1 µg/m^3.[67]

William H. Sutherland found Sharp's report in agency files in 1980, after he was named to take over as chief of the division. Sharp's findings prompted Sutherland to recommend to LaMonica, who had been elevated to deputy administrator of the Coal Division, that MSHA should put more resources into assuring that dust exposures were kept at a safe level. This was when inspectors spent just 10% of their time overseeing dust tests. Sutherland lost this argument.[67]

When Boden's report came out in 1984, Sutherland again urged LaMonica—by then administrator of the Coal Division—to have inspectors increase tests of coal mine dust. Again, Sutherland lost his argument. LaMonica left MSHA in 1986 to become a vice president of BCOA.[67]

10.10.3. Abnormal White Centers

In the early 1990s, MSHA discovered "abnormal white centers" (AWCs) in the dust sample filters in one-third of the nation's coal mines; it looked like dust had been blown off the filters in order to reduce their weight. Lynn Martin, Secretary of Labor under President George HW Bush, accused the industry of having an "addiction to cheating." Soon after MSHA announced that AWC samples would be rejected on March 26, 1991, their occurrence fell off rapidly from 6.5% to less than 1% of all samples. At some particular mines, the percentage of AWC samples dropped from 25% to zero. MSHA proceeded to issue citations based solely on the occurrence of an AWC and, in concert with the U.S. Department of Justice, investigate possible criminal violations at the mines from which AWCs were identified.[69]

After MSHA issued citations, a group of mine operators challenged their citations. The MSHRC's administrative law judge hearing the case required MSHA to prove that AWC samples could only occur by someone blowing on the filter. Failing this, the administrative law judge stipulated that MSHA could not issue a citation based solely on the occurrence of an AWC. To this end, industry experts were successful in testimony that created sufficient doubt for the administrative law judge to reject MSHA's citations since it had failed to carry its burden of proof.[69]

However, the administrative law judge allowed MSHA to bring a case against Keystone's Urling mine in Pennsylvania in 1995. Ironically, the company acknowledged possible carelessness in taking dust samples that could have resulted in AWC samples. Although under this argument the company was culpable in submitting inaccurate samples, this defense of carelessness worked for the company on the narrow issue of tampering with the samples. In 1998, MSHA lost the case, which went all the way to the Court of Appeals in Washington, DC.[69]

However, success for MSHA came from the joint investigation with the Justice Department of sampling practices. MSHA gathered enough evidence to convict more than 200 mine operators and their contractors on criminal charges of submitting fraudulent samples, but in these cases, the AWC samples were treated merely as one piece of evidence. The convictions resulted in withdrawing training certifications, issuing fines, and placing the violators under house arrest.[69] Federal records describe 103 cases resulting in criminal convictions for fraudulent dust sampling from 1980 through 2002. Criminal fines totaled $2.2 million, and some mining company officials went to jail.[68]

In 2009, President Barack Obama named Joseph A. Main as MSHA Administrator. Between 2009 and 2012, an MSHA enforcement effort called "dust busters" targeted mines with coal dust problems. In 96 different inspections, MSHA found 531 mine dust violations, and many violators were large mining companies.[68]

Under Main's leadership, MSHA has proposed several changes to overhaul the current standards and reduce miners' exposure to unhealthy dust. These changes include cutting coal mine dust limits in half to 1.0 µg/m^3 because of the silicosis hazard, sampling to reflect actual exposure, and ending a practice of mining companies demonstrating compliance by averaging five dust samples. However, mining companies still collect their own samples with the threat of criminal prosecution based on acts of fraud.[68]

THE INCENTIVE NARRATIVE

In the mid-1980s, a coal mining company hired a new CEO to improve its safety record. The new CEO was a retired military officer with no prior mining experience. He mounted a major and highly touted company safety program with a competition among the many different mine section crews to achieve zero lost-time injuries over a full year. The crew that could attain this record would receive a sizable end-of-year cash bonus plus other gifts. One mine section crew achieved the record of no lost-time injuries for the year. To celebrate their accomplishment, the CEO hosted a fancy luncheon for the 12 miners on the crew. Food was plentiful, and popular recorded music was played. Helpers (all young women in alluring dress) handed out the cash bonus envelopes and other prizes to each miner. Then the helpers brought out a large bowl. Each miner drew a numbered slip of paper from that bowl. More gifts were handed out to each miner by the helpers. Then the helpers brought out another bowl filled with ignition keys. The miners then lined up in the order of the numbers that they had drawn from the first bowl. A loud engine roar was heard just outside the door to the room. The door was opened to reveal a new pickup truck. Its engine was turned off, and its ignition key removed. In the order of their numbers the miners lined up. Each inserted his key into the ignition switch. The fourth miner's key started the engine, and he won the truck. Later that day, two mine safety consultants who attended the celebration met with the mine section crews. Miners in the winning crew reported that they had worked with no lost time injuries until near the end of the year. Then one miner in their crew broke his ankle while unloading supplies. In order to remain eligible for the award his buddies covered for him for nearly half a shift. He rode out on the mantrip and got to his vehicle with help from his buddies. He called in to work the next morning and reported that he broke his ankle when he was home while playing basketball. His time away from work was not recorded as a lost-time injury.

The CEO's strategy resulted in lowering the mine's lost-time injury rate largely because miners tried to work safely to avoid injuries. It was also likely because other injury events may have been concealed by miners and their section foremen in order to receive the incentive awards. In subsequent years, the number of half-day lost-time injury rates increased.

Research has reported that safety incentives that involve competition among workers and work crews can reduce injury rates, but not always. The competition often results in higher injury rates for a mine, factory, or plant. The most effective injury reduction programs involve collaborative efforts by workers and managers across all sections of an operation. This is especially the case when the collaborative efforts include identifying workplace hazards, tracking and documenting close calls and minor injury events, and putting in place immediate preventive measures to mitigate the hazards identified.[6,76,77]

REFERENCES

1. Black CC. Role of the Department of Health, Education, and Welfare in the administration of Public Law 91-173. In: Papers and Proceedings of the National Conference on Medicine and the Federal Coal Mine Health and Safety Act of 1969, Public Law 91-173; June 15–18, 1970; Washington, DC.

2. Ison YD. The Scofield mine disaster in 1900 was Utah's worst. *History Blazer.* January 1995. Available at: http://historytogo.utah.gov/utah_chapters/mining_and_railroads/thescofieldminedisasterin1900wasutahsworst.html. Accessed December 13, 2012.

3. Government Accountability Office. Mine safety: questions regarding enforcement at Wilberg Coal Mine. Briefing report to the ranking minority member, Senate Committee on Labor and Human Resources. November 1987. Available at: http://www.gao.gov/assets/80/76908.pdf. Accessed December 13, 2012.

4. Gorrell M. Remembering the Wilberg Mine disaster. *Salt Lake Tribune.* December 19, 2004. Available at: http://www.sltrib.com/news/ci_2491518. Accessed December 16, 2012.

5. Sauer B. The dynamics of disaster: a three-dimensional view of documentation in a tightly regulated industry. *Tech Comm Q.* 1994;3(4):393–419.

6. Cole H, Wasielewski R, Lineberry GT, et al. Miner and trainer responses to simulated mine emergency problems. In: Proceedings, Mine Safety Education and Training Seminar; 1988; Pittsburgh, PA. Information Circular Report 9185.

7. Brnich MJ, Wiehagen WJ, Cole HP, et al. *An Overview of Research on Self-Contained Self-Rescuer Training.* Pittsburgh, PA: U.S. Department of the Interior; 1993. Bureau of Mines, B-695.

8. Curran DJ. *Dead Laws for Dead Men: The Politics of the Federal Coal Mine Health and Safety Legislation.* Pittsburgh, PA: University of Pittsburgh Press; 1993.

9. Barrett R. Retrospect: We've come a long way. *MESA: The Magazine of Mining Health and Safety.* Mining Enforcement and Safety Administration, U.S. Department of the Interior. Available at: http://www.msha.gov/FocusOn/40thAnniversary/MESAArticle.pdf. Accessed December 14, 2012.

10. Merchant JA, Taylor G, Hodus TK. Coal workers' pneumoconiosis and exposure to other carbonaceous dusts. In: Merchant JA, Boehlecke BA, Taylor G, et al., eds. *Occupational Respiratory Diseases.* Cincinnati, OH: Department of Health and Human Services, Public Health Service;1986:329–384. NIOSH Publication 86-102.

11. Nichting AT, Beverage LE, Johnson KL. Mine safety and health law. In: Kogel JE, Trivedi NC, Barker JM, eds. *Industrial Minerals and Rocks: Commodities, Markets, and Uses.* Englewood, CO: Society for Mining Metallurgy and Exploration; 2006:109–119.

12. Rabinowitz RS. *Occupational Safety and Health Law*. 2nd ed. Washington, DC: Bureau of National Affairs;2002.

13. Mine Safety and Health Administration. History of mine safety and health legislation. Available at: http://www.msha.gov/mshainfo/mshainf2.htm. Accessed December 17, 2012.

14. Anonymous. Uncovering Okla. mining accidents. *The Lawton Constitution*. August 26, 2012. Available at: http://www.swoknews.com/styles-new/miscellaneous/item/751-uncovering-okla-mining-accidents. Accessed December 17, 2012.

15. Dillon LA. *They Died in the Darkness*. Parsons, WV: McClain Printing Company;1976.

16. Page AW. Safety first underground: The new Bureau of Mines and its life saving campaign in the coal fields. *The World's Work: A History of Our Time*. 1912;23:549–563.

17. Brnich MJ, Kowalski-Trakofker KM. Underground coal mine disasters 1900-2010: events, responses, and a look to the future. In: Brune JF, ed. *Extracting the Science: A Century of Mining Research*. Englewood, CO: Society of Mining, Metallurgy, and Exploration;2010:363–372.

18. Bokat SA, Thomson HA. *Occupational Safety and Health Law*. Washington, DC: Bureau of National Affairs;1988.

19. Derickson A. *Black Lung: Anatomy of a Public Health Disaster*. Ithaca, NY: Cornell University Press;1998.

20. Weeks JL. What you need to know about the Mine Safety and Health Administration. In: Levy BS, Wegman DH, eds. *Occupational Health: Recognizing and Preventing Work-Related Disease*. Boston: Little, Brown and Co.;1988:48–50.

21. Hartley RE, Kenny D. *Death Underground: The Centralia and West Frankfort Mine Disasters*. Carbondale, IL: Southern Illinois Press;2006.

22. Grayson RL, Watzman B. History and overview of mine health and safety. In: Karmis M, ed. *Mine Health and Safety Management*. Littleton, CO: Society for Mining, Metallurgy, and Exploration, Inc.;2001:1–13.

23. National Archives. Records of the U.S. Bureau of Mines. Record Group 70, 1860–1996 (Bulk 1910-90). 1995. Available at: http://www.archives.gov/research/guide-fed-records/groups/070.html. Accessed December 29, 2012.

24. Derickson A. *Workers' Health, Workers' Democracy: The Western Miners' Struggle, 1891-1825*. Ithaca, NY: Cornell University Press;1988.

25. Seltzer C. Moral dimensions of occupational health: The case of the 1969 Coal Mine Health and Safety Act. In: Bayer R, ed. *The Safety and Health of Workers: Case Studies in the Politics of Professional Responsibility.* New York, NY: Oxford University Press;1988:242–270.

26. Olsen G. *The Dark Deep: Disaster and Redemption in America's Richest Silver Mine.* New York, NY: Three Rivers Press;2005.

27. McAteer JD. *Miner's Manual.* Washington, DC: Crossroads Press;1981.

28. Breslin JA. *One Hundred Years of Federal Mining Safety and Health Research.* Pittsburgh, PA, Pittsburgh Research Laboratory;2010. Available at: http://www.cdc.gov/niosh/mining/UserFiles/works/pdfs/2010-128.pdf. Accessed December 29, 2012.

29. Weeks JL. Tampering with dust samples in coal mines (again). *Am J Indust Med.* 1991;20(2):41–144.

30. Boden LI. Government regulation of occupational safety: underground coal mine accidents 1973-75. *Am J Public Health.* 1985;75(5):497–501.

31. Parobeck PS, Jankowski RA. Assessment of the respirable levels in the nation's underground and surface coal mining operations. *Am Ind Hyg Assoc J.* 1979;40(10):910–915.

32. Secretary of Labor. Interagency agreement between the Mine Safety and Health Administration, U.S. Department of Labor, and the Occupational Safety and Health Administration. March 29, 1979. Available at: http://www.osha.gov/pls/oshaweb/owadisp.show_document?p_table=MOU&p_id=222. Accessed December 23, 2012.

33. Postgate R. *The Outline of History of Life and Mankind by H.G. Wells, Revised and Brought Up to the End of the Second World War.* Vol. 2. Garden City, NY: Garden City Book;1949:765.

34. Aldrich M. Preventing "The needless peril of the coal mine": the Bureau of Mines and the campaign against coal mine explosions, 1910-1940. *Technol Cult.* 1995;36(3):483–518.

35. Smith GO. Letter from Director, U.S. Geological Survey, to Surgeon General Walter Wyman; May 10, 1910; letter in response (on behalf of the Surgeon General) from Dr. John F. Anderson, Director, Hygienic Laboratory, Public Health and Marine-Hospital Service, to Dr. Smith; May 14, 1910.

36. Doyle HN. *The Federal Industrial Hygiene Agency: A History of the Division of Occupational Health, U.S. Public Health Service.* Cincinnati, OH: American

Conference of Governmental Hygienists;1974. Report prepared for History of Industrial Hygiene Committee.

37. Graebner W. *Coal-Mining Safety in the Progressive Period: The Political Economy of Reform.* Lexington, KY: University Press of Kentucky;1976.

38. Tuchman RJ, Brinkley RF. A history of the Bureau of Mines Pittsburgh Research Center. 1990. Available at: http://www.cdc.gov/niosh/mining/works/coversheet1609.html. Accessed July 22, 2014.

39. Holmes JA. Letter from Director, Bureau of Mines, to Surgeon General Walter Wyman; November 22, 1910; and responding letter from Dr. Wyman to Dr. Holmes; December 2, 1910.

40. Williams RC. *The United States Public Health Service: 1798-1950.* Richmond, VA: Whittet and Shepperson;1951.

41. Mock HE. Industrial medicine and surgery—a resume of its development and scope. *J Ind Hyg.* 1914;1(1):1–8.

42. Brodeur P. *Outrageous Misconduct: The Asbestos Industry on Trial.* New York, NY: Pantheon Books;1985.

43. Vilensky JA. *Dew of Death: The Story of Lewisite, America's World War I Weapon of Mass Destruction.* Bloomington, IN: Indiana University Press;2005.

44. Vilensky JA, Sinish PR. Dew of death: the story of lewisite, America's World War I weapon of mass destruction. *Q J Mil Hist.* and originally published in the Spring 2005 edition. Available at: http://www.historynet.com/weaponry-lewisite-americas-world-war-i-chemical-weapon.htm. Accessed January 7, 2013.

45. Held BJ. History of respiratory protective devices in the U.S. Report prepared at: Lawrence Livermore Laboratory, Livermore, CA, under the auspices of the U.S. Energy Research and Development Administration under contract no. W-7405-Eng.-48; 1977:23.

46. Smart JK. History of the Army protective mask. NBC Defense Systems, Aberdeen Proving Ground, MD. DSN: 584-2566. Available at: http://www.dtic.mil/cgi-bin/GetTRDoc?AD=ada376445. Accessed January 2, 2013.

47. Edgewood Chemical Biological Center. 90-year timeline. 2007. Available at: http://www.ecbc.army.mil/about/old_files/history.htm. Accessed July 22, 2014.

48. McGerr M. *A Fierce Discontent: The Rise and Fall of the Progressive Movement in America.* New York, NY: Oxford University Press;2003.

49. Agricola G. *De Re Metallica.* Hoover HC, Hoover LH, trans. New York, NY: Dover Publications, Inc.;1950.

49a. Rose VE, Cohrssen B, eds. *Patty's Industrial Hygiene.* 6th ed. Hoboken, NJ: John Wiley & Sons, Inc.;2010.

50. Rosen G. *The History of Miners' Diseases: A Medical And Social Interpretation.* New York, NY: Schuman;1943.

51. Rosner D, Markowitz G. *Deadly Dust: Silicosis and the Politics of Occupational Disease in Twentieth-Century America.* Princeton, NJ: Princeton University Press;1991.

52. Seltzer C. *Fire in the Hole: Miners and Managers in the American Coal Industry.* Lexington, KY: University of Kentucky Press;1985.

53. Cherniack M. *The Hawk's Nest Incident: America's Worst Industrial Disaster.* New Haven, CT: Yale University Press;1989.

54. Goldsmith F, Kerr LE. *Occupational Safety and Health: The Prevention and Control of Work-Related Hazards.* New York, NY: Human Sciences Press, Inc.;1982.

55. Stockinger HE. What are governmental agencies doing in occupational health? In: Proceedings of the President's Conference on Occupational Safety; June 23-25, 1964; Washington, DC:141-153.

56. Corn JK. *Environment and Health in Nineteenth Century America: Two Case Studies.* New York, NY: Peter Lang;1989.

57. Derickson A. The United Mine Workers of America and the recognition of occupational respiratory diseases, 1902-1968. *Am J Public Health.* 1991;81(6):782-790.

58. Berkes H. As mine protections fail, black lung cases surge. NPR and the Center for Public Integrity. July 9, 2012. Available at: http://www.npr.org/2012/07/09/155978300/as-mine-protections-fail-black-lung-cases-surge. Accessed January 13, 2013.

59. Koplin AN. Government and health: the significance of the coal strike and contract in retrospect. *Am J Public Health.* 1979;69(2):154-156.

60. Mulcahy RP. *A Social Contract for the Coal Fields: The Rise and Fall of the United Mine Workers of America Welfare and Retirement Fund.* Knoxville, TN: University of Tennessee Press;2000.

61. Lorin Edgar Kerr. Available at: http://en.wikipedia.org/wiki/Lorin_E._Kerr. Accessed July 22, 2014.

62. Dotson-Lewis B. Dr. Donald Rasmussen, a doctor devoting his life to defeating black lung. Oral history interview with Dr. Donald L. Rasmussen, 2002. COAL: Blog about coal mining, black lung, and the culture of Appalachia. September 12, 2012. Available at: http://dotson-lewis.blogspot.com/2011/04/black-lung-dr-donald-rasmussen.html. Accessed December 30, 2012.

63. Armbrister T. *Act of Vengeance: The Yablonski Murders.* New York, NY: Saturday Review Press;1975.

64. Kerr LE. Black lung. *J Public Health Pol.* 1980;1(1):50–63.

65. Centers for Disease Control and Prevention. Occupational respiratory disease surveillance: NIOSH/DRDS/CWHSP celebrate the 35th anniversary of the Federal Coal Mine Health and Safety Act. 2011. Available at: http://www.cdc.gov/niosh/topics/surveillance/ords/CoalMineHealthSafetyAct35Years.html. Accessed January 11, 2013.

65a. Congress clears comprehensive coal mine safety bill. *CQ Almanac.* 1969. Available at: http://library.cqpress.com/cqalmanac/cqal69-1246794. Accessed January 30, 2015.

66. Mclaughlin RF. Mine safety legislation: A history of neglect. *Boston Coll Law Rev.* 1969;11(1):31–45.

67. Harris G. U.S. mine agency ignored fraud: Dust cheating finally addressed, but response slow. *The Courier-Journal.* April 20, 1998. Available at: http://www.courier-journal.com/cjextra/dust/frame_govt_ignored.html. Accessed January 13, 2013.

68. Berkes H. Black-lung rule loopholes leave miners vulnerable. NPR and the Center for Public Integrity. July 10, 2012. Available at: http://www.npr.org/2012/07/10/155981916/black-lung-rule-loopholes-leave-miners-vulnerable. Accessed January 13, 2013.

69. Weeks JL. The fox guarding the chicken coop: Monitoring exposure to respirable coal mine dust, 1969–2000. *Am J Public Health.* 2003;93(8):1236–1244.

70. Government Accountability Office. *Mine Safety and Health Tampering Scandal Led to Improved Sampling Devices.* Washington, DC: Government Accountability Office;1993. GAO/HI&D-98-63, Mine Health Improved Sampling Devices.

71. Peluso RG. Continuous monitoring of environmental parameters in underground coal mines. Mine Safety and Health Administration. 1994. Available at: http://www.msha.gov/S&Hinfo/techrpt/dust/CONMON.pdf. Accessed January 11, 2013.

72. Government Accountability Office. *Improvements Still Needed in Coal Mine Dust-Sampling Program and Penalty Assessments and Collections.* Washington, DC: Government Accountability Office;1975. Available at: http://www.gao.gov/assets/120/114174.pdf. Accessed June 4, 2014.

73. Sharp G. Dust *Monitoring and Control in the Underground Coal Mines of Eastern Kentucky* [master's thesis]. Lexington, KY: University of Kentucky;1978.

74. Boden LI, Gold M. The accuracy of self-reported regulatory data: the case of coal mine dust. *Am J Ind Med.* 1984;6(6):427–440.

75. Seixas NS, Robins TG, Rice CH, et al. Assessment of potential biases in the application of MSHA respirable coal mine dust data to an epidemiologic study. *Am Ind Hyg Assoc J.* 1990;51(10):534–540.

76. Cole HP, Berger PK, Garrity TF, et al. Medical compliance behavior and miner health and safety. *Ann Am Conf Gov Ind Hyg.* 1986;14:425–433.

77. DeJoy DM, Schaffer BS, Wilson MG, et al. Creating safer workplaces: assessing the determinants and role of safety climate. *J Safety Research.* 2004;35(1):81–90.

11

Other Worker Protections and Exclusions

There will always be greedy, careless people in this world, and some of them will gain a good deal of power. It is your job as our elected officials to protect U.S. citizens and our fragile earth from the likes of them.

—Marilyn Sewell[1]

THE DEEPWATER HORIZON NARRATIVE

On April 20, 2010, a blowout on a well attached to the Deepwater Horizon drilling rig in the Gulf of Mexico exploded, causing 4.9 million barrels of oil to flow from the well, making it the worst offshore spill in U.S. history. BP leased the drilling rig Deepwater Horizon from the Swiss firm Transocean Ltd. The rig was located about 50 miles southeast of the Louisiana coast. BP was the majority owner of the well. On the morning of April 12—after burning for about a day and a half—the Deepwater Horizon sank. It rests now about a mile below the gulf's surface. The resulting oil spill caused widespread environmental and economic damage, affecting not only the Gulf of Mexico but also the coastlines and estuaries of Louisiana, Alabama, Mississippi, and Florida. On June 16, 2010, BP agreed to an escrow fund of $20 billion to settle economic injury claims by commercial fishers and various gulf industries.[1a] The report from President Barack Obama's National Commission on the BP Deepwater Horizon Oil Spill and Offshore Drilling addressed the occupational safety and health issue as well as the environmental consequences of the spill.[2]

Lest one forget, the explosion took 11 workers' lives and injured 17 others who suffered burns, broken legs, and smoke inhalation. None of the dead worked directly for BP. Two were employed by M-I Swaco, a division of the oilfield services company Schlumberger. The rest of the decedents worked for Transocean. Here is a list of the 11 workers who died after the blast; no bodies were recovered.[1,2]

- Jason Anderson, 35, of Texas. Married and father of two.
- Aaron Dale "Bubba" Burkeen, 37, of Mississippi. Married with two children.
- Donald Clark, 49, of Louisiana. Scheduled to leave the rig on April 21.
- Stephen Ray Curtis, 40, of Louisiana. Married with two teenagers.
- Gordon Jones, 28, of Louisiana. Married, and his son was born three weeks later. Arrived on the rig the day before the explosion.
- Roy Wyatt Kemp, 27, of Louisiana. Married with a daughter and scheduled to leave the rig on April 21.
- Karl Kleppinger Jr., 38, of Mississippi. A first Gulf War veteran and married with one child.
- Keith Blair Manuel, 56, of Louisiana. Married with three daughters.
- Dewey A. Revette, 48, of Mississippi. Married for 26 years and scheduled to leave the rig on April 21.
- Shane M. Roshto, 22, of Mississippi. Married and scheduled to leave the rig on April 21.
- Adam Weise, 24, Texas. Scheduled to leave the rig on April 21.

Environmental damage claims by the federal government and Gulf Coast states are still pending against BP and its partners on the Deepwater Horizon drilling rig: Switzerland-based rig owner Transocean Ltd. and Houston-based cement contractor Halliburton. Civil claims could total more than $40 billion if BP is found "grossly negligent" by a federal judge, much of which could come from fines under violations of the Clean Water Act. Regarding criminal charges in December 2012, BP has agreed to pay $4.5 billion in a settlement with the U.S. government to plead guilty to felony counts related to the deaths of the 11 workers and lying to Congress. In addition, BP's former vice president of exploration for the Gulf of Mexico has been indicted for obstruction of Congress and making false statements. Two other BP employees were indicted on manslaughter charges in connection with the deaths of the 11 workers. The federal indictment claims that they acted negligently in their supervision of key safety tests performed on the drilling rig before the deadly explosion when they failed to phone engineers onshore to alert them of problems in the drilling operation.[1,3] At the time of this writing, this was the situation.

11.1. INTRODUCTION

Nothing in this Act shall apply to working conditions of employees with respect to which other Federal agencies, and State agencies acting under section 274 of the Atomic Energy Act of 1954, as amended (42 U.S.C. 2021), exercise statutory authority to prescribe or enforce standards or regulations affecting occupational safety or health.

—Section 4(b)(1), Occupational Safety and Health Act of 1970

Based on judicial decisions, the primacy for agencies other than the Occupational Safety and Health Administration (OSHA) for protecting the occupational safety and health of employees under other statutes consistent with § 4(b)(1) of the OSHAct rests on four criteria:

1. The employer must be covered by another federal statute.
2. The federal statute must address the safety and health of employees.
3. A responsible agency under the federal statute must have exercised its authority to prescribe or enforce occupational safety and health standards or regulations.
4. The specific working conditions must be covered by the agency's standards.

Five general areas are covered by these preemptions. One is offshore work on the continental shelf, a second is working conditions regarding nuclear energy, another concerns transportation-related work, fourth are conditions covered by consumer and environmental law, and fifth are rules applied to specific conditions under labor law outside of the Occupational Safety and Health Act (OSHAct; see Appendix). State and local government employees are also excluded from coverage by OSHA. Another area covered by the OSHAct but excluded by appropriation riders includes situations of an employer with a small number of employees in small businesses. A final category of workers not covered by the OSHAct is the self-employed worker, for whom there is no employer-employee relationship.

The previous chapter served as a clear example of the Mine Safety and Health Administration having primacy of authority over the safety and health of miners by the preemption criteria. This chapter addresses other worker populations that are not covered by OSHA. These populations are included under other agencies that exercise authority in the protection of workers, state and local government employees, workers in particular workplaces where employment is less than 11 employees, and self-employed workers. To distinguish overlapping authorities regarding other agencies, OSHA maintains a system of Memorandums of Understanding (MOUs).

11.2. EXCLUSIVE ECONOMIC ZONE

The Secretary of the Interior shall, by regulation, provide for judicial enforcement of this Act by the courts established for areas in which there are no United States district courts having jurisdiction.

—Section 4(a), Occupational Safety and Health Act of 1970

In 1983, President Ronald Reagan proclaimed the sovereign rights and jurisdiction of the United States in an Exclusive Economic Zone (EEZ) that extended to 200 nautical miles of sea contiguous to the United States, Puerto Rico, and the Northern Mariana Islands. The proclamation gave rights to the United States to exploit and conserve the natural resources within the EEZ and establish a jurisdiction for construction of structures at sea within the EEZ, and it extended the legal reach of the U.S. Coast Guard (USCG) within the EEZ.[4] The outer continental shelf is included within the EEZ.

OSHA has authority to enforce standards and regulations on the outer continental shelf, but both the USCG and the U.S. Department of the Interior (DoI) have established worker protection standards that preempt OSHA authorities. While the OSHAct confers authority to OSHA for the outer continental shelf, the Outer Continental Shelf Lands Act of 1953, as amended, confers authority to the USCG for safety in this area. Thus, OSHA is preempted by § 4(b) of the OSHAct from enforcement of standards where the USCG and DoI exercise occupational safety and health authorities. However, OSHA retains authority in two areas. One area is worker discrimination under § 11 of the OSHAct, and the other is shared responsibility by the USCG and OSHA on "uninspected" vessels. An example of shared responsibility is fish processing vessels, where the USCG protects the safety of seamen but OSHA protects the safety and health of fish processing workers. In these cases, an OSHA compliance officer may accompany a USCG boarding party onto a fish processing vessel.

11.2.1. Outer Continental Shelf Lands Act of 1953 As Amended in 1978

The Outer Continental Shelf Lands Act of 1953 established a policy for the management and exploitation of oil and natural gas in the outer continental shelf, and for protecting the marine and coastal environment. The Submerged Lands Act passed earlier in the year gave states jurisdiction three miles out from the shoreline, except for Texas and western Florida, which had jurisdiction out to nine miles. Federal agencies must notify the DoI regarding their activities that will have a direct and significant effect on the outer continental shelf or its development. This act expanded the USCG's role for safety and health on the outer continental shelf as well as continuing the present role it exercises for safety of vessels, diving, artificial islands, fixed drill rigs, and so on. Section 208 of the 1953 Act as amended in 1978 states: "Nothing in this Act shall affect the authority provided by law to the Secretary of Labor for the protection of Occupational Safety and Health." Under § 4(b)(1) of the OSHAct, OSHA has responsibility for any hazardous working condition for which the USCG has yet to promulgate enforceable standards. Moreover, the Secretary of Commerce, in cooperation with the Secretary of Homeland Security and the Director of the National Institute for Occupational Safety and Health (NIOSH), has the responsibility to conduct studies of underwater diving techniques and equipment suitable for the protection of human safety.[2,4]

11.2.2. Offshore Oil Rigs

OSHA did not investigate the April 2010 explosion on the Deepwater Horizon in the Gulf of Mexico that killed 11 workers and injured 17 others. The agency lacks jurisdiction over this workplace since it is beyond the three-mile state boundary, but it is within the 100-nautical-mile EEZ, over which the DoI and USCG have joint jurisdiction. The joint jurisdiction applies to offshore floating facilities that are tethered to the sea floor.[5] The drilling platform was a vessel (motored from Korea, where it was constructed), and the USCG has the responsibility to investigate vessel-related incidents. Since the DoI's Minerals Management Service (MMS) manages resources within the EEZ, provides oil drilling permits, and collects revenue for the permits, its responsibility to investigate work-related injuries and deaths on the rigs that it permits may potentially be compromised. One month after the spill, President Obama established the National Commission on the BP Deepwater Horizon Oil Spill and Offshore Drilling to develop options to guard against and mitigate the impact of oil spills associated with offshore drilling in the future. The commission issued its report in January 2011. It recommended reform to assure "political autonomy, technical expertise, and their full consideration of environmental protection concerns. In October 2011, Secretary of the Interior Ken Salazar divided the MMS into three entities, one of which was the Bureau of Safety and Environmental Enforcement, to enforce safety and environmental regulations.[6] The new bureau has regional offices in Anchorage, Alaska; Camarillo, California; and New Orleans, Louisiana.

11.2.3. Commercial Fishing Industry Vessel Safety Act of 1988

Congress had enacted the Commercial Fishing Industry Vessel Safety Act (CFIVSA) in 1988. It required the USCG to issue new regulations for safety equipment and operating procedures for fishing, fish tender, and fish processing vessels. It also increased casualty reporting requirements and provided for penalties of up to $5,000 and imprisonment for violators.[7]

In October 2010, President Obama signed a CFIVSA amendment, which changed requirements for the industry and authorities for the USCG, including treating documented and state-registered vessels under its authority; making dockside safety examinations mandatory; adding new equipment and training requirements; expanding stability, classification, and load line requirements for fishing vessels; establishing grant programs for training and research; and reauthorizing and expanding the Commercial Fishing Industry Vessel Safety Advisory Committee.[8]

11.2.4. Deep Water Missions Regarding Shipping Vessels

The USCG has statutory authority to prescribe and enforce regulations affecting the safety and health of seamen on board vessels inspected and certified by the agency. Since the USCG has issued comprehensive standards for working conditions on inspected vessels, OSHA may not enforce the OSHAct with respect to seamen on inspected vessels. The USCG also regulates commercial diving conducted from inspected vessels. Types of inspected vessels include freight vessels, nautical school vessels, off-shore supply vessels, passenger vessels, sailing school vessels, seagoing barges, seagoing motor vessels, small passenger vessels, steam vessels, tank vessels, fish processing vessels of more than 5,000 gross tons, and fish tender vessels of more than 500 gross tons.

11.3. DEPARTMENT OF ENERGY

Created predominantly to deal with the energy crisis of the 1970s, the U.S. Department of Energy's (DoE) mission and budget priorities have changed dramatically over time. By the early 1980s, its nuclear weapons production had grown substantially, and following revelations about environmental mismanagement in the mid- to late 1980s, DoE's cleanup budget began to expand, overshadowing other activities. With the Cold War's end, DoE found new or expanded missions in industrial competitiveness and science.[9]

In 1967, based on a U.S. Public Health Service study, the interagency Federal Radiation Council—which advises the president on standards drawn from the expertise of several agencies for the protection of human health from radiation exposure—reported that uranium miners were dying of lung cancer from exposure to radon "daughters" to which thousands of miners were exposed.[10] Public attention focused on the federal inaction regarding the protection of these miners. At the center of this attention was the radiation council, which was created by executive order in 1959 to advise the president on protective measures to take against all types of radiation hazards.[11] The council was expected to recommend a standard, but it could not reconcile differences between an Atomic Energy Commission (AEC) recommended standard and a tougher standard advocated by Secretary of Labor W. Willard Wirtz. With no decision by the council, the next day, a frustrated Secretary Wirtz was jarred into announcing his version of the standard under the Walsh-Healey Public Contracts Act.[12]

In 1974, OSHA recognized the AEC's authority to establish and enforce occupational safety and health standards at AEC-sponsored contractor facilities. The AEC (Marcus Rowden and Dixie Lee Ray) and the DoL (Secretary John T. Dunlop) exchanged letters agreeing to AEC authority over contractor employees based upon the exceptions in the OSHAct.[13] In the 20 years that have intervened since the signing of the original 1974 agreement, DoE has exercised its authority over working conditions at its government-owned, contractor operated facilities by developing and promulgating DoE orders and conducting an extensive program of internal oversight at these facilities. However, in May 1993, Secretary of Energy Hazel R. O'Leary announced that DoE would immediately begin the process of shifting from internal oversight of occupational safety and health to external enforcement by OSHA.

In early 1996, DoE began several initiatives to address budget reductions and to facilitate local community stability and revitalization as the DoE weapons production mission diminished following the end of the Cold War. These initiatives resulted in the privatization, reindustrialization, or commercialization of many facilities and operations through various mechanisms, such as leases or subleases, and property sales. Some privatized facilities and operations were engaged in private commercial enterprise, and thus should no longer be subject to DoE worker safety and health regulatory authority under § 4(b)(1), which exempts employers whose occupational safety and health is protected by other federal agencies from OSHA enforcement. Therefore, DoE and OSHA established a formal protocol for the transfer of jurisdiction from DoE to OSHA for the regulation of occupational safety and health requirements.[14]

Beginning in 1990, the DoE had sponsored research under the Worker and Public Health Activities Program conducted by the U.S. Department of Health and Human Services. Within this program, NIOSH created the Occupational Energy Research Program (OERP) to conduct occupational studies previously conducted by the DoE, including occupational health research among workers at DoE and other energy-related facilities. This research assesses the incidence and prevalence of acute and chronic disease among nuclear workers, evaluates associations of work-related exposures and disease, and determines the nature and extent of occupational exposures to physical, chemical, and radiological agents in energy-related industries.[15]

In 2000, President Bill Clinton signed into law the Energy Employees Occupational Illness Compensation Program, which is designed to compensate individuals who worked in nuclear weapons production and as a result of occupational exposures contracted certain illnesses.[15]

11.4. TRANSPORTATION STATUTES

The OSHAct permitted federal agencies other than OSHA to assert jurisdiction over specific categories of employees. Transportation was an early sector for the federal government to regulate worker safety and health for because the test of interstate commerce was evident, such as regarding interstate transport on navigable streams. The USCG was located within the U.S. Department of Transportation (DoT) but was transferred to the U.S. Department of Homeland Security (DHS) upon its creation in 2002.

11.4.1. Railway Safety Appliance Act of 1893

The Railway Safety Appliance Act of 1893, which went into effect on January 1, 1898, was upheld by the Supreme Court in 1904. The original act made it unlawful for a railroad company engaged in interstate commerce to run any train without having a sufficient number of cars equipped with train brakes (such as air brakes) so that the engineer on the locomotive could control the speed of the train without requiring brakemen to use a hand brake. The act also prohibited interstate carriers from hauling on or using a railroad line in moving interstate traffic on any car not equipped with couplers that could be coupled and uncoupled automatically. Later amendments extended the coverage to other safety appliances.[16]

11.4.2. Boiler Inspection Act of 1911

The federal Boiler Inspection Act of 1911 was enacted for the safety of employees. Thus, after July 1, 1911, it became unlawful for any interstate common carrier to use any steam locomotive engine unless the boiler was kept in safe operating condition to prevent peril to life or limb, and it required that all boilers be inspected in accord with the act.[4]

11.4.3. Rail Safety Act of 1970

The Federal Railroad Administration, within the DoT, exercises jurisdiction over all aspects of railroad safety as mandated in the Rail Safety Act of 1970. The primary objective of federal law pertaining to railroad safety is to promote the safety of railroad employees, passengers, and the public.[4]

11.4.4. Federal Aviation Act of 1975

In 1975, the Federal Aviation Administration (FAA) claimed safety and health jurisdiction over crew members, including flight attendants. Five years later, in 1980, the House Committee on Government Relations expressed concern that aviation employees remained uncovered by OSHA and strongly encouraged FAA and OSHA to develop an MOU between the two agencies.

In a 2000 MOU with OSHA, FAA claimed control of the safety and health of employees on an aircraft "in operation from the time the aircraft is first boarded by a crew member, preparatory to a flight, to the time the last crew member leaves the aircraft after the completion of that flight, including stops on the ground during which at least one crew member remains on the aircraft, even if the engines are shut down." OSHA enforces standards that protect other aviation industry employees, such as maintenance and ground support personnel.[17]

11.4.5. Hazardous Materials Transportation Act of 1975

The objective of the Hazardous Materials Transportation Act of 1975 (HMTA) as amended in 1990 was "to improve the regulatory and enforcement authority of the Secretary of Transportation to protect the Nation adequately against risks to life and property which are inherent in the transportation of hazardous materials in commerce." The HMTA empowered the Secretary of Transportation to designate as hazardous material any "particular quantity or form" of a material that might "pose an unreasonable risk to safety and health or property." Regulations applied to "any person who transports, or causes to be transported or shipped, a hazardous material; or who manufactures, fabricates, marks, maintains, reconditions, repairs, or tests a package or container which is represented, marked, certified, or sold by such person for use in the transportation in commerce of certain hazardous materials."[18] Enforcement of the HMTA was shared by each of the following administrations under delegations from the Secretary of Transportation:

- The Research and Special Programs Administration was responsible for container manufacturers, reconditioners, and retesters and shared authority over shippers of hazardous materials.
- The Federal Highway Administration was responsible for motor carriers.
- The Federal Railroad Administration was responsible for rail carriers.
- The FAA pertained to air carriers.

The USCG is responsible for inspecting shipments by water. DoE and EPA regulate the transport of radioactive materials, while the U.S. Nuclear Regulatory Commission regulates nuclear power plant radioactive wastes. OSHA is responsible for the protection of workers employed for hazardous waste operations and emergency response to hazardous waste spills. The amendment to HMTA—the Hazardous Materials Transportation Uniform Safety Act of 1990[19]—included authorization for the National Institute of Environmental Health Sciences of the National Institutes of Health to administer a program of grants to qualified nonprofit organizations to provide training and education to hazardous materials employees regarding the safe unloading, loading, handling, storage, and transportation of hazardous materials and regarding emergency preparedness for responding to incidents involving the transportation of hazardous materials. The amendment also established consistency of hazardous waste transport rules between states.

11.4.6. Pipeline Safety Improvement Act of 1979

The DoT sets safety standards for onshore liquid natural gas (LNG) facilities. The DoT's authority originally stemmed from the Natural Gas Pipeline Safety Act of 1968 and the Hazardous Liquids Pipeline Safety Act of 1979, which were combined as the Pipeline Safety Act of 1994 and amended again in 2002 by the Pipeline Safety Improvement Act. Under the resulting statutory scheme, the DoT is charged with issuing minimum safety standards for the siting, design, construction, and operation of LNG facilities.[4]

11.4.7. Surface Transportation Act of 1982

Under the Surface Transportation Act of 1982, OSHA administers a discrimination-complaint investigation program for employees in the trucking industry. In addition to similar authorities under § 11(c) of the OSHAct and with a 180-day rather than a 30-day statute of limitations, OSHA has the authority for cases with merit to order an employer to reinstate a discharged worker—including independent contractors—with back pay and compensatory damages rather than taking the case to court.[4]

11.4.8. Motor Carrier Safety Improvement Act of 1999

Two federal agencies that are part of the DoT—the Federal Motor Carrier Safety Administration (FMCSA) and the National Highway Traffic Safety Administration (NHTSA)—develop and enforce safety standards related to vehicle design and operation. Motor carrier safety is the responsibility of the FMCSA, established by the Motor Carrier Safety Improvement Act of 1999. Regulations under FMCSA cover commercial motor carriers, including long-haul trucking, while NHTSA regulations set minimum design and safety performance requirements to which all vehicle manufacturers must conform.[4]

Federal motor carrier safety regulations cover businesses that operate commercial motor vehicles in interstate commerce. Intrastate motor carriers are subject to state regulations, which must be identical to or compatible with the federal regulations in order for states to receive motor carrier safety grants from FMCSA.[19] Three other agencies play roles in protecting workers who operate motor vehicles on the job. First, the U.S. Department of Labor's (DoL) Employment Standards Administration (ESA) enforces child labor provisions of the Fair Labor Standards Act that define conditions under which workers age 17 and under may operate a motor vehicle. Second, OSHA has regulations covering certain industries that address vehicle and equipment operation, primarily the operation of machinery and equipment off the highway. Finally, the National Transportation Safety Board (NTSB) investigates selected roadway crashes and develops safety recommendations directed at federal and state agencies and other groups.

11.5. BOARD INVESTIGATIONS

Two independent boards investigate catastrophes but lack regulatory authority except for access to incident sites. However, they recommend regulatory actions based upon their investigations. One of these boards is the NTSB, and the other is the Chemical Safety and Hazard Investigation Board (CSB).

11.5.1. Independent Safety Board Act of 1974

The NTSB is an independent federal agency that began operations in 1967, and in 1974, Congress enacted the Independent Safety Board Act to investigate every civil aviation incident in the United States and significant incidents in the other modes of transportation—railroad, highway, marine, and pipeline—and issue safety recommendations aimed at preventing future incidents. Although independent, it relies on the DoT for funding and administrative support but it is not part of DoT or affiliated with any of its modal agencies. Many safety features currently incorporated into airplanes, automobiles, trains, pipelines, and marine vessels had their genesis in NTSB recommendations. The NTSB also serves as the "court of appeals" for any aviator, mechanic, or mariner whenever certification action is taken by the FAA or the USCG Commandant, or when civil penalties are assessed by the FAA.[19a]

11.5.2. Chemical Safety and Hazard Investigation Board

Both OSHA and the U.S. Environmental Protection Agency (EPA) have a responsibility to investigate major chemical catastrophes to determine whether any violations of their laws occurred and, if so, to require correction of these violations and ensure compliance with their laws. These functions are similar to some of the responsibilities of the Chemical Safety and Hazard Investigation Board (CSB), created by the Clean Air Act of 1990.

The CSB is an independent federal agency created by the Clean Air Act of 1990. Its mission is to ensure the safety of workers and the public by preventing or reducing the effects of chemical incidents. The CSB is the lead federal agency in the conduct of investigations dedicated to identifying the cause or causes of chemical incidents, advises industry and labor on actions they should take to improve safety, and makes regulatory recommendations to EPA and OSHA. The board is composed of five members who are appointed by the president and confirmed by the Senate, and members serve fixed terms of five years. OSHA and CSB cooperate while carrying out their respective statutory responsibilities. In addition, CSB and OSHA investigators work with other federal, state, and local investigatory and response groups to reduce duplication of effort and to ensure that response and investigation activities do not compromise worker or public safety and health.[20]

11.6. ENVIRONMENTAL AND CONSUMER PROTECTION

The creation of the Environmental Protection Agency in 1970 and the passage shortly thereafter of statutes giving the new agency broad powers to reduce pollution were political moves informed by a theory of how to best prevent a regulatory agency from being "captured" by industry or afflicted with bureaucratic sloth.

—Alfred Marcus[21]

11.6.1. Federal Hazardous Substances Act of 1960, As Amended

The Consumer Product Safety Commission (CPSC) regulates the manufacture, transportation, and sale of hazardous substances under the Federal Hazardous Substances Act. The commission is empowered to define a hazardous substance, require labeling, inspect manufacturers, and control the sales of hazardous substances. The CPSC can also regulate hazardous substances under the Consumer Product Safety Act of 1972. A CPSC regulation can supersede labeling under OSHA's hazard communication standard, but the CPSC cannot regulate for injury prevention if an OSHA standard eliminates or reduces the risk to workers sufficiently.[22]

11.6.2. Federal Insecticide, Fungicide, and Rodenticide Act of 1947

The Federal Insecticide, Fungicide, and Rodenticide Act (FIFRA) was enacted in 1947. Since then, pesticide products have been subject to federal regulation under FIFRA. In 1972, FIFRA was amended by the Federal Environmental Pesticide Control Act. The amendments broadened federal pesticide regulatory authority by making it "unlawful for any person to use any registered pesticide in a manner inconsistent with its labeling," and they provided civil and criminal penalties for violations of FIFRA.

The primary focus of FIFRA is to provide federal control of pesticide distribution, sale, and use. The EPA was given authority under FIFRA not only to study the consequences of pesticide usage but also to require users (farmers, utility companies, and others) to register when purchasing pesticides. Through later amendments to the law, users also must take examinations for certification as applicators of pesticides. All pesticides used in the United States must be registered (licensed) by the EPA. Registration assures that pesticides will be properly labeled and that if used in accordance with specifications, they will not cause "unreasonable" harm to the environment. In 1988, Congress amended the Federal Environmental Pesticide Control Act, requiring the EPA to reregister or cancel up to 50,000 products that had been allowed to remain on the market (grandfathered) under the 1972 law.[23]

In 1974, the EPA promulgated a set of workplace safety standards covering pesticide use on farms. However, farmworker groups wanted standards from OSHA rather than the EPA because of OSHA's greater experience and tougher enforcement powers and challenged these regulations. The court disagreed with the farmworkers in 1975. In *Organized Migrants in Community Action, Inc. v. Brennan,* the appellate court held that Congress had given the EPA broad statutory authority under FIFRA to regulate farmworker safety.

Under § 4(b)(1) of the OSHAct, the court acknowledged that OSHA had broad enforcement powers but found that Congress must have intended for the EPA to preempt OSHA regarding farmworker protection. However, OSHA retained authority for the regulation of pesticides in other work environments, such as pesticide formulation.[23]

The EPA implemented comprehensive regulations intended to protect farmworkers from the harmful effects of pesticides in the workplace. The Worker Protection Standard (WPS) mandated that farmworkers receive training in the avoidance of pesticide exposure and what to do if an exposure occurred. A revised WPS was proposed by the EPA in 1988, was adopted in 1992, and went into effect in 1995. The revised WPS requires that farmworkers receive training in how to avoid pesticide poisoning. These requirements are accompanied by parallel regulations requiring that worker protection information be provided on the label of pesticide containers. Providing the WPS training is the responsibility of the farmer or employer, and providing accurate information on the pesticide label on how to safely handle that pesticide and how to avoid exposures to farmworkers is the responsibility of the chemical company manufacturing the pesticide. The WPS is enforced as labeling requirements vis-à-vis workplace safety requirements.[21] The Federal Food Quality Protection Act of 1996 did not change the WPS.

11.6.3. Toxic Substances Control Act of 1976

Congress enacted the Toxic Substances Control Act (TSCA) of 1976 to give the EPA the ability to track the 75,000 industrial chemicals currently produced or imported into the United States. The EPA screens these chemicals and can require reporting or testing of those that may pose an environmental or human health hazard. The agency can ban the manufacture and import of those chemicals that pose an unreasonable risk. In addition, EPA has mechanisms in place to track the thousands of new chemicals that industry develops each year with either unknown or dangerous characteristics. The agency then can control these chemicals as necessary to protect human health and the environment. The TSCA supplements other federal statutes, including the OSHAct. Asbestos Hazard Emergency Response Act (AHERA) amendments to the TSCA provide for worker protection regulations, which the EPA has promulgated. Under a MOU, OSHA has access to confidential business information submitted to the EPA under the TSCA.[4]

11.6.4. Asbestos Hazard Emergency Response Act of 1986

Since the late 1970s, the EPA had focused its attention on the disease-causing potential of exposure to airborne asbestos in schools. According to a 1984 EPA survey, about 34,800 schools were believed to have friable asbestos-containing materials, potentially exposing an estimated 15 million students and 1.4 million school employees. Congress introduced the Asbestos Hazard Emergency Response Act in spring 1986 to "provide for the establishment of Federal regulations which require inspection for asbestos-containing material and [which ensure] implementation of appropriate response actions . . . in the Nation's schools in a safe and complete manner."[24] The act was presented to President Reagan for signature on October 14, 1986. It required regulations for inspections, abatement, response actions, periodic surveillance of asbestos, transport and disposal, and management plan requirements for schools.

The EPA issued this final rule under § 6 of the TSCA in 2000.[25] In this, EPA amended both the Asbestos Worker Protection Rule (WPR) and the Asbestos-in-Schools Rule. The WPR amendment protects state and local government employees from the health risks of exposure to asbestos to the same extent as private sector workers by adopting for these employees the OSHA asbestos standards. The WPR's coverage is extended to state and local government employees who are performing construction work, custodial work, and automotive brake and clutch repair work. This final rule cross-references the OSHA Asbestos Standards for Construction and for General Industry, so that future amendments to these OSHA standards are directly and equally effective for employees covered by the WPR. The EPA also amended the Asbestos-in-Schools Rule to provide coverage under the WPR for employees of public local education agencies who perform operations, maintenance, and repair activities.

11.6.5. Superfund Amendments and Reauthorization Act of 1986

Congress enacted the Comprehensive Environmental Response, Compensation, and Liability Act (CERCLA), commonly known as Superfund, on December 11, 1980. This law created a tax on the chemical and petroleum industries and provided broad federal authority to respond directly to releases or threatened releases of hazardous substances that might endanger public health or the environment. The Superfund Amendments and Reauthorization Act of 1986 reauthorized CERCLA to continue cleanup activities around the country. Several site-specific amendments, definitions clarifications, and technical requirements were added to the legislation, including additional enforcement authorities. Hazardous waste workers are protected by rules under CERCLA.[4]

11.7. LABOR AND EMPLOYMENT STANDARDS STATUTES

In the 1930s, workers had begun to organize in a militant fashion, and in 1933 and 1934, a great wave of strikes occurred across the nation in the form of general strikes and factory takeovers. Violent confrontations occurred between workers trying to form unions and the police and private security forces defending the interests of antiunion employers. The Supreme Court declared the National Industrial Recovery Act of 1933 unconstitutional in 1935, after which organized labor was again looking for relief from employers who had been free to spy on, interrogate, discipline, discharge, and blacklist union members. The National Labor Relations Board (NLRB) administers the first statute shown below, and the ESA administers the other laws shown below under the umbrella of the DoL.

11.7.1. National Labor Relations Act of 1935

A Congress sympathetic to labor unions passed the National Labor Relations Act (NLRA) in July 1935. The broad intention of the act, commonly known as the Wagner Act after Senator Robert R. Wagner (D) of New York, was to guarantee employees "the right to self-organization, to form, join, or assist labor organizations, to bargain collectively through representatives of their own choosing, and to engage in concerted activities for the purpose of collective bargaining or other mutual aid and protection."[26] The NLRA is applied to all employers involved in interstate commerce except airlines, railroads, agriculture, and government.

In order to enforce and maintain those rights, the act included a provision for the NLRB to arbitrate deadlocked labor-management disputes, guarantee democratic union elections, and penalize unfair labor practices by employers. The board of five members is appointed by the president and is assisted by 33 regional directors. The NLRB further determines proper bargaining units, conducts elections for union representation, and investigates charges of unfair labor practices by employers. Unfair practices, by law, include such things as interference, coercion, or restraint in labor's self-organizing rights; interference with the formation of labor unions; encouragement or discouragement of union membership; and the refusal to bargain collectively with duly chosen employee representatives. Working conditions, including safety, are negotiable in collective bargaining.

11.7.2. Fair Labor Standards Act of 1938

The Fair Labor Standards Act (FLSA) exempts agricultural workers from overtime premium pay but requires the payment of the minimum wage to workers employed on larger farms (farms employing more than seven full-time workers). The act has special child-labor regulations that apply to agricultural employment; children younger than 16 years are forbidden to work during school hours and in certain jobs deemed too dangerous. The ESA administers this law.

The restrictions shown in Table 11-1 do not apply to youth who are employed by their parents on a farm owned or operated by their parents.[26a,26b] A few states rely solely on the federal laws found in the FLSA. States may have

Table 11-1. Federal Child Labor Requirements Under the Fair Labor Standards Act

	Nonagricultural Employment	Agricultural Employment
Age	The minimum age for employment is 14. There are some exceptions such as newspaper delivery; performing in radio, television, movie, or theatrical productions; and work for parents in their solely owned nonfarm business (except in manufacturing or in hazardous jobs).	▶ 10- and 11-year-olds may perform jobs on farms owned or operated by parent(s), or with a parent's written consent in nonhazardous jobs. ▶ 12- and 13-year-olds may work in nonhazardous jobs with a parent's consent. ▶ 14- and 15-year-olds may perform any nonhazardous farm job. ▶ 16-year-olds and older may perform any job.
Hazardous employment	There are 17 prohibited jobs for youths younger than 18, such as manufacturing or storing explosives or coal mining. There are additional prohibited occupations for 14- and 15-year-olds.	Youths younger than 16 are prohibited from certain occupations and activities that the Secretary of Labor has determined to be hazardous.

different minimum ages for employment, different hours of work restrictions, and additional occupations identified as hazardous. If the employment falls under FLSA jurisdiction, then both federal and state laws apply—and the most restrictive law (whether it is the state or the federal) is enforced.

11.7.3. Migrant and Seasonal Agricultural Worker Protection Act of 1983

The Migrant and Seasonal Agricultural Worker Protection Act of 1983 regulates the hiring and employment activities of agricultural employers, farm labor contractors, and associations using migrant and seasonal agricultural workers. The act prescribes wage protections, housing and transportation safety standards, farm labor contractor registration requirements, and disclosure requirements.[4]

11.7.4. Longshore and Harbor Workers' Compensation Act of 1927, as amended in 1984

The Longshore and Harbor Workers' Compensation Act is administered by the ESA. This law requires employers to assure that workers' compensation is funded and available to eligible employees.[4]

11.8. STATE AND LOCAL GOVERNMENT EMPLOYEES

The term "employer" means a person engaged in a business affecting commerce who has employees, but does not include the United States (not including the United States Postal Service) or any State or political subdivision of a State.
    —Section 3(5), Occupational Safety and Health Act of 1970

State and local government workers are excluded from federal coverage under the OSHAct. However, states operating their own occupational safety and health programs under OSHA-approved plans as described in Chapter 8 are required to extend their coverage to public sector (state and local government) workers in the state. States without approved plans are permitted by OSHA to develop plans that cover only public sector workers, while private sector employment remains under federal OSHA jurisdiction. The Bureau of Labor Statistics publishes annual fatality data for all public administration workers, but only 24 states and three other jurisdictions submit data on public employee occupational injuries and illnesses, which are recorded on an OSHA log.[26c] States without OSHA-approved state plans may voluntarily provide safety and health protection to their governmental workers.

However, NIOSH has nonregulatory authority under other statutes than the OSHAct for research and public health. The institute has established a research program for one particular category of state and local employees: public safety workers. It has an estimated nearly two million career public safety workers employed in the fire service, law enforcement, corrections, and emergency medical services. Volunteers add to this number, nearly matching a total of the employed workers who provide firefighting and emergency medical services in many locations throughout the country.[27] The institute has conducted comprehensive fatality investigations of firefighter deaths for years with recommendations for preventing future fatalities.

11.9. APPROPRIATION RIDERS

That none of the funds appropriated under this paragraph [OSHA funds] shall be obligated or expended to prescribe, issue, administer, or enforce any standard, rule, regulation, or order under the Occupational Safety and Health Act of 1970 which is applicable to any person who is engaged in a farming operation which does not maintain a temporary labor camp and employs ten or fewer employees....

—Public Law 102-170, November 22, 1991, 105 Stat 1107

In the annual appropriations for OSHA funding, Congress can restrict the expenditure of funds on specified activities. Appropriation riders have prohibited the OSHA inspection—and inspection by the ESA in enforcing OSHA's Field Sanitation and Temporary Labor Camp standards—of employers who employ 10 or fewer employees, listed below. These riders address two conditions of employers with 10 or fewer employees and which are also shown in more detail regarding OSHA activities in Table 11-2. However, OSHA is not restricted by the riders from inspecting workplaces employing more than 10 workers.[28]

- Farms with 10 or fewer employees (at any time) *and* no temporary labor camp activity within the last 12 months
- Nonfarm employers with 10 or fewer employees within the last 12 months *and* in a two-digit industry sector below average lost-day injury rate

Table 11-2. Exemptions and Limitations established by Appropriation Riders for Occupational Safety and Health Administration Enforcement

OSHA Activity	Nonfarm Employers < 11 Employees and in an Industry Sector With Below Average Lost-Day Injury Rate	Farms With > 10 Employees or an Active Temporary Labor Camp	Farms < 11 Employees
• Programmed safety inspections	Cannot inspect	Can inspect	Not permitted
• Programmed health inspections	Can inspect	Can inspect	Not permitted
• Fatality or catastrophe investigations	Can inspect	Can inspect	Not permitted
• Imminent danger	Can inspect	Can inspect	Not permitted
• Discrimination	Can inspect	Can inspect	Not permitted
• Employee complaint	Can inspect*	Can inspect	Not permitted
• Consultation and technical assistance	Permitted	Permitted	Not permitted
• Education and training	Permitted	Permitted	Not permitted
• Conduct surveys and studies	Permitted	Permitted	Not permitted

Note: OSHA = Occupational Safety and Health Administration.
*Limits on citations and penalties.

11.10. THE SELF-EMPLOYED

The term "employee" means an employee of an employer who is employed in a business of his employer which affects commerce.
—Section 3(6), Occupational Safety and Health Act of 1970

Self-employed workers account for 7.4% of the civilian workforce but account for nearly 20% of occupational fatalities.[29] Self-employed workers are not regulated under the OSHAct except indirectly in multiemployer worksites when a general contractor has responsibility for subcontractors on a worksite. In a 2004 study, the self-employed fatality rate was 11.4 deaths per 100,000 full-time workers, compared with 4.2 deaths per 100,000 full-time employees for the seven-year period 1995–2001.[29] As shown in Figure 11-1, these rates are shown to be higher across many sectors of the economy, with the exception of the construction sector. These data do not include children younger than age 16 and self-employed workers who are incorporated, which is explained in the next few paragraphs.

Over this period, the number of fatalities of self-employed workers exceeded those of wage and salary workers in the agriculture, forestry, and fishing industry by 3,231 and 2,190 deaths, respectively.[29] Indeed, the high death rate

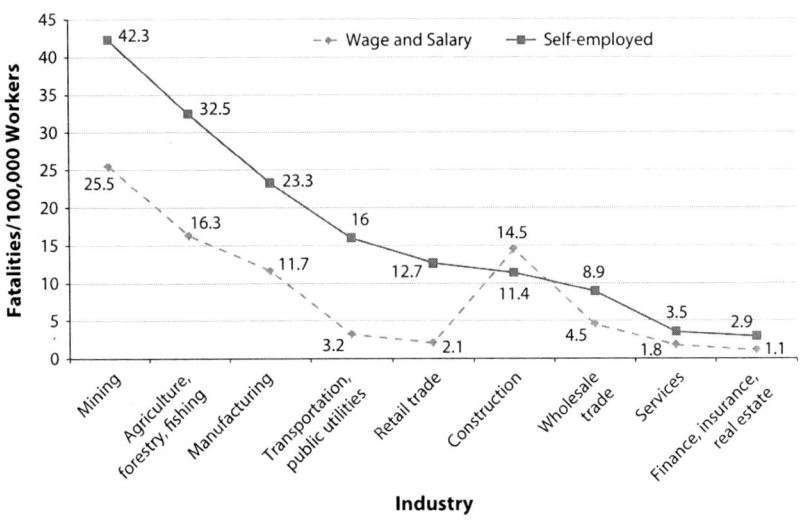

Source: Pegula.[29]

Figure 11-1. Fatality rates of self-employed workers compared with wage and salary workers, 1995–2001.

in this industry, where self-employed workers dominate in individual states, can become an important consideration in preventing occupational fatalities. In Kentucky, where agriculture is a large industry, the fatality rate was 27.6 deaths per 100,000 self-employed workers in a 2004 study.[30]

In 2009, of 149.9 million workers, 15.3 million individuals (10.2%) were self-employed. Of all self-employed persons, 9.8 million, or nearly two-thirds, were unincorporated; the remaining 5.5 million were incorporated. Self-employed workers typically incorporate their businesses in order to receive benefits that include limited liability, tax considerations, and the enhanced opportunity to raise capital through the sale of stocks and bonds.[31] Regarding agriculture, OSHA and the U.S. Department of Agriculture Extension Service have an MOU that provides for the state cooperative extension services to diffuse occupational safety and health information from OSHA into the farming community. Moreover, NIOSH has an agricultural safety and health research and public health program for reaching farmers and their families.

The principal interventions to protect self-employed workers are product safety and education. Governmental policies can address product safety through transportation statutes, environmental laws such as FIFRA or TSCA, some Food and Drug Administration-regulated electronic products regarding radiation, or CPSC-regulated consumer products. The federal government can also regulate unsafe products that are imported into the United States.[32]

11.11. THE OCCUPATIONAL OBSCENITY[33]

If we cannot develop a U.S. model for a proven intervention on a single most important cause of agricultural mortality, how can we succeed in addressing less dramatic yet still important causes of agricultural diseases and injuries?

—Dr. James A. Merchant[34]

In 1993, NIOSH published a report from which the following account is quoted:[33]

> Each year, an average of 132 American farm workers are crushed to death as tractors overturn during operation. Nearly all of these fatalities can be prevented, according to a report released this week by 'NIOSH.' NIOSH Director J. Donald Millar calls tractor rollovers an "occupational obscenity." According to Millar, "There is no scientific excuse for the persistence of this problem. This is something we know how to prevent." The key to prevention is the presence of a rollover protective structure (ROPS) on every tractor in use. A ROPS is a structural component attached to vehicles (like a roll-bar) which is designed to protect the operator if the vehicle overturns during operation. ROPS can be either unenclosed, as shown in the picture below, or enclosed, as part of a tractor cab. Safety restraints, such as seat belts, should be used in conjunction with the ROPS to keep the operator within the space protected by the device.
>
> NIOSH urges all tractor owners to install ROPS on their tractors. . . . The use of ROPS could substantially reduce the national toll of occupational fatalities associated with tractors. To encourage the use of ROPS, at least one manufacturer has reduced the price of ROPS and is selling them at manufacturer's cost. An article in this week's edition (January 1993) of the Centers for Disease Control and Prevention's (CDC) Morbidity and Mortality Weekly Report (MMWR) describes the magnitude of this problem and explores the effectiveness of ROPS in preventing these tragic injuries. Agriculture remains one of this nation's most hazardous industries, ranking fourth among industries in the United States at highest risk for work-related fatalities. One of the biggest killers on the farm today is the tractor,

and by far the leading cause of tractor-related deaths is the tractor rollover. "A tractor without a ROPS is a fatality waiting to happen," said Melvin L. Myers, coordinator for the agricultural safety and health program at NIOSH, which estimates that more than half of the 4.61 million tractors in use in the United States lack ROPS and safety belts. Of these, 61% were manufactured before 1971, the year ROPS first became available as optional equipment on farm tractors. Tractors manufactured before 1971 generally were not designed to accommodate the addition of ROPS. If tractors without ROPS are not retrofitted, NIOSH estimates that 2,800 rollover-related deaths could occur during the period that these tractors remain in use (an estimated 31 years). The potential public health benefit of retrofitting tractors with ROPS could be substantial.

Each day preventable rollover injuries are reported across the country. Tragically, incidents such as these are neither unusual nor unique:

September 30, 1992, a 35-year-old man was crushed to death on a family farm in Winslow, Arkansas. He was bush hogging when his tractor overturned and pinned him underneath.

On October 9, 1992, a 69-year-old man was killed beneath a tractor in Russellville, Arkansas. It overturned while he was backing it off a trailer.

On November 13, 1992, a 45-year-old woman was crushed beneath a tractor in Belgrade, Minnesota. She was unloading corn with a tractor and wagon, when the wagon hit an elevator, tipping the tractor over on top of her.

On December 5, 1992, a 65-year-old man lost his life when his tractor overturned in Holman, Texas. He was pushing a round bale of hay with his tractor, when the tractor apparently went up the bale, causing the tractor to overturn on top of him.

Since 1967, a series of tractor rollover incidents has been investigated in Nebraska. Forty percent of the 250 persons involved in unprotected tractor rollover incidents died. In contrast, the study found that only 2%, or one person died, of the 61 persons operating ROPS-equipped tractors that rolled over. The one fatal victim was not personally restrained and was thrown from the ROPS protective zone during rollover. This incident emphasizes the need to use safety restraints, such as seat belts, in conjunction with ROPS in order to keep the operator within the space protected by the ROPS. Between 1961 and 1983, a 92% reduction in tractor rollover fatalities followed a requirement to install ROPS on all tractors in Sweden.

National and community-based injury-prevention programs should include plans for retrofitting or refurbishing farm tractors with ROPS to prevent fatalities associated with tractor rollover. These programs may include: A buy-back of older, unprotected tractors; Interventions tailored to the needs of specific farming regions (e.g., dairy, grain, and orchard); Effectiveness studies of community- and demonstration-project intervention initiatives. In addition, guidelines should be developed for design of ROPS for tractors manufactured before 1971.

The NIOSH Agricultural Health and Safety Initiative is supporting surveillance, research, and intervention efforts directed at farmers, farm families, and farm workers nationwide. As part of this initiative, NIOSH convened the Surgeon General's Conference on Agricultural Safety and Health in 1991.

The proceedings of that conference, which brought together experts in agricultural safety and health from across the country, have just been released. Not surprisingly, the results confirm that tractor rollovers are a serious problem which continues to plague the agricultural population. Twenty-seven speakers at the conference referred to this preventable problem. "Amidst expressions of anguish and pleas for reason, there was an overwhelming interest in a particular issue, namely the need to reduce the risk of fatalities related to tractor rollovers," said NIOSH Director Dr. J. Donald Millar, summarizing the conference.

THE LONG HAUL NARRATIVE

Summer jobs in Alaska held the lure of adventure and of a share in the payment of the fish catches aboard fishing vessels in the 1980s.[35] Peter Barry took one of these jobs while on summer break from college. In August 1985, he was part of a six-man crew aboard the fishing vessel Western Sea, a 70-year-old purse seiner that departed Kodiak, Alaska, to fish for salmon. Then on August 20, another fishing vessel, the Dusk, came across the floating body of Peter Barry in the frigid waters near Kodiak. Until the recovery of his body, there was no report that the vessel was in peril. The USCG launched an intensive search with cutters and aircraft but failed to locate any survivors. Twenty-one days after Peter's body was recovered, two more crewmembers were recovered, floating lifeless. All three bodies wore USCG-approved life jackets.

Peter's parents, Robert (the U.S. Ambassador to Bulgaria) and Peggy Barry, immediately sought answers to questions regarding Peter's death.[36] They learned that fishing vessels were not required to carry available safety equipment such as survival craft, immersion suits, and emergency position–indicating radio beacons to inform and guide the USCG for a rescue. Robert and Peggy Barry organized safety advocates, government officials, the legislators, and the surviving families of other commercial fishers lost at sea to campaign for mandatory safety regulations. Three bills were introduced in the House in 1986. At the hearings on these bills, Peggy Barry and other family members of the crew lost on the Western Sea testified passionately for legislation to require emergency rescue equipment on commercial fishing vessels. A compromise bill, The Commercial Fishing Vessel Liability and Safety Act, was sent to the full House, but two issues blocked its enactment: (1) the USCG argued for voluntary requirements, and (2) trial lawyers attacked a limited liability clause for vessel owners at $500,000 for cases of permanent injury.

Try and try again: In March 1987, on behalf of Robert and Peggy Barry, Representative Mike Lowry (D) of Washington introduced a bill in the House dealing with fishing vessel safety (H.R. 1836). The bill called for the licensing of operators of commercial fishing vessels and the training of all crew members. It established uniform casualty reporting and an advisory committee to make recommendations to the Secretary of Transportation that related to fishing safety.

Meanwhile, Representative Gerry E. Studds (D) of Massachusetts, Chairman of the Subcommittee on Fisheries and Wildlife Conservation and the Environment, introduced an alternative bill (H.R. 1841) that had two titles. Title I dealt with compensation for temporary injuries on fishing industry vessels, and Title II applied to safety on all fishing vessels. There was little difference between the safety proposals in the Studds and Lowry bills. Hearings were held in June 1987 on these bills, and in September and December on a companion Senate bill introduced by Senator John H. Chafee (R) of Rhode Island (S. 849).

The USCG remained convinced that the voluntary approach was viable, and it did not support the proposed advisory committee. However, the NTSB came to the Barrys' rescue with testimony based on its comprehensive 1987 study, *Uninspected Commercial Fishing Vessels*.[37] The NTSB recommended safety measures consistent with those advocated by the Barrys.

The House committee revised the Studds bill by dropping Title I, which contained liability and compensation issues, but kept Title II, which contained the safety issues. On September 9, 1988, the Commercial Fishing Industry Vessel Safety Act, which contained the legal authority for the CFIVSA, became law. This was the first safety legislation enacted in the United States applying specifically to commercial fishing vessels.[38,39] Peggy Barry became a member of the first Commercial Fishing Industry Vessel Safety Advisory Committee.[35]

REFERENCES

1. Sewell M. Who's responsible for the Deepwater Horizon oil spill? May 26, 2010. Available at: http://www.marilynsewell.com. Accessed January 30, 2015.
1a. Associated Press. Gulf Oil spill deaths: The 11 rig workers who died during the BP Deepwater Horizon explosion. *Huffington Post*. Posted on November 15, 2011. Available at: http://www.huffingtonpost.com/2012/11/15/gulf-oil-spill-deaths_n_2139669.html. Accessed December 26, 2012.
2. National Commission on the BP Deepwater Horizon Oil Spill and Offshore Drilling. Deep water: the gulf oil disaster and the future of offshore drilling. Final report. 2011. Available at: http://cybercemetery.unt.edu/archive/oilspill/20121210200431/http://www.oilspillcommission.gov/final-report. Accessed June 12, 2014.
3. Jervis R, Johnson K. 3 BP executives indicted over Gulf oil spill: BP agrees to pay $4.5 billion in fines in the largest such settlement in U.S. history. *USA Today*. November 15, 2012. Available at: http://www.usatoday.com/story/money/business/2012/11/15/bp-near-settlement-with-us-over-gulf-spill/1706209. Accessed December 26, 2012.
4. Blosser F. *Primer on Occupational Safety and Health*. Washington, DC: Bureau of National Affairs;1992.
5. Minerals Management Service. Memorandum of agreement between the Minerals Management Service, U.S. Department of Interior and the U.S. Coast Guard, Department of Homeland Security. MMS/USCG MOA: OCS-04. February 28, 2008. Available at: http://www.uscg.mil/hq/cg5/cg522/cg5222/docs/mou/floating_offshore_facilities.pdf. Accessed January 19, 2013.
6. U.S. Department of the Interior. The reorganization of the former MMS. Bureau of Safety and Environmental Enforcement. 2011. Available at: http://www.bsee.gov/About-BSEE/BSEE-History/Reorganization/Reorganization.aspx. Accessed January 16, 2013.
7. Steinman AM. Protective clothing in cold water survival. In: Myers ML, Klatt ML, eds. *Proceedings of the National Fishing Industry Safety and Health Workshop*. Anchorage, AK: U.S. Department of Health and Human Services, National Institute for Occupational Safety and Health;1994. DHHS (NIOSH) Publication No. 94-109.

8. Christensen E, Kemerer J. Fishing vessel safety. *Proceedings.* 2010-2011;67(4):6-13.

9. Hearing before the House Subcommittee on Energy and Environment, Committee on Science and the Subcommittee on Energy and Power, Committee on Commerce (July 13, 1999) (testimony of V Rezendes, Department of Energy). Available at: http://www.gpo.gov/fdsys/pkg/GAOREPORTS-T-RCED-99-255/pdf/GAOREPORTS-T-RCED-99-255.pdf. Accessed January 19, 2013.

10. Tompkins PC, Palmiter CC. Guidance for the control of radiation hazards in uranium mining. Federal Radiation Council Staff Report No. 8 [revised]. September 1967. Available at: http://www.epa.gov/rpdweb00/docs/federal/frc_rpt8.pdf. Accessed October 14, 2012.

11. Flemming AS. The Federal Radiation Council. *Public Health Rep.* 1959;74:1107-1108.

12. MacLaury J. The job safety law of 1970: its passage was perilous. *Monthly Labor Rev.* 1981;104(3):18-24.

13. Wirtz WW. Memorandum of Understanding. Letter to Dixie Lee Ray, U.S. Atomic Energy Commission; February 4, 1974. Available at: https://www.osha.gov/pls/oshaweb/owadisp.show_document?p_table=MOU&p_id=215&p_table=MOU. Accessed June 4, 2014.

14. Office of Environment, Safety, and Health. Memorandum of Understanding between the U.S. Department of Labor, Occupational Safety and Health Administration, and the U.S. Department of Energy Office of Environment, Safety and Health on safety and health enforcement at privatized facilities and operations. July 25, 2000. Available at: http://energy.gov/sites/prod/files/2014/07/f18/MOU_DOE_OSHA2000.pdf. Accessed January 22, 2013.

15. National Institute for Occupational Safety and Health. The NIOSH occupational energy research program: evidence for the National Academy's "Review of the Worker and Public Health Activities Program Administered by the Department of Energy and the Department of Health and Human Services." Cincinnati, OH: Department of Health and Human Services, NIOSH;2005. Available at: http://www.cdc.gov/niosh/nas/oerp/pdfs/OERP-NAS.pdf. Accessed November 29, 2012.

16. Usselman SW. Air brakes for freight trains: technological innovation in the American railroad industry, 1869-1900. *Bus Hist Rev.* 1984;58(1):30-50.

17. Federal Aviation Administration. Memorandum of Understanding between the Federal Aviation Administration, U.S. Department of Transportation, and the Occupational Safety and Health Administration, U.S. Department of Labor. August 9, 2000. Available at: http://www.osha.gov/pls/oshaweb/owadisp.show_document?p_table=MOU&p_id=283. Accessed January 19, 2013.

18. Hazardous Materials Transportation Act, 49 U.S.C. §§ 5101-5127 (1975).

19. Pratt SG. *Work-Related Roadway Crashes: Challenges and Opportunities for Prevention.* Cincinnati, OH: National Institute for Occupational Health and Safety;2003. DHHS (NIOSH) Publication No. 2003-119, NIOSH Hazard Review.

19a. National Safety Transportation Board. Wikipedia. January 7, 2015. Available at: http://en.wikipedia.org/wiki/National_Transportation_Safety_Board. Accessed January 30, 2015.

20. Chemical Safety and Hazard Investigation Board. Memorandum of Understanding between U.S. Department of Labor, Occupational Safety and Health Administration, and the U.S. Chemical Safety and Hazard Investigation Board on Chemical Incident Investigations. September 24, 1998. Available at: http://www.osha.gov/pls/oshaweb/owadisp.show_document?p_table=MOU&p_id=247. Accessed January 19, 2013.

21. Marcus A. Environmental Protection Agency. In Wilson JQ, ed., *The Politics of Regulation*. New York, NY: Basic Books, Inc.;1980.

22. Rabinowitz RS. *Occupational Safety and Health Law*. 2nd ed. Washington, DC: Bureau of National Affairs;2002.

23. Gold LJ. Pesticide laws and Michigan's migrant farmworkers: are they protected? Michigan State University, Research Report No. 12. 1995. Available at: http://www.jsri.msu.edu/pdfs/rr/rr12.pdf. Accessed January 18, 2013.

24. Asbestos Hazard Emergency Response Act, 15 U.S.C. § 2641–2656 (1986).

25. Environmental Protection Agency. Asbestos Worker Protection, Final Rule. 40 CFR Part 763-Asbestos (2000). Available at: http://www2.epa.gov/asbestos/code-federal-regulations-chapter-40-part-763-asbestos. Accessed June 12, 2014.

26. National Labor Relations Act, 29 U.S.C. § 151–169 (1935).

26a. U.S. Department of Labor. Child labor requirements in agricultural occupations under the Fair Labor Standards Act. Child Labor Bulletin 102. WH-1295. Revised June 2007. Available at: http://www.dol.gov/whd/regs/compliance/childlabor102.pdf. Accessed February 19, 2015.

26b. U.S. Department of Labor. Fact sheet #43: youth employment provisions of the Fair Labor Standards Act for nonagricultural occupations. FS 43. July 2010. Available at: http://www.dol.gov/whd/regs/compliance/whdfs43.pdf. Accessed February 19, 2015.

26c. U.S. Department of Labor. Chapter 9: occupational safety and health statistics. BLS Handbook of Methods. September 5, 2012. Available at: http://stats.bls.gov/opub/hom/pdf/homch9.pdf. Accessed January 30, 2015.

27. National Institute for Occupational Safety and Health. National public safety agenda for occupational safety and health research and practice in the U.S. public safety subsector. National Occupational Research Agenda [revised]. April 2009. Available at: http://www.cdc.gov/niosh/nora/comment/agendas/pubsafsub/pdfs/PubSafSubApr2009.pdf. Accessed January 18, 2013.

28. Occupational Safety and Health Administration. Enforcement exemptions and limitations under the Appropriations Act. Directive No. CPL 2-0.51 I.

October 15, 1997. Available at: http://www.osha.gov/pls/oshaweb/owadisp.show_document?p_id=1518&p_table=directives. Accessed January 19, 2013.

29. Pegula SM. Occupational fatalities: self-employed workers and wage and salary workers. *Monthly Labor Rev.* 2004;127(3):30–40.

30. Bunn T, Costich J, Slavova S. Identification and characterization of Kentucky self-employed occupational injury fatalities using multiple sources, 1995-2004. *Am J Ind Med.* 2006;49(12):1005–1012.

31. Hipple SF. Self-employment in the United States. *Monthly Labor Rev.* 2009;132(9): 17–32.

32. Myers ML, Purschwitz MA. ROPS deficiency of gray-market tractors. *J Agric Saf Health.* 2012;18(2):129–140.

33. National Institute for Occupational Safety and Health. NIOSH reports on the preventability of tractor rollovers. DHHS (NIOSH) Publication No. 93-119. January 29, 1993. Available at: http://www.cdc.gov/niosh/updates/93-119.html. Accessed May 29, 2014.

34. Merchant JA. Research for agricultural safety and health. In: Myers ML, Herrick RF, Olenchock SA, et al., eds. *Papers and Proceedings of the Surgeon General's Conference on Agricultural Safety and Health.* Cincinnati, OH: National Institute for Occupational Safety and Health;1992. DHHS (NIOSH) Publication No. 92-105.

35. Barry P. Keynote: The long haul. In: Myers ML, Klatt ML, eds. *Proceedings of the National Fishing Industry Safety and Health Workshop.* Cincinnati, OH: National Institute for Occupational Safety and Health;1994:23–27.

36. Wendland J. Saving lives at sea through advocacy: the Commercial Fishing Industry Vessel Safety Advisory Committee. The Coast Guard proceedings of the Marine Safety and Security Council. *J Saf Sea.* 2010–2011. Available at: http://www.uscg.mil/proceedings/archive/2010/Vol67_No4_Wint2010-11.pdf. Accessed December 26, 2012.

37. National Transportation Safety Board. Uninspected commercial fishing vessels. NTSB/SS-87/02. September 1987. Available at: http://www.ntsb.gov/doclib/recletters/1987/M87_68_69.pdf. Accessed December 26, 2012.

38. Spitzer JD. Living to fish, dying to fish. U.S. Coast Guard Fishing vessel casualty task force report. March 1999. Available at: http://www.ntsb.gov/news/events/2010/fishing_vessel/background/USCG%20Task%20Force%20Report-%20Dying%20to%20Fish%201999.pdf. Accessed December 26, 2012.

39. Hiscock RC. *Fishing Vessel Safety in the United States: The Tragedy of Missed Opportunities.* Orleans, MA: Marine Safety Foundation;2000. Available at: https://www.ntsb.gov/news/events/2010/fishing_vessel/presentations/1-Hiscock-Tragedy-of-Missed-Oppportunies-Study-2000.pdf. Accessed July 22, 2014.

12

International Policy

The big issues in the world now are questions of standards and regulations. This is a huge debate. In Europe, there has always been this protest over "American imperialism." Now Americans finally cannot believe that there might be what they think is "EU imperialism" when it comes to setting those standards.

—Nicolas Théry[1]

BUILDING SUSTAINABILITY NARRATIVE

Dr. Kenneth Bridbord of the National Institutes of Health (NIH) Fogarty International Center conceived of a way to bridge the education and science gap between developed and developing nations in the mid-1990s. With his background at the U.S. Environmental Protection Agency (EPA), the National Institute for Occupational Safety and Health (NIOSH), and NIH, he was able to assemble grant funding from the Fogarty Center, NIOSH, and the National Institute of Environmental Health Sciences (NIEHS) for the International Training and Research in Environmental and Occupational Health program. Over a 16-year period, the program supported 22 projects that linked U.S. academic scientists with scientists from low- and middle-income countries and conducted training to enhance the research capabilities of scientists at 75 institutions in 43 countries in Asia, Africa, Eastern Europe, and Latin America. Through research between these scientists and their U.S. partners, they published articles that covered advanced basic sciences, developed methods, and informed policy outcomes. Because of the changing nature of the health sciences, institutional capacity building focused on data-driven science through the synthesis of technology and informed knowledge.[2]

With sustainability in mind, Dr. Mastafa A. El Batawi, director of the former Office of Occupational Health at the World Health Organization (WHO), sought the development of professional associations separate from the influence of developed nations in order to grow peer groups among developing nations. As an example, in the region of the Americas he stimulated associations apart from the potential dominance by the United States and Canada. Consistent with this approach, the Fogarty Center, NIOSH, and NIEHS program focused on sustainability by building networks of multiple national and international partners. Accordingly, the program supported the development of multinational networks of regional hubs for Global Environmental and Occupational Health Sciences (GEOHealth). The investment in the program enabled the scientists to advance important health science, train and attract quality scientists, and provide evidence critical to informed policy discussions both locally and internationally.[2] The announcement of availability of funds for this program closed in 2011.

12.1. INTRODUCTION

Environmental justice affirms the right of all workers to a safe and healthy work environment, without being forced to choose between an unsafe livelihood and unemployment. It also affirms the right of those who work at home to be free from environmental hazards.
 —First National People of Color Environmental Leadership Summit, Principles of Environmental Justice No. 8[3]

International organizations offer a framework for international cooperation. They are important in providing a mechanism for translating agreed-to values into rights and duties[4] and then into international law in order to change norms. This change in norms qualifies as a law only if the norms have moved through a lawmaking process.[5]

International lawmaking can take one or more perspectives: doctrinal, policy, and explanatory approaches. Lawyers are familiar with the doctrinal perspective that follows precedence to understand the source of law. Customary law described in Chapter 4 follows the doctrinal perspective. This is a case law approach for the task is to determine the particular norms that are the basis of law.

The policy perspective is about change and is used when existing norms are unsatisfactory and moves from what law is to what law should be. Variables addressed in the policy approach include the following:[5]

- What should be the policy goal? This may address complexity, long-term problems, or disparity.

- Who should act on the policy? This addresses the appropriate forum and whether that forum is public or private or both (e.g., an international organization).
- What legal form should be used? This could be a treaty or revised treaty or action by an international organization or a private standard-setting organization.
- What type of policy instrument should be used? A variety of instruments are available, including government mandates, market approaches, technology innovations, or voluntary programs.
- To whom should the policies be directed?

The doctrinal perspective requires action based on established norms, whereas the policy perspective proffers a change in norms. However, the two perspectives are similar in that they represent the participants in the legal system. The explanatory perspective differs from these approaches since observers outside of the legal system investigate the emergence of international norms and the effectiveness of these norms. Political scientists may address this perspective viewed from different schools: (1) realists—the role of power, (2) institutionalists—the role of interests, (3) liberals—the role of domestic politics, and (4) constructionists—the role of values and knowledge. To understand international law, all three perspectives are important. The doctrinal perspective would defend the status quo, the policy approach would argue for keeping but changing existing law, and the explanatory perspective would consider factors that influence the law's development and effectiveness.[5]

Later in this chapter, the reader sees these perspectives revealed in controversies regarding asbestos disagreements in which a World Trade Organization (WTO) dispute resolution settlement involved the doctrinal perspective, which maintains primacy with market approaches, and the policy perspective, which advocates the protection of human life. The explanatory perspective on this issue is exemplified by an organization of scientists and health professionals, the Collegium Ramazzini.

Norms of international law aim to guide or influence the behavior of states and also institutions and individuals.[5] The sources of norms in international law are shown in Table 12-1.

This chapter begins with a general overview of global work-related diseases and injuries, followed by an explanation of the Occupational Safety and Health Administration's (OSHA) international activities. Next, the United Nations (UN) and a number of its specialized agencies are described. These

Table 12-1. Legal Forms of International Law as Sources of Norms

Legal Forms	Source of International Norms
Intergovernmental agreements	Treaties are the principal source of international norms.
Decisions of treaty bodies	From treaties, institutions are created to supplement and interpret norms.
Decisions of international organizations	United Nations specialized agencies adopt many resolutions that may be routine or rules that have a significant effect.
Conference resolutions and declarations	International conferences adopt resolutions and declarations that affect the behavior of states.
Claims by states	States can claim justifications for their actions or criticisms of another's actions either with other states or within international forums.
Judicial and arbitral decisions	Although rare, international judicial decisions affect norms; national judicial decisions can affect international norms.
Business codes of conduct	Self-regulation by business groups includes standards.
Legal scholars and experts	Individuals or teams publish results of studies.

agencies include the International Labour Organization (ILO), including its recommendations and conventions, and the WHO and its occupational health endeavors, including its International Agency for Research on Cancer (IARC). Four other UN agencies with a role in occupational safety and health include the International Maritime Organization (IMO), the International Atomic Energy Agency (IAEA), the Food and Agriculture Organization (FAO), and the UN Environment Programme (UNEP). Other international groups that have a role in protecting occupational safety and health include the World Bank, the Organisation for Economic Co-operation and Development (OECD), and organizations and agreements that are involved in international trade, including the WTO and the North American Free Trade Agreement (NAFTA). The European Union (EU) system to protect occupational safety and health and its emergent international leadership in occupational and environmental health policy is described. Although there are countless nongovernmental organizations involved in protecting occupational safety and health, two that serve an important role in occupational safety and health are the International Organization for Standardization (ISO) and the Collegium Ramazzini. Two additional sections address the export of hazards: one deals with the global pandemic of asbestos-related diseases, and the other addresses the transfer of risk by transnational corporations of factory work to emerging economies. The penultimate section describes a catastrophe in India emanating from a leak of a lethal chemical at a transnational facility that killed thousands of people. The final section addresses child labor, forced labor, and human trafficking.

12.2. GLOBAL BURDEN OF WORK-RELATED DISEASES AND INJURIES

At the trial there arose considerable discussion as to whether the "haves" or the "have nots" were the more ambitious, for the appetites of both might easily become the cause of no small disturbance. Actually, however, such disturbances are more often caused by the "haves," since the fear of losing what they have arouses in them the same inclination we find in those who want to get more, for men are inclined to think that they cannot hold securely what they possess unless they get more at the others' expense. Furthermore, those who have great possessions can bring about changes with greater effect and greater speed.

—Niccolo Machiavelli[6]

A way to measure the prosperity of a population is its average life expectancy. The 32 countries with the longest life expectancy have an average age before death ranging from 68 years in Hungary to more than 73 years in Norway. Even though the United States has the highest per capita gross domestic product in the world, it is number 16 in life expectancy in the world, at 69.8 years. In the next quintile with 50 nations, the average life expectancy ranges from 54.2 years in South Korea to 68 years in Uruguay. The third quintile of 46 nations ranges from 43.5 years in Mauritania to 53.4 years in the Arab Emirates. The penultimate range for 42 nations spans from 31.3 years in Afghanistan to 42.8 years in Bolivia. Data are unavailable from 15 nations, including Russia.[7]

Great advances have occurred in the developed nations over the last two centuries, when the average life expectancy around the world and for past millennia was close to that of Afghanistan. Much of the rise in life expectancy is attributed to the control of infectious diseases, but thousands have died from work-related injuries and diseases (including infectious diseases), which remains a problem particularly where there is a lower life expectancy. Between 1950 and 1990, life expectancy in developing countries increased from 40 to 63 years, accompanied by a rise in the incidence of noncommunicable diseases in adults and the elderly.[7]

Establishing the global burden of occupational injuries and diseases is hampered by fragmented and dissimilar reporting systems in developed countries

Table 12-2. Global Burden of Occupational Injury and Disease

Annual cases	Leigh et al. 1999*		Driscoll et al. 2005**
	Direct Method[†]	Indirect Method[‡]	Estimates Review
Nonfatal injuries	45,696,000	100,000,000	
Fatal injuries	141,813	101,000	350,000
Disease incidence	4,240,7000-10,010,000	11,000,000	
Disease mortality	583,700-704,200	700,000	1,650,000

*Source: Leigh et al.[9]
**Source: Driscoll et al.[11]
[†]Derived from ILO and WHO data and extrapolation between similar countries where data were available.
[‡]Calculated based on a study by age/gender/specific disease rates and mapped against the representative countries in each of eight World Bank regions with multipliers from known country-level burdens to countries in those regions.

and almost no reporting in many developing countries. Using available country data, worldwide occupational nonfatal injuries are estimated to total 45,696,000 injuries per year and fatal injuries are estimated to total 141,813 deaths per year. Using available data for occupational diseases as of 2004, the estimated annual incidence ranges from 4,240,700 to 10,010,800 cases per year, and associated mortality ranges from 583,700 to 704,200 deaths per year.[8]

However, when the estimates are calculated based on a study by age/gender/specific disease rates and mapped against the representative countries in each of eight World Bank regions with multipliers from known country-level burdens to countries in those regions, the aggregated estimates differ as shown in Table 12-2.[9] These data are what was available prior to 1994, even though the study was conducted in 1999, and no comparable study has been undertaken up to the time of this writing. The nonfatal and fatal annual injuries were 100 million and 101 thousand, respectively, and disease incidence and disease mortality were 11 million and 700 thousand, respectively. The classification of the cause of occupational disease outcomes is shown in Figure 12-1, as measured by Disability-Adjusted Life-Years (DALYs).[8] The numbers refer to DALYs, and the percentages show the relative magnitude of DALYs by disease outcome. The outcomes were associated with selected occupational risk factors.

WHO uses DALYs to measure the global burden of injury and disease. A DALY is a weighting system based on the age of a full and healthy life of 80 years for men and 82.5 years for women. The weighting follows a present

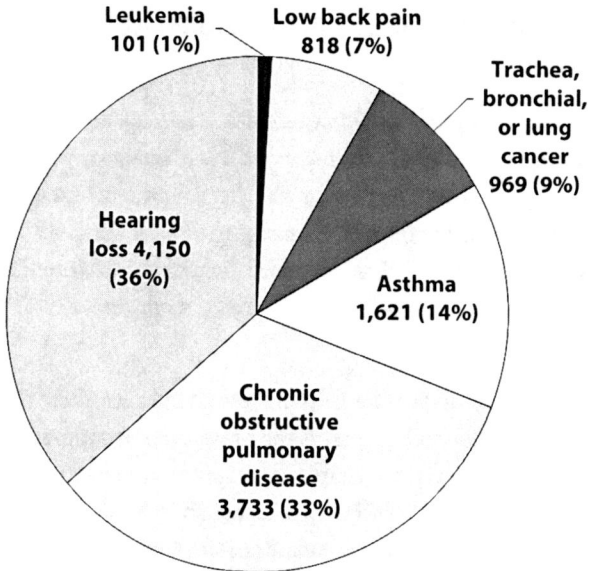

Figure 12-1. Distribution of six types of occupational diseases worldwide, 2004.

value scale of less weighting from birth to early adulthood and peak weighting during adulthood that declines gradually into old age.[10] Present-value calculations are described in Chapter 13.

A later review of several studies determined that the estimates for fatal injuries were more than three times higher at 350,000, and the disease mortality rates were more than double at 1.65 million deaths.[11] These estimates are also shown in Table 12-2. Estimates from the EU in 2009 demonstrate the stark disparity in understanding the global burden of occupational injuries and diseases.[12] The EU estimate places the number of occupational fatalities globally at 357,948, more than three times those calculated by the results shown in Table 12-2; but the estimate of work-related diseases estimated in the EU report is 1.9 million, which is a significantly lower number by more than fivefold than shown in Table 12-2.

A 1999 study estimated 38 million DALYs per year lost from occupational injuries and diseases, representing 2.7% of all DALYs lost worldwide from all causes of early disability and death.[8] Another study suggested that this percentage should be doubled because of the exclusion of outcomes and risk factors.[10]

12.3. OCCUPATIONAL SAFETY AND HEALTH ADMINISTRATION INTERNATIONAL

The growth of multinational corporations, the needs of new and vulnerable migrant and immigrant workers, the increased use of temporary or leased workers, often uneducated in terms of safety and for whom local management has passed off responsibility, the impact of emerging technologies that present new and often unknown hazards—these divergent forces can either pull us apart or bring us together; it is our choice, our challenge, and our future.

—David Michaels[13]

OSHA's authority is limited to the United States. However, three factors draw OSHA into international policy. First is the presence of immigrant workers in the United States for whom the Occupational Safety and Health Act (OSHAct; see Appendix) applies. Thus, OSHA has established a system of agreements and alliances with other country consulates in the United States to assure that immigrants understand their rights. As part of the agreements, OSHA emphasizes compliance with standards for those immigrants at high risk of injury or occupational disease.

Second, OSHA is involved in cooperation with other governments in the exchange of information and technical assistance where needed. Third, OSHA participates in the harmonization of systems between nations that affect occupational safety and health. As an example, the harmonization of industrial classification with Canada and Mexico resulted in a shift from the Standard Industrial Classification system established in the United States in 1937 to the adoption of the North American Industry Classification System in 1997. A more recent effort was the Globally Harmonized System for Hazard Communication, which was adopted by the UN in 2003 and by OSHA in 2012; this system is described in Chapter 14. A description of OSHA's international activities follows.

12.3.1. Mexico

In 2007, OSHA and the Minister of Foreign Affairs of the United Mexican States (through its embassy and consulates) agreed to the well-being of Mexican workers in the United States through a joint declaration. This agreement described an information campaign and opportunities to train Mexican workers regarding their rights under the OSHAct to protect their safety and health.[14]

The role of OSHA is to assure the safety and health of workers that include immigrants in the United States by setting and enforcing standards; providing training, outreach, and education; establishing partnerships; and encouraging continual improvement in workplace safety and health. The U.S. Department of Labor's (DoL) Wage and Hour Division is also collaborating with Mexican consulates to protect workers in the United States. Mexico has 47 consulates in 24 states and Washington, DC: 11 in Texas, 10 in California, five in Arizona, two in Florida, one in Washington in addition to the embassy located there, and one in each of the following states—Alaska, Arkansas, Colorado, Georgia, Idaho, Indiana, Illinois, Louisiana, Massachusetts, Michigan, Minnesota, Missouri, Nebraska, Nevada, New Mexico, New York, North Carolina, Oregon, Pennsylvania, and Utah.[15]

12.3.2. Latin America

The United States has Letters of Agreement with several other Latin American and Caribbean consulates similar to the agreements with Mexican consulates. These agreements are with the consulates of Costa Rica, the Dominican Republic, El Salvador, Guatemala, Nicaragua, Ecuador, Honduras, and Peru. Regional OSHA offices have also established alliances with Latin American consulates located in the United States. These alliances stress an OSHA regional office commitment to improving information, guidance, and access to education and training resources so as to promote workers' rights in protecting their occupational and safety and health as their country's nationals working in that region in the United States. The alliances also emphasize particular hazards to be addressed such as falls from elevations. The New York regional office has alliances with consulates from El Salvador, Guatemala, Nicaragua, Ecuador, Argentina, Brazil, Chile, Columbia, and Venezuela. The Philadelphia regional office has an alliance with the consulate from the Dominican Republic, and the Atlanta regional office has an alliance with the consulate from Guatemala.[15]

12.3.3. Europe

In 1995, the United States and the EU signed the New Transatlantic Agenda, followed by a meeting of the Joint Working Group on Employment and Labor-Related Issues. This working group of officials from the DoL and the

EU has sponsored meetings, workshops, and conferences that address employment topics including occupational safety and health. Subsequently, OSHA engaged in the "Joint U.S. and European Union Cooperation in Workplace Safety and Health" program with the EU European Agency for Safety and Health at Work (EU-OSHA). This cooperation emphasizes the importance of U.S.–EU transatlantic engagement in sharing ideas, leveraging resources, and finding solutions to address occupational safety and health hazards of common concern.[15]

At the foundation of this cooperation is the series of EU/U.S. Joint Conferences on Occupational Safety and Health, with the first conference held in Luxembourg in 1998. Alternating between the United States and Europe, the seventh joint conference was held in 2012 in Brussels, Belgium. Topics at this conference included chemicals, the prevention of catastrophic events, nanotechnology, and occupational safety and health in a green economy. The conference was also a forum to establish EU/U.S. collaboration to launch a global wiki on occupational safety and health that was launched in 2013.[15]

12.3.4. China

After the first China International Forum on Work Safety convened in 2002 regarding mine safety, the second forum convened in Beijing, China, in 2004. The DoL and China's State Administration of Work Safety (SAWS) signed a letter of understanding in 2004 with the common objective of ensuring economic growth, creating employment, raising living standards and supporting widely shared prosperity, and providing workers with safe work environments. The provision of safety aimed to be in accord with relevant international safe work principles and respect for the national laws and legal provisions of each country. The third of these forums convened in Beijing in 2006, and the China International Forum on Workplace Emergency Management and Rescue was convened in Beijing in 2007. At that meeting, OSHA Administrator Edwin G. Foulke Jr. listed lessons learned regarding emergency preparedness and response:[15]

1. Every employer needs to develop and implement an emergency response plan to protect employees against catastrophic events, including those employees responding in an emergency.
2. Establish an "incident command system" that organizes responders from various levels of government and expertise to increase effectiveness and reduce the duplication of response operations and planning.

3. Include in every business emergency response plan procedures to facilitate the arrival of external responders such as firefighters, medical personnel, and police.
4. Coordinate the employer's emergency response plan with the plans drawn up by local officials in their communities.
5. Include test exercises that engage all levels of government and the private sector and apply the lessons learned forward.

The DoL and SAWS entered into a Memorandum of Understanding regarding work safety and health in 2011. The aim of this agreement is to expand cooperation to improve occupational safety and health, including an exchange of information on laws, regulations, policies, industrial standards, science and technology, and supervision and enforcement.[16]

12.3.5. Philippines

In 2012, OSHA entered into a Letter of Agreement with the Department of Foreign Affairs of the Philippines aimed at informing Filipino workers in the United States about their labor rights. Also in 2012, three OSHA area offices in Florida entered into an alliance with the consular section of the Philippine Embassy. In this alliance, the OSHA area offices provide Filipino workers and employers with information, guidance, and access to education and training resources to promote workers' rights in protecting their occupational safety and health. The topics for this information outreach include common workplace safety and health hazards, chemical safety, bloodborne pathogens, electrocutions, falls, and struck-by and caught-in/between hazards. In addition, information is provided to help the workers understand their rights and the employer duties under the OSHAct.[15]

12.3.6. American National Standards Institute

The American National Standards Institute (ANSI) promotes the use of U.S. standards internationally, advocates U.S. policy and technical positions in international and regional standards organizations, and encourages the adoption of international standards as national standards as needed for the user community. The institute provides OSHA with draft international safety and health standards, and OSHA provides ANSI with comments on the proposed international standards. The institute provides these comments to the Technical Advisory Group developing the U.S. position on these standards.[17]

The OSHA and ANSI have worked together under mutual agreements since 1976. These agreements focus on coordinating voluntary national consensus standards in the United States as well as supporting ANSI in its role in the international arena, such as participation in the ISO. Through ANSI, OSHA comments on the international consensus standards, which may or may not be consistent with OSHA standards after adoption by the international community. In 2001, OSHA and ANSI signed an agreement to continue their joint efforts to improve safety and health standards for workers around the world.[17]

12.4. UNITED NATIONS

Workers around the world—despite vast differences in their physical, social, economic, and political environments—face virtually the same kinds of workplace hazards.

—Linda Rosenstock, Mark R. Cullen, Marilyn Fingerhut[18]

In 1941, Prime Minister of Great Britain Winston Churchill and U.S. President Franklin D. Roosevelt signed the Atlantic Charter, which declared, "that all men in all lands may live out their lives in freedom from fear and want." This declaration expressed the intent of the UN Charter, which applied to all men and women in nations large and small four years later. Its constitution declared that world peace depended upon international social and economic justice. In 1948, the UN General Assembly adopted the Universal Declaration of Human Rights.[19]

The UN is made up of several specialized agencies. These agencies include the ILO, WHO, IMO, IAEA, FAO, and UNEP.[20]

12.4.1. International Labour Organization

The ILO was an early international institution that addressed occupational safety and health and predated the UN. It was founded in 1919 as a product of the Treaty of Versailles and signed an agreement in 1946 to become a specialized agency of the UN. The ILO is ruled by a tripartite approach in which its governing body is composed of worker, employer, and government representatives from each member country.[21]

The ILO is governed by the International Labour Conference with 185 member states, a governing body (described above), and the International Labour Office. The conference meets annually and establishes ILO standards and policies. Based on ILO policy, the governing body meets three times per year in Geneva, Switzerland, and proposes the ILO program and budget that it submits to the conference for adoption. The ILO headquarters is based in Geneva, where the International Labour Office comprises a secretariat, research center, and publishing house. A director-general is elected every five years by the governing body and directs the International Labour Office.[22]

The ILO has regional, area, and branch offices in more than 40 countries under the leadership of the director-general. Five regional offices are located in Addis Ababa, Ethiopia, for the Region of Africa; Lima, Peru, for the Region of the Americas in addition to an office in Washington, DC; Beirut, Lebanon, for the Arab States Region; Bangkok, Thailand, for the Asia and Pacific Region; and Geneva for the Europe and Central Asia Region, which is colocated with the ILO headquarters.[22]

Beginning in 1919, occupational safety and health has been at the heart of the ILO's work, including its standards-setting activities. Accordingly, in 2003, the International Labour Conference adopted the Global Strategy on Occupational Safety and Health. The conference action confirms the role of ILO instruments as a central pillar for the protection of occupational safety and health around the world. The strategy calls for action to better connect ILO standards with other actions, such as advocacy, awareness raising, knowledge development, management, information dissemination, and technical cooperation. The strategy emphasizes a preventive approach and a safety culture as key to achieving sustainable safety and health at work.[22]

The ILO enacts two types of standards: a convention and a recommendation. A convention is considered a matter of treaty obligation if it is adopted by a member state. A recommendation is submitted to members for their consideration to enact laws at a member state's level. A list of ILO conventions and recommendations regarding occupational safety and health is shown in Table 12-3. Beyond this list, ILO also addresses child labor, servitude, social security, and other conditions of employment.[23]

The *ILO Encyclopaedia of Occupational Health and Safety* provides information on occupational safety and health problems and their technical and social solutions. The first edition of the *Encyclopaedia* was published in 1930, followed by editions in 1971, 1983, and 1998. More than 2,000 experts

Table 12-3. International Labour Organization Conventions and Recommendations Regarding Occupational Safety and Health, Year of Effect, and Assigned Number

Conventions	Recommendations
White Lead (Painting), 1921 (No. 13)	Anthrax Prevention, 1919 (No. 3)
Underground Work (Women), 1935 (No. 45)	Lead Poisoning (Women and Children), 1919 (No. 4)
Safety Provisions (Building), 1937 (No. 62)-outdated	White Phosphorus, 1919 (No. 6)
	Prevention of Industrial Accidents, 1929 (No. 31)
Radiation Protection, 1960 (No. 115)	Power-Driven Machinery, 1929 (No. 32)
Guarding of Machinery, 1963 (No. 119)	Safety Provisions (Building), 1937 (No. 53)-replaced
Hygiene (Commerce and Offices), 1964 (No. 120)	Co-operation in Accident Prevention (Building), 1937 (No. 55)-replaced
Maximum Weight, 1967 (No. 127)	Protection of Workers' Health, 1953 (No. 97)
Benzene, 1971 (No. 136)	Welfare Facilities, 1956 (No. 102)
Occupational Cancer, 1974 (No. 139)	Occupational Health Services, 1959 (No. 112)-replaced
Working Environment (Air Pollution, Noise, and Vibration), 1977 (No. 148)	Radiation Protection, 1960 (No. 114)
	Guarding of Machinery, 1963 (No. 118)
Occupational Safety and Health, 1981 (No. 155)	Hygiene (Commerce and Offices), 1964 (No. 120)
	Maximum Weight, 1967 (No. 128)
Protocol of 2002 to Occupational Safety and Health, 1981 (No. 155)	Benzene, 1971 (No. 144)
	Occupational Cancer, 1974 (No. 147)
Occupational Health Services, 1985 (No. 161)	Working Environment (Air Pollution, Noise, and Vibration), 1977 (No. 156)
Asbestos, 1986 (No. 162)	Occupational Safety and Health, 1981 (No. 164)
Safety and Health in Construction, 1988 (No. 167)	Occupational Health Services, 1985 (No. 171)
	Asbestos, 1986 (No. 172)
Chemicals, 1990 (No. 170)	Safety and Health in Construction, 1988 (No. 175)
Prevention of Major Industrial Accidents, 1993 (No. 174)	Chemicals, 1990 (No. 177)
	Prevention of Major Industrial Accidents, 1993 (No. 181)
Safety and Health in Mines, 1995 (No. 176)	Safety and Health in Mines, 1995 (No. 183)
Safety and Health in Agriculture, 2001 (No. 184)	Safety and Health in Agriculture, 2001 (No. 192)
	List of Occupational Diseases, 2002 (No. 194)
Promotional Framework for Occupational Safety and Health, 2006 (No. 187)	Promotional Framework for Occupational Safety and Health, 2006 (No. 197)

worldwide share their knowledge within the *Encyclopaedia* so as to improve working conditions and the safety and health of the world's workers.[24]

The International Social Security Association (ISSA) is headquartered at the International Labour Office in Geneva. Founded in 1927, the ISSA is the principal international institution bringing together social security agencies and organizations. The ISSA's aim is to promote excellence in social security administration in a globalizing world. The ISSA partners with the ILO and with other international bodies active in the field of social security. An aim of the ISSA is the prevention of social risks as an important aspect of social security. The association addresses the prevention of occupational risks through 11 committees on industries including chemistry, mining, iron and metal industry, construction, agriculture, and machine safety. It provides access to information, expert advice, business standards, practical guidelines, and platforms for members to promote dynamic social security systems worldwide. The ISSA facilitates the collection and exchange of good practices and the improvement of social security through knowledge transfer and advocacy.[25]

12.4.2. World Health Organization

A UN conference in San Francisco adopted a declaration in 1945 regarding the need for an international health organization. A year later, representatives from 61 nations met in New York City at the International Health Conference and signed the WHO constitution, and the WHO became a specialized agency of the UN in 1948. Predating the WHO, the Pan American Sanitary Bureau was established in 1902, became the WHO Regional Office of the Americas in 1949, and was renamed the Pan American Health Organization (PAHO) in 1958.[21]

The WHO is governed by the World Health Assembly and by a 24-member executive board. The assembly meets annually in Geneva and elects eight members to the executive board annually for three-year terms. Regional offices are located in Brazzaville, Congo, representing Africa; Washington for PAHO; Alexandria, Egypt, representing the eastern Mediterranean; Copenhagen, Denmark, representing Europe; New Delhi, India, representing Southeast Asia; and Manila, Philippines, representing the western Pacific.[20] The WHO is responsible for providing leadership on global health matters, shaping the health research agenda, setting norms and standards, articulating evidence-based policy options, providing technical support to countries, and monitoring and assessing health trends.[26]

Member countries of the UN may become members of the WHO, which has 194 member states, by accepting its constitution. Other countries may be admitted as members when their application has been approved by a simple majority vote of the World Health Assembly. Territories that are not responsible for the conduct of their international relations may be admitted as associate members upon application made on their behalf by the member or other authority responsible for their international relations.[26]

Dr. Mastafa A. El Batawi, director of the WHO's Office of Occupational Health while it existed in the 1980s, established Collaborating Centers for Occupational Health around the world that followed a model used more broadly by WHO. Currently there are 65 Collaborating Centers on Occupational Health, one of which is NIOSH. In 2007, the World Health Assembly endorsed the Global Plan of Action on Workers' Health 2008–2017. Several factors led to this endorsement:

- Recommendations of the World Summit on Sustainable Development in Johannesburg, South Africa, in 2002 on strengthening WHO action on occupational health and linking it to public health.
- The functions mandated in Article 2 of the WHO constitution include promoting the improvement of working conditions and other aspects of environmental hygiene.
- The ILO Promotional Framework for Occupational Safety and Health Convention in 2006.
- Other ILO instruments in the area of occupational safety and health adopted by the International Labour Conference.
- The health of workers is determined not only by occupational hazards, but also by social and individual factors and access to health services.
- Interventions exist for primary prevention of occupational hazards and for developing healthy workplaces.
- Major gaps exist between and within countries in the exposure of workers and local communities to occupational hazards and in their access to occupational health services.
- The health of workers is an essential prerequisite for productivity and economic development.

The WHO's work on occupational health is governed by the Global Plan, with a Plan of Action that has the following five objectives:[27]

1. Devise and implement policy instruments on workers' health.
2. Protect and promote health at the workplace.
3. Improve the performance of and access to occupational health services.
4. Provide and communicate evidence for action and practice.
5. Incorporate workers' health into other policies.

Based on a French initiative, the World Health Assembly established IARC in 1965, headquartered in Lyon, France. As a WHO agency, IARC follows the general governing rules of the UN with a governing council, a scientific council, and a secretariat. The governing council directs the general policy of IARC and is composed of the representatives of participating states and of the WHO director-general. The governing council elects IARC's director, who normally serves for a five-year term. The council meets annually the week prior to the World Health Assembly annual meeting. The scientific council consists of experts selected for their technical competence in cancer research and allied fields. The council reviews the research program and recommends permanent activities to the governing council. The secretariat consists of a director and the technical and administrative staff. The director of IARC is elected by and reports to the governing council. The director developments and implements the scientific program and oversees the day-to-day operations of the agency. Among other publications, IARC produced 100 monographs from 1972 to 2012 in a series called the *Evaluation of Carcinogenic Risks to Humans*, most of which have subjects with a significant bearing on occupational health, such as polynuclear organic compounds and wood dust.[28]

The WHO, ILO, and UNEP formed the WHO International Programme on Chemical Safety (IPCS) in 1980 to promote the development, harmonization, and use of scientifically sound methodologies to evaluate risks to human health and the environment from chemical exposure. IPCS named eight chemicals that endanger occupational health as public health concerns: arsenic, asbestos, benzene, cadmium, dioxin and dioxin-like substances, lead, mercury, and highly hazardous pesticides. The IPCS also promotes the building of poison centers around the world. In a joint activity of the WHO, ILO, and UNEP, an IPCS peer review committee developed International Chemical Safety Cards, which summarize health and safety information on chemicals for use by workers and employers in factories, agriculture, construction, and other workplaces.[29]

12.4.3. International Maritime Organization

A UN maritime conference convened in Geneva in 1948. This conference led to the International Maritime Consultative Organization Convention, which was ratified by 21 nations in 1958, and was headquartered in London.[21] In 1982, it was renamed the IMO.

The IMO enacted the International Convention for the Safety of Life at Sea (SOLAS) in 1960.[30] A 1947 explosion of two vessels docked at Texas City, TX, that were loaded with ammonia nitrate killed 468 people and left more than 100 missing and 3,000 injured. Property damage was estimated at $491 million (in 2013 dollars).[31] Because of this explosion, delegates to the 1960 SOLAS developed the nonmandatory Code of Safe Practice for Solid Bulk Cargoes that focused on preventing incidents related to damage to the vessel due to improper cargo distribution, loss of stability during the voyage, and chemical reactions or hazards. Further revisions made the code mandatory in 2011.[32]

A 1974 amendment consolidated several amendments to SOLAS. SOLAS requires certification of inspections to ensure that the vessel has met required standards. The SOLAS Convention states that "the officer carrying out the control shall take such steps as will ensure that the ship shall not sail until it can proceed to sea without danger to the passengers or the crew." It has addressed crew safety regarding fishing vessels as recently as 1996.[30]

In 1983, IMO's Maritime Safety Committee adopted the International Bulk Chemical Code to establish safe chemicals carriage. The code lists dangerous chemicals and noxious liquid substances transported in bulk by sea and their carriage and equipment requirements to minimize risk to the ship, crew, and environment.[31]

12.4.4. International Atomic Energy Agency

A statute conference with representatives from 81 nations was convened in New York City in 1956, and attendees unanimously agreed to establish the IAEA, with a headquarters in Vienna, Austria. The purpose of the IAEA is to promote the peaceful use of atomic energy. The agency is governed by a general conference meeting annually, a board of governors composed of 25 government members that meets four times per year, and a secretariat headed by a director-general. The secretariat proposes programs and budgets and carries out approved programs.[33]

From the beginning, the agency has addressed nuclear waste management, publishing 27 technical documents on this subject from 1961 through 1971. Figure 12-2 shows the process for creating IAEA standards.[21]

Radiation risks may transcend national borders, and international cooperation serves to promote and enhance safety globally by exchanging experience and improving hazard controls, incident prevention, emergency response, and mitigation of harmful consequences. The IAEA safety standards are binding international instruments. The preparation and review of safety standards

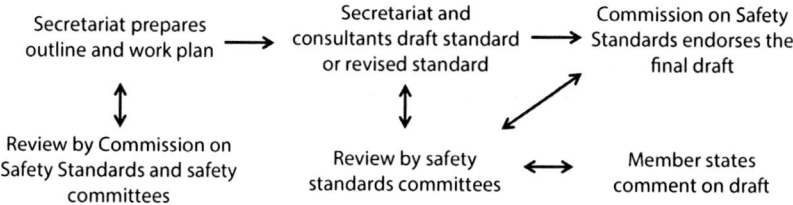

Figure 12-2. The process for developing and issuing IAEA standards.

involves the secretariat and four safety standards committees covering (1) nuclear safety, (2) radiation safety, (3) the safety of radioactive waste, and (4) the safe transport of radioactive material.[33]

The IAEA Commission on Safety Standards oversees the entire safety standards program. The members of the commission are appointed by the director-general and include senior government officials with responsibility for establishing national standards. The agency's safety standards apply throughout the lifetime of facilities and activities that are used and conducted for peaceful purposes. Under these standards, safety requirements use "shall" statements that are mandatory, while recommendations use "should" statements that are advisory.[33]

International experts were convened by the IAEA and the nuclear agency of the OECD to develop the International Nuclear and Radiological Event Scale (INES) in 1990. Created as a tool for promptly communicating to the public in consistent terms the safety significance of reported nuclear and radiological incidents and accidents, INES is a seven-point scale with levels 1–3 relating to "incidents," and the final four levels relating to "accidents." Events without safety significance are called "deviations" and are classified as a level 0. The scale can be applied to any event associated with nuclear facilities, as well as the transport, storage, and use of radioactive material and radiation sources. It is shown below:[33]

Deviations
- 0: Events without safety significance

Incidents
- 1: Anomaly
- 2: Incident
- 3: Serious incident

Accidents
- 4: Accident with local consequences
- 5: Accidents with wider consequences
- 6: Serious accidents
- 7: Major accident

The 1986 Chernobyl (Soviet Union) event was assigned the highest level, 7, of "safety significance." The 1979 event at Three Mile Island in Pennsylvania was a 5 on the INES scale, but the 2011 Fukushima (Japan) event was soon upgraded from 5 to 7.[33a]

12.4.5. Food and Agriculture Organization

In 1945, the first session of the FAO Conference convened in Quebec City, Canada, and established the FAO as a specialized agency of the UN. Representatives of FAO members meet at a biennial conference and elect council members to serve three-year rotating terms to oversee program and budgetary activities. The conference also elects a director-general to a four-year term of office that is renewable one time. The FAO has 191 member states, two associate members, and the EU as a member organization.[34] Its headquarters is in Rome, Italy.

In 1994, 49% of the world's population was engaged in agriculture. Of this agricultural population, 76% were located in Asia, 13% in Africa, and 4% each in Latin America and the Near East, and the remaining 3% were located in Europe and North America.[35] Agriculture is among the most hazardous industries in the world. The FAO provides information to the agriculture industry about the hazards and their control through bulletins.

In India, 70% (950 million) of the population works in agriculture. In the three Indian states of Haryana, Punjab, and Up, 5,000 to 10,000 agricultural fatalities occur annually, half of which are attributable to pesticide poisoning. In addition, 150,000 to 200,000 serious injuries occur in the three states each year, and when extrapolated to the whole nation, 16 million agriculture-related injuries occur each year.[8]

Worldwide, acute pesticide poisoning affects an estimated two to five million people every year, of whom 40,000 die from exposures to toxic products and from rudimentary conditions of pesticide use and storage. Pesticides are routinely stored in homes in developing countries so as to secure them from theft. According to the WHO, while developing nations accounted for 20% of all pesticide use in the early 1990s, they accounted for more than 99% of pesticide poisonings.[36]

Hazards to agricultural workers include powered machinery, sharp tools, snake bites, and zoonotic diseases. Millions of injuries occur, from which 170,000 agricultural workers are killed annually. The FAO promotes greater organization and empowerment of the agricultural workforce and ways for small farmers to control exposure to hazards. Guidelines from the ILO and WHO exist for hazard reduction in agricultural work, as do occupational health services for agricultural workers, but they lack enforcement. The FAO suggests that the agriculture and health sectors should work together.[36]

12.4.6. United Nations Environment Programme

The UN created UNEP in 1972, with a governing council, an environment secretariat, and an environment fund. Its headquarters was established in Nairobi, Kenya, in 1973.[19] One of the requirements placed on UNEP was to collaborate with organizations of workers and employers on the working and living environment of workers. In its collaboration with the WHO and ILO on the International Program on Chemical Safety, UNEP maintains the International Register of Potentially Toxic Chemicals. This register aims to bridge the gap between knowledge of the world's chemicals and the potential use of these chemicals.[37]

12.5. WORLD BANK GROUP (WORLD BANK)

When the highly privileged (in developing countries) are few and the desperately poor are many—and when the gap between them is worsening rather than improving—it is only a question of time before a decisive choice must be made between the political costs of reform and the political risks of rebellion.

—Robert McNamara[38]

The World Bank, which began as the International Bank for Reconstruction and Development, was established in 1944 to facilitate post–World War II reconstruction and development and has moved to a mandate to alleviate worldwide poverty. The World Bank Group is composed of five organizations, as shown in Table 12-4. The World Bank Group is an exception to the "one

Table 12-4. The World Bank Group

Organization	Mission
International Bank for Reconstruction and Development (the original World Bank)	Lends to governments of middle-income and creditworthy low-income countries.
International Development Association (affiliated with the World Bank in 1960)	Provides grants and interest-free loans (credits) for up to 50 years to governments of the poorest countries.
International Finance Corporation	Provides loans to the private sector to help developing countries achieve sustainable growth by financing investment, mobilizing capital in international financial markets, and providing advisory services to businesses and governments.
Multilateral Investment Guarantee Agency (created in 1988)	Promotes foreign direct investment into developing countries to support economic growth, reduce poverty, and improve people's lives; offers political risk insurance (guarantees) to investors and lenders.
International Centre for Settlement of Investment Disputes	Provides international facilities for conciliation and arbitration of investment disputes.

nation, one vote" principle. Its voting power is proportional to the contributions to the World Bank's capital. The World Bank is headquartered in Washington, DC, with more than 100 offices worldwide, and since the United States is its principal contributor, the World Bank's presidents have all been U.S. citizens.[21,39]

The powers of the World Bank are vested in a board of governors, with one governor and one alternate governor from each member state. The operation of the World Bank lies in the hands of 12 executive directors—five of whom represent the major contributors to the World Bank, and the others who are elected by the board. The president of the World Bank serves as the head of each of the organizations within the World Bank Group. While the World Bank continually bargains with its borrowers, it rejects bargaining for consensus. Rather, it depends upon economic rationality based upon routine decision making founded on engineering and economic analysis.[40]

In the late 1980s, the World Bank initiated a review of priorities for the control of specific diseases and used this information as input for comparative cost-effectiveness estimates of interventions addressing most conditions of importance in developing countries. This process resulted in the 1993 publication of the now classic book, *Disease Control Priorities in Developing*

Countries, and its companion document, the *World Development Report 1993: Investing in Health.*[41]

The World Bank has classified the world's nations into eight regions. The 1999 study referred to earlier in Table 12-2 and Figure 12-1 also reported injuries and diseases by World Bank region based on 1994 data.[8] Table 12-5 shows injuries, fatal injuries, occupational disease incidence, and working population in the eight regions for that year.[41] Figure 12-3 shows the 1994 gross rate of injuries per 1,000 workers by World Bank region in ascending order. The worldwide rate is 48.8 injuries per 1,000 workers each year. Two regions are below this worldwide rate: Formerly Socialist Economies of Europe and Established Market Economies. The injury rate is above the average in the remaining six regions, with the Middle Eastern Crescent region at the highest rate, 64.0 injuries per 1,000 workers.

While the World Bank has established a priority for environmental protection that includes occupational safety and health, its policies are swayed by economic considerations. Indeed, a double standard is apparent when nations are bifurcated into either banning a hazardous substance such as asbestos or not banning asbestos. In another disparity between nations, the World Bank has applied a gradient approach to standards in which less stringent standards are applied for the less affluent populations. Information from a former chief economist within the World Bank supported the migration of (risk transfer of)

Table 12-5. Global Burden of Occupational Injuries and Diseases by World Bank Region, 1994

Region	Injuries*	Fatal Injuries	Disease Incidence*	Working Population*
China	24.42	83,950 (26.9%)	2.53	432
Established Market Economies	10.35	15,392 (4.9%)	1.18	364
India	18.30	48,441 (15.5%)	1.85	324
Other Asian & Islands	14.71	70,341 (22.5%)	1.49	260
Formerly Socialist Economies of Europe	4.85	16,652 (5.3%)	0.50	188
Latin America & Caribbean	9.89	42,379 (13.6%)	1.02	179
Sub-Saharan Africa	9.02	115,971 (37.1%)	1.06	155
Middle Eastern Crescent	9.15	68,101 (21.8%)	1.04	143
Total	100.69	312,481	10.68	2,063

Source: Leigh et al.[9]
Note: Fatal injuries applied proportion from direct method to the indirect method.
*Millions.

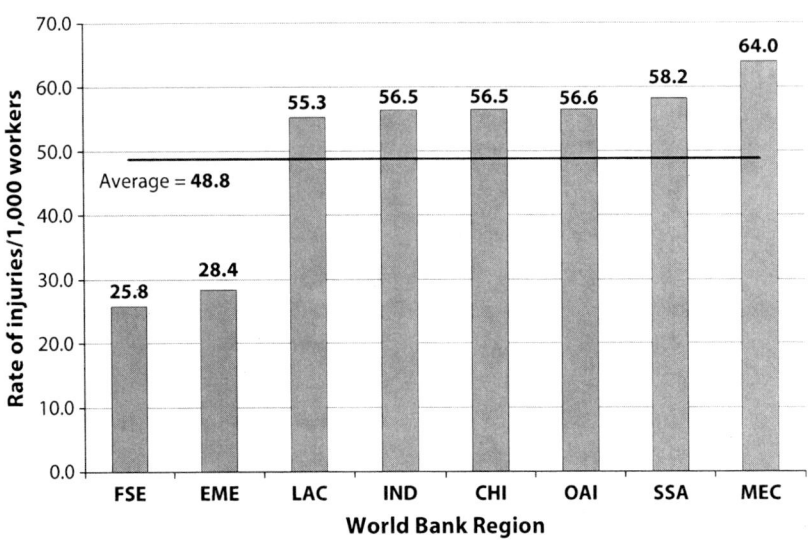

Note: FSE = Formerly Socialist Economies of Europe; EME = Established Market Economies; LAC = Latin America and Caribbean; IND = India; CHI = China; OAI = Other Asian and Islands; SSA = Sub-Saharan Africa; MEC = Middle Eastern Crescent.
Source: Leigh.[9]
Figure 12-3. Injuries per 1,000 workers by World Bank region.

"dirty" industries to developing countries. By his logic, in 1993, the costs of health-impairing pollution depended on the foregone earnings of those directly affected by increased morbidity and mortality (e.g., the death of those with lower wages is less costly).[42] This is a common practice: to devalue the lives of those with lower wages, which is discussed in Chapter 13.

12.6. THE ORGANISATION FOR ECONOMIC CO-OPERATION AND DEVELOPMENT

What are the sufferings? What is needed? What can best be done? What must be done?

—George C. Marshall, Marshall Plan Speech, 1947[43]

In 1948, the Organization for Europe on Economic Cooperation was created to administer support provided by the United States and Canada to Europe under the Marshall Plan. After the United States and Canada joined 18 other nations of the organization in 1960, it was renamed the Organisation for Economic

Co-operation and Development (OECD) in 1961, with its headquarters located in Paris. An executive committee of the organization prepares decisions and recommendations for the OECD Council, which has representatives from all member states, and a secretariat executes the council's decisions.[21] Growing to 34 member states in 2013, with the European Commission participating, the OECD's aim is to build strong economies for its member states.

The OECD had created a system of safety codes and schemes in the late 1950s (before its renaming) that was available to any member nation of the UN or the WTO. Among the earliest codes was the testing of tractors, begun in 1959, to facilitate trade and import procedures by updating international rules to certify tractors. In 1967, operator safety became a factor for certification, which addressed noise exposure and protection in the event of a tractor overturn or from a falling object by developing rollover protective structures (ROPS) and falling object protection structures (FOPS). As of 2013, 10,000 tractor models have been tested for noise exposure, and ROPS and FOPS on more than 3,000 tractor models have been tested by certified testing facilities.[44]

The OECD has addressed other issues that relate to occupational safety and health. In 1989, it compared injury frequency rate and severity between industries in its member states, and in 1990, it conducted a like comparison regarding occupational illnesses.[45,46] In 2003, the OECD published guiding principles for chemical-related incidents followed by reports from a series of workshops: the OECD Environment, Health and Safety Publications Series on Chemical Accidents No. 10.[47] The OECD maintains the Database on Research into Safety of Manufactured Nanomaterials as a resource that collects information about research projects that address human health and safety and environmental issues of manufactured nanomaterials. As described in Chapter 4, OECD established a code of conduct and guidelines in 2008 for multinational companies that included taking adequate steps to ensure occupational health and safety in their operations. In 2010, the OECD compared the risks of nuclear power generation with the risks of other energy sources.[48]

12.7. INTERNATIONAL TRADE

Even free trade's First Cheerleader, [President] Bill Clinton, confesses that most people think the World Trade Organization is "some rich guys' club where people get in, talk in funny language and make a bunch of rules that help the people that already have and stick it to the people that have not."

—Margot Horn Blower[49]

Shortly after World War II in 1948, the international community created the General Agreement on Tariffs and Trade (GATT) to peacefully negotiate trade. The participants in GATT were called "contracting" parties, which meant that when they affirmed the agreement, they were bound by contract to honor its provisions.[50]

This section addresses the occupational safety and health relationship to international trade by describing the activities of the WTO, the Basel Convention of 1989 on the Control of Transboundary Movements of Hazardous Wastes, NAFTA, and the Rotterdam Convention. The unregulated movement of transnational companies and the lack of protection for workers who cross borders seeking work are two core aspects of globalization that affect labor rights and workers' health and safety.[51]

12.7.1. World Trade Organization

The WTO was created in 1995 through the 1986–1994 Uruguay Round of GATT and earlier negotiations. World Trade Organization (WTO) agreements, negotiated and signed by most of the world's trading nations, provide the legal ground rules for international commerce. There were 159 member states of WTO in 2013.

The WTO's purpose is to help trade flow as freely as possible with no undesirable side effects as a path to economic development and human well-being. Free trade means removing obstacles and ensuring stability and trade rules around the world that are transparent and predictable. The WTO's primary decision-making body is the Ministerial Conference, which meets at least once every two years. A general council meets several times a year in the Geneva headquarters and comprises ambassadors, delegation heads in Geneva, and officials sent by member states. The general council also serves as the Trade Policy Review Body and the Dispute Settlement Body. A goods council, services council, and intellectual property council report to the general council. Specialized committees, working groups, and working parties deal with the individual agreements and special areas such as the environment, development, and regional trade agreements. The headquarters located in Geneva is headed by a director-general.[52]

Article 20 of GATT allows governments to protect human, animal, or plant life or health, provided they do not discriminate or use this as disguised protectionism. In addition, there are two specific WTO agreements dealing with food safety and animal and plant health and safety, and with product standards in general. Both try to identify how to meet the need to apply standards and at the same time avoid protectionism in disguise. These issues are becoming more important as tariff barriers fall. In both cases, if a country applies international standards, it is less likely to be challenged legally in the WTO than if it sets its own standards.

The WTO has a dispute-settlement apparatus that when one member nation claims a violation against another nation of articles under the 1995 GATT or a Technical Barriers to Trade agreement of 1994, the WTO implements a dispute settlement procedure. The 1995 GATT established the Appellate Body to hear appeals of decisions from panels that were part of the process previously under the Dispute Settlement Body. The Appellate Body also provides legal advice to the panels. In this procedure, consultation and mediations are attempted within 60 days of the complaint. Failing a settlement, a panel is appointed to determine if the plaintiff's claim is valid.[53-55]

The panel is composed of trade diplomats who are typically retired.[56] The work of the panel is to be concluded within one year following the complaint. Either of the parties can appeal a decision from the panel to the Appellate Body, and its decision is final with one exception: All WTO member nations sitting as the Dispute Settlement Body can overturn an Appellate ruling with a unanimous vote, which is inconceivable since one of the parties would not vote against its own interest, thus the Appellate Body decision is most certainly final. If the defendant is found to be in violation of the agreements, penalties attached to its international movement of goods can be established.[53,55]

Of the WTO agreements, just one addresses human health, and that agreement regards food safety (sanitary and phytosanitary measures). To date, no agreement has been reached regarding occupational safety and health as a trade issue. When labor standards in trade agreements were a topic at the 1999 Seattle Ministerial Conference, developing nation members claimed that arguments for including labor standards in trade agreements were made contrary to free trade by one of two groups: either politically powerful lobbying groups that were protectionist (e.g., unions), or morally driven human rights groups. They contended that the morally driven groups were misguided because their actions might force poor workers out of their jobs without providing a viable alternative. In sum, their argument against trade-based labor standards, whether protectionist or morally motivated, was to protect developed country firms from developing country competition.[57]

An International Confederation of Free Trade Unions statement of 2001 proposed a reorientation of the multilateral trading system to promote sustainable world economic growth and development. This reorientation would create decent jobs and a broader spread of the benefits of globalization for all people in both developed and developing countries. According to this proposal, development priorities must come second to protecting the environment and safety and health, including the working environment and occupational safety and health. This would require recognition of the precautionary principle in cases involving both consumers' and workers' safety and health and to render impossible any repeat of the type of challenge at the WTO that France and the EU has faced over its ban on trade in asbestos, which is described further in Section 12-10.[58]

12.7.2. The Basel Convention on the Control of Transboundary Movements of Hazardous Wastes

The Basel Convention of 1989 on the Control of Transboundary Movements of Hazardous Wastes was based upon an earlier decision by the OECD to control the trade in hazardous wastes. Radioactive wastes were covered concurrently under a parallel IAEA agreement. The developing nations at the Basel meeting wanted an absolute ban on waste exports, while most of the developed nations advocated for no ban. The compromise was that exporters would manage the waste in a safe manner and that no waste could be exported to a nation that banned the importation of hazardous waste. The Basel Convention became a starting point for the control of transboundary movements of hazardous wastes. Following the ratification of the convention, it became law in 1992.[59]

12.7.3. North American Free Trade Agreement

Bilateral agreements emerged in 1965 as the Maquiladora Program under the U.S.-Mexico Border Industrial Program with the aim of generating employment and stimulating industry by capitalizing on the abundant and low-cost labor in Mexico. The program provided a duty-free zone for those components from the country of origin of products that pass over the border. A condition of the program was that any hazardous waste generated in production would go back to the country of origin of the materials that were the source of the wastes. This policy is understood as a failure.[59]

In 1989, Canada and the United States agreed to the bilateral Free Trade Agreement in 1994, and the pact became NAFTA with Mexico added.[60] The North American Free Trade Agreement (NAFTA) was the countries' first experience in addressing labor rights including occupational safety and health in a trade agreement through its "labor side agreement," the North American Agreement on Labor Cooperation (NAALC). The three signatory nations agreed to improve working conditions and living standards through cooperative activities and to promote 11 basic labor principles, including principle number 9, "prevention of occupational injuries and illnesses: prescribing and implementing standards to minimize the causes of occupational injuries and illnesses." Another principle, number 7, addresses compensation for occupational injuries and illnesses. The NAALC provides for the public to submit a complaint to any of the three member nations alleging the failure of another member nation to enforce its labor standards. Under the agreement, violations of worker health and safety standards can ultimately result in fines and trade sanctions. The NAALC recognizes each nation's sovereignty and its right to establish its own labor laws and regulations.[51]

A two-level structure is used to resolve complaints: the international level and the national level. The Commission for Labor Cooperation is at the international level, created under the NAALC. The commission is composed of the Council of Ministers and a secretariat. The council sets policy and makes decisions for the NAALC and consists of the three labor ministers or their representatives. The secretariat provides support to the council.[61]

The council also promotes international cooperative activities on a broad range of issues involving labor law, labor standards, labor relations, and labor markets. In 2007, Mexico suggested a cooperative activity, Occupational Safety and Health in Mining Safety in North America. The NAALC council instructed the Secretariat of the Commission for Labor Cooperation as well as the National Administrative Offices (NAOs) to organize this cooperative activity.[61]

The NAO within each member nation's labor ministry is the second level. Labor law matters arising in the territory of another member nation may be raised by the NAO or by members of the public through the submission of a complaint or public communication.[61]

When a complaint is made, it is submitted to the NAO as a "communication" from the nation from which it is made. The NAO then consults with the NAO in the nation against which the complaint is made. If a resolution is made at this level, then the process is complete. If resolution fails, the complaint is submitted to an independent evaluation committee of experts named by the council. If resolution fails at this step, the complaint is passed on to an arbitral panel for dispute resolution that is established by the Council, as shown in Figure 12-4.[62] The secretariat of the commission provides support for the evaluation committee of experts and the arbitral panel. If unresolved, the council administers fines and trade sanctions. As shown in Table 12-6, of a total of 13 complaints filed regarding occupational injuries and illnesses, seven cases regarding the prevention of injuries were filed with the United States or Canadian NAO alleging failure of the Mexican government to enforce its regulations, five were filed in Mexico against the U.S. government, and one was filed in the United States against Canada.[63] Of these 13 complaints, none have made it beyond the consultation step.[61,63] The typical resolution was issued as a press release with no notification to the party submitting the complaint, and there was no time limit for coming to a resolution.[51]

Several problems led the side agreements to fail by design. There was no participation by workers for whom the side agreement was designed to protect, there were no deadlines and no procedure for being informed of resolutions, transparency was absent, no political will was present, and the sanctions were against the government and not the offending parties. The NAALC was not designed to improve or create standards where none existed, and it established no enforcement mechanism to ensure that the principles were promoted.[51] To address the protection of workers' safety and health, one author expressed

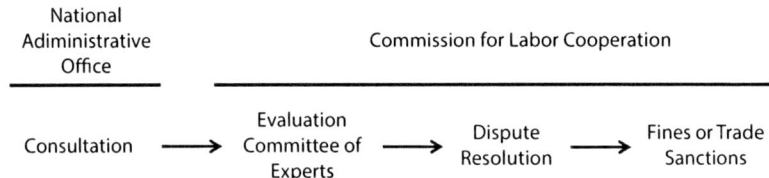

Figure 12-4. Process for resolving a complaint or a public communication under the North American Free Trade Agreement.

Table 12-6. Thirteen Public Communications Seeking National Administrative Office Labor Laws Review of Two Occupational Injuries and Illnesses Principles Under the North American Free Trade Agreement Labor Side Agreement

| Year | Recipient NAO (Number) | Regarding | Occupational Injuries and Illnesses Principle* | | Resolution |
			Prevention	Compensation	
1997	United States (9702)	Mexico	X		U.S.-Mexico cooperation on health and safety information
1997	United States (9703)	Mexico	X		
1998	Canada (98-1)	Mexico	X		Canada to participate in the Working Group of Government Experts on Occupational Safety and Health
1998	Mexico (9801)	United States	X	X	Government-to-government meeting, public outreach by DoL, Secretariat Guide
1998	Mexico (9802)	United States		X	
1998	Mexico (9803)	United States	X	X	
1998	United States (9704)	Canada	X	X	Not accepted for review
1999	United States (9901)	Mexico	X		Bilateral working group of government experts on workplace health and safety
2000	United States (2000-01)	Mexico	X	X	
2001	Mexico (2001-1)	United States	X	X	Recommendation that DoL undertake action to remedy procedural problems
2003	United States (2003-1)	Mexico	X		Accepted for review, follow-up unreported
2003	Mexico (2003-1)	United States	X	X	
2003	Canada (2003-1)	Mexico	X		Unreported

Note: NAO = National Administrative Office; DoL = U.S. Department of Labor. No record of additional cases after 2004; *n* = 28.
*There are 11 labor principles, and the request in most cases addresses additional principles.

lessons learned to overcome the weaknesses of NAFTA in subsequent trade treaties:[62]

1. A minimum floor of occupational safety and health regulations.
2. An "upward harmonization" of regulatory standards and actual practice.
3. Formal responsibility and liability of employers for violations of the standards.
4. Effective enforcement of national regulations and international standards.
5. Transparency and public participation.
6. Recognition of disparate economic conditions among trading partners.
7. Provision of financial and technical assistance to overcome economic disincentives and lack of resources.

A 2004 study of the side agreement concluded that the NAALC has failed to protect workers' rights to safe jobs and is in danger of fading into oblivion.[51] That study was prophetic, for all positions in the secretariat are vacant at this writing in 2013.[61]

12.7.4. The Rotterdam Convention

The FAO Council (in 1994) and the UNEP Governing Council (in 1995) mandated their executive heads to launch negotiations to provide the world's most vulnerable countries with the necessary information to enable them to assess the risks of hazardous chemicals and to make informed decisions on their future import. The resulting Rotterdam Convention is an international agreement intended to regulate global trade in dangerous chemicals that have been banned or severely restricted because of their hazards to human health or the environment. The text of the Rotterdam Convention on the Prior Informed Consent Procedure for Certain Hazardous Chemicals and Pesticides in International Trade was adopted at a diplomatic conference held in Rotterdam in 1998 by 170 countries and became legally binding for its parties. The convention facilitates information exchange among parties for a very broad range of potentially hazardous chemicals. The convention requires each party to notify the convention's secretariat when taking a domestic regulatory action to ban or severely restrict a chemical. One incentive for this convention was an estimated 200,000 people killed annually from pesticide poisoning, and 73% of the chemicals covered by the Rotterdam Convention are pesticides.[64]

Currently, prior informed consent is required on 45 chemicals, including four forms of asbestos, but not chrysotile—the principal form of asbestos that moves in international trade. The convention's Chemical Review Committee recommended the listing of chrysotile, but Kazakhstan, Kyrgyzstan, Vietnam, Russia, and Zimbabwe thwarted the will of more than 100 other countries by opposing listing chrysotile in 2008. The convention's requirement for unanimity allowed for this stonewalling.[64,65]

12.8. EUROPEAN UNION

Treaties, as Bismarck reminded us, are harder to enforce than sovereign laws. The member nations of the EU exert far more influence over Brussels than do the U.S. states over Washington.

—Randall Baker[66]

Three treaties established the European Community: the 1951 European Coal and Steel Community, the 1957 European Economic Community, and the 1957 European Atomic Energy Community treaties, comprising Belgium, the Federal Republic of Germany, France, Italy, Luxembourg, and the Netherlands. A fourth treaty brought the United Kingdom, Denmark, and Ireland into the European Community in 1972. The European Community structure of governance includes a European Parliament, Council of Ministers, the European Commission, and the Court of Justice. This structure can be compared to the U.S. checks-and-balances system—respectively, the House of Representatives, the Senate, the Executive Branch, and the Supreme Court. The European Parliament provides democratic control in the form of members from member states elected by universal suffrage. The Council of Ministers represents the member states and makes unanimous decisions regarding powers given to it by the treaty. The European Commission is the executive branch of the European Community, headed by the Secretariat-General. The Court of Justice provides for judicial control through nine judges with the authority to rule on compliance with the law consistent with the treaty.[21] A separate president is named to head the parliament, the council, and the commission.

The Single European Act (SEA) of 1987 was a treaty revision that aimed to harmonize laws and resolve policy discrepancies among European Community member states. An article in this act authorized the council to uphold the minimum requirements for "encouraging improvements, especially in the working environment, as regards the health and safety of workers." The treaty entrusted the commission to develop a dialogue between management and labor at the European level.

In 1992, the Treaty on European Union, known as the Maastricht Treaty, created the EU. The popular political concept behind this treaty was subsidiarity, which means centralization where necessary, decentralization where possible. Since 1992, several treaty revisions have changed the power of EU institutions and provided for accession of more European states into the EU, as can be seen in Table 12-7.[67] Treaty revisions reflect a process for the EU that

Table 12-7. European Union Countries

Current Members		Potential Member States	
Entry Year	Member State		
1952	Belgium	Acceding country	Croatia
	France		
	Germany		
	Italy		
	Luxembourg		
	Netherlands		
1973	Denmark	Candidate countries	Iceland
	Ireland		Montenegro
	United Kingdom		Serbia
1981	Greece		Former Yugoslav Republic of Macedonia
1986	Portugal		Turkey
	Spain		
1995	Austria	Potential candidates	Albania
	Finland		Bosnia and Herzegovina
	Sweden		Kosovo
2004	Cyprus		
	Czech Republic		
	Estonia		
	Hungary		
	Latvia		
	Lithuania		
	Malta		
	Poland		
	Slovakia		
	Slovenia		
2007	Bulgaria		
	Romania		

is evolutionary—not like the constitutional system in the United States, which was revolutionary. The EU process has required patience.[68] The Maastricht Treaty also introduced another important element of governance in which environmental policy would be "based on the precautionary principle and on the principles that preventive action should be taken, that environmental damage should as a priority be rectified at the source and that the polluter should pay."[69]

The commission has the exclusive right to make policy proposals, the parliament provides advice on these proposals, and the council makes its decisions based upon the proposals. However, over time, the council has become a source of ideas for policies and substance and the commission as a channel for these policies, but the influence of the parliament cannot be underestimated. Since the parliament must give advice before a policy moves to the council, it can delay and frustrate a policy. However, the parliament provides an important bridge to the parliaments of the member states in their actions on EU decisions. Council decisions were designed originally as needing unanimous assent, but because of the veto power of just a single member, decisions were stymied. Thus, the council has moved to using a majority vote.[68]

After the council makes a decision, the policy moves to the commission for implementation, which is the responsibility of the individual state members. The commission does not have police powers,[68] but it can sue a member in court if a state fails to act on the policy. Figure 12-5 shows the logic of EU policy making.

EU policies are either EU-wide regulations to be implemented by member states or financial support for specific purposes. These policies are of three forms: decisions, regulations, and directives. Decisions have a direct legal effect upon a recipient. Regulations have a direct legal effect on a category of

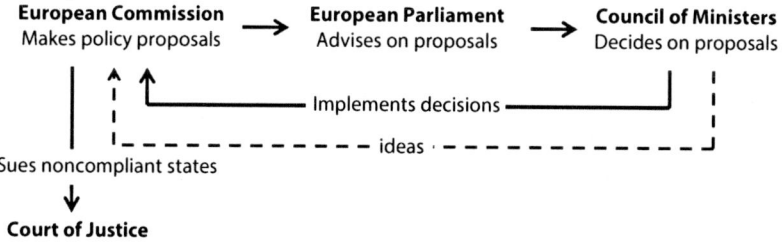

Figure 12-5. The European Union structure for policy making.

people or organizations within the EU. Directives are a statement of goals to be achieved with an order for member states to enact laws accordingly. The directives are the most popular policy form since they allow member states a large role in their implementation. Moreover, directives as EU policy remain invisible to the public since the perceived source of law is at the member state level through "letterhead" governments. Because of the characteristic of this policy form, directives have given the EU an ever stronger hand in policy making.[70] EU policies attempt to integrate policy goals into a broad policy-making system. In contrast with the United States, the EU has voluntary compliance with directives without a binding compliance mechanism.[66]

Early directives issued by the commission were developed by a committee system. Sometimes an ad hoc committee would be established, comprising a representative from each member state (there were nine members prior to 1981) and chaired by a commission representative to address a specific issue. In the 1980s, standing committees were given the task to develop directives for action. One was the Economic and Social Committee, and another was the Committee on Harmonization. Proposals were presented by the commission and reviewed with advice from the parliament before the council issued a directive. Prior to 1987, directives addressed safety signs, vinyl chloride, carcinogens, lead, asbestos, noise, and labeling. With the advent of the SEA in 1987, an emphasis was placed on creating a level playing field. The SEA was relevant to occupational safety and health in two important ways:[71]

- A shift in policy occurred from single-issue directives to directives that addressed general duties and minimum standards.
- A change away from unanimous vote in the council to a two-thirds "qualified majority" to avoid a blocking minority vote. Council votes were allocated "roughly" by country size (e.g., 10 votes by France, three votes by Denmark).

Four EU institutions involved in occupational safety and health policy are described below: the Economic and Social Committee of the Commission (EESC), the European Foundation for the Improvement of Living and Working Conditions, the European Agency for Safety and Health at Work, and the European Chemical Agency. They are presented in order of their creation. The European Chemical Agency is discussed in the context of the Regulation on Registration, Evaluation, Authorization, and Restriction of Chemicals (REACH) regulation, which it administers. At the UN level and at the EU, "economic and social" implies becoming a civil society through the rule of law.

12.8.1. Economic and Social Committee of the Commission

The EESC is a consultative body for the EU that was established in 1958. Its assembly is composed of employer, worker, and other stakeholder representatives. Its headquarters is located in Brussels. It is mandatory for the EESC to be consulted on issues stipulated in the treaties and regarding cases that the institutions deem appropriate. It can issue opinions to the three larger institutions: the council, the commission, and the European Parliament (see Figure 12-5). The EESC may also be consulted on an exploratory basis by one of the other institutions and can issue opinions on its own initiative (about 15% are own-initiative opinions).[72]

Exploratory opinions requested by other institutions enable the various stakeholders represented within the EESC to express their expectations, concerns, and needs before the commission drafts its proposals. Own-initiative and exploratory opinions often raise the awareness of decision-making bodies, particularly the commission, about subjects that have attracted little attention. The EESC adopts on average 170 opinions per year on a range of subjects concerning European integration, playing an active role in shaping EU policies, and preparing EU decisions.[72] After the enactment of the SEA, the Advisory Committee on Safety, Hygiene, and Work became active in developing the substance of proposed directives in tandem with the EESC.

12.8.2. European Foundation for the Improvement of Living and Working Conditions

In 1974, the council decided on a resolution that established a social action program for workers, aimed at humanizing living and working conditions. The European Foundation for the Improvement of Living and Working Conditions (Eurofound is its current designation) is one of the first bodies to be established to work in specialized areas of EU policy. The council established the foundation to contribute to the planning and design of better living and working conditions in Europe, and its work has informed EESC proposals.

In 1992, the foundation's European Work Survey identified differences among member states regarding working conditions related to safety and health. The differences were attributed to the types of strategies followed by public and company policies in the 13 member states. The foundation initiated an assessment of these differences in 1993 with the following conclusions:[73]

- The states differ primarily by the age of previous control strategies, some dating back a century.
- Those states, in which occupational safety and health is a recent concern, have found directives helpful as a ready-made upgrade of old policies.
- There is a potential deterioration of protective standards in those states where higher standards are the norm in order to maintain competitiveness within the EU.
- Available data are inadequate for assessing performance of occupational safety and health policies.
- Occupational diseases identified today reflect exposures from the past, which presents a handicap for current policies since these exposures change.
- Strengths identified include cooperation between management and unions and the inspector, which are key for improving working conditions.
- Weaknesses identified include the jeopardy presented by deregulation and budget-driven constraints on inspection, weak social partner relationships (e.g., unions), inadequate training, policies addressing large companies and not small companies, and researchers' lack of concern for applied research.
- Insurance schemes should emphasize prevention.

In 2005, a regulation established the governing and management structure of the Eurofound, comprising a governing board, a bureau, and a director and deputy director. The governing board establishes guidelines for the Eurofound, and the bureau as established by the governing board monitors the implementation of governing board decisions between the governing board meetings. In particular, the Eurofound is directed to cooperate with the European Agency for Safety and Health at Work. (i.e., EU-OSHA), which is described below and is closely associated with the European Commission.[74]

The Eurofound provides facts and figures, shows trends, and analyzes policies and practices as the basis of evidence-based advice for the development of policy recommendations. Eurofound's strategy for 2013–2016 focuses on policies in four priority areas:[75]

1. Increase labor market participation and combat unemployment by creating jobs, improving labor market functioning, and promoting integration.
2. Improve working conditions and make work sustainable throughout the course of life.
3. Develop industrial relations to ensure equitable and productive solutions in a changing policy context.
4. Improve standards of living and promote social cohesion in the face of economic disparities and social inequalities.

12.8.3. European Agency for Safety and Health at Work

National programs within the EU address five principles for occupational safety and health to their laws: (1) protection and prevention, (2) adjustment of work, (3) health promotion, (4) cure and rehabilitation, and (5) primary health care. Addressing all five principles is considered to be a comprehensive approach for providing for occupational safety and health.[76]

An EU policy field addresses the continuous improvement of safety and health at work as a matter of social and employment policy. The range and diversity of occupational safety and health issues in Europe go beyond the resources and expertise of a single member state or institution. Thus, in the spirit of subsidiarity, a council regulation in 1994 established the European Agency for Safety and Health at Work (EU-OSHA).[77]

The mission of EU-OSHA is to provide the European Community bodies, the EU member states, and those involved in the occupational safety and health field with useful technical, scientific, and economic information. The EU-OSHA was mandated to establish a network in which the member states were to inform the agency of the main components of their national health and safety policies in work information networks, including institutions that could assist the agency. This network brings together and shares the region's pool of knowledge and information on occupational safety and health-related issues such as good prevention practices.[75]

EU-OSHA acts as a catalyst to develop, analyze, and disseminate information to improve occupational safety and health in Europe as well as develop a network of safety and health websites. The agency also mounts campaigns and operates a publications program that produces specialist information reports and fact sheets.[77]

In 2003, a council decision provided that the EU-OSHA director establish the Advisory Committee on Safety and Health at Work. In 2005, a council regulation established three governing bodies for the agency: first, a Director as the legal representative of EU-OSHA; second, a governing board made up of three representatives from each of 27 member states and comprising one representative each from government, employers, and workers (like the ILO tripartite structure) and including representatives of the European Commission; and third, an 11-member bureau established by the governing board that monitors the implementation of the governing board's decisions between board meetings.[78]

12.8.4. European Chemical Agency

Congress enacted the Toxic Substances Control Act (TSCA) in 1976 as a way to anticipate chemical hazards and control them prior to their introduction into widespread use. However, the TSCA had a loophole. More than 60,000 chemicals were already in widespread use and were not required under the TSCA to undergo testing. The European Commission issued a proposal in 2003 for the REACH program (mentioned above in Section 12.8). The aim of this proposal was to fill the breach in the TSCA by requiring the registration, evaluation, and authorization of chemicals so that they would be permitted to remain in the market. This proposal reversed the burden of proof from the presumption of "safe until proven hazardous" to a burden upon manufacturers to prove the chemicals safe before they were used in production; safety focused upon carcinogens, mutagens, and reproductive toxins.[1]

The European Chemical Agency, headquartered in Helsinki, Finland, administers the REACH program. The required registration of chemicals is based on the seriousness of risk and the amount of the chemical produced each year. By the end of 2008, 65,000 chemicals had been preregistered. Consistent with the precautionary principle, manufacturers or importers of chemicals must estimate human exposure by all routes for each potential use as part of a chemical risk assessment and generate risk management measures for each application. Placing the responsibility on the manufacturer or importer overcomes placing the responsibility of risk assessment on the employer and overcomes the slow pace of EU interventions in chemical safety. REACH is a regulation and not a directive; thus, it is a requirement directly from the EU. Directives in place remain important, such as the control of exposure from welding fumes or where an employer needs to control unique working conditions that are overlooked in the risk management measures provided.[79]

12.9. NONGOVERNMENTAL ORGANIZATIONS

Many organizations arise outside of government and influence policy. These nongovernmental organizations (NGOs) include unions, trade associations, professional organizations, and interest groups across the international policy spectrum. From among these many organizations, four are described below.

12.9.1. International Organization for Standardization

The ISO story began in 1946, when delegates from 25 countries met at the Institute of Civil Engineers in London and decided to create a new international organization "to facilitate the international coordination and unification of industrial standards." In 1947, ISO began operations. It is the world's largest developer of voluntary international industrial standards. International standards give specifications for products, services, and good practice, helping to make industry more efficient and effective. Developed through global consensus, the standards ease barriers to international trade and provide for safety through cross border commonality. Developing ISO standards is a consensus-based approach, and comments from stakeholders are taken into account. The ISO has published more than 19,500 international standards for products.[80]

The International Organization for Standardization (ISO) responds to a request from industry or other stakeholders such as consumer groups for standards development. Typically, an industry sector or group communicates the need for a standard to its national member, which then contacts the ISO. Standards are developed by groups of experts from across the world that are part of larger groups called technical committees. These experts negotiate all aspects of the standards, including their scope, key definitions, and content. The technical committees are made up of experts from the relevant industry but also include experts from consumer associations, academia, NGOs, and government.[81] Many ISO standards address occupational safety and health.

Examples include machinery safety, ergonomics, and fire safety.[81] Insurance companies look to these standards as a way to understand the risk of exposure to occupational hazards.

12.9.2. International Commission on Occupational Health

The International Commission on Occupational Health (ICOH) is an international nongovernmental professional society whose aims are to foster the scientific progress, knowledge, and development of occupational health and safety in all its aspects. It was founded in 1906 in Milan as the Permanent Commission on Occupational Health. Today, ICOH is the world's leading international scientific society in the field of occupational health with a membership of 2,000 professionals from 93 countries. It is recognized by the UN as an NGO and has close working relationships with ILO, WHO, UNEP, and ISSA. The most visible activities of ICOH are the triennial World Congresses on Occupational Health, which are usually attended by some 3,000 participants. The commission has 33 scientific committees and sponsors the *International Journal of Occupational and Environmental Health*.[82,83]

In its role in the development of some scientific documents and policy recommendations, ICOH has not always been scientifically objective, particularly in regard to asbestos and other fibers and some chemicals and pesticides. Many ICOH members serve multinational corporate interests to influence public health policy, most likely deliberately.[84]

12.9.3. International Association of Labour Inspection

The International Association of Labour Inspection was organized in 1972 to provide a forum for inspectors to exchange information about their work. It meets every three years, concurrent with the World Congress on Occupational Health. At its triennial meeting, results of surveys are presented, information is exchanged regarding the changing world of work, and skills are developed for prevention especially as industries change in each nation.[85]

12.9.4. Collegium Ramazzini

Independent of commercial interests, the Collegium Ramazzini is an international academic society that evaluates public health issues in occupational and environmental health. It has 180 clinicians and scientists from around the world elected to membership. The Collegium derives its name from Bernardino Ramazzini, the "father" of occupational medicine (see Chapter 5). The Collegium is an independent, international academy founded in 1982 by Irving J. Selikoff, Cesare Maltoni, and other eminent scientists. Its mission is to advance the study of occupational and environmental health issues and to be a bridge between the world of scientific discovery and the social and political centers that must act on the discoveries of science to protect public health. The Collegium focuses on the identification of preventable risk factors. By holding conferences, symposia, and training courses; publishing statements and research papers; and publicizing its views, the Collegium Ramazzini seeks to inform legislators, regulators, and other decision makers about the policy implications of scientific findings.[86]

12.10. THE GLOBAL PANDEMIC

As it became obvious that France would ban the use of white asbestos and imports from Canada, the Asbestos Institute, which was set up to promote the safe use of asbestos on a global scale and to defend use of asbestos and to lobby for the industry, sprung into action.

—K. Ravi Srinivas[87]

Asbestos exposure is widely recognized as an occupational hazard. A correlation between national asbestos consumption and the incidence of asbestos-related diseases, including mesothelioma, has been observed. Toward the end of the 20th century, governments in many developed countries banned or seriously restricted the use of asbestos. As a result, global asbestos producers have engaged in aggressive marketing campaigns to sell asbestos to developing countries. Consumption of white asbestos is increasing in Asia, Latin America, and the Commonwealth of Independent States (Azerbaijan, Armenia, Belarus, Georgia, Kazakhstan, Kyrgyzstan, Moldova, Russia, Tajikistan, Turkmenistan, Uzbekistan, and Ukraine). In most of the countries in these areas, there is little control of asbestos exposures. It is likely that the lethal effects of asbestos exposure, which are occurring in the United States, the United Kingdom, and Australia, will be replicated in the developing world.[88]

As asbestos increasingly became the focus of government oversight in industrialized countries, continued capital accumulation efforts necessitated risk transfer to developing countries. "Risk transfer" is characterized by the movement of hazardous production processes and products outside of industrialized countries as transnational corporations seek a more amenable context in which to continue capital accumulation efforts. In 2007, asbestos consumption in developing countries was more than two million metric tons but negligible elsewhere in the world economy.[42]

In the following sections, the asbestos-related diseases pandemic and two lobby efforts by Canada are described and demonstrate the implications of transnational corporations' pursuit of business and influence beyond the borders of one country to other parts of the world. The first lobby effort regards international influence through the IPCS, and the second lobby effort concerns a dispute settlement at the WTO.

12.10.1. The Social Production of Disease

Asbestos-related diseases are still a major public health problem. The WHO has estimated that 107,000 people worldwide die annually from mesothelioma, lung cancer associated with asbestos exposure, and asbestosis.[89] About 125 million people worldwide are exposed to asbestos in their work environments, and millions more have been exposed to asbestos in years past. In 2000, an estimated 43,000 deaths worldwide resulted from malignant mesothelioma, and population-attributable risk for lung cancer among males exposed to asbestos ranges between 10 and 20%.[61] Although the pandemic of asbestos-related disease has plateaued or is expected to plateau in most of the developed world, little is known about the pandemic in developing countries. Increased asbestos use by these countries is expected to result in an increase in asbestos-related diseases in the future.[89]

If the global use of asbestos was to cease today, a decrease in the incidence of asbestos-related diseases would become evident only two or more decades from now.[90] In the current pandemic, four waves of illness and death follow wherever asbestos is mined, transported, processed, used, or dumped as waste.[91]

- First, asbestos-related deaths occur among workers in the mining and milling of asbestos fiber and the manufacture of asbestos products.
- Second, asbestos-related diseases affect people who use asbestos-containing products, such as shipyard insulators and construction workers.

- Third, the disease occurs among people exposed to asbestos-containing products in situ in buildings, such as schoolteachers, nurses, and factory inspectors.
- Fourth, the disease occurs among bystanders such as family members who are exposed when another family member brings particles home on clothing or who are exposed to dust from asbestos mine spoils.

Across each phase of this pandemic, bystanders are exposed to asbestos, including wives who wash their husbands' asbestos-covered work clothes or people who live near asbestos mines, factories, or dumps.[91] The profound tragedy of the asbestos pandemic is that virtually all illnesses and deaths related to asbestos are preventable. Safer substitutes for asbestos exist, and they have been introduced successfully in many nations. The asbestos cancer pandemic may take as many as 10 million lives before asbestos is banned worldwide and all exposure is brought to an end.[65]

12.10.2. The Double Standard

Scientists have estimated that between 1995 and 2019, more than a half-million people in Europe would die as a result of exposure to asbestos;[92] thus, the EU banned the use of asbestos in all of its member states in 2005.[41] Moreover, a total of 52 countries where safer alternatives have replaced asbestos products have banned asbestos. However, many countries still import and export asbestos and asbestos-containing products.[93] Countries that still mine asbestos include Brazil, Canada, China, India, Kazakhstan, Russia, and Zimbabwe. The greatest importers of asbestos include India, Thailand, South Korea, Indonesia, Algeria, and Mexico and 30 more.[42]

A double standard emerges when some countries ban a dangerous product and others do not.[94] While the dangers of asbestos are widely known, the complex interaction of asbestos industry stakeholders, government officials, diplomats, politicians, and professional advisors stymie uniform action in eliminating asbestos exposure and reducing exposures to asbestos already in place.[88]

Transnational corporations have shifted the use of asbestos to developing countries and use an argument that one form of asbestos is less of a risk than other forms of asbestos. The issue has come down to the difference between two forms of asbestos: amphiboles and serpentine. The former are stronger and stiffer, while serpentine—chrysotile—asbestos is more flexible and softer. Thus—so the argument goes—chrysotile can potentially be dissolved or expelled from the body more readily; therefore, chrysotile is deemed safer than amphibole forms of asbestos. Early claims that chrysotile might be less dangerous than other forms of asbestos have not been substantiated.[90]

Chrysotile is essentially the only form of asbestos produced today and the only form involved in international trade in the 21st century, and it represents 95% of all the asbestos ever used worldwide. Despite a demonstrated link between exposure to chrysotile and mesothelioma, the asbestos industry claims that chrysotile is safe under "controlled use" conditions. However, even relatively low levels of asbestos exposure, including to chrysotile, can lead to cancer including mesothelioma; thus, there is no safe level of exposure to chrysotile. Workers exposed to chrysotile fibers alone have excessive risks of lung cancer and mesothelioma.[42,90]

In 1977, the IARC issued a monograph on asbestos. This document concluded that all forms of asbestos were carcinogenic and that it was "not possible to assess whether there is a level of exposure in humans below which an increased risk of cancer would not occur."[93] The ILO and WHO have adopted resolutions that define all types of asbestos as carcinogenic and have called for a global ban on the production and use of asbestos. There is general agreement among scientists and physicians, and widespread support from numerous national health agencies in countries around the world and UN agencies, that chrysotile causes various cancers, including mesothelioma and lung cancer.[42]

Numerous epidemiologic studies, case reports, controlled animal experiments, and toxicological studies refute the assertion that chrysotile is safe. While the risks of exposure to asbestos cannot be controlled by technology or by regulation of work practices, some countries have banned other forms of asbestos, but the so-called controlled use of chrysotile asbestos is exempted from the ban, an exemption that reflects the political and economic influence of the asbestos mining and manufacturing industry lobbies.[94]

Scientists and responsible authorities in countries allowing the use of asbestos should have no illusion that "controlled use" of chrysotile asbestos is an effective alternative to a ban on all uses of asbestos. Even the best workplace controls cannot prevent occupational and environmental exposures to products in use or as waste.[90] Nonetheless, asbestos exporter Russia was able to lobby to keep the Rotterdam Convention from restricting the trade of chrysotile by using labels to inform workers about the safe handling of chrysotile.[94]

12.10.3. Influence Peddling

The Canadian Medical Association, the Canadian Cancer Society, and Canada's leading health experts oppose the export of asbestos to developing countries. The National Public Health Institute of Quebec has published 15 reports, all of them showing a failure to achieve "controlled use" of asbestos within Quebec. Pat Martin, a member of Canada's parliament and former asbestos miner, has asked, "If we in the developed world haven't found a way to handle chrysotile safely, how can we expect them to do so in developing nations?"[90]

Nonetheless, consultant experts of the Canadian chrysotile asbestos industry contend that "exposure to chrysotile in a pure form seems likely to present a very low if any risk of mesothelioma." The Chrysotile Institute, a registered lobby group for the Quebec asbestos mining industry, takes the position that chrysotile can be handled safely through control measures.[90]

M.E. Meek, a Canadian government official, appeared in 1986 as a witness for Canada and the asbestos industry at EPA hearings on the proposed asbestos ban in the United States. Following 10 years of preparation, EPA issued a final rule in 1989 that prohibited the manufacture, importation, processing, and distribution in commerce of most asbestos-containing products.[95] The 5th Circuit Court (New Orleans) ruled against the standard in 1991 because no intermediate level of risk was assessed compared with banning asbestos and no assessment was made regarding substitute products. The court also found that EPA had not conducted a cost-benefit analysis.[96] These lobbying efforts are shown in the timeline shown in Figure 12-6.

An IPCS working group that met in 1986 that included Meek (in the same year that she offered testimony regarding the EPA ban on asbestos) was responsible for the first IPCS expert report on asbestos: *Asbestos and Other Natural Mineral Fibres*. The report went through two drafts, the second of which was prepared by Meek, J. Corbett McDonald, Fedor Valic, and two other scientists. McDonald had conducted epidemiological research on asbestos that began in the 1960s under the sponsorship of the Canadian asbestos industry. Valic, a professor from Croatia, was the secretary of the task group. The report acknowledged that asbestos could cause cancer and asbestosis but dismissed the problem, stating that "Adequate control measures should significantly reduce these risks."[94]

Seven members of another IPCS working group convened in 1988 that included Meek and McDonald of Canada. This group concluded that

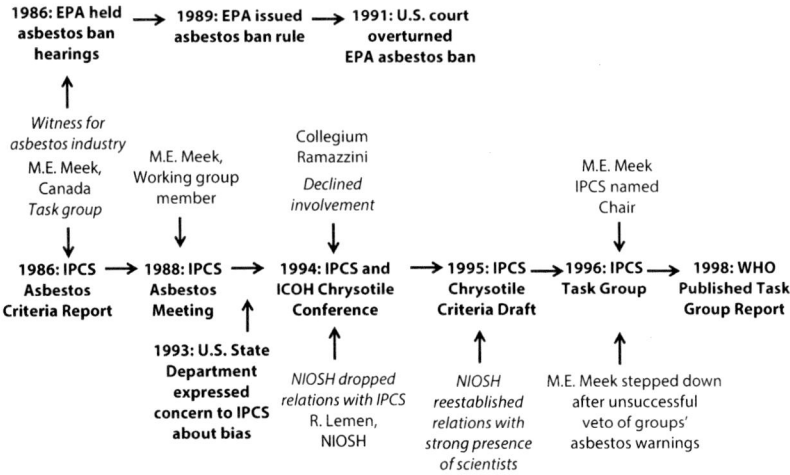

Note: EPA = U.S. Environmental Protection Agency; IPCS = International Program for Chemical Safety; ICOH = International Commission on Occupational Health; NIOSH = National Institute for Occupational Safety and Health; WHO = World Health Organization.

Figure 12-6. Timeline of Canadian influence on international asbestos policies.

automotive friction products made from chrysotile asbestos "provided good work practices were followed . . . detectable risks in vehicle maintenance and repair workers were not expected," in *A Report of an IPCS Working Group Meeting on the Reduction of Asbestos in the Environment*.[94]

In 1993, the IPCS launched an effort to prepare an updated Environmental Health Criteria document on chrysotile asbestos. This brought a strong response from Dr. Richard Lemen, acting director of NIOSH. Expressing "deep concern about the apparent lack of objectivity" with which the IPCS was evaluating chemicals, Lemen said, "This concern initially arose when IPCS sponsored the development of a criteria document on chrysotile asbestos, which was written by individuals with known ties to the asbestos industry. Subsequently, IPCS, along with the ICOH, co-sponsored a conference on chrysotile asbestos with the same group of scientists."[94]

Citing similar problems with a number of reports on chemicals, Lemen concluded, "Because of our concern about the apparent disregard for scientific objectivity, we believe it is inappropriate for NIOSH to continue participation in IPCS activities." The following month, the IPCS went ahead with the chrysotile meeting with "financial assistance from various industry organizations towards the costs of holding the workshop." Proceedings of this conference were edited by industry consultants Graham W Gibbs and K. Browne, along with IPCS consultant Valic.[94]

Dr. Philip J. Landrigan of the Mount Sinai School of Medicine wrote to Timothy Wirth, Undersecretary of the Environment at the U.S. Department of State (State Department), expressing concern about industry's unfettered influence in the important role of IPCS reports on international trade. As a result, the State Department met with agencies involved with the IPCS, which led to a letter from the State Department to the chief of the IPCS conveying unease regarding the influence of the industry consultants.[94]

In 1995, NIOSH reestablished relations with IPCS but was critical of a draft Environmental Health Criteria document on chrysotile asbestos that was based on the 1994 conference proceedings that were produced following NIOSH's earlier departure from IPCS. The institute claimed that the draft had serious omissions regarding results from epidemiology studies. The IPCS task group on chrysotile criteria met in Geneva in 1996 with Meek as chair. Observers at the meeting included Gibbs, representing the ICOH, and Daniel Bouige of the Asbestos International Association. Valic was the secretary for the meeting. Landrigan and other notable epidemiology experts were on the panel. Meek stepped down as chair of the task group in a controversy after unsuccessfully attempted to veto the task group's decision to include a warning against asbestos use in construction materials. The task group also refused Gibbs's participation in writing the conclusions and recommendations of the document since he was an observer and not a member of the task group.[93] In 1998, WHO published the document, *Environmental Health Criteria 203: Chrysotile Asbestos,* which concluded that no threshold of exposure had been identified for the carcinogenic risk of chrysotile and recommended the use of safer substitutes.[97]

12.10.4. The Dispute

The first nation to ban asbestos-containing products was Iceland in 1983, followed by eight more European nations prior to 1997. France banned chrysotile asbestos imports and asbestos-containing products and use, effective on the first day of 1997. In that same year, the EU banned its production and use effective in 2005, the gap in years likely in order to accommodate member nations' transition to alternative products and uses. Since Canada was a major producer of chrysotile asbestos mined for export to other nations, it sought consultations in 1998 with France and the EU regarding the ban. The EU refused to accept Canada's safe use principle regarding chrysotile asbestos and its desire for access to French markets.[87] The EU acted on behalf of France in this case.

Canada lodged a complaint with the WTO Dispute Settlement Body against France, claiming that its export product, chrysotile, could be used safely with proper controls. The burden of proof was at first upon Canada in this case. A previous ISO standard in 1984 provided for controlled use of asbestos in the manufacture of reinforced cement products. Once Canada presented its testimony, the burden shifted to the EU to present evidence contrary to the Canadian claim.[51] The timeline for this case is shown in Figure 12-7. Four issues that were considered in the case are shown in Table 12-8.[53,54]

In 2000, the WTO convened a hearing regarding the dispute and named a panel to evaluate and decide whether the French ban was a violation of WTO rules. The panel upheld the ban based upon a clause in GATT that rested on the issue of risk to human life (see Table 12-8).[53]

Canada then appealed the decision to the WTO Appellate Body, claiming that asbestos substitutes for chrysotile were like products and as a result were in violation of WTO rules. The Appellate Body disagreed with this logic and determined that health risk is a factor in determining likeness. Two members of a three-member board of the Appellate Body said that toxicity is a physical property under the first criterion (of four criteria) and were able to distinguish chrysotile as carcinogenic from its substitutes. The third member concurred but stated that rather than being a physical property, carcinogenic risk should be a fifth criterion. The other two declined to adopt carcinogenicity as a fifth criterion since GATT Article III.4 does not specify the protection of human

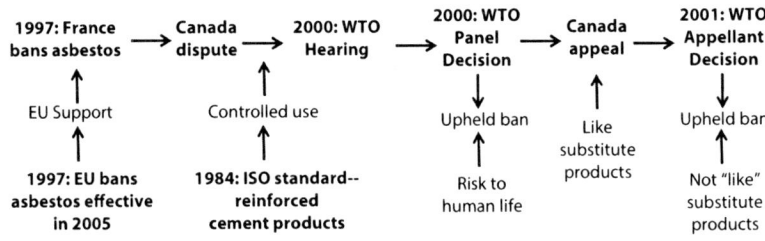

Note: EU = European Union; WTO = World Trade Organization; ISO = International Organization for Standardization.

Figure 12-7. Timeline of Canadian attempt to reverse French asbestos ban.

Table 12-8. Summary of World Trade Organization Findings Regarding Claims by Canada Against France's ban on Asbestos

Issues	WTO Panel (2000)	Appellate Body (2001)
1. GATT Article III.4: Like products	Found a violation since chrysotile is like its substitutes.	Reversed the panel's finding since Canada had failed to prove likeness and considered carcinogenicity a physical property in determining likeness.
2. GATT Article XI: Nontariff barriers	Not considered since a violation was found.	Declined to rule.
3. GATT Article XX(b): Exceptions: public health	French ban authorized because no other reasonable measure existed against the threat to human life.	Upheld panel's finding; French ban on imports was justified.
4. Technical barriers to trade: Technical regulation	Inapplicable since a ban is not a regulation.	Reversed the panel's finding regarding inapplicability, but judged as inadequate basis for a ruling.

Source: Cone;[53] Howse.[54]
Note: GATT = General Agreement on Tariffs and Trade.

health but rather economic and competitive relationships. As for the other three criteria, the Appellate Body was critical of the panel's interpretations of the second and third criteria but had little to add regarding the fourth criterion. The EU had to demonstrate that the French ban was for the protection of human life or health and that the ban was not a trade-protectionist measure under the guise of the protection of human life or health.[53]

The WTO rendered a decision in 2001 supporting the French ban against the Canadian arguments regarding the safe use controls of chrysotile and the likeness of chrysotile and its substitute. The decision recognized toxicity as a physical property and the public health exception for the protection of human life and health.[53]

12.11. THE EXPORT OF FACTORY HAZARDS

There is one record to which our transatlantic cousins may lay claim without fear of emulation; for in the matter of safeguarding its workmen, the United States enjoys the unenviable reputation of being the most backward of the civilized nations.

—*The Colliery Guardian*[98]

While the previous section discusses the risk transfer of a hazard with chronic consequences, this section addresses the acute consequence of the export of work by transnational corporations to developing nations where labor and life are cheap. The lack of institutional protections in the nations to which the risk is transferred follows a pattern of neglect that the developed nations experienced more than a century ago. This pattern demonstrates the inattention to the safety and health of workers in nations attempting to grow from poverty into affluence.

In China, a great wave of migration occurred from the rural areas of the country to urban areas for people to find jobs as China emerged as the world's factory.[99] Following staggering economic growth along with its own spate of disasters in mines and suicides in high-technology factories, the demand for workers has outstripped the supply, leading to a private sector rise in wages by 14% in 2012.[100] Moreover, popular movements in China are challenging the production of hazardous chemicals.[101] As a result, transnational corporations seeking the lowest cost of manufacturing have moved to suppliers in Vietnam, Bangladesh, and Cambodia.[100]

After 1880, an earlier great wave of migration occurred from Europe to the United States, where jobs were plentiful. Immigrants filled these jobs, whether on the railroads or in the steel mills, mines, or factories.[102] During 1910, braid and embroidery factory fires occurred weekly in New York City. In late 1910, a fire started in a lamp factory on the third floor of a 50-year-old building in Newark, New Jersey. A garment factory was situated on the fourth floor, six girls were burned to death there, and 19 more died when they jumped from the fourth-story windows to the pavement below.[102] Four months later in March 1911, a great fire occurred at the Triangle Shirtwaist Company in New York City, killing 146 workers, most of whom were immigrant women. Many died in the fire, others from collapsing fire escapes, and more from jumping from the eighth and ninth floors of the building. Another 23 women died within days from injuries that resulted from the fire. This fire generated major changes in fire safety codes and inspections in buildings. Elsewhere, one insurance company had paid out damages for 11 shirtwaist factory fires in Paris, France, by the end of 1911.[103]

A century later, similar tragedies continue as a result of risk transfers of industries to less developed countries. Low wages are the driver for garment factory work contracted by transnational corporations accompanied by the exploitation of the safety and health of workers. Bangladesh is the world's second-largest clothing exporter after China. The average wage for garment workers in Bangladesh in 2013 was 10 to 30 cents an hour. A century after the Triangle Shirtwaist Company fire, garment factory fires have been a recurring problem in Bangladesh and have killed about 700 people since 2006, according to an NGO called the Clean Clothes Campaign. In 2012, at least 110 people were killed in a fire at the Tazreen Fashions factory, and eight died in January 2013 in another garment factory fire.[104]

On April 24, 2013, Rana Plaza, a massive building that housed five garment factories and a shopping complex outside Dhaka (Bangladesh), collapsed and killed 1,127 people, most of whom were apparel workers. More than 1,800 were hospitalized and more than 300 required major surgeries. More than 30 injured victims required amputation, affecting their ability to find work.[105] Then two weeks later, a blaze swept through another Bangladesh apparel factory, killing another eight people.[104]

Bangladesh has 5,000 factories, but the government had only 11 factory inspectors in 2012. European retailers signed a pact on May 13, 2013, to commit to improved safety in Bangladesh garment factories. These companies agreed to contract only with factories that met fire and safety standards and that paid for repairs and renovations. The Bangladesh government announced that it would raise the minimum wage and make unionization easier. Large U.S. companies have been absent from making commitments, with the exception of two companies that agreed to join the pact made by the European retailers. U.S. companies are hesitant to sign the pact because of potential liability within the courts, commitments of up to $2.5 million to making fire and safety improvements in Bangladesh, and agreements with labor.[106,107]

The ILO will administer the program with three members of a governing board from the signers of the pact.[107] Because of the loss of life and serious injuries caused by the collapse of the Rana Plaza building and the recent factory fires, an ILO delegation visited Bangladesh to meet with tripartite partners from government, labor, and industry. The partners resolved to do everything possible to prevent further tragedy and agreed to develop an action plan with the ILO focused on the following steps:[108]

- Submit to Parliament in Bangladesh a labor law reform package that includes occupational safety and health.
- Assess the structural safety and fire safety of all active export-oriented garment factories in Bangladesh, and initiate remedial actions by the end of 2013.

- The ILO launched a skills and training program for workers injured in the recent tragedies that resulted in disability.
- Bangladesh agreed to recruit 200 additional inspectors within six months and upgrade its inspectorate to a directorate with a regular budget to enable the recruitment of at least 800 inspectors and the development of an adequate infrastructure.
- Improve safety and health by implementing the National Tripartite Plan of Action on Fire Safety in Bangladesh, which will include the structural integrity of buildings.
- Improved protection, in law and practice, for the fundamental rights to freedom of association and the right to collective bargaining, as well as occupational safety and health and progress on trade union registration.

The tripartite partners resolved to increase their efforts to provide every single worker in Bangladesh with a safe workplace and to ensure workers' rights and representation, regardless of whether the workplace is a garment factory, a retail shop, or a bank.[108]

Wal-Mart Stores Inc. took a unilateral approach by banning about 250 Bangladesh factories in an attempt to be more transparent with whom it contracts. Less transparent are the criteria that it uses, which complicates uniformity in the standards with which a company must comply. Some of the Wal-Mart banned factories appear on approved factory lists of other retailers. Multiple standards are a problem when one requirement may conflict with another requirement, such as where to place fire extinguishers. Moreover, the Wal-Mart approach goes beyond safety and health to address child labor, human rights abuses, bribery, and corporal punishment.[108]

Beyond Bangladesh, the global market includes Cambodia, which is experiencing growth in its garment industry. In May 2013, three workers died in a collapse of a factory floor there.[109]

More broadly, researchers espousing the "explanatory perspective" of international law have encouraged one global standard for transnational corporations across the world. Furthermore, they recommended three key principles for countries to create incentives and sustainable mechanisms for improving working conditions in factories: (1) transparency—disclose the names, locations, and conditions of factories, including contracted factories; (2) verifications—employ third-party monitors for the factories; and (3) worker participation—involve workers in improving working conditions and practices.[110]

12.12. THE BHOPAL CATASTROPHE

If Bhopal helped to crystallize a single issue for policy makers, that issue was the drastic inadequacy of compensation for victims of mass disasters in Third World countries.

—Sheila Jasanoff[111]

In 1984, a chemical leak from a pesticide manufacturing plant in Bhopal, India, exposed 520,000 people to the lethal gas methyl isocyanate, killing 8,000 during the first weeks after the incident.[112] This toll mounted to 15,000 as latent effects took hold. Another 300,000 people have suffered lifelong misery from the exposure.[113] The pesticide manufactured there was Sevin, also known as Carbaryl, for which methyl isocyanate was an intermediate chemical in its production. The plant was owned by Union Carbide India Ltd., in which the Union Carbide Corporation owned a controlling interest.[112]

Prior to the leak at the plant, signals of problems loomed. In 1976, two trade unions expressed concern about toxic exposures in letters sent to the plant management and to the Ministry of Labor of Madhya Pradesh, the Indian state where Bhopal is located. They received no reply. In 1981, a plant worker died from an exposure to phosgene gas, for which management blamed the victim for lack of personal protection. In 1982, 24 workers were hospitalized after exposure from a leak of phosgene. Later in 1982, 18 workers were affected by an exposure to a methyl isocyanate leak, and in another exposure incident, the gas burned more than 30% of a chemical engineer's body. Also in 1982, there was another leak of methyl isocyanate, methylcarbaryl chloride, chloroform, and hydrochloric acid; and in still another, an operator opened a valve in a methyl isocyanate pipeline in which a joint broke and the gas exposure burned a supervisor and caused severe health effects in two other workers. During 1983 and 1984, various leaks of methyl isocyanate, chlorine, monomethylamine, phosgene, and carbon tetrachloride occurred, sometimes in combination.[112]

During a recession in 1984, Union Carbide experienced a decline in profits in its international operations, and agricultural production was on the decline around Bhopal; thus revenues were reduced further. Workers were laid off, shift size was reduced from 11 to five workers, maintenance crews were cut in half, refrigeration units were shut down, and safety flares and washing towers were left unrepaired. Meanwhile, the workers, and the general public, were uninformed about the toxicity of methyl isocyanate gas.[113]

Minutes after midnight on December 3, 1984, while the residents of Bhopal slept, about 40 tons of methyl isocyanate gas leaked into the city's air from the Union Carbide plant. A supervisor at the plant turned off the alarm of the leak so as not to panic the public. Straightaway, the leak killed an estimated 4,000 people, which rose to 8,000 dead within weeks; many of the victims were children. More than 25 years later, activists said that thousands of children were born later with brain damage, missing palates, and twisted limbs as a result of their parents' exposure to the gas or methyl isocyanate–contaminated water.[114]

In 1989, Union Carbide settled with the Indian government for $470 million as compensation for this catastrophe.[115] Over the decades since then, groups of survivors have emerged and continued to agitate for fair compensation beyond this paltry settlement and against injustices in the Indian courts.[116] In 2010, an Indian court convicted seven former senior employees of Union Carbide's Indian subsidiary for their roles in the 1984 leak. They each received a two-year prison sentences and were fined $2,175. The American CEO had escaped from India and prosecution following a brief detention in 1984 by the police.[114]

Evident in this catastrophe was the asymmetry of law and science between developed and developing countries and of power and knowledge between producers, workers, and the public regarding transnational risks.[117] Asymmetries become manifest when known technologies in developed countries emerge as new technologies in developing countries accompanied by emergent risks where the workforce is less educated and skilled regarding safety technologies. Emblematic of this asymmetry was when management at the Bhopal plant encouraged its workers to drink several glasses of milk a day and eat a high-protein diet of fish and eggs so as to develop resistance against toxic substance exposure.[112] In contrast with developed countries, developing countries have yet to develop layers of controls to protect against risk and to deal with the aftermath of hazard control failures, as follows:[118]

- First layer—inherently safer technology with preventive design, procedures, and worker training. Ironically, an inherently safer design for pesticide production at the Bhopal plant was later found in which a different reaction route for producing the pesticide eliminated the intermediate chemical, methyl isocyanate.[119]
- Second layer—governmental standards and enforcement to assure safety and uniform compliance across society.

- Third layer—infrastructure to cope with injury and disease.
- Fourth layer—compensation as a matter of law though insurance or tort claims.

Countries face copious hurdles in developing these controls. These hurdles involve contradictions in which opposing tendencies or forces place competing or irreconcilable demands on a system's performance.[120] While there are many possible contradictions across technology, organizational objectives, and situations, one stands out above all else. It regards a contradiction of capitalism: namely, externalities (see Chapter 13). In Bhopal, Union Carbide had reduced costs with cutbacks in maintenance and labor, which externalized risk and magnified the catastrophe. Externalizing the risk led not only to catastrophic death in Bhopal but also to inadequate compensation for the sick survivors and the affected families of the dead.

Nonetheless, the Bhopal disaster was a prescient event that should have forewarned of other leaks of methyl isocyanate soon thereafter in the United States. Leaks there led to OSHA's egregious enforcement policy as described in Chapter 8. Furthermore, Bhopal is discussed in Chapter 14 regarding the expansion of right-to-know policies across the United States.

12.13. CHILD LABOR, FORCED LABOR, AND HUMAN TRAFFICKING

We remain committed to ending child exploitation—including child soldiering, child trafficking, and any work that harms the health, safety, or morals of children.

—Hillary Clinton[121]

In addition to OSHA and the Mine Safety and Health Administration, the DoL has an Office of Child Labor, Forced Labor, and Human Trafficking in its Bureau of International Labor Affairs. In response to a request from Congress, this office was created in 1993 to investigate and report on child labor around the world. Starting in 2002, the office has published an annual report entitled *Findings on the Worst Forms of Child Labor*, as mandated by the Trade and Development Act of 2000.[122]

The worst forms of child labor include work that is likely to harm the health, safety, or morals of children because of working conditions. They include all forms of slavery or practices similar to slavery, such as the sale or trafficking of children, debt bondage, and serfdom, or forced or compulsory labor, including forced or compulsory recruitment of children for use in armed conflict; the use, procuring, or offering of a child for prostitution, for the production of pornography, or for pornographic purposes; and the use, procuring, or offering of a child for illicit activities, in particular for the production and trafficking of drugs.[122]

President Clinton signed Executive Order 13126, "Prohibition of Acquisition of Products Produced by Forced or Indentured Child Labor," in 1999. The purpose of this order is to ensure that federal agencies do not procure goods made by forced or indentured child labor. It requires the DoL, in consultation with the Departments of State and todays Homeland Security, to publish and maintain a list of products, by country of origin, believed to be mined, produced, or manufactured by forced or indentured child labor. Table 12-9 shows the number of goods identified as being produced by child labor or forced labor by country, as recorded by the DoL in 2013.[122]

For example, the countries that produced the following goods on the list are shown in parentheses: bricks (Afghanistan, Burma, China, India, Nepal, and Pakistan), cotton (Benin, Burkina Faso, China, Tajikistan, and Uzbekistan), and gold (Burkina Faso and the Democratic Republic of Congo). The DoL identified a total of 37 goods that were manufactured by child and/or forced labor.[122]

Companies that engage in practices of servitude are conducting business outside of the norms of the OECD Code of Conduct and in violation of a tenet of capitalism, not to mention moral behavior. The Code of Conduct was addressed in Chapter 4 regarding law and, more specifically, transnational companies. The tenet regarding capitalism, which is founded on a worker freely working for an employer (e.g., no slavery or serfdom), is discussed next in Chapter 13.

DIBROMOCHLOROPROPANE: EXPORTING HAZARDS NARRATIVE

In preparing for U.S. Food and Drug Administration (FDA) approval of the nematicide dibromochloropropane (DBCP) in 1961, Shell Chemical Company and Dow Chemical Company had the chemical tested on rats, which resulted in organ damage and reduced the size of the testes in the male rats; at higher concentrations, the male rats were sterile. Despite requests for inquiries by the

Table 12-9. Number of Goods Produced by Child and/or Forced Labor by Country in Violation of International Standards, 2013

Country	Child Labor	Forced Labor	Country	Child Labor	Forced Labor	Country	Child Labor	Forced Labor
Afghanistan	4	1	Guatemala	6		Niger	5	1
Angola	1	1	Guinea	5		Nigeria	5	3
Argentina	11	1	Honduras	3		North Korea		7
Azerbaijan	1		India	21	7	Pakistan	6	
Bangladesh	13	1	Indonesia	6		Panama	3	
Belize	4	1	Iran	1		Paraguay	5	1
Benin	2		Jordan		1	Peru	5	5
Bolivia	10	5	Kazakhstan	1	1	Philippines	13	
Brazil	13	5	Kenya	7		Russia	1	1
Burkina Faso	2	2	Kyrgyz Republic	2		Rwanda	1	
Burma	11	13	Lebanon	1		Senegal	1	
Cambodia	7		Lesotho	1		Sierra Leone	5	1
Cameroon	1		Liberia	2		South Sudan	1	1
Central African Republic	1		Madagascar	2		Suriname	1	
Chad	1		Malawi	2	1	Tajikistan	1	1
China	7	11	Malaysia		2	Tanzania	8	
Columbia	8	1	Mali	3	1	Thailand	4	3
Côte d'Ivoire	2	2	Mauritania	2		Turkey	8	
Congo	7	4	Mexico	11		Turkmenistan	1	1
Dominican Republic	5	1	Mongolia	3		Uganda	10	
Ecuador	4		Mozambique	1		Ukraine	2	
Egypt	2		Namibia	1		Uzbekistan	1	1
El Salvador	4		Nepal	4	4	Vietnam	2	1
Ethiopia	3	1	Nicaragua	7		Zambia	5	
Ghana	4	2						

Source: U.S. Department of Labor.[122]

U.S. Department of Agriculture and the FDA concerning workers' exposure, the companies' stonewalling and assurances that DBCP was not a danger to human health led to the FDA's grudging approval of the use of DBCP. In 1977, workers in DBCP manufacturing plants were found to have low sperm counts, and some were sterile. OSHA promulgated a standard to restrict exposure to a very low level in California, where the hazard was brought to light, and EPA banned the use of DBCP but with restricted use in Hawaii. However, production was not banned.[123,124]

In 1969, DBCP manufacturers started marketing DBCP internationally, in particular to the Standard Fruit Company (which became Dole in 1991). Standard Fruit and other international companies began full-scale commercial use of DBCP in Costa Rica and at their banana plantations around the world, including in the Caribbean, West Africa, and the Philippines. Workers who formulated the chemical in warehouses and applied it in the field or through irrigation towers were heavily exposed to DBCP. No protections were used. After the banning of DBCP in the United States, Standard demanded that Dow continue providing DBCP for its operations. Although Dow hesitated, it relented under threat by Standard of a suit for breach of contract. Standard promised Dow that it would follow stringent safety precautions and would indemnify Dow against any liability related to the use of DBCP. Over the next 10 years, Standard neither provided personal protective equipment for its workers nor instructed workers and managers on the safe handling of DBCP. Precautions requested by Dow based upon the Hawaiian restriction by EPA were ignored. Labels on the drums of DBCP were written in English rather than the local languages. Storage drums used for DBCP were reused for other applications without cleaning. Disregard for worker safety at the highest level at Standard created a culture of neglect for protecting workers from DBCP exposures. Learning of the hazards, Costa Rica banned the use of DBCP despite Standard's lobbying for the contrary. Standard continued using DBCP until 1982 in Honduras and in the Philippines into the late 1980s.[123,124]

While the U.S. victims received compensation for their diseases through the tort system, workers in foreign nations ran into a stone wall in U.S. courts because of a doctrine of a "more convenient forum" in their home country, despite the lower worker protections there. However, a Texas law negated this doctrine by recognizing common law in these cases, and a suit by Costa Rican workers under that law led to a $20 million settlement by Standard for 1,000 workers ($20,000 each). Business interests soon launched a lobbying campaign to change the Texas law. They were successful in 1993. The defendant companies then battled to move the cases to federal court, where the "more convenient forum" doctrine can be applied. Nevertheless, in 1997, 26,000 workers in Latin America and elsewhere were compensated with $41 million in a settlement ($1,577 each) in a case that entered the Texas court before 1993. In 2002, a Nicaraguan tribunal sentenced multinational companies to pay $89 million to 450 workers for damages and interest because of DBCP poisoning ($197,777 each), and in 2007, Amvac Chemical agreed to compensate 14 sterile banana plantation workers in Nicaragua with $300,000 ($23,077 each).[123,124]

REFERENCES

1. Schapiro M. *Exposed: The Toxic Chemistry of Everyday Products and What's at Stake for American Power*. White River Junction, VT: Chelsea Green Publishing;2007.

2. Rosenthal J, Jessup C, Felknor S, et al. International environmental and occupational health: From individual scientists to networked science hubs. *Am J Ind Med*. 2012;55(12):1069–1077.

3. Johnson BL. *Environmental Policy and Public Health*. Boca Raton, FL: CRC Press;2007.

4. Coppée GH. International occupational health: the role of international organizations. In: Stellman JA, ed. *ILO Encyclopaedia of Occupational Health and Safety*. Vol 1. Geneva, Switzerland: International Labour Office;1998:23.36–23.46.

5. Bodansky D. *The Art and Craft of International Environmental Law*. Cambridge, MA: Harvard University Press;2010.

6. Machiavelli N. *The Prince*. Marriott WK, trans. In: Hutchins RM, ed. *Great Books of the Western World*. Vol. 23. Chicago, IL: William Benton;1952:1–38.

7. WorldLifeExpectancy. The history of life expectancy. WorldLifeExpectancy Live Longer Live Better. Available at: http://www.worldlifeexpectancy.com/history-of-life-expectancy. Accessed May 14, 2013.

8. Concha-Barrientos M, Nelson DI, Driscoll T, et al. Selected occupational risk factors. In: Ezzati M, Lopez AD, Rodgers A, et al., eds. *Comparative Quantification of Health Risks*. Geneva, Switzerland;2004:1651–1801.

9. Leigh J, Macaskill P, Kuosma E, Mandryk J. Global burden of disease and injury due to occupational factors. *Epidemiol*. 1999;10(5):626–631.

10. Culyer AJ, Tompa E. Equity. In: Tompa E, Culyer AJ, Dolinschi R, eds. *Economic Evaluation of Interventions for Occupational Health and Safety: Developing Good Practice*. New York, NY: Oxford University Press;2008:215–234.

11. Driscoll T, Takala J, Steenland K, et al. Review of estimates of the global burden of injury and illness due to occupational exposures. *Am J Indust Med*. 2005;48(6):491–502.

12. Takala J, Hämäläinen P. Globalization of risks. *Afr News Occup Health Saf.* 2009;19:70–73.

13. Michaels D. Remarks. XIX world congress on safety and health at work. September 11, 2011. Available at: http://www.osha.gov/pls/oshaweb/owadisp.show_document?p_table=SPEECHES&p_id=2626. Accessed May 16, 2013.

14. Michaels D, Sarukhan A. Joint declaration between the Department of Labor of the United States of America and Ministry of Foreign Affairs of the United Mexican States concerning workplace laws and regulations applicable to Mexican workers in the United States. May 4, 2010. Available at: http://www.osha.gov/international/docs/MexicoLOA2009.pdf. Accessed May 7, 2013.

15. U.S. Department of Labor. OSHA International website. Available at: http://www.osha.gov/international. Accessed May 7, 2013.

16. Solis HL, Lin L. Memorandum of Understanding between the Department of Labor of the United States of America and the State Administration of Work Safety of the People's Republic of China regarding cooperation on work safety and health. May 27, 2011. Available at: http://www.osha.gov/international/docs/2011-MOU-with-SAWS.pdf. Accessed May 7, 2013.

17. Office of Communications. OSHA and American National Standards Institute agree to expand international roles [news release]. January 19, 2001. Available at: http://www.osha.gov/pls/oshaweb/owadisp.show_document?p_table=NEWS_RELEASES&p_id=197. Accessed May 7, 2013.

18. Rosenstock L, Cullen MR, Fingerhut M. Advancing worker health and safety in the developing world. *J Occup Environ Med.* 2005;47(92):132–136.

19. Eichelberger CM. *UN: The First Fifteen Years.* New York, NY: Harper & Brothers; 1960.

20. International Labour Office. The United Nations and specialized agencies. In: Stellman JA, ed. *ILO Encyclopaedia of Occupational Health and Safety.* Vol. 1. Geneva, Switzerland: International Labour Office;1998:23.42–23.46.

21. Myers ML. *A Survey of International Intergovernmental Organizations: The Strategies That They Use to Abate Pollution.* Washington, DC: U.S. Environmental Protection Agency;1978. EPA 600/9-78-033.

22. International Labour Organization. About ILO. 2013. Available at: http://www.ilo.org/global/about-the-ilo/lang--en/index.htm. Accessed May 9, 2013.

23. Kliesch GR. International Labour Organization. In: Stellman JA, ed. *ILO Encyclopedia of Occupational Health and Safety.* Vol. 1. Geneva, Switzerland: International Labour Office;1998:23.46–23.52.

24. Stellman JA, ed. *ILO Encyclopedia of Occupational Health and Safety.* Geneva, Switzerland: International Labour Office;1998.

25. Meertens DJ. International Social Security Association. In: Stellman JA, ed. *ILO Encyclopaedia of Occupational Health and Safety.* Vol. 1. Geneva, Switzerland: International Labour Office;1998:23.55–23.58.

26. World Health Organization. Countries. 2013. Available at: http://www.who.int/countries/en. Accessed May 10. 2013.

27. Sixtieth World Health Assembly. *Global Plan of Action on Workers' Health 2008–2017.* 2007. Available at: http://www.who.int/occupational_health/WHO_health_assembly_en_web.pdf. Accessed May 7, 2013.

28. International Agency for Research on Cancer. About IARC. 2013. Available at: http://www.iarc.fr/en/about/governance.php. Accessed May 10, 2013.

29. World Health Organization. International Programme on Chemical Safety. 2013. Available at: http://www.who.int/ipcs/en. Accessed May 11, 2013.

30. International Maritime Organization. Conventions. 2013. Available at: http://www.imo.org/About/Conventions/Pages/Home.aspx. Accessed May 12, 2013.

31. National Fire Protection Association. The Texas City disaster. *NFPA Q.* 1947;41(1):24–57. Available at: http://www.nfpa.org/assets/files/pdf/texascity.pdf. Accessed May 12, 2013.

32. Bornhorst R, Min J. Hazardous materials carriage: the history of vessel safety standards. *Proceedings.* 2012;69(2):63–67.

33. International Atomic Energy Agency. IAEA safety standards: the global reference for protecting people and the environment from harmful effects of ionizing radiation. June 2009. Available at: http://www-ns.iaea.org/downloads/standards/iaea-safety-standards-brochure.pdf. Accessed May 11, 2013.

33a. Kiger PJ. Fukushima leak's 'level 3' rating: what it means. National Geographic. August 29, 2013. Available at: http://news.nationalgeographic.com/news/energy/2013/08/130829-fukushima-level-3-serious-incident-rating. Accessed January 30, 2015.

34. Food and Agriculture Organization. About FAO. 2013. Available at: http://www.fao.org/about/en. Accessed May 9, 2013.

35. Myers M. Agriculture and natural resource-based industries: general profile. In: Stellman JA, ed. *ILO Encyclopaedia of Occupational Health and Safety.* Vol. 3. Geneva, Switzerland: International Labour Office;1998:64.2–64.5.

36. Cole D. Understanding the links between agriculture and health: occupational health hazards of agriculture. Washington, DC: International Food Policy

Research Institute;2006. Focus 13, Brief 8. Available at: http://lib.icimod.org/record/12427/files/4397.pdf. Accessed May 9, 2013.

37. Huismans JW. The international register of potentially toxic chemicals (IRPTC): its present state of development and future plans. Ambio. 1978;7(5/6):275–277.

38. Reid E. McNamara's World Bank. *Foreign Affairs.* 1973;51(4):794–810.

39. World Bank. The World Bank. 2013. Available at: http://www.worldbank.org. Accessed May 12, 2013.

40. Le Prestre P. *The World Bank and the Environmental Challenge.* Selinsgrove, PA: Susquehanna University Press;1990.

41. Jamison DT, Mosley WH, Measham AR, et al., eds. *Disease Control Priorities in Developing Countries.* New York, NY: Oxford University Press;1993.

42. Rice J. The global reorganization and revitalization of the asbestos industry, 1970–2007. *Int J Health Serv.* 2011;41(2):239–254.

43. Marshall GC. The "Marshall Plan" speech at Harvard University, 5 June 1947. Available at: http://www.oecd.org/general/themarshallplanspeechatharvarduniversity5june1947.htm. Accessed July 22, 2014.

44. Organisation for International Co-operation and Development. OECD tractor codes brochure. 2013. Available at: http://www.oecd.org/els/emp/3888265.pdf. Accessed April 23, 2013.

45. Organisation for International Co-operation and Development. Occupational accidents in OECD countries. In: *Employment Outlook 1989.* Paris, France: OECD Publications Service;1989:133–159. Available at: http://www.oecd.org/els/emp/3888265.pdf. Accessed April 23, 2013.

46. Organisation for International Co-operation and Development. Occupational illnesses in OECD countries. In: *Employment Outlook 1990.* Paris, France: OECD Publications Service;1990:105–122. Available at: http://www.oecd.org/els/emp/4343111.pdf. Accessed April 23, 2013.

47. Organisation for International Co-operation and Development. *OECD Guiding Principles for Chemical Accident Prevention, Preparedness, and Response.* Paris, France: OECD Publications Service;2003.

48. Organisation for International Co-operation and Development. Comparing nuclear accident risks with those from other energy sources. 2010. Available at: http://www.oecd-nea.org/ndd/reports/2010/nea6862-comparing-risks.pdf. Accessed April 23, 2013.

49. Horn Blower M. Antiglobalization forces are threatening to turn the WTO's meeting on free trade into a free-for-all. November 22, 1999. Available at: http://www.cnn.com/ALLPOLITICS/time/1999/11/22/seattle.battle.html. Accessed May 21, 2013.

50. World Trade Organization. Text of the General Agreement on Tariffs and Trade. July 1986. Available at: http://www.wto.org/english/docs_e/legal_e/gatt47_e.pdf. Accessed May 14, 2013.

51. Delp L, Arriaga M, Palma G, et al. NAFTA's Labor Side Agreement: *Fading into Oblivion? An Assessment of Workplace Health and Safety Cases.* Los Angeles, CA: UCLA Center for Labor Research and Education;2004. Available at: http://www.labor.ucla.edu/publications/pdf/nafta.pdf. Accessed May 16, 2013.

52. World Trade Organization. Understanding the WTO: Who we are. 2013. Available at: http://www.wto.org/english/thewto_e/whatis_e/who_we_are_e.htm. Accessed May 19, 2013.

53. Cone SM. The asbestos case and dispute settlement in the World Trade Organization: the uneasy relationship between panels and the appellate body. *Michigan J Int Law.* 2001;23(1):103–142.

54. Howse R, Türk E. The WTO impact on internal regulations: a case study of the *Canada-EC Asbestos* dispute. In: Berman GA, Mavroidis PC, eds. *Trade and Human Safety.* New York, NY: Cambridge University Press;2006.

55. Marceau G, Trachman JP. A map of the World Trade Organization law of domestic regulation of goods. In: Berman GA, Mavroidis PC, eds. *Trade and Human Safety.* New York, NY: Cambridge University Press;2006:9–76.

56. Castleman B. WTO confidential: the case of asbestos. *Int J Health Serv.* 2002;32(3):489–501.

57. Vandaele DA. *International Labour Rights and the Social Clause: Friends or Foes.* Nottingham, UK: Cameron May;2004.

58. International Confederation of Free Trade Unions. ICFTU statement on the agenda for the 4th ministerial conference of the World Trade Organization. November 2001. Available at: http://search.wto.org/search?q=occupational+health&site=English_website&client=english_frontend&proxystylesheet=english_frontend&output=xml_no_dtd&numgm=5&proxyreload=1&ie=ISO-8859-1&oe=ISO-8859-1. Accessed May 21, 2013.

59. Asante-Duah DK, Nagy IV. *International Trade in Hazardous Waste.* New York, NY: Routledge;1998.

60. Walker C. NAFTA and occupational health: a Canadian perspective. *J Public Health Pol.* 1997;18(3):325–333.

61. Secretariat of the Commission for Labor Cooperation. The Commission for Labor Cooperation. Available at: http://new.naalc.org/commission.htm. Accessed May 18, 2013.

62. Commission for Labor Cooperation. The North American agreement on labor cooperation. North American Free Trade Agreement. Summary of public communications (as of March 2004). Available at: http://www.naalc.org/naalc.htm. Accessed May 3, 2014.

63. Brown G. Why NAFTA failed and what's needed to protect workers' health and safety in international trade treaties. *New Solut.* 2005;15(2):153–180.

64. Rotterdam Convention. How it was formed. 2010. Available at: http://www.pic.int/TheConvention/Overview/Howitwasdeveloped/tabid/1045/language/en-US/Default.aspx. Accessed May 12, 2013.

65. LaDou J, Castleman B, Frank A, et al. The case for a global ban on asbestos. *Environ Health Perspect.* 2010;118(7):897–901.

66. Baker R. The rationale behind this study. In: Baker R, ed. *Environmental Law and Policy in the European Union and the United States.* London, UK: Praeger;1997:5–17.

67. European Union. List of countries. Available at: http://europa.eu/about-eu/countries. Accessed May 5, 2013.

68. von Hasselt WG. European and American political decision making. In: Baker R, ed. *Environmental Law and Policy in the European Union and the United States.* London, UK: Praeger;1997:21–30.

69. Jordan A, O'Riordan T. The precautionary principle: a legal and policy history. In: Martuzzi M, Tickner JA, eds. *The Precautionary Principle: Protecting Public Health, the Environment, and the Future of Our Children.* Copenhagen, Denmark: World Health Organization Regional Office for Europe;2004: 31–48.

70. Hoetjes BJS. The European Union: evolution, nature, and trends. In: Baker R, ed. *Environmental Law and Policy in the European Union and the United States.* London, UK: Praeger;1997:31–44.

71. Dalton AJP. *Safety, Health and Environmental Hazards at the Workplace.* New York, NY: Cassell;1998.

72. Ledune B. *The European Economic and Social Committee: 50 Years of Participatory Democracy, 1958–2008*. Brussels, Belgium: European Economic and Social Committee;2008.

73. Piotet F. *Policies on Health and Safety in Thirteen Countries of the European Union, Volume II: The European Situation*. Dublin, Ireland: European Foundation for the Improvement of Living and Working Conditions;1996. EF/96/14/EN.

74. Eurofound. About Eurofound. December 21, 2012. Available at: http://www.eurofound.europa.eu/about/index.htm. Accessed May 5, 2013.

75. Eurofound. From crisis to recovery: Better informed policies for a competitive and fair Europe—Four-year work programme 2013–2016. November 21, 2012. Available at: http://www.eurofound.europa.eu/publications/htmlfiles/ef1252.htm. Accessed May 5, 2013.

76. Rantanen J, Lehtinen S, Iavicoli S. Occupational health services in selected International Commission on Occupational Health member countries. *Scand J Work Environ Health*. 2013;39(2):212–216.

77. European Union. European Agency for Safety and Health at Work (EU-OSHA). Available at: http://europa.eu/agencies/regulatory_agencies_bodies/policy_agencies/osha/index_en.htm. Accessed May 5, 2013.

78. European Union. Council Regulation (EC) No 1112/2005 of 24 June 2005 amending Regulation (EC) No 2062/94 establishing a European Agency for Safety and Health at Work. Available at: http://eur-lex.europa.eu/LexUriServ/site/en/oj/2005/l_184/l_18420050715en00050009.pdf. Accessed May 5, 2013.

79. Ogden T. REACH—How is it going? *Ann Occup Hyg*. 2009;54(1):1–4.

80. International Standards Organization. ISO website. 2013. Available at: http://www.iso.org/iso/home.htm. Accessed May 15, 2013.

81. Eicher LD. International Organization for Standardization. In: Stellman JA, ed. *ILO Encyclopaedia of Occupational Health and Safety*. Vol. 1. Geneva, Switzerland: International Labour Office;1998:23.52–23.55.

82. Jeyaratnam J. The International Commission on Occupational Safety and Health. In: Stellman JA, ed. *ILO Encyclopaedia of Occupational Health and Safety*. Vol. 1. Geneva, Switzerland: International Labour Office;1998:23.58–23.59.

83. International Commission on Occupational Health. ICOH website. 2013. Available at: http://www.icohweb.org/site_new/ico_about.asp. Accessed May 17, 2013.

84. Ashford NA, Castleman B, Frank AL, et al. The International Commission on Occupational Health (ICOH) and its influence on international organizations. *Int J Occup Environ Health*. 2002;8(2):156–162.

85. Snoball D. International Association of Labour inspection. In: Stellman JA, ed. *ILO Encyclopaedia of Occupational Health and Safety.* Vol. 1. Geneva, Switzerland: International Labour Office;1998:23.60.

86. Collegium Ramazzini. Collegium Ramazzini website. 2013. Available at: http://www.collegiumramazzini.org/index.asp. Accessed May 14, 2013.

87. Srinivas KR. WTO and asbestos: dispute settlement at work. *Econ Polit Week.* 2001;36(36):3442–3447.

88. Kazan-Allen L. Asbestos and mesothelioma: worldwide trends. *Lung Cancer.* 2005;49(Suppl 1):S3–8.

89. Stayner L, Welch LS, Lemen R. The worldwide pandemic of asbestos-related diseases. *Annu Rev Public Health.* 2013;34:205–216.

90. Collegium Ramazzini. Asbestos is still with us: repeat call for a universal ban. 2010. Available at: http://www.collegiumramazzini.org/download/15_Fifteenth-CRStatement(2010).pdf. Accessed May 19, 2013.

91. Kazan-Allen L. Asbestos: from magic mineral to killer dust. Presented at: First Public Asbestos Workshop; April 28, 2013; Istanbul, Turkey. Available at: http://www.ibasecretariat.org/lka-paper-asbestos-from-magic-mineral-to-killer-dust-apr-28-2013.pdf. Accessed May 18, 2013.

92. Brophy JT, Keith MM, Schieman J. Canada's asbestos legacy at home and abroad. *Int J Occup Environ Health.* 2007;13(2):235–242.

93. Castleman BI. The double standard in industrial hazards. In: Ives JH, ed. *The Export of Hazards: Transnational Corporations and Environmental Control Issues.* Boston, MA: Routledge & Kegan Paul;1985:60–89.

94. Castleman BI. Controversies at international organizations over asbestos industry influence. *Int J Health Serv.* 2001;31(1):193–202.

95. Asbestos manufacture, importation, processing, and distribution in commerce prohibitions. Final rule. *Fed Regist.* 1989;54(132):29462–29513.

96. *Corrosion Proof Fittings v. EPA,* 947 F.2d 1201 (5th Cir. 1991).

97. International Programme on Chemical Safety. *Environmental Health Criteria 203: Chrysotile Asbestos.* Geneva, Switzerland: World Health Organization;1998.

98. Aldrich M. Preventing the "needless peril of the coal mine": the Bureau of Mines and the campaign against coal mine explosions, 1910–1940. *Technol Cult.* 1995;36(3):483–518.

99. Chang LT. *Factory Girls: From Village to City in a Changing China.* New York, NY: Spiegel & Grau;2009.

100. Chu K. Rising wages pose dilemma for China. *Wall Street Journal.* May 18–19, 2013;261(116):A7.

101. Zhang K, Lin L, Murphy C. Behind Chinese protests, Growing dismay at pollution. *Wall Street Journal.* May 18–19, 2013;261(116):A7.

102. Hopkins MA. 1910 Newark factory fire. *McClure's Magazine.* 1911;36(6). Available at: http://www.oldnewark.com/histories/factoryfire01.htm. Accessed May 17, 2013.

103. von Drehle D. *Triangle: The Fire that Changed America.* New York, NY: Grove Press;2003.

104. Kapner S, Larhiri T, Zimmerman A. Promises in Bangladesh. *Wall Street Journal.* May 14, 2013;261(112):B1, B7.

105. Fairclough G. Bangladesh amputees face tests of survival. *Wall Street Journal.* May 23, 2013;261(120):A10.

106. Cheng A. Abercrombie & Fitch teen retailer joins Bangladesh pact. *Wall Street Journal.* May 16, 2013;261(114):B7.

107. International Labor Organization. Conclusions of the ILO's high-level mission to Bangladesh. May 4, 2013. Available at: http://www.ilo.org/global/about-the-ilo/activities/statements-speeches/WCMS_212463/lang--en/index.htm. Accessed May 7, 2013.

108. Zimmerman A, Lahira T, Johnson K, et al. Standards clash in Bangladesh reforms. *Wall Street Journal.* May 17, 2013;261(115):B1–B2.

109. Narin S. Three die in Cambodia factory. *Wall Street Journal.* May 17, 2013; 261(115):A8.

110. O'Rourke D, Brown GD. Experiments in transforming the global workplace: incentives for and impediments to improving workplace conditions in China. *Int J Occup Environ Health.* 2003;9(4):378–385.

111. Jasanoff S. Introduction: Learning from disaster. In: Jasanoff S, ed. *Learning from Disaster: Risk Management after Bhopal.* Philadelphia, PA: University of Pennsylvania Press;1994:1–21.

112. Eckerman I. The Bhopal disaster 1984—working conditions and the role of the trade unions. *Asian-Pacific Newsletter on Occupational Health and Safety.* 2006;13(2):48–49.

113. Gupta JP. The Bhopal gas tragedy: could it have happened in a developed country? *J Loss Prev Proc Ind.* 2001;15(1):1-4.

114. 7 guilty in Bhopal tragedy that killed 15,000. NBC news services. June 7, 2010. Available at: http://www.nbcnews.com/id/37551856/ns/world_news-south_and_central_asia/t/guilty-bhopal-tragedy-killed/#.Ux0YaPldVu4. Accessed March 9, 2014.

115. Broughton E. The Bhopal disaster and its aftermath: A review. *Environ Health.* 2005;4(6). Available at: http://www.ncbi.nlm.nih.gov/pmc/articles/PMC1142333/pdf/1476-069X-4-6.pdf. Accessed June 12, 2014.

116. Scandret E, Mukherjee S. Globalization and abstraction in the Bhopal survivors' movement. *Interface.* 2011;3(1):195-209.

117. Jasanoff S. Bhopal's trial of knowledge and ignorance. *Hist Sci Soc.* 2007;98(2): 344-350.

118. Galander M. The transnational traffic in legal remedies. In: Jasanoff S, ed. *Learning from Disaster: Risk Management after Bhopal.* Philadelphia, PA: University of Pennsylvania Press;1994:133-157.

119. Myers ML. 2006. Emerging technologies: inherently safer designs. *Prof Saf.* 51(10):20-26.

120. Shrivastave P. Societal contradictions and industrial crises. In: Jasanoff S, ed. *Learning from Disaster: Risk Management after Bhopal.* Philadelphia, PA: University of Pennsylvania Press;1994:248-267.

121. Clinton HR. Remarks to: Working Together to Combat Child Labor Conference; June 8, 2010; U.S. Department of State, Washington, DC. Available at: http://www.state.gov/secretary/20092013clinton/rm/2010/06/142789.htm. Accessed June 5, 2014.

122. U.S. Department of Labor. Office of Child Labor, Forced Labor, and Human Trafficking. Bureau of International Labor Affairs. Available at: http://www.dol.gov/ilab/programs/ocft. Accessed March 9, 2014.

123. Siegel CS, Siegel DS. The history of DBCP from a judicial perspective. *Int J Occup Environ Health.* 1999;5:127-135.

124. Bingham E, Monforton C. The pesticide DBCP and male infertility. In: *Late Lessons from Early Warnings: Science, Precaution, Innovation.* Copenhagen, Denmark: European Environmental Agency;2013:235-271. EEA Report No 1/2013. Part A—Lessons from Health Hazards.

III. INSTRUMENTS OF POLICY

In Part III of the book, I cover four chapters that address instruments of policy. These instruments add to the armamentarium addressed in Part I, which included law and advocacy, respectively, in Chapters 4 and 6. In Part III, Chapter 13, I discuss economics, which has emerged as an important policy tool and demands attention. This attention relates not only to the traditional compensation principle and workers' compensation but also to issues of trade-offs and externalities in the world of occupational safety and health. The public health professional needs to attend to economics for two reasons: first is an awareness of compensation policies, and second is an understanding of the arguments and counter-arguments regarding economic analysis, typically applied as a foil to improved occupational safety and health rather than applied as a means for preventive action, which will be addressed further in Chapter 16.

In Chapter 14, I address the Occupational Safety and Health Administration (OSHA) hazard communication standard (HazCom) and workers' right-to-know. HazCom is extremely important for it informs employers and workers alike of potential chemical hazards in the workplace. Both were previously kept in the dark about most of these potential hazards. Moreover, the standard is not static like many other occupational safety and health standards that are held in place with the science of the time when they were promulgated. HazCom is a generic standard that addresses not only hazards of current chemicals but also the hazards of new chemicals as they emerge into the workplace. In Chapter 14, I also address right-to-know issues that include environmental laws and the discovery process in tort law.

In Chapter 15, the penultimate chapter, I inquire into the important issue of leadership and ethics. Closely aligned with Chapter 6 regarding advocacy, I place a spotlight on past leadership failures of managers and corporate physicians to protect the safety and health of workers. In this chapter, I dwell into the situations that drive these failures and the important role that OSHA has to change these situations. In the chapter, I also address the ethics of leadership from both business and public health perspectives and the use of informal leadership within organizations.

In Chapter 16, I address the role of policy analysis regarding occupational safety and health in the context of policy formulation and implementation. Policy analysis also offers an opportunity for bringing together and reviewing many concepts described previously in this book. I review OSHA policy over time, legislative attempts at OSHA reform, and the role of politics and special interests in policy development. I also describe different analytical approaches—both qualitative and quantitative—and the troubling problem of economic analysis employed as a guiding principle rather than as a technique for determining feasibility for the implementation of occupational safety and health policies. At the end of this chapter, I address the issue of globalization and the challenge that it brings for which answers remain to be understood.

13

Workers' Compensation and Work as an Economic Activity

Each loss has its compensation
There is healing for every pain,
But the bird with a broken pinion
Never soars so high again.

—Hezekiah Butterworth[1]

THE MEXICAN IMMIGRANT NARRATIVE

Martin Zempoaltecatl was born in Mexico, and at age 19 he moved to New York City. He worked at first as a dishwasher and then trained to be a cook. He became an apprentice cook at two different restaurants, and then at age 22, he was hired as an assistant chef at a restaurant in the World Trade Center. Martin sent most of his wages to his parents in Mexico so that they could build a new home. His salary in 2000 was $20,589. He lived with two of his brothers, and both of them covered most of their living expenses in New York. In 2001, Martin's parents had completed half of the construction of their new home when Martin died at work in the World Trade Center on September 11 as a result of the terrorist attacks. His parents were compensated by the U.S. government for his death with more than $250,000, which allowed them to complete the house in Mexico in his memory.[2]

13.1. INTRODUCTION

I reject the idea that we need to ask people to choose between their jobs and their safety.

—President Barack Obama, 2010[3]

Table 13-1. Economics Glossary Shown in Dichotomy

Macroeconomics: Deals with large-scale economic phenomena, especially inflation, unemployment, and economic growth.

Microeconomics: Deals with the choices and actions of small economic units: households, business firms, and governmental units.

Positive externalities: The benefit generated by one party and used by other parties without payment.

Negative externalities: The costs generated by an economic agent that affects other parties are not recognized as market transactions.

Fixed costs: The portion of total costs of a program incurred even when output is nil, such as costs associated with overhead, facilities, and overhead salaries.

Variable costs: The portion of the total cost that increases with greater output, such as the costs associated with increasing the number of persons seen in an education program.

Human capital: An approach that incorporates direct and indirect costs but excludes pain and suffering regarding the value of a health outcome.

Willingness to pay: An approach for determining the value of a health outcome based on society's valuation of (willingness to pay for) that outcome.

Direct costs: Costs associated with prevention activities and the healthcare system.

Indirect costs: Costs not directly associated with prevention and healthcare activities that accrue to individuals (e.g., loss of time from work), society (e.g., disability payments), or employers (e.g., decreased productivity).

Incentive: Something, such as the fear of punishment or the expectation of reward, that induces action or motivates effort.

Disincentive: Something that prevents or discourages action; a deterrent.

Economies of scale: more units of a good or a service can be produced on a larger scale, yet with less average input costs.

Diseconomies of scale: Production is less than in proportion to inputs, resulting in inefficiencies within the firm or industry and rising average costs.

Supply: How much of something is available.

Demand: How much of something people need or want.

Wants: Something someone would like to have that is not absolutely necessary, but it would be a good thing to have.

Needs: Something necessary to survive and a person cannot do without.

Goods: Something that you can use or consume.

Services: Something that someone does for a person.

Explicit costs: Payments that are made for a good or service outside of the enterprise.

Implicit costs: Incurred internally, in which a transaction does not occur outside of the enterprise.

Tangible costs: Objective costs or benefits expressed in dollars or in units.

Intangible costs: Subjective costs or benefits that are difficult to measure because different people place different values on them.

While a one-dimensional measure of work, "paid employment," is used in practically all analyses of the cost of occupational safety and health, it misses the broader and multidimensional sense of work that includes household and subsistence work. Work is the means that people use to provide goods and services for themselves and for others. Within a social context it is an activity that produces something of value for other people.[4] Nonetheless, paid employment is evaluated in this chapter since it is a widely used measure, and it is the object of protection under the Occupational Safety and Health Act (OSHAct; see Appendix). A glossary of economic terms used in this chapter is listed in Table 13-1.

In contrast with the idea of "governance," which is about sharing scarce resources, the idea of economics is about making choices when presented with scarce resources, including a person's time. Economics is the study of the choices people make and the actions they take in order to make the best use of scarce resources in meeting their wants and needs. However, another determinant regarding choices is uncertainty (e.g., risk).[5]

This chapter views economics from the perspective of cost. First, it examines the burden of occupational injuries and diseases upon the economy. Second, a section describes the nexus of occupational safety and health between macroeconomics and microeconomics, a realm named mesoeconomics. Third, the compensation principle and the policy of workers' compensation systems is explained, followed by an analysis by a national commission mandated by the OSHAct of the effectiveness of workers' compensation as a prevention strategy. Next, workers' compensation strategies are described in detail to inform readers who need to manage these systems, including a description of several compensation systems. Another section addresses the process that victims use to seek compensation through tort law measures. The penultimate section discusses an economic analysis of interventions to prevent occupational injury or disease. The final section addresses the issue of workers' compensation fraud.

13.2. THE ECONOMIC BURDEN OF OCCUPATIONAL INJURIES AND DISEASES

The Congress finds that personal injuries and illnesses arising out of work situations impose a substantial burden upon, and are a hindrance to, interstate commerce in terms of lost production, wage loss, medical expenses, and disability compensation payments.

—Occupational Safety and Health Act, Section 2(a)

Understanding the total human and economic burden of occupational injuries and diseases is crucial to setting priorities for the occupational safety and health agenda. The cost of work-related injuries and diseases includes the direct cost of health care and indirect costs such as the inability to work.

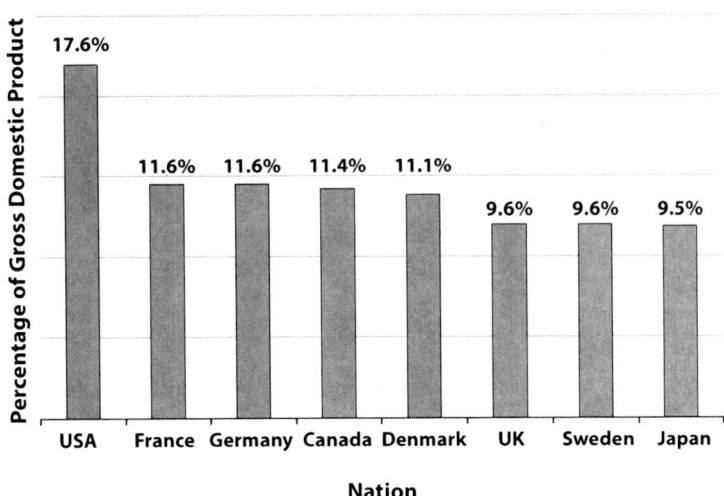

Source: Organisation for Economic Co-operation and Development.[7]

Figure 13-1. Healthcare spending as a percentage of gross domestic product, 2010.

Financing the health care of U.S. citizens is a costly affair. Moreover, the United States is a model of inefficiency when compared with other industrialized nations, as shown in Figure 13-1.[6,7] A health policy book names solutions to the high cost of health care:[8]

- Reducing medical errors and improving care coordination,
- Public reporting of cost and quality data,
- Paying for provider performance on quality and efficiency,
- Development and promulgation of clinical guidelines and quality standards,
- Better management of high-cost patients,
- Improved administrative efficiency,
- Automatic and affordable health insurance for all.

A part of this cost is the burden of occupational injuries and diseases. Workers' compensation is a response to these injuries and diseases, but its cost also includes indirect costs of lost wages resulting from disabilities associated with work-related injuries and diseases (i.e., indemnity). Direct costs are associated with the health care or funeral expense associated with the incident that has resulted in the injury or disease. Another dimension of direct costs is the investment in an intervention to prevent the injury or disease.[9]

Table 13-2. Direct (Medical) and Indirect (Lost Earnings, Fringe Benefits, Home Production) Costs of Occupational Injuries and Diseases, 2007

Injury, Disease, Cost	Injuries		Diseases		Total		
	Fatal	Nonfatal	Fatal	Nonfatal	Fatal	Nonfatal	Total
Number	5,600	8,559,000	33,000	427,000	38,600	8,986,000	9,0246,000
Direct Cost	$0.31	$45.95	$17.66	$3.17	$18.0	$49.0	$67.0
Indirect Cost	$5.68	$139.89	$27.89	$9.09	$34.0	$149.0	$183.0
Total Cost	$5.99	$185.84	$45.55	$12.26	$51.54	$191.1	$250.0

Source: Leigh.[10]
Note: Dollars in billions.

Each year, millions of occupational injuries and illnesses occur in the United States, as shown in Table 13-2. In a 2011 study of occupational injuries and diseases in 2007, investigators reported 5,600 fatalities, 8.6 million nonfatal injuries, and 427,000 and 33,000 disease-related illnesses and deaths, respectively, related to work. The direct and indirect cost of these injuries and diseases totaled $250 billion, which was 2% of the gross domestic product (GDP). Direct costs—medical costs—were estimated to total $67.0 billion, while indirect costs—lost production—were estimated to total $183.0 billion.[10]

When the costs of occupational injuries and diseases are compared with the national costs of other diseases and disabilities, their magnitude is significant.[11] The cost of occupational injuries and diseases compares to 87% of the cost of cardiovascular diseases including stroke and 94% of the cost of cancers,[12–16] and an estimated 5–10% and 6–10% of these disease categories (respectively) are work-related. The cost of occupational injuries and diseases compared with the cost of musculoskeletal disorders—mostly from arthritis—and injuries is 82 and 50%, respectively.[17–19] See Table 13-3 for further detail. For these two conditions, 38–45% and 38% respectively are estimated to be work-related. Occupational injuries and diseases cost relates to 83% of the estimated cost of Alzheimer's disease.[20]

In addition to the direct costs of health care related to occupational injury and disease, there are numerous indirect economic costs. Employers sustain some of these, including additional hiring and training costs, disruption of work processes by workplace incidents, and the effects of workplace injuries or exposures on the productivity of coworkers who may feel at heightened risk. Other indirect costs are borne by the injured workers and their families—for example, loss of income, depletion of savings, and a reduced standard of living;

Table 13-3. Cost of Diseases and Injuries Nationwide Adjusted to 2013 Dollars in Billions

Condition	Cost (billions)			% Work-Related[c]	Source
	Indirect[a]	Direct[b]	Total		
Cardiovascular	$129.0	$213.7	$342.7	5–10	Go et al.[12]
Cancer	$164.0	$134.7	$298.7	6–10	Bradley et al.[15] and Mariotto et al.[16]
Occupational	$202.1	$80.3	$282.4	100	Leigh[10]
Musculoskeletal	$144.6	$199.9	$344.5	38–45[d]	USBJI[17]
Injuries	$434.7	$129.1	$563.8	38[e]	Finkelstein et al.[19]
Alzheimer's	$151.6[f]	$186.0	$337.6	NA	Alzheimer's Association[20]

Note: NA = not applicable; USBJI = U.S. Bone and Joint Initiative.
[a]Adjusted to 2013 by the Consumer Price Index.[13]
[b]Adjusted to 2013 by medical care.[14]
[c]Source: Leigh et al.[11]
[d]Based on a 1999 estimate (explicit costs only).[18]
[e]Based on 2012 occupational total injury cost ($216.6) divided by the total 2012 cost of injuries.
[f]Unpaid care (implicit cost).

increased expenditures for professional counseling and purchased caregiver services in the home; home modifications and equipment related to disability; and deferral or loss of education for family members. Other costs may fall on the community in the form of increased need for social service programs.

While the cost of workers' compensation is enormous and to be described later in this chapter, the cost extends to other health insurance systems as well, including Social Security disability, Medicare, and Medicaid payments. Tort liability is yet another response for underpayment of compensation for work-related injuries and diseases, which includes compensation for pain and suffering. It appears that the cost of work-related illness and disability in both human and economic terms justifies the allocation of substantial resources for the control of workplace hazards.

13.3. MESOECONOMICS

The term mesoeconomics has been applied to the area of economics that lies between and embraces both macro and micro considerations. It draws upon the theories proposed to explain the relationships among aggregate units of the economy and upon principles that suggest the behavior of specific economic units.

—James L. Riggs[21]

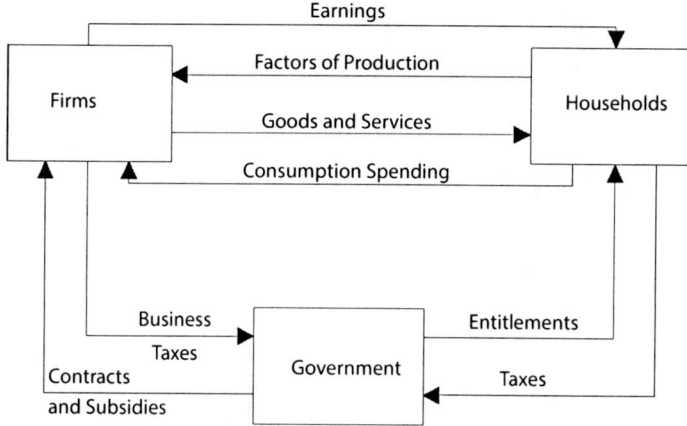

Figure 13-2. Macroeconomic model.

The fundamental classifications of economics are macroeconomics and microeconomics.[22] These classifications have evolved into separate economic explanations of monetary and fiscal policies of governments at the macro level and explanations of the behavior of individual firms and households at the micro level.

Macroeconomics refers to large-scale phenomena typically at the national or global level, which is illustrated as a system in Figure 13-2. The GDP is calculated from the flows—either way—through this system, which is a macroeconomic measure of the nation's production. Macroeconomics deals with inflation, unemployment, and economic growth as well as fiscal and monetary policy.

Microeconomics deals with small economic units including households, business firms, and units of government. Households supply inputs for the economy such as labor and consume goods and services produced by the economy. Business firms produce goods and services using inputs from the households and subsidies from the government. The actions of governmental units are also studied by microeconomists.

While economics addresses free market considerations in the choices and actions that people take, market imperfections argue for the regulation of firms down to the individual level for the protection of workers' safety and health.[23] Regulations bring together macroeconomics and microeconomics into a nexus called mesoeconomics. To better explain this nexus, several concepts are described. These concepts include the meaning of opportunity costs, labor as a factor in production, capitalism, contradictions of capitalism, externalities, and incentives.

13.3.1. Opportunity Costs

An opportunity cost is the cost of forgoing the opportunity of one thing in order to have another thing. When a worker is injured, a cost is incurred at the expense of a foregone opportunity of not getting or doing something else.

When workers are injured, they may forgo time with their families as they heal, and they are likely to delay purchases at home because of lost wages. They may suffer pain with an opportunity cost of time without pain. When workers are killed, they lose their opportunity for life, and their families forgo companionship and acceptable financial support. Workers who die from occupational diseases lose the opportunity for a long life and likely lose the freedom from pain and suffering while sick.

The employer of an injured worker will incur possible increased insurance expenses with funds that could have been used to invest in new equipment. The direct and indirect costs of an occupational injury to an employer, whether explicit (cash outlay) or implicit (noncash cost), means funds or time will be spent related to the injury rather than in a productive activity.

13.3.2. Labor as a Factor of Production

An important concept in the economics of work is the division of labor, which refers to the phenomenon that virtually no one produces all or most of what they consume. The economy divides the production of goods and services through specialization, in which individual workers contribute to a part of the economy while others contribute to other parts. This division of labor makes it possible for society to produce a variety of goods and services for consumption, and the worker's contribution arises because of differences in talents, education, skills, locations, entrepreneurship, and other factors. Specialization also provides for increased production because of focused learning. Moreover, specialization leads to economies of scale in which productivity increases as the size of the enterprise increases, feeding off of labor specialization. The downside of specialization in the extreme is to diminish the work to a repetitive, unthinking process that diminishes the value of work. One occupational safety and health result of the repetitive process in the design of work is the potential for musculoskeletal disorders, the antithesis of good ergonomic design.

13.3.3. Capitalism

Two economic systems have been in conflict for more than a century. One system is the planned economy, which has been shown to be able to muster massive resources to attack mutual problems, such as the response by the United States to World War II by organizing the economy into a war machine or the U.S. response to the Soviets' lead in the space race by placing a man on the moon in a decade. The other system is capitalism, which has been associated with economic growth that has sometimes increased the per capita standard of living at staggering rates.[24] Capitalism's success in the Cold War christened it as the universal approach for riches in the world. A major detractor to capitalism is the issue of occupational safety and health because of the tragic circumstances of death, maiming, and poisoning of workers around the world. A reaction to these tragedies is public advocacy in pluralistic societies by unions and interventions into the workplaces by government. Indeed, one of the early architects of institutions of regulatory bodies, pluralism, and compensation systems was the economist John Commons, in an effort to "save Capitalism by making it good."[25] Capitalism has three characteristics: sociopolitical, institutional, and administrative.[5]

First, the sociopolitical characteristic is capital accumulation. Capital is an active process of reinfusing investment into an economy for financial gain and accumulation. This process differs from wealth accumulation that is passive, whereby the gain is hoarded for personal use or display (i.e., conspicuous consumption) and not dispersed. Karl Marx described capital accumulation as the cycle of money that begets commodities that begets more money (the M-C-M circuit). This dynamic process entails the owners of capital buying objects and labor and combining them to create commodities that are sold at a price higher than their cost. Driven by the possible failure to expand so as to avoid absorption by a more successful capitalist, the firm innovates, mounts aggressive competitive strategies, and harbors self-protection policies (e.g., in competition with worker safety). Apart from rational economics present in small-scale decisions, a suprarational and political drive for capital accumulation motivates a capitalist to rise higher in the social strata above the working class.[5]

Second, the institutional characteristic is market allocation. The market is the organization of production and distribution by unregulated competition. Market allocation relates to Adam Smith's famous reference to the "invisible hand" that depends upon self-interest to maximize personal welfare, notwithstanding that from a broader reading of his writings, he regarded explanations of human action based on self-interest and self-love as absurd. This institution drives the processes of investment (i.e., capital) and of consumption that spread goods and services to the population. Markets are necessary for capital accumulation but are insufficient as an independent system for the public good.[5] In a free job market, institutions are necessary to fully inform workers about the hazards of their jobs, but they must not create externalities, they must be perfectly competitive (e.g., workers can easily quit one job for another), and the level of occupational risk must be socially acceptable.[26] Moreover, in the ideal market, exchange is guaranteed between legally free individuals (e.g., under neither serfdom nor slavery), with no corruption and no extraction of labor by political superiority,[27] notwithstanding that human trafficking remains a problem in the global economy, as addressed in Chapter 12.

Third, the administrative characteristic involves two symbiotic but opposing realms. One realm is the private sector, which encompasses economic activity that differs from noneconomic activity such as custom-based or command-and-control authority. These economic activities include the labor process. The other realm is the public sector, which includes the enactment and enforcement of laws such as the protection of property and contracts, the support of the prerogatives of the dominant class, and the national defense of territory.[5] Indeed, corporations are creatures sanctioned by the public sector. Critical to capitalism is government's protection of private property.[28] The public realm is necessary to preserve capitalism, while the exclusion of the government from the private sector arguably fosters the opportunity for democracies to develop.[5]

13.3.4. Capitalism's Contradictions

Mesoeconomics comes into play through two contradictions of capitalism. One contradiction regards decreased demand generated by capitalism in society, which spawned Keynesian economics. This contradiction risks a "realization crisis" in which a quantitative gap expands between lower consumption because of lower relative wages (and thus reduced buying power) and overproduction because of reduced labor costs, ending in the inability to sell commodities at their value within the macro-market (e.g., the housing bubble). Microlevel capitalists Henry Ford and J.R. Simplot recognized this gap and accommodated their workers with living wages and improved working conditions for a time so as to improve the macroeconomy. In the realization crisis, the unintended consequence of capitalism is the reduction in market demand for commodities because of cost reduction to preserve profits, which is contingent on a lot of power over labor (i.e., exploitation). The result is a reduction in purchasing power by labor within society. Costs continue to be lowered "in every imaginable way" (and potentially investments in safety), thus reducing consumption at the macroeconomy level.[29]

The second contradiction regards the drive to reduce costs. This contradiction is generated by externalizing production costs so as to preserve or increase profits. The consequence is to raise costs to society beyond a firm such as shifting the cost of health care away from the firm, including workers' compensation benefits, by lobbying for changes in the law (e.g., loopholes). This cost shifting may apply to the workforce, the environment, or social services, or it may result in social subsidies for the firm. Nonetheless, this shift of private into social costs results in a market failure to account for all production costs (i.e., the cost of doing business).[29]

13.3.5. Externalities

The problem of cost externalization is central to the economic analysis of occupational safety and health. Externalities are those costs not included within the prices paid in the market. In 2007, the cost of workers' compensation was $78.9 billion, which included the medical cost of injured workers, cash indemnity to provide for part of injured workers' lost wages, and the transaction cost incurred in administering the system, as shown in Figure 13-3. Also shown in the figure is the additional cost outside of the workers' compensation market of occupational injuries and illnesses (i.e., an externality), which was $26.9 billion, paid either by Medicaid or Medicare or by other insurance.[30,31]

The total of $105.8 billion falls short of the estimated annual cost of $250.0 billion shown earlier in Table 13-2,[10] neither of which includes compensation

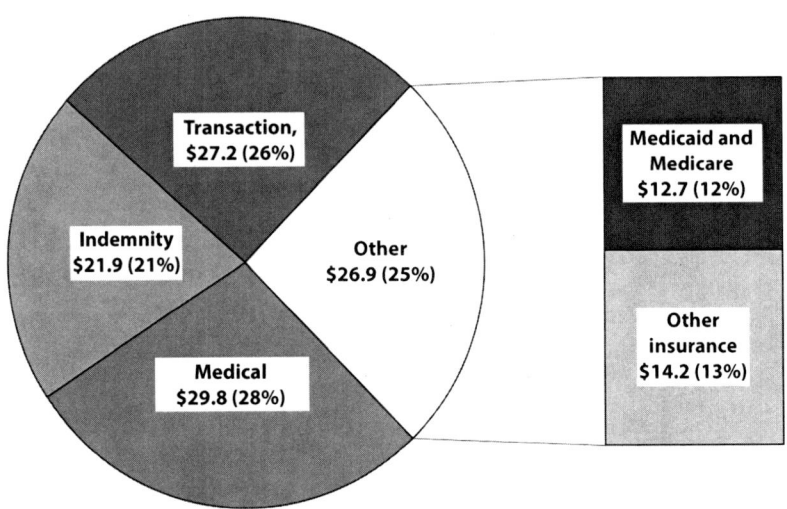

Source: Sengupta et al.;[30] Leigh et al.[32]
Note: Figure is in billions of dollars.
Figure 13-3. The social cost of work-related injury compensation.

for pain and suffering. Not counting the transaction costs, workers' compensation pays less than 25% of the shortfall. The reasons are many:[10]

- Workers' compensation misses between 23 and 53% of medically attended nonfatal injuries.
- It misses at least 91% of occupational disease deaths.
- It does not cover 40% of occupational injuries and diseases because of statutory exclusions (e.g., agriculture, small businesses) and exclusions of self-employed workers.
- The system underestimates indirect costs, including lost wages, fringe benefits, and home production.
- It misses delayed onsets of disabilities (or suicides) that are a consequence of occupational injuries or exposures.

Externalities can be positive or negative and are transactions that occur outside of the market system. Externalities occur when the buying or selling of goods and their consequences affects third parties who were not part of the original transaction. In the case of negative externalities (e.g., the cost is incurred by the taxpayer for a work injury rather than being borne by the employer), regulation is a way to bring control over the external consequence. An example of a negative externality is a machine design that results in injuries of self-employed workers who have no workers' compensation. The workers and their families incur the cost of the resulting injuries from a defective design, which were not part of the free market transaction. An example of a positive externality is the creation of a safety procedure at a cost by one firm that is adopted by many other firms that do not share in that cost.

Few studies address which groups in the economy pay for occupational injury and illness when workers' compensation does not. However, a 2011 study based on 2007 data estimated total workers' compensation benefits to be $51.7 billion, with $29.8 billion for medical benefits and $21.9 billion for indemnity benefits. For medical costs not covered by workers' compensation, other (nonworkers' compensation) insurance covered $14.22 billion; Medicare covered $7.16 billion, and Medicaid covered $5.47 billion. This distribution of cost is shown in Figure 13-3, in which 66% of the cash outlay is covered by workers' compensation and the remaining cost is externalized. This cost is for compensation and does not include the "in-kind" implicit cost borne by families and social services beyond the compensation systems.[30]

Another study investigated the interaction between workers' compensation and the Social Security Disability Insurance (DI) systems. The investigators found that 3 and 7% of all DI claims were awarded after five and 10 years of a precipitating workplace injury, respectively. The source of the DI funds is the federal Social Security tax paid into the federal Disability Trust Fund.[32]

This DI program supplements workers' compensation when it pays benefits for disabled workers younger than 65 for whom a disability is expected to extend beyond 12 months or result in death. A worker is eligible after the minimum number of quarters of employment covered by Social Security. The benefits paid are based upon wages and allowances for a spouse and children. The combination of Social Security disability and workers' compensation benefits cannot exceed 80% of the average current earnings prior to the disability.[32] Social Security disability benefits are offset by the amount of workers' compensation benefits.

In 2010, 70,000 workers nationwide were awarded DI benefits 10 years after an injury at an average award of $13,500 each, totaling $945 million, but with offsets because of continued workers' compensation payments, the total was $889 million. This total was for new awardees and did not include the continuing award for qualified disabilities before or after the 10-year period, nor did it count the cost burden into the future for the first-year awards. With an estimated duration of awards over 13.5 years, the burden upon the DI system in 2010 was $12 billion for the accumulated cohorts from previous years. This analysis only counted the cohorts with a 10-year delay of disability onset and not cohorts with work-related disabilities before or after the 10-year waiting period.[33]

The concept of moral hazard is associated with the concept of externalities. Moral hazard is the potential of parties who are insulated from risk behaving differently from the way they would if they were fully exposed to the risk. As an example, if an employer is not at financial risk of compensating an employee for a latent disease resulting from employment, the employer may ignore controlling the exposure to the hazard causing the disease. The insulation from risk may be because of ignorance of the hazard by both the employer and the worker.

13.3.6. Incentives

Incentives have been a focus of renewed interest among policy makers because they are more compatible with economic efficiency objectives. Perhaps the most promising approaches today are those that link protective measures and incentives. Various instruments can be designed to internalize the economic costs of hazardous working conditions.

In the early years of the 19th century, enlightened industrialists recognized that deaths and injuries could be prevented. They combined with others to establish the National Safety Council in 1913. Through the work of this organization many technological interventions were identified and used to prevent pernicious and persistent injuries, especially in American factories. While these voluntary interventions were encouraged, employers fought any changes in the employer-employee relationship (i.e., unions).[34]

From an economic standpoint, expenditures to improve working conditions are investments; they incur an initial cost in order to produce a flow of future benefits. Experience demonstrates that the value of these investments is usually greater than initially thought, due not only to the intangible and long-run benefits of worker health and well-being, but also to the ability of enterprises to innovate in ways that enhance product quality, reduce waste, and improve working conditions simultaneously. At an economy-wide level, this is an essential component of the development process. Nevertheless, enterprises that would benefit from these investments may still fail to make them, due to the potential for competitive disadvantage. In the end, while investments in better working conditions should not be made only on economic grounds, decision makers are increasingly interested in measuring their net economic costs—the economic costs of preventive activities minus the economic costs avoided by prevention.

An in-depth retrospective on the cost and feasibility of the Occupational Safety and Health Administration's (OSHA) standards conducted by the Office of Technology Assessment (OTA) in 1995 found that OSHA correctly judged the technological feasibility for seven of eight of the standards evaluated and correctly judged the economic feasibility for six of the eight. In fact, for a number of the standards, the OTA determined that OSHA had significantly overestimated actual compliance costs, usually because employers developed new technologies or found substitutes that cost much less than predicted control measures (an example of technology forcing incentives). The OTA found that the actual costs of control were far lower than those predicted by industry, which usually were based on unrealistic assumptions, inflated estimates, and failures to take into account process improvements and other efficiencies gained through experience, not to mention the benefits of reduced injuries and illnesses.[35]

The higher costs of providing workers' compensation benefits in risky occupations are an incentive that should lead employers to improve safety in order to lower their insurance costs. The compensation for an injury must be high enough to provide an incentive for the employer to take corrective action and avoid future injury costs.[36]

13.4. THE COMPENSATION PRINCIPLE

Employers and entrepreneurs who enjoy the economic benefits of businesses should bear the cost of the injuries and deaths that are incident to the manufacture, preparation, and distribution of goods and services.

—J.W. Little, T.A. Eaton, G.R. Smith[36]

The compensation principle applies to business payments for the repairs and losses for which its activities result in the destruction of equipment or other property, regardless of fault. The same principle applies to the compensation of work-related injuries or diseases through a system of workers' compensation insurance as a cost of doing business. In the theory, the cost borne by the business is added to the cost of the product or service produced uniformly across competitors so that one business entity garners no competitive advantage over another enterprise. However, if one business pays a lower compensation than another, then the idea of compensation uniformity is lost.[36]

Two conditions can result in the lack of uniformity. One example is the statute of one state requiring less compensation or coverage than another, and the other example is the systemic denial of benefits for particular conditions as a condition of either the state statute or the policy of the insurer. When a state court in New York of a century ago found a compensation system unconstitutional as a "deprivation of property without due process of law," other states placed limits on coverage to assuage lobbying groups. These limits included exclusions of coverage, mandatory waiting periods, maximum indemnity benefits, and benefits proportional to earnings and limits on a maximum payment.[36]

The compensation movement for work-related injuries or illnesses emerged first in Germany in 1884, and was limited to the hazardous industries of mining, manufacturing, and transportation. Great Britain followed in 1897, with compensation coverage of particularly hazardous industries, leading to coverage of all employment in 1906. By 1911, workers' compensation in Germany covered all forms of employment. In 1908, workers' compensation was present in nearly all developed countries with the exception of the United States, where initial attempts by states were declared unconstitutional in the courts.[36]

In 1911, Wisconsin became the first state to enact a workers' compensation system that was not declared unconstitutional. In that same year, Washington State enacted a workers' compensation system in which the state was the monopoly provider. Alarmed by the Washington approach, private insurance companies lobbied in other states against monopoly systems. The lobbying efforts led to many states using a market-driven approach to insurance that was unique among all nations. Initially, Canada followed the Washington model, but starting in 1914, the provinces started incorporating market-driven provisions like those in the United States.[37] As of 2013, six states have monopoly systems: West Virginia, Ohio, Nevada, Washington, North Dakota, and Wyoming.

13.4.1. The Compromise

To address the problem of workers and their families bearing the cost of the injuries, the great workers' compensation compromise was struck between workers and employers. State legislators enacted statutes that were constituted on four doctrines:[34]

1. The remedy was exclusive.
2. Benefits were paid to the injured worker regardless of fault.
3. Employers could insure against the risk of workplace injuries.
4. Employers retained control of internal decision making.

Today, the workers' compensation systems maintain the same basic structure as originally enacted.[34] Workers' compensation statutes were considered revolutionary at the time of their passage because they ignored the element of blame.[33]

All 50 states have workers' compensation laws, as does the District of Columbia, American Samoa, Guam, Puerto Rico, and the U.S. Virgin Islands. Each Canadian province or territory has also enacted workers' compensation laws. Every state except Texas and Oklahoma require employers to purchase workers' compensation insurance, which covers an injured employee's medical expenses and lost wages. There are different state rules regarding how much coverage a firm must buy, what percentage of an injured employee's wages a firm must pay if the employee is unable to work, and how long a firm must cover an injured employee. Some policies include liability insurance that protects employers against lawsuits related to a workplace death or injury.[33]

The laws cover virtually all industrial employment. Some cover all private and public employment, while others exempt employers with a small number of employees. Most laws exclude farm labor, domestic servants, and casual employees. However, most of these laws provide for voluntary coverage for these excluded workers. Conversely, many states provide for coverage of civil defense and voluntary firefighters who are injured in the line of duty. Confusion arises at times when a worker's occupation takes him or her outside of a jurisdiction such as across a state line. Reconciliation of this confusion depends upon the provisions in the statute and the circumstances of the injury.[33]

Legislators established two different approaches for state workers' compensation insurance funds to provide a stable source of insurance coverage. They aimed to protect employers from underwriting uncertainties by making it possible to have continuing availability of coverage. Compensation laws are either compulsory or elective,[33] and either universal or variable services are provided by workers' compensation systems,[38] which are described in Table 13-4.

Table 13-4. Types of State Workers' Compensation Insurance Funds

Approach	State funds: Designed to be nonprofit to keep premiums at the lowest possible cost for employers and were established solely to provide one type of insurance: workers' compensation. State funds can operate at an exclusive or competitive level. States with exclusive funds require all employers to procure their workers' compensation insurance from the state fund or, in some jurisdictions, to self-insure. Exclusive state funds develop their own rates and experience by using the services of in-house actuaries or actuarial firms. Administrative costs are low because they do not issue renewal policies and have no marketing programs.	Competitive funds: A ready market to employers for this insurance. Depending on the state, employers may insure with the state fund or a private carrier, or be self-insured. Competitive state funds offer an available market that is not dependent on the size of the employer's premium, nature of business, or loss history. Most competitive funds pay dividends to policyholders. Overhead expense ratios of both exclusive and competitive funds are consistently lower than expense factors for private carriers.
Type of Law	Compulsory law: Requires that each employer under its scope accept its legal provisions and provide benefits as established by statute.	Elective law: The employer can elect to accept or reject coverage, but if it rejects coverage, it loses the three common law defenses (the fellow-servant, assumption of risk, and contributory negligence). In effect, the elective law is, thus, compulsory.
Type of Service	Universal system: Provides medical services for injured workers and income replacement for either temporary or permanent disability. This system also provides survivor benefits in the event of an occupational fatality.	Variable system: Variable and involves rehabilitation and retraining.
Trade-offs	Employer: No fault, exclusive remedy (cannot be sued for cost of injury), insurance available.	Employee: No fault, immediate and complete medical coverage, common law defenses forfeited.

There are also a wide variety of state laws regarding what types of employees qualify for workers' compensation benefits. Some states exclude contractors and consultants, volunteer workers, farm workers, domestic servants, and certain other groups. States also enforce different rules about whether part-time employees qualify for benefits. In addition, insurance sales methods vary from state to state. A few states require employers to purchase insurance through a single state agency, while others allow private insurers to offer workers' compensation policies.[33]

13.4.2. Administration

Workers' compensation laws were designed for prompt and effective disposition of injury cases. Even though the workers' compensation system was thought to be self-administering within the marketplace, the complexity of the system has resulted in the states taking a role in its administration. The state depends upon the courts, a special commission or board, or a combination of both. Insurance is provided by either a private provider, the state, or both. Statutes also provide for an appeal procedure.[33]

When an injury occurs, the worker files a claim typically by informing the supervisor or the employer in serious situations. The employer is required to immediately file a workers' compensation claim with the insurance carrier, which then notifies the appropriate state agency. Although it varies by state, a state agency typically reviews cases to determine whether a claim is valid and what benefits the injured worker should receive. The claim can be accepted, leading to compensation for direct costs and a portion of indirect costs. However, the insurer may deny the claim, such as for low back pain or psychological stress. The worker may abandon the claim or seek a lawyer to advance the claim. The lawyer may choose to take or decline the case. If the lawyer takes the case, the lawyer bargains with the insurer's lawyer for a settlement. Failing a settlement, the case is argued before an administrative law judge employed by the state who rules for either the worker or the insurer (and employer).[39] While state statutes include settlement conditions and regulate attorney fees, pay for attorneys engaged by the victim to defend claims is most often taken out of the benefits paid to the victim.[34]

Second injury funds have been established in some states to encourage employers to hire physically disabled people who have been previously injured, whether work-related or not. Following a claim paid by a workers' compensation insurer, employers can request reimbursement from the secondary fund if the compensation includes care for the initial injury. In the absence of such a fund, the employers are usually liable for the total injury, which may lead to not hiring the disabled person.

State governments, along with private insurers, also investigate possible insurance fraud and keep detailed statistics on workplace injuries and compensation claims. Fraud will be discussed in detail in Section 13.10. Statutes include requirements for the employers to report the injury and associated penalties if they fail to make the report.[33]

13.4.3. Coverage

Workers' compensation benefits provide coverage for medical expenses as well as reimbursement for lost wages when employees are injured on the job. A principle of the compensation movement is that coverage of the law is virtually universal, although no state law covers all forms of employment. Another principle is to provide compensation for all work-related injuries and diseases. To distinguish the work-related injuries and diseases from other health problems, statutory definitions and tests have been adopted in each state. Typically, benefits are limited to "personal injury caused by accidents arising out of and in the course of employment." Coverage also varies based upon interpretations of the laws. Occupational diseases can elude statutory definition because of the variety of exposures, risk factors, and disease manifestations. Thus, states typically cover all occupational diseases, which are then left for administrative interpretations.[33]

Coverage by workers' compensation systems vary. The systems usually cover employees of firms with more than a few employees. Special compensation systems—national in scope—cover maritime workers, railroad workers, and federal employees. Several other categories of workers are typically not covered by the national system and include agricultural workers, self-employed workers, business owners, domestic workers, and volunteers.[34]

Most laws require employers to purchase insurance in which there are penalties for failure to insure. The law may specify conditions under which self-insurance is permitted. Large companies may be the only enterprises that can self-insure, and they prefer this choice to avoid the administrative costs associated with insurance policies, especially when business operations cross many state jurisdictions. Self-insurance is allowed in 47 states and is most effective when the risk can be spread across a large number of employees.[34]

13.4.4. Occupational Diseases and Latent Effects

Initial laws did not address occupational diseases, but now they all cover these diseases. These laws cover all diseases that arise out of and in the course of employment. Compensation is typically the same as that for injury.[33] However, compensation under most of these laws does not cover ordinary diseases of life or those that are not peculiar to or characteristic of the worker's occupation. Moreover, chronic diseases may not become manifest until years after a workplace exposure. Figure 13-4 shows this lag of the manifestation of a disease

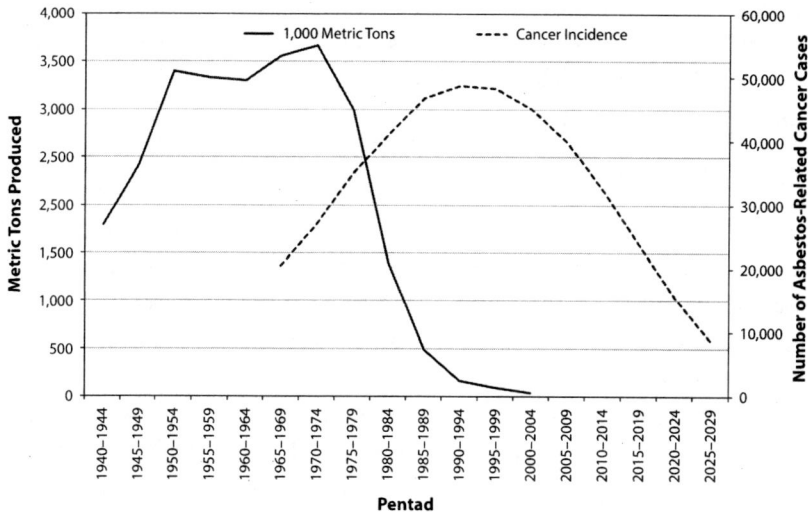

Source: Virta;[40] Carroll et al.[41]

Figure 13-4. The lag of asbestos-related cancers years after potential exposure to friable asbestos fibers at work.

35 years after the potential exposure.[40,41] Special restrictions may relate to latent diseases resulting from exposure to coal mine dust, other dust, asbestos, silica, or radiation. Some states have provided coverage for heart attacks or respiratory conditions for police officers and firefighters.[33]

Compensation for occupational injury is substantially higher than for occupational disease. A government report published in 1980 addressed this discrepancy. Compared with occupational injury claims, occupational disease claims are not reported as quickly and take longer to be established in the workers' compensation system. Workers with occupational diseases wait twice as long from the "date of injury" for their first income replacement benefits to begin than do those with occupational injuries. Claims resulting from occupational disease are open longer than occupational injury claims, suggesting that injured workers with occupational diseases require medical treatment and/or income replacement benefits for longer periods of time than those who have occupational injuries. Occupational disease claims are more likely to be contested on the grounds of compensability compared with occupational injury claims.[42]

Occupational diseases are underreported and underrepresented in claims. The latency period diminishes claims since an ailment often arises during retirement and is difficult to attribute to a responsible employer. The disease may also be multifactorial, and compensation may depend upon an "objective finding." Moreover, information may be lacking because of missing data, incomplete differential diagnosis, inadequate exposure history, and irrelevant data.[38]

Nearly 80% of occupational disease claims can be categorized into four general groups: disorders resulting from repetitive trauma, skin disorders, toxic effects of chemicals, and respiratory disorders. Repetitive trauma disorders account for more than 40% of all occupational disease claims. The most severe cases of occupational disease, as measured by impairment rating, are vascular conditions, diseases of the lung, mental disorders, and conditions of the nervous system.[38]

Special revisions to state workers' compensation systems have been provided regarding noise-induced hearing loss since this disability can be caused by both occupational and nonoccupational exposures. Thresholds for compensation may be established by statute, as may be deductions for age-related prebycusis.[33]

13.4.5. Benefits

The benefits paid to injured employees are designed to cover most of their economic loss, including both loss of earnings and extra expenses associated with the injury. Benefits include cash indemnity for loss of income or earning capacity, medical benefits without dollar or time limits, and rehabilitation in the case of severe disabilities. Four disability classifications are used in determining cash benefits: temporary total, permanent total, temporary partial, and permanent partial as shown in Table 13-5.[33] There are three requirements to qualify for workers' compensation:

1. Personal injury or disease,
2. Disability (see Table 13-5),
3. Work-relatedness (causation).

Table 13-5. Four Classifications of Disability for Injured Workers Under Workers' Compensation Systems

	Temporary	Permanent
Total	temporary-total	permanent-total
Partial	temporary-partial	permanent-partial

Most cases involve temporary total disability in which the employee is totally disabled but is expected to recover and return to employment. A formula computed based upon a percentage of weekly wages is used for determining cash benefits, and limitations are placed on the minimum and maximum level (e.g., no more than two-thirds of the average wage in the state). In addition, some states limit the time for payment and the amount of award for the disability. Permanent total disability indicates that the employee is totally and permanently unable to perform gainful employment, which is the most costly condition for compensation and is more than 12 times the cost of a fatal injury, as shown in Figure 13-5. For permanent total disability, most states provide for payments through the employee's lifetime but with a cap on indemnities as allowed in the statute.[10,33]

There are three approaches for rating permanent disability. First is the impairment model, which is based upon schedules and guidelines such as the American Medical Association's (AMA) *Guides to the Evaluation of Permanent Impairment*.[43] Second is a wage-loss formula that calculates actual loss of wages due to injury. Third is the loss of earnings capacity in the loss of future wages based on an actuarial model.[38]

The AMA's *Guides* is a tool that often gives a range yet achieves some consistency. The evaluation is based upon expert consensus and validity in terms of relative impairment within functional systems. The downsides of the *Guides*

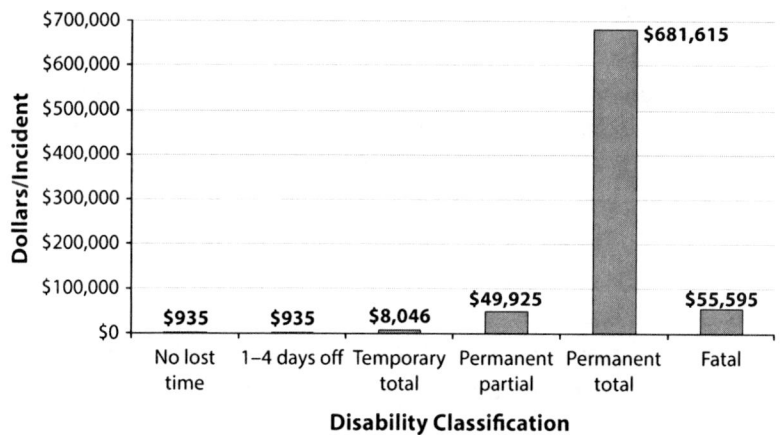

Source: Leigh.[10]

Figure 13-5. Estimated costs per incident for different classes of disability, 2007.

are that it includes no objective validation, is often used indiscriminately as a formula for disability, and avoids many important types of disability. These disabilities include chronic pain; mental changes such as depression; reversible conditions such as airway reactivity and dermatitis; and stress-related disorders including irritable colon. The *Guides* have become a self-perpetuating industry involving complicated revisions, guides to the *Guides,* training programs, and a certification scheme.[38]

Medical benefits are normally unlimited and are specified in a statute or by administrative discretion. Regarding the choice of a physician, about half of the states give the decision of the physician to the employer, and the other half provides this choice to the employee. In some states physicians must be chosen from an approved list provided by the state. Although compensation for medical and hospital care is provided immediately, statutes likely provide a waiting period before income benefits are paid.[33] The laws provide for payment of temporary disability benefits after a waiting period of three to seven days.[44]

Who picks a physician is a factor, and thus the right of choice of physician becomes an issue. In half of the states and Washington, DC, workers can choose the physician—usually the family physician. In the other half of the states, the employer or insurer can select the physician from a list of approved physicians. This approach gave rise to preferred provider organizations and other managed care models. In such a system, control over medical records is lost by the worker.[38]

Rehabilitation is considered a part of medical treatment, but it may take more time and include vocational rehabilitation and retraining. Rehabilitation is provided for in all states even though it is not specified in some statutes. The Federal Vocational Rehabilitation Act funds aid to all states for the vocational rehabilitation of industrially disabled employees.[33]

In the case of a fatality, benefits pay for a burial and provide a proportion of the worker's former weekly wages to the spouse and children. The economic loss associated with death is often less than that related to a permanent total disability. Benefits are typically paid to the surviving spouse until (and if) they remarry and to children until they reach a specified age. Some states place limits on these awards.[33]

Scheduled injuries are listed in the statute by specific body parts in which the loss results in a presumed loss in wages (e.g., loss of a leg or the loss of a finger). As an example, Georgia had a scheduled payment of $96,626 for the loss of an arm at the shoulder in 2004, whereas in Illinois and Puerto Rico, the scheduled payments for the same injury were $305,919 and $12,000, respectively. The statutes limit the number of weeks that these payments are made, and the length of this limitation depends upon the severity of the injury.[33]

13.5. THE NATIONAL COMMISSION ON STATE WORKMEN'S COMPENSATION LAWS

[T]hat the threat of or, if necessary, the enactment of Federal mandates will remove from each State the main barrier of effective workmen's compensation reform: the fear that compensation costs may drive employers to move away to markets where protection for disabled workers is inadequate but less expensive.

—Report of the National Commission on State Workmen's Compensation Laws[45]

The OSHAct states that nothing in the act will affect any workers' compensation law (§ 4(b)(4)). Nonetheless, § 27 of the OSHAct established the National Commission on State Workmen's Compensation Laws in 1972 to investigate inadequacies in the state systems and whether these systems should be federalized.

The commission's purpose was to issue a report based on its findings, the first time a federal-level agency examined individual workers' compensation laws. Upon its establishment in 1972, the commission stated that a workers' compensation system should: (1) provide broad coverage of employees and work-related injuries and diseases, (2) provide substantial protection against interruption of income, (3) provide sufficient medical care and rehabilitation services, (4) encourage workplace safety, and (5) deliver benefits in an efficient and effective manner.[36]

President Richard Nixon appointed the members of the commission. During summer 1972, the commission issued two publications: *Supplemental Studies of National Commission on Workmen's Compensation Laws* and *Compendium on Workmen's Compensation Laws*. In addition, the commission submitted the *Report of the National Commission on Workmen's Compensation* to the President and Congress, as specified in the OSHAct. As a result, a number of states reexamined their workers' compensation laws and made revisions and improvements.[46]

The commission concluded that state laws were not achieving their potential. It made 84 recommendations, 19 considered essential, for improving the system, although the focus was on coverage and benefits and not on prevention.

The commission recommended maintaining the states' systems with an expansion of benefits and eligibility and improvement of the administrative design of the systems. The 19 essential recommendations did little more than acknowledge improving workplace safety. The commission also recommended that if, by 1975, the states failed to adopt the recommendations, then federal legislation should be adopted to ensure compliance.[33] Four of the 19 essential recommendations are listed below:

- Coverage by workmen's compensation laws [should] be compulsory.
- All states [should] provide full coverage for work-related diseases.
- Temporary total disability benefits [should] be at least 66.66% of the worker's gross weekly wage.
- Right to medical and physical rehabilitation benefits does not terminate by the passage of time.

In January 1976, members of the Interagency Workers' Compensation Task Force, composed of federal government departments and agencies (including the Departments of Labor (DoL); Health, Education, and Welfare; Commerce; and Housing and Urban Development as well as the Office of Management and Budget), reported on needs to reform the state-based systems. Their report warned that without reform the system would become more expensive, less equitable, and less effective.[34]

Consistent with the commission's recommendations, 12 states have mandatory coverage for all employees: Alaska, Washington, Oregon, Idaho, Montana, California, Arizona, Kansas, Ohio, New Hampshire, Massachusetts, and Connecticut. Contrary to the commission's recommendations, Texas has no mandatory coverage for workers' compensation, and the remaining states have exemptions for small employers or agricultural workers or both.[30]

Another troubling aspect of the state systems is the inequity in the costs to employers between the states. The average manual rate, which is the cost to the employer per $100 of payroll, varied widely from a low in Texas of $0.66 to more than four times higher in Montana at $2.73 in 2010, as shown in Figure 13-6. The average manual rate across all industries nationwide was $1.19 in that year.[30] The states with a lower rate have a competitive advantage in drawing employers

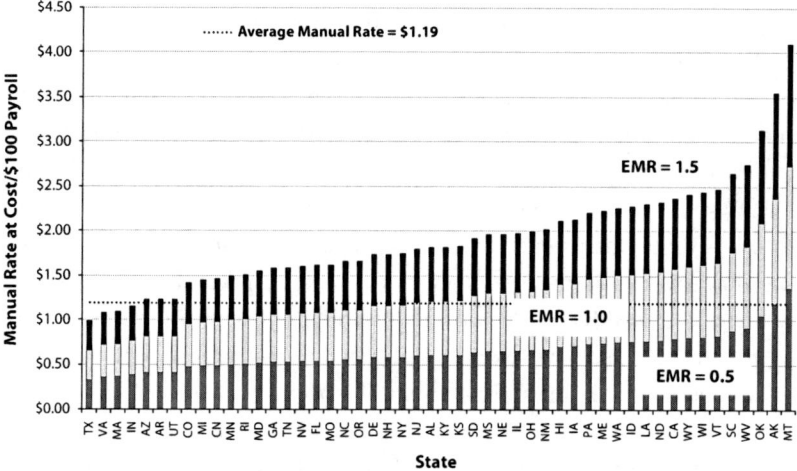

Figure 13-6. The cost to employers of workers' compensation by state per $100 of payroll, and the potential effect of the experience modification rating (EMR) on this cost, 2010.

into their states; moreover, this practice violates the idea of compensation uniformity discussed earlier under the compensation principle.

13.6. COMPENSATION STRATEGIES

Consider the ends which the several rules seek to accomplish, the reasons why those ends are desired, what is given up to gain them, and whether they are worth the price.

—Oliver Wendell Holmes[47]

Compensation laws are designed as an incentive to reduce the frequency and severity of occupational injuries in two ways. First, insurers or government programs such as casualty insurance carriers, employers, state funds, and safety agencies provide technical assistance that includes safety engineering. Second, incentives through the insurance premium structure are designed to stimulate preventive actions, so employers can reduce their premiums by improving their safety record.[33]

13.6.1. Manual Rate

In establishing rates for workers' compensation, states calculate their average premium rate and class rates for different industrial groups typically averaged over the three previous years. This rate—expressed as a premium at a cost per $100 of payroll—is known as the manual rate, which can vary a lot between industries. Workers' compensation premiums depend upon the nature of the business, the jobs performed, and the number of hours that employees work.

Each type of occupation is assigned a risk classification. Risk is determined by two factors: the frequency of on-the-job injury and the severity of injury. Severity is measured by both medical payments and indemnity benefits.[36] Riskier work is assigned a higher premium. As an example, an employer may pay 48¢ in premiums for every $100 in payroll that goes to a clerk in a retail store compared with a truck driver's premiums that may cost $9 per $100 of payroll. To arrive at a base rate for workers' compensation insurance, each classification is translated into a dollar amount, which is then multiplied by a percentage per $100 of the total payroll for that employee. For example, the office clerk classification in California is roughly $1.25 per $100. So if that employee is paid $500 per week, the workers' compensation insurance premium for that employee costs roughly $6.25 per week. Each state uses this basic process to calculate base rates.[36]

Nonetheless, there are ways to control costs, such as through workers' compensation insurance boards in each state. In the state of Washington, premiums are paid against the hours of work rather than the payroll, which provides a measure to evaluate exposure regarding injuries or illnesses experienced based on hours rather than wages. Conversely, insurance companies have an incentive to index premiums to wages so that when wages increase, so do the premiums.

13.6.2. Experience Modification

Experience rating is based upon an employer's workers' compensation claims record for the previous three years in comparison to its industrial classification. From this comparison, an insurance company calculates an experience modification rate (or experience factor). Employers with low claims have a factor of less than 1.0 and pay less, whereas employers with high claims have a rate above 1.0 and pay more. A merit rating corrects for inequities between occupations by modifying the manual rate (the inherent risk of injury associated with an occupation), provides for competition between insurance companies, and has the potential to stimulate injury prevention.[34] The formula for a workers' compensation insurance premium (WCIP) is shown below:

WCIP = Experience Modification Rating × Manual Rate × Payroll Units

The influence of the experience modification rating (EMR) is shown in Figure 13-6. The norm for the EMR is 1.0 (the average for the industry), but a rating of 0.5, based on a poor safety record, or 1.5, based on a good safety record, can influence the cost of WCIP dramatically. Insurance companies adjust the EMR based upon past claims and thus anticipate future risk. Moreover, the rating methodology clouds the incentive to reduce hazards:

1. The premium is calculated based upon the product of total payroll and the employer's calculated rate. Thus, low-wage firms pay less than high-wage firms, which can encourage the hiring of less skilled, low-wage workers, which may lead to more injuries.
2. The three-year averaging technique dampens immediate results from safety upgrades; the accompanying short-run perceptions of these improvements do not affect the bottom line.
3. The rating schemes measure trivial incidents in combination with severe incidents. The schemes are based upon injury frequency rather than severity, thus two minor injuries count for more than one fatality.

Employer ignorance of the EMR system is an impediment to its use as an incentive to reduce costs by reducing injuries. This ignorance feeds the lack of emphasis on primary prevention of injuries.[34]

Furthermore, a firm does not become fully experience rated until it employs 1,000 or more workers. The only way for small employers to reduce their rate is if the whole industry experiences an injury reduction. Small employers are required to pay the manual rate with no experience rating adjustment since they do not have enough employees to provide statistical validity by the insurance actuaries. Self-insurance is the purest form for experience rating, in which payment reflects the actual costs.[34]

13.6.3. Insurance Pools

Many states operate insurance pools for firms that cannot afford standard coverage, such as those with poor safety records or a long history of workers' compensation claims. Some states allow certain types of firms to self-insure if they have the financial resources to cover potential claims.[33] In addition, 24 states have high-risk insurance pools at increased insurance premiums for employers.[38] These pools are EMR based on the classification of the pool, either as high hazard or a collection of small employers within an industry, and thus do not internalize costs of claims to individual employers.

13.6.4. Compensation Paradox

Evidence indicates that the focus has been on reducing costs without a focus on reducing injuries and illnesses. A paradox in the workers' compensation system is that while the costs of workers' compensation have increased rapidly, the frequency of lost-time injuries has not decreased.[34]

Of the four categories of beneficiaries, temporary total disability represents about three-fourths of the number of claims, but the highest cost category is permanent disability. This high cost is not limited to lost time of the victim, but a substantial amount goes to healthcare providers and lawyers. In recent years, inflation of the medical costs in workers' compensation has exceeded the general increase in medical costs nationwide.[34]

In addition, occupational diseases have been underreported. Diseases comprise ailments that are not the result of a single traumatic event and include cumulative trauma disorders. The majority of reported injuries and illnesses include maladies that have been around for some time and for which preventive interventions are recognized (e.g., strains and sprains, struck by objects, falls, machinery-related injuries). Three issues contribute to the paradox of cost escalation and the persistence of occupational injuries and illnesses.[34]

1. Cost escalation relates to the persistence of occupational hazards, broader coverage of the compensation system, worker behavior, changes in demographics and economic sectors, and the validity of data, which is affected by changes in reporting requirements.
2. Employers and insurers focus on cost-cutting strategies in contrast to preventing occupational injuries and diseases. This focus involves insurance market changes and cost containment attempts (e.g., loss control and political action).
3. If employers take work-related injuries and illnesses seriously, they can reduce their incidence whether cost control is a motivator or not. This

issue was addressed by a 1993 study in California with the following conclusions:[34]

- Employers can reduce the severity and rate of injuries by as much as 40%.
- Employees can often identify cost-effective interventions.
- Large claims are predominantly caused by commonplace injuries.
- Many effective primary prevention actions are inexpensive.
- Many improvements in safety and health can also improve productivity.
- Proven interventions can prevent the most significant injuries, which are caused by known hazards.

The traditional conflict in the compensation dialogue has been between employers and employees, but the dialogue has moved to a contest between insurers and trial lawyers as depicted in Figure 13-7. In political negotiations about the high and rising cost of workers' compensation, employers wish to reduce cost while workers wish to receive adequate compensation or, more important, suffer no injury. Meanwhile, insurance companies wish to charge profitable rates and avoid costly claims as trial attorneys aim to represent the worker or other parties with a wish to win benefits in contested cases.

These strategies move beyond the idea that costs alone will reduce injuries and illnesses. In the late 1980s and early 1990s, Oregon and Texas were successful in reducing employers' premium costs. Oregon's success was over a longer period of time. Incidence rates there dropped 21% from 1989 to 1991, and fatality rates dropped from 7.1 to 4.9 deaths per 100,000 workers from 1987 to 1992. Disabling injuries dropped by 33%. These reductions followed substantial

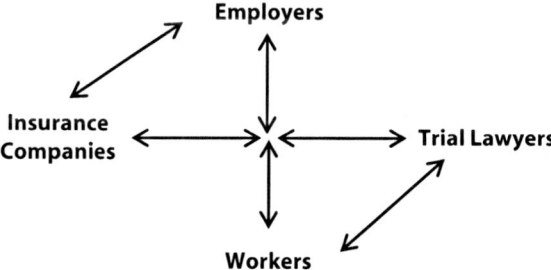

Figure 13-7. The interaction of interested parties that influence workers' compensation statutes.

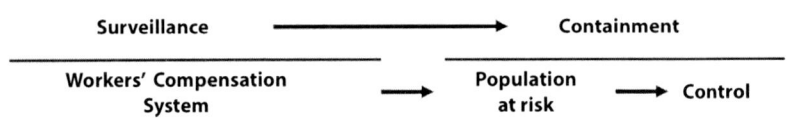

Figure 13-8. The use of the workers' compensation system as a surveillance tool in the surveillance-containment model.

strengthening of the state OSHA office, with an increase in employees there from 90 to 243. Moreover, the state OSHA staff shifted their approach from posters to ergonomics and engineering controls. Penalty assessment rose from $1 million in 1987 to $3.0 million in 1992. As a result, employers increased their requests for voluntary consultations through an approach of workers' compensation as a prevention institution by providing technical assistance to employers. In addition, safety committees became part of the employer-employee fabric at workplaces, increasing nearly eightfold over the period.[34]

Oregon follows the surveillance-containment model discussed in Chapter 2. Workers' compensation data provide for the surveillance arm of the model by identifying and reporting the injury or illness. These data feed the containment arm of the model by allowing the state plan agency to define the population at highest risk and intervene with OSHA inspections. These inspections focus on the abatement of hazards. The application of this model is depicted in Figure 13-8. This model was also followed by OSHA's Maine 200 Pilot Program, which was described in Chapter 7.

Conversely, cost reductions are also attributable to more stringent rules for compensation for chronic diseases; where a problem emerges from a combination of work and nonwork exposure, the compensation is denied. On top of this, the Oregon state fund that was responsible for about one-third of the state's employees reduced the claims paid through administrative rules from 153,000 in 1988 to 108,000 in 1992. The interlocking effect of the enforcement actions and the policies for the reduction of compensable claims is difficult to sort out; nonetheless, the injury rate reduction occurred after the increased enforcement actions and before the change in claims policies.[34]

13.6.5. The Inspection Incentive

An additional strategy consistent with the surveillance-containment model is increased OSHA inspections that were found in a 2012 study to reduce injuries by 9.4% and workers' compensation costs by 26%.[48] While three studies from 1979 to 1991 found no relationship of OSHA inspections to injury reduction,[49-51] more recent studies from 1992 to 2012 predicted that OSHA inspections led to declines in injuries.[52-56] Except for the 2012 study, none of these studies used a randomized design or other method that ensured that the inspected firms were similar to those in the comparison group, but the 2012 study did as described earlier in Chapter 8. Moreover, the firms that were inspected were uncompromised by sales reductions or credit ratings. The study was conducted in California, where the state OSHA office randomizes inspections. It used a matched data set of 409 inspected firms and 409 controls matched by industry and size. The lower rates experienced by the inspected firm were sustained for several years.[48,57]

13.6.6. Healthcare Reform

A study by the RAND Corporation in 2012 on the effect of the Patient Protection and Affordable Care Act of 2010 on the workers' compensation system investigated the impact of a similar 2006 law in Massachusetts. The results of the investigation found a drop in emergency room volume by 5 to 10%, but fees paid were unaffected. The study did not examine other care services for pharmaceuticals, but claims in Massachusetts were less than claims in surrounding states. Evidence from this study suggests that healthcare reform may reduce medical costs borne by the workers' compensation system.[58]

13.6.7. Other Compensation Statutes

Several federal laws that provide compensation for workers' injuries and diseases based upon statutes enacted by Congress are listed in Table 13-6. These laws include the District of Columbia Workers' Compensation Act and the Federal Employees' Compensation Act (FECA). Congress has enacted laws for injury compensation of interstate railroad workers under the Federal Employers' Liability Act, workers on navigable water through the Longshore and Harbor Workers' Compensation Act, and sailors on the high seas through the Merchant Marine Act. Other federal laws address special populations that have suffered significantly from occupational exposures, including coal miners under the Black Lung Benefits Act and nuclear workers and uranium miners under the Radiation Exposure Compensation Act, as well as victims of the

Table 13-6. Other Compensation Statutes in the United States

Statute	Description
Federal Employers' Liability Act of 1908	Assures railroad employees a safe workplace and gives them and their families the right to recover compensation for a railroad-related injury, but the injured party must prove negligence of the employer.
Federal Employees' Compensation Act (FECA) of 1916	Protects all civilian federal employees and their dependents from the cost of workplace injury and death; administered by the U.S. Department of Labor (DoL).
Merchant Marine Act of 1917 (Jones Act)	Allows injured sailors on U.S. flag vessels to obtain damages from their employers for the negligence of the ship owner, the captain, or fellow members of the crew like that allowed for recoveries by railroad workers.
Longshore and Harbor Workers' Compensation Act of 1927	Requires insurance for compensation and medical care to employees disabled from injuries that occur on the navigable waters of the United States, or in adjoining areas customarily used in loading, unloading, repairing, or building a vessel.
District of Columbia Workers' Compensation Act	Used language from the Longshore and Harbor Workers' Compensation Act for employers to provide workers' compensation for any employee in the District of Columbia.
Social Security Disability Act of 1956	Provides disability benefits for employees who have paid into Social Security but begins after a five-month waiting period. Established Medicare and Medicaid. Medicare begins 29 months after a medically verified inability to work.
Black Lung Benefits Act of 1969	Provides monthly payments and medical benefits to coal miners totally disabled from coal worker's pneumoconiosis (CWP), or black lung disease, arising from employment in or around the nation's coal mines and provides monthly benefits to a miner's dependent survivors if CWP caused or hastened the miner's death.
Radiation Exposure Compensation Act of 1990	Compensates workers who contracted cancer and other work-related diseases as a result of exposure to U.S. atmospheric nuclear testing or to high levels of radon while working in uranium mines.
Health Security Act in 1993	This bill failed passage, but it aimed to establish a relationship between workers' compensation and national health care reform.
Air Transportation Safety and System Stabilization Act of 2001	Provides full, fair, and reasonable compensation, without regard to fault, for the entire loss suffered by each victim and each family from the terrorist attacks of September 11, 2001.
9/11 Health and Compensation Act of 2010	Provides for long-term, comprehensive health care and compensation for first responders and others exposed to toxins at Ground Zero.

2001 terrorist attacks on the United States through the Air Transportation Safety and System Stabilization and 9/11 Health and Compensation Acts.

The DoL's Employment Standards Administration adjudicates and processes claims filed by coal miners and their survivors under the Black Lung

Benefits Act—Title IV of the Federal Mine Safety and Health Act of 1977—as amended. The 1978 amendments set up the Black Lung Disability Trust Fund, which is financed by an excise tax on coal production to pay for claims for those miners last employed prior to 1970 and for whom no responsible coal mine operator could be identified.[33] The National Institute for Occupational Safety and Health (NIOSH) establishes the standards for X-ray reading and performs autopsies related to this program.

The DoL (OSHA) and the Departments of Health and Human Services (NIOSH), Justice, and Energy (DoE) administer the Radiation Exposure Compensation Act. Congress amended the Act—the Energy Employees' Occupational Illness Compensation Program Act of 2000—to add uranium mill and ore workers as eligible claimants, geographic regions to the "down-winder" provisions, recognized illnesses, and the threshold radiation exposure for uranium miners.[59,60]

The 9/11 Health and Compensation Act established a World Trade Center (WTC) Health Program within NIOSH to provide medical monitoring and treatment for WTC attack responders and community members. The program pays for medical treatment costs at a rate based upon FECA treatment rates, like those set for black lung, longshoremen, and congressional members. The payment is offset by workers' compensation payments and is limited to 55,000 responders and community members. In addition to the WTC screening and monitoring programs, the Agency for Toxic Substances and Disease Registry (ATSDR) maintains the WTC Health Registry. In 2003, ATSDR, in collaboration with the New York City Department of Health and Mental Hygiene, established the WTC Health Registry to identify and track the long-term health effects of tens of thousands of residents, schoolchildren, and workers (located in the vicinity of the WTC collapse, as well as those participating in the response effort) who were the most directly exposed to smoke, dust, and debris resulting from the WTC collapse.[61]

13.7. TORT LIABILITY

The asbestos saga suggests that the worse the failure for regulation, the more likely that the courts will respond with high liability. This is because the callous behavior of producers in consciously exposing workers and product users to danger tends to make judges and juries very sympathetic to plaintiffs.

—Michelle J. White[62]

Workers' compensation is an exclusive remedy for employees so that they cannot sue their employer, but this restriction does not bar common law tort suits against third parties. These parties include the manufacturer of the equipment or substance that is associated with an injury, including illness.[39]

Tort liability supplements the market in a more decentralized way, making injurers pay for the harm they cause by compensating victims, but it also gives injurers incentives to reduce the harm. The different liability standards used by courts aim to achieve those goals in different ways: in particular, under the doctrine of negligence, injurers are responsible only if their actions fail to meet a standard of due care, whereas under the doctrine of strict liability, injurers are responsible regardless of how much care they exercise in trying to minimize injuries.[63]

13.7.1. Workplace Torts

Since workers' compensation systems have limitations in compensating victims, workers have increasingly sought compensation for occupational injuries and diseases with the use of tort lawsuits. Workplace tort suits tend to involve serious injury or disease because of the high cost of bringing such a suit in both time and money. Results of these suits vary between states and between cases. In the common law tort system, the burden of proof lies with the plaintiff and requires the injured party—the plaintiff—to prove three facts:[26]

1. The defendant is liable for the injury (either by negligence or strict liability),
2. The actions of the defendant proximately caused the injury, and
3. The plaintiff suffered actual damages because of the injury—economic, physical, and/or psychological.

The plaintiff must carry the burden by a preponderance of the evidence. If the plaintiff is successful, the trier of fact—either a jury or the judge—must place a monetary value on the plaintiff's damages.

A defendant is liable for negligence if the plaintiff shows that the defendant has a duty to the plaintiff, the defendant breached that duty, the defendant's negligent conduct was the cause of the harm to the plaintiff, and the plaintiff was harmed. The convergence of the law of negligence and of warranties has led to strict liability law. Under strict liability the plaintiff does not have to prove that the defendant was negligent or directly at fault for causing damage to life, limb, or property by a hazardous activity or a defective product. Strict liability arises from the fact of the activity or product being inherently hazardous or defective and not from any wrongdoing, and it aims to protect consumer expectations. Japan and the European Union have adopted the strict liability criteria as well.[64]

Under joint-and-several liability, one or more injurers can be held responsible for paying all of the damages caused by a number of injurers. Under the collateral-source rule, the amount of damages owed by a defendant does not take into account any benefits that an injured plaintiff has received from an insurance policy or other independent source. Class action suits regard many claims that cover similar factual ground and are combined into a single larger case.

Subrogation is the right of an insurer to reclaim funds from a settlement awarded to an insured party that the insurer had previously paid to that party for the same injury. This right provides an incentive for insurers to refer their injured policy holders to trial attorneys to seek damages with possible recovery of awards.

Different than workers' compensation, noneconomic damages can be awarded under tort law and are losses for physical and emotional pain, suffering, inconvenience, physical impairment, mental anguish, disfigurement, loss of society and companionship, loss of consortium (other than loss of domestic service), hedonic damages (compensation for the loss of "enjoyment of life"), injury to reputation, and all other nonpecuniary losses of any kind or nature.

13.7.2. The Cost of Tort Liability

From an economic perspective, the tort system can be examined against two criteria: (1) efficiency—minimizing the system's total cost to the economy, and (2) equity—treating all parties fairly. Data about the overall costs and benefits of tort liability are too scarce to allow economists to judge the efficiency of the current system; thus, justifications for it must be based on its effects on deterring injuries, promoting equity, or both. The efficiency of the tort system is measured by how well it minimizes the sum of several types of costs: (1) direct cost of injuries or diseases, (2) intervention cost, (3) transaction costs such as attorney fees, and (4) friction costs associated with disruptions in the economy such as plant closings and bankruptcies.[48]

Congress has considered bills to address concerns that critics have raised about the tort system or types of tort cases. Among those concerns are that the "transaction costs" of the system—particularly attorneys' fees—are too high, punitive damages and compensatory damages for pain and suffering are often awarded arbitrarily with no beneficial effect on safety, the class action suit is easily abused by plaintiffs' attorneys, and in suits over exposure to asbestos, too much money and court time are being devoted to people who do not yet show any signs of physical impairment. Conversely, supporters of the existing tort system argue that it serves important policy goals, such as compensating victims, holding injurers responsible for their actions, and improving safety. Supporters also say that critics overstate the extent and severity of the perceived problems with the system.[63]

Transaction costs are for attorney fees, which are shown earlier in Figure 13-3. For the defendant, the fees are paid whether the case is won or lost at trial, whereas the claimant's attorney fees are only paid in the event that the case is found for the claimant.

In efficiency terms, the primary benefits of the tort system are measured by reductions in injury costs. Those benefits arise indirectly, through precautions taken by potential injurers. What constitutes equity in relation to the tort system is ultimately subjective. However, there is consensus that compensating victims for their injuries is equitable.[63]

13.7.3. Asbestos Torts

From 1940 through 1979, an estimated 27.5 million U.S. workers were potentially exposed to asbestos. As of 1982, an estimated 8,200 asbestos-related cancer deaths were occurring each year, which was expected to rise to 9,700 annually by 2000, after which a downturn in the mortality rate was expected while remaining substantial for an additional three decades.[65] The dangers of exposure to asbestos were known prior to World War II, but nevertheless, many manufacturers of asbestos products failed to warn their employees of the risks of exposure or to protect them. These failures led to the worst occupational health disaster in U.S. history.[41]

In 1973, an insulation worker won damages in a liability suit from large asbestos manufacturers in *Clarence Borel v. Fibreboard Paper Products Corporation, et al.* Within the next 10 years, other victims filed another 25,000 product liability suits. Many of these suits were successfully challenged, but over time, evidence proved that the major asbestos producers knew of the health hazards of exposure to asbestos dating back to the 1930s. By the end of 2002, 730,000 people had filed lawsuits against more than 8,400 defendants, and 85 corporations had filed for bankruptcy. The estimated cost to defendants and insurers was $70 billion by 2002, but the estimated eventual number of claims ranged from 1.0 to 3.0 million at a cost of $200 to $265 billion.[62]

While the asbestos exposure to millions of Americans has had a tragic effect upon their lives and the cohesion and livelihood of their families, these suits also have a far-reaching impact on insurers for the asbestos production companies. When Clarence Borel sued 11 asbestos companies in Beaumont, Texas, in 1969 for failure to warn him about the hazards of handling asbestos, the suits that followed brought down large companies such as Johns-Manville. Lloyd's of London, an insurer of last resort that underwrote insurance for other companies, reported a loss of $980 million in 1991 resulting from covering asbestos claims, and in 1992, Lloyd's reported a loss of $3.85 billion, including losses associated with the Exxon Valdez oil spill and the 1989 San Francisco earthquake. In 1993, their losses rose to $4.4 billion. The British Parliament enacted protective legislation for Lloyd's, and Lloyd's set up a separate corporation to deal with its pre-1993 obligations.[66] Nonetheless, by the late 1970s, litigation costs proved more effective than regulation in eliminating asbestos in most products in the United States.[62]

13.8. COST ANALYSIS

Congress itself defined the basic relationship between costs and benefits, by placing "benefit" of worker health above all other considerations save those making attainment of this "benefit" unachievable.

—U.S. Supreme Court[67]

For some time, public health professionals shunned the idea of putting a price on health and, more specifically, on human life. However, cost analysis is now a necessary part of evaluating the costs and benefits of alternative intervention policies. Indeed, making a business case for an intervention has emerged as an intervention in and of itself. As a tool, cost analysis techniques have advantages as well as limitations:[26]

Advantages
- Systematic and rational techniques are used to evaluate and clarify choices among possible alternatives.
- The process makes the estimates of costs and benefits and assumptions used explicit.
- The method allows analysis of time effects between when an intervention is used and its future effects.

Limitations
- The measures and metrics may be inappropriate for some policy effects.
- Assumptions can distort results.
- Defects in the market can affect the estimates of the costs and benefits of an intervention.

The analytical techniques described below—cost-benefit analysis (CBA) and cost effectiveness analysis (CEA)—are addressed further in Chapter 16 regarding policy analysis. In addition, the different metrics that are used in these analyses are explained, as is the effect of time measurement on the analysis. Last, the difficult area of the worth of a life is discussed.

13.8.1. Human Capital

In the early 1700s, Daniel Bernoulli introduced the idea of human capital, the sum of education, talent, training, and experience possessed by people. The human capital method has been applied to the cost analysis of a variety of injuries and illnesses. It includes two categories of costs: direct and indirect.

Direct costs are the dollars spent on medical care, pharmaceuticals and medical supplies, rehabilitation, and ambulance services. They also include administrative costs including insurance, Medicare, Medicaid, Veteran's Administration, and workers' compensation. Indirect costs represent forgone opportunities for the injured or ill person. Lost earnings and fringe benefits are included, as well as related costs of unpaid caregivers and other actions by coworkers, family, and the employer. They do not compensate for pain and suffering.

13.8.2. Willingness to Pay

The willingness-to-pay (WTP) method is an alternative way to determine the cost of injuries and illnesses. Rather than splitting costs into indirect and direct costs, the WTP approach attempts to include costs that reflect market transactions including pain and suffering. It depends upon a person's willingness to pay for an intervention (e.g., a hard hat) to reduce a risk by a certain amount. People are surveyed to determine this willingness. The WTP approach captures the notion of opportunity cost by measuring what individuals are willing to forgo to enjoy a particular benefit.[68]

13.8.3. Cost–Benefit Analysis

Cost–benefit analysis is an economic analysis in which all costs and benefits are converted into monetary values and results are expressed as dollars of benefit per dollars expended. It is a framework to help decision makers keep their thinking straight and transparent. In addition, CBA is a policy-making tool by which the costs of imposing a regulation are weighed against the potential benefits of reducing the harm. It systematically organizes the impacts of policy proposals, forces explicit assignment of values to the impacts, and forces judgments into the open. It evolved from the field of welfare economics.[68] Cost-benefit analysis (CBA) is often described as a neutral tool in policy making, but recent studies by legal scholars show that CBA is inherently political and may even advise against public protections.[69]

13.8.4. Cost-Effectiveness Analysis

In the public health arena, controversies over valuing human life in monetary terms have moved attention from CBA to CEA as the principal method for evaluating the costs and effects of different healthcare strategies. Cost-effectiveness analysis (CEA) evolved from cost engineering, decision analysis, and operations research and generates a cost-effectiveness ratio in which monetary values are in the numerator and an outcome is in the denominator. While CBA can accommodate multiple outcomes since they are given monetary values, CEA is limited to a single outcome. It is useful for ranking the cost-effectiveness of alternative strategies for preventing or reducing a negative health outcome.[70]

13.8.5. Health Metrics

The World Bank developed a measure that integrated years of life lost and years lived with a disability into the disability-adjusted life-year (DALY). The DALY allows the integration of mortality and morbidity regarding injury, illness, and risk factors based on value judgments of disability and resource allocation. The World Health Organization has adopted the DALY as a measure of public health around the world. Another metric is the quality-adjusted life-year (QALY), which accounts for both quality of life and survival benefits. The QALY uses utility theory by measuring a health state quantified on a scale between 0 and 1, representing death and the best imaginable health, respectively.[71]

13.8.6. Temporal Considerations

Three time effects are considered when conducting a cost analysis: discounting, inflation, and the analytic horizon. When the time frame of the intervention and the related outcomes differ, discounting is a way to assure that the cost is adjusted to a present value to assure constancy in the costs and benefits used in the calculation. The discount rate reflects the present value of costs and benefits, and at a personal level, this rate can vary greatly. It can be understood as, for example, a person's time preference in investing in interest-bearing accounts such as in a savings account. It relates to people valuing resources today as higher than the value they may place on the same resources in the future. Individuals can differ in how they may discount an investment preference into the future (e.g., the time-value of money), but in public health studies, a social discount rate is used as a way to compare the results of one intervention to another, thus the discount rate should be the same. The current annual social discount rate used for this purpose is 3% (i.e., the present value of $1.00 next year is $0.97). When the discounting of the dollar is used in a calculation, the outcome (e.g., injuries averted) must also be discounted at the same rate, although using the same discount rate has been questioned.[72]

The choice of a discount rate can have a significant effect on the present value of future earnings as shown in Figure 13-9.[73] At the peak present value, the difference can be half a million dollars with no discounting at 0% and discounting at 3%.

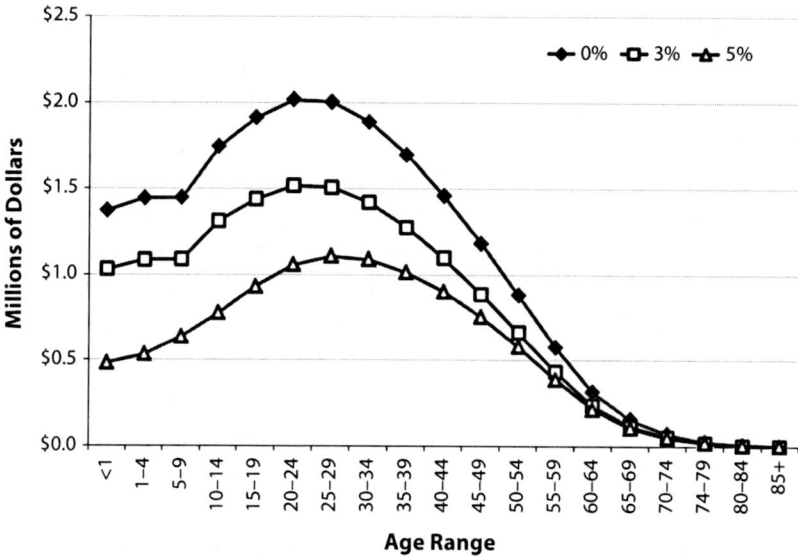

Source: Max et al.[72]
Note: Numbers are in 2000 dollars.
Figure 13-9. The present value of male earnings discounted at 0%, 3%, and 5% over a lifetime.

Inflation, the second time consideration, is the devaluing of a dollar over time. As an example, $100 in 2000 had the same buying power as $134 in 2013: with 2000 as the index year, the index for 2013 is 1.34. All numbers used from the past need to be adjusted for inflation to the study year.

The third time consideration is the analytic horizon: how far into the future to conduct the analysis. This is important for an investment in an intervention today that may prevent injuries well into the future. The investment may be in a machine guard with a onetime expenditure in the first year, but it will protect workers from injury into the future. If the life of the machine with a guard installed will last for 10 years, then it is reasonable to choose a 10-year analytic horizon against which positive outcomes will accrue over that time period.

13.8.7. What Is a Life Worth?

Life is a different metric than dollars; thus, placing a financial value on life must look at the costs involved with injury, illness, and death, including both direct and indirect costs into future costs. Placing a financial value on life is nothing new. A medieval system of restitution for one person's physical harm to another emerged out of decentralized Germanic societies as wergild, meaning "man money." In those societies, every person had a monetary value based on status and importance. As an example, women of childbearing age were valued more highly than women not of childbearing age. Restitution also varied by the severity of the injury, and failure to pay restitution meant shunning by the clan and uncertain survival alone in the wilderness. This system found its way to England in the medieval migrations, evolving eventually into the common law tort system.[74] Today, these calculations can result in different values depending upon potential earnings and the severity of the injury or disease.

In 2005, Kenneth Feinberg published his book *What Is a Life Worth?* documenting his experience as the Special Master for compensating the 9/11 victims and their families for physical injuries and deaths from the 9/11 Victim Compensation Fund.[2] The fund distributed $7.0 billion based upon the direct and indirect costs of fatal or nonfatal injuries. This amount reflected $2.9 billion in offsets for other compensations such as life insurance and workers' compensation. The average award for deceased victims was $2.1 million ($n = 2,880$) and an average award of $392,968 ($n = 2,680$) for physical injury victims.[2] The indirect cost awards were based on the family size and extant earnings of the victims. Figure 13-10 shows the distribution of the awards by age and gender of the decedents.[2] As can be seen, there is a disparity in compensation to families of decedents related to both age and gender.

Consistent with Figure 13-10, based upon lifetime earnings, age and gender discrimination can result, as shown in Figure 13-11. The same type of graph could be shown for different races and ethnic groups. Thus, differentiating populations based upon the present value of earnings can lead to discrimination.

The government has assigned a common cost of an injury based upon severity regardless of age, gender, or race. The severity scale used is the Maximum Abbreviated Injury Scale. The U.S. Department of Transportation led this approach, seen in Table 13-7, which is based upon cases seen in hospital emergency departments.[75] These cost figures are vastly different from those documented by workers' compensation.

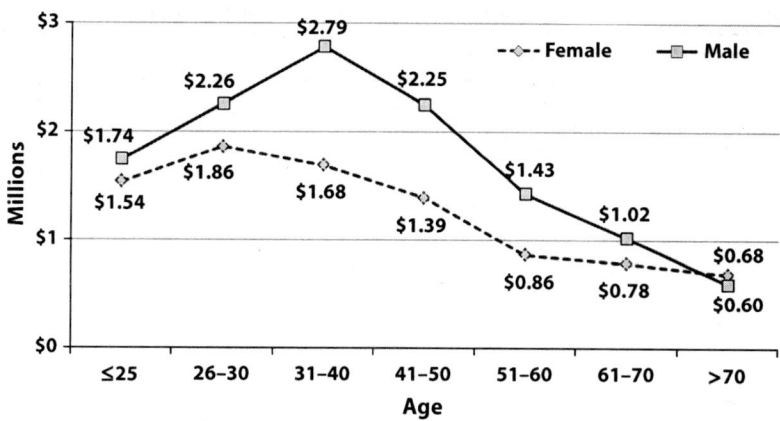

Source: Feinberg.[2]

Figure 13-10. Average awards provided to the families of each 9/11 decedent.

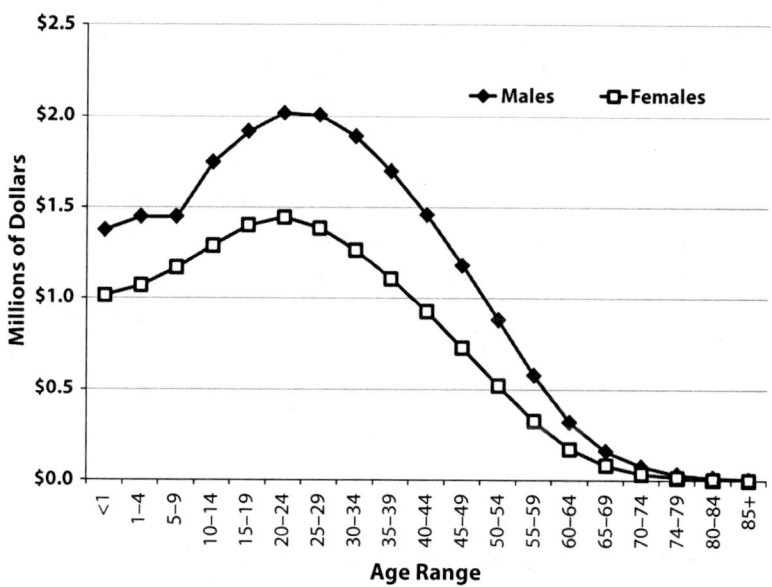

Source: Max et al.[72]
Note: Numbers are in 2000 dollars.

Figure 13-11. Present value at 3% discount rate of lifetime earnings by gender over a lifetime.

Table 13-7. Maximum Abbreviated Injury Scale and Associated Cost of Injury

Severity	Total Cost
No injury	$0
Minor	$20,123
Moderate	$211,664
Serious	$421,033
Severe	$980,250
Critical	$3,220,016
Untreatable (Death)	$4,510,960

Source: Blincoe et al.[75]
Note: Numbers are in 2013 dollars, adjusted with the Consumer Price Index.

13.9. THE DIMENSIONS OF FRAUD IN WORKERS' COMPENSATION

In every study that has been done on fraud in workers' compensation, employer, insurer, and provider fraud are found to be a dramatically greater problem than claimant fraud.

—Robert Stern, AFL-CIO[76]

It all comes down to incentives. Any participant in the workers' compensation system can engage in fraud when he or she can benefit from the crime of fraud. This incentive can be indirect regarding workers' compensation. For example, as described in Chapter 10, mine operators may engage in coal mine dust sampler tampering to avoid the cost of dust control, which likely leads to continued cases of CWP and the resulting compensation for black lung. However, workers' compensation fraud can occur in more direct ways, as listed below.[77]

- A worker may file a false claim.
- An employer may misclassify workers into less hazardous categories of work to reduce premium costs (i.e., premium fraud).
- An attorney may conspire with healthcare providers to provide false information for legal proceedings.
- An insurer may engage in fraud by overcharging employers, hoarding excessive reserves, issuing bogus policies, or denying or delaying justifiable claims.

- A healthcare provider may increase its income by prescribing unnecessary treatments, overcharging for services, or accepting a kickback from an attorney.

Each of these participants in the workers' compensation system is described below regarding fraud. In addition, an additional injustice is discussed, which involves the government's complicity in "legal" fraud from the perspective of the compensation principle. It is important to note that fraud is not a large problem regarding workers' compensation. State-level studies have shown that the cost of fraud is between 1 and 2% of the cost of all claims in Ohio, for example.[76]

For better information, the "red flags" used by the Fraud and Compliance Unit of the Georgia State Board of Workers' Compensation are shown in Table 13-8. Also shown are the percentage of arrests and monetary losses associated with each category of participants. A total of 598 investigations were conducted that resulted in 135 arrests.[78]

13.9.1. Claimant Fraud and Fundamental Attribution Error

Worker fraud—also known as claimant fraud—has many faces. A claimant may falsely allege that an injury is work-related or that an injury is more serious than it is, or a legitimate injury may turn fraudulent after a period of time. A worker may file a claim for a nonexistent injury, or a worker may work at a second job while drawing compensation from another job.[77]

As reported in 2000 in California, claimant fraud was less than 0.3% of all claims, and in Wisconsin, claimant fraud failed to exceed 0.1% of all claims there.[76] Nonetheless, in a review covering 42 states regarding all types of workers' compensation fraud, 78% of completed investigations were of claimant fraud.[77] Most investigations of claimants result in no convictions, and those that do involve

Table 13-8. Workers' Compensation Fraud Arrests, Monetary Losses Involved, and Red Flags for Investigations in Georgia, 1995–1999

Participants	Red Flags
Claimant: 67% of arrests and 16% of monetary losses	• The injury is not witnessed by a coworker. • Injury occurs immediately after a vacation day, a Monday, or seasonal activities. • The injury is inconsistent with job duties. • Claimant is disgruntled, facing firing, layoff, soon to retire, or seasonal work is about to end. • The claimant has a history of short-term employment. • Claimant has moved out of state or the immediate area. • Description of incident varies from the first report of injury and the medical history received by the physician. • Knowledge among employees that claimant is active in sports or has another job. • Claimant is never home to answer the phone or is always sleeping and cannot be disturbed. • Claimant is reported to be suntanned, muscular, has callused hands, or grease under the fingernails. • Claimant requests a change in physician when receives a "Release for Work" form. • Details of accident are vague and/or are not promptly reported to supervisor. • Claimant is experiencing financial difficulties.
Employer: 24% of arrests and 27% of monetary losses	• Failure of employer to carry workers' compensation insurance. • Claim filed for health insurance instead of workers' compensation insurance. • Failure to file "First Report of Injury." • Information on "First Report of Injury" is incorrect or falsified. • Advises employee to file under Company "b" instead of Company "a." • Employer changes employee's job classification.
Attorney for claimant: No arrests	• Attorney lien or representation letter dated the day of the reported incident. • Same doctor/lawyer pair previously observed to handle this kind of injury. • Claimant initially wants to settle with insurer, but later retains an attorney with increased subjective medical demands. • Pattern of occupational type claims for industries, i.e., black lung, asbestosis; multiple class action suits. • Attorney threatens further legal action unless a quick settlement is made. • Attorney inquires about a settlement or buyout early in the life of the claim.
Insurer: 3% of arrests and 5% of monetary losses	• None reported
Medical provider: 9% of arrests and 52% of monetary losses	• Repeat incidents where the same doctor and attorneys are involved together on claims of questionable merit. • Claims that appear to be boilerplate copies from the same provider involving different claimants. • Injuries are all subjective, such as stress, inability to sleep, headaches, nausea, etc.

Table 13-8. (Continued)

Participants	Red Flags
Medical provider: 9% of arrests and 52% of monetary losses	• Diagnosis is inconsistent with treatment. • Medical bills submitted without adequate descriptions of office visits and other treatment. • Medical bills submitted are photocopies of original bill. • Claimant appears to be getting better until visit with a new provider, followed by unexpected regression. • Treatment dates coincide with holidays or weekends. • Provider type is inconsistent with injury. • Workers' compensation insurer and health carrier are billed simultaneously; payment is accepted from both. • Treatment directed to a separate facility in which the referring physician has a financial interest without disclosure.

Source: Atkins.[78]
Note: For arrests, n = 135; for monetary losses, n = $5.3 million; for red flags, n = 598.

relatively small amounts of money. The investigations are more costly than the alleged money at stake, and the focus of the investigations is diverted from large-scale fraud by others. For example, prior to 1998, in the first four cases prosecuted in Maine for workers' compensation fraud, three involved claimants who were fined $1,000 each, and one was an employer that was fined $1.6 million.[77]

Nevertheless, news stories proliferate about workers committing fraud, fed by skepticism regarding the validity of claims. While there is worker fraud, this proliferation of news stories may be driven by "fundamental attribution error" in which people in power tend to place an undue emphasis on internal characteristics to explain a victim's injury in a given situation, rather than considering external factors.[78a] This error is discussed further in Chapter 15 regarding the phenomenon of "blaming the victim." Publicity regarding fraud is easier when pictures matter, such as secret videos of an injured worker fishing or of a claimant receiving benefits for back pain and seen lifting loads into the trunk of his car. Fraud of the white-collar kind does not grab the attention of reporters when pictures are unavailable and do not tell the story.

13.9.2. Employer Premium Fraud

Employers that engage in fraud gain a competitive advantage by externalizing costs to other employers, workers and their families, and the public. As shown in Table 13-8, one-fourth of those arrested in Georgia for fraud were employers, representing just over one-fourth of monetary losses. An employer may avoid or minimize the cost of insurance by several means. Examples of employer fraud include falsified certificates of insurance, "charging" employees for workers' compensation premiums, and misleading workers about the existence of insurance coverage. In the calculation of premiums, an employer may classify a worker into a less hazardous job to reduce the premium payment. An employer may underreport its payroll, or it may underreport injuries so as to reduce its experience modification ratio. It may require an injured worker (e.g., with an amputated finger) to return to work to avoid reporting a lost day injury. In addition, an employer may claim an employee as an independent contractor to avoid paying premiums.[77,78]

Employer fraud is less investigated than claimant fraud, but millions of dollars are at stake regarding premium fraud. One of the few reviews of this type of fraud cites four cases. In the mid-1990s, an audit in Ohio of 4% of employers resulted in the recovery of $19 million. In 1995, an audit in New York uncovered a failure by employers to pay $525 million in premiums, which represented 30% of all premiums collected in that year. Between 1993 and 1995, one Rhode Island investigator identified 136 companies that qualified for workers' compensation but illegally avoided paying premiums. Prior to 1998, Montana collected about $550,000 from employers attempting to avoid premium payments annually.[77]

In addition, a compliance audit conducted in 1995 and 1996 in Florida found that 13.1% of 22,758 employers were illegally operating without mandated workers' compensation insurance. The auditors stated that these employers had also not purchased workers' compensation insurance, other employers intentionally reported or misclassified its payroll units, and others falsely claimed that many employees were independent contractors.[76]

13.9.3. Attorney Fraud

Table 13-8 shows no arrests of attorneys in Georgia for the period covered regarding fraud. However, an attorney may recruit and help workers file bogus claims, or an attorney may participate in illegal medical mills (discussed below) comprising chiropractors, doctors, and employee recruiters, including unwary workers, to file fraudulent claims.[77,78]

13.9.4. Insurer Fraud and Benefits Denial

Insurance carriers' fraud at the expense of workers is likely significant.[78] Carrier fraud takes place when an insurer makes false statements about a worker's eligibility to collect payments in an effort to pay reduced benefits. Indeed, as a matter of routine, some carriers deny claims for invisible disorders such as low back pain or upper-limb musculoskeletal disorders.[79]

As shown before in Table 13-8, one red flag for worker fraud is an injury complaint on a Monday. However, a Canadian study found that Monday is the most likely day for strains and sprains to occur, when workers are more susceptible to an injury after a weekend of rest.[79] In addition, symptoms of byssinosis in U.S. textile mills earlier in the 20th century were manifest on Mondays with shortness of breath and chest tightness when sensitized workers were reexposed to cotton dust after a weekend off, which may have been the origin of the term "red flag."[80]

In a dire twist to the no-fault insurance system, a claim denial results in the burden of proof shifting to the worker. A worker may give up and abandon attempts to be compensated or may engage an attorney to pursue compensation. Attorney fees potentially dilute the possible benefits to the worker and add to the transaction costs involved in resolution of the claim. Adjusters and agents may engage in fraud by refusing payment or by issuing bogus policies. A carrier may encourage a claimant to engage an attorney to bring third-party suits against others and thereby potentially collect a portion of liability awards under subjugation rules.

13.9.5. Healthcare Provider Fraud and Medical Mills

Healthcare fraud can amount to substantial sums as reflected in Table 13-8, which shows that with 9% of the arrests in Georgia, more than half of the financial losses arose from this type of fraud. A healthcare specialist can provide kickbacks for referrals from authorized treating physicians and engage in "creative" billing practices. A given treatment may be more expensive than needed, or clinics may order more treatments than necessary. A provider can charge for services not performed or give referrals to clinics in which the referring doctor has a financial interest, or a pharmacist may bill fraudulent workers' compensation insurance claims for prescription drugs. As an example, a pharmacist collected more than $600,000 by overcharging for prescribed drugs over a four-year period in California.[79]

A clinic may bill an insurance carrier for a treatment of injuries that never happened. This clinic may be a shell company for bogus workers' compensation claims with no licensed physicians, minor medical equipment, and little or no needed treatment. These sorts of establishments may be well-organized criminal activities known as medical mills, sometimes involving an unscrupulous attorney.[78]

13.9.6. Legal Fraud

Legal fraud refers to a government's complicity in avoiding paying workers' compensation. Governments can be complicit in at least three ways. One way is the violation of the uniformity tenet of the compensation principle, in which no state gains a competitive advantage over other states for attracting employers by legislating lower compensation premiums. This type of legal fraud is made clear by Figure 13-6, in which there is a significant lack of uniformity between states regarding compensation costs and the relative lack of benefits to injured workers.

Another factor regarding complicity is state-level legislatures rolling back benefits, narrowing the definition of injuries covered by compensation, and introducing impediments to collecting compensation. All of these legal changes reflect a fundamental attribution error, shifting costs to the victims. Such moves lead to the free rider problem that benefits employers and insurance companies by shifting the cost burden of work-related injuries and diseases to workers and their families and other insurance systems including Medicare, Medicaid, and Social Security. This legislated shift is estimated to be six times the cost of workers' compensation fraud.[76]

The third way that governments are complicit in legal fraud is the protection of employers from an obligation to pay compensation for workers' injuries. Perhaps one of the greatest injustices in this regard was the indifference given to uranium miners and their families during the "uranium frenzy." Chapter 14 addresses worker protection provided by the DoE; however, the injustices experienced by uranium miners under the earlier jurisdiction of the U.S. Atomic Energy Commission (AEC) goes much deeper. These mines were operated under contract with the AEC. Because of national security concerns and Cold War imperatives, the AEC denied any effect to animal and human health from radiation exposures and then fought any claims for compensation from damages arising from radiation exposure to avoid setting a precedent. While the AEC had the authority to enforce safe conditions in the mines from radon and its derivatives through ventilation, they obfuscated the problem and any responsibility through propaganda and denial. Patient Zero, a Colorado uranium miner, died in 1956 of a unique cancer of the lungs that was associated with radiation exposure. Workers' compensation was denied to the widow through collusion between the mine employer and the AEC. Controls recommended in 1950 by the U.S. Public Health Service were still not implemented by 1964. More miners died, and many were of the Navajo tribe. Relief did not come until the passage of the Radiation Exposure Compensation Act of 1990.[81]

THE VINYL CHLORIDE NARRATIVE

In 1974, when OSHA sought to regulate vinyl chloride monomers (VCM; the term is shortened to "vinyl chloride" in the OSHA standard), substantial evidence existed about its toxicity—especially its link to a rare form of liver cancer, angiosarcoma—but little was known about the safe level of exposure or how many people had or would die from angiosarcoma through exposure to VCM. At the time, there were only 13 known cases of angiosarcoma deaths from VCM exposure. Still, OSHA chose to take a precautionary stance and sought to lower the allowable exposure level to 1 ppm over an 8-hour period. Previously, industry had allowed an exposure of 200 ppm "time-weighted average" with a maximum allowable exposure of 500 ppm. By statute, OSHA does not perform CBA and must enforce a policy of feasibility. If OSHA had performed CBA when determining an exposure limit for VCM with the knowledge available at the time, CBA would have come out in favor of a much weaker standard. Heinzerling, Ackerman, and Massey compared the estimated cost of compliance at the time with the estimated value of a life in order to determine how many lives would be saved to justify the OSHA regulatory standard.[82] The estimated cost of compliance with the VCM regulation was thought to be $200 million per year (though it turned out to be much lower). For the value of a human life, the authors used two different estimates: the highest value of a life based on current U.S. Environmental Protection Agency calculations and adjusted for inflation, which was $1.81 million, and the much lower value of life used in the Ford Pinto controversy that occurred around the same time, which estimated the value of a statistical life at $200,000. Only 7,000 people worked in the VCM industry. Using the Ford Pinto value, one out of every seven workers would have had to die to justify the stringent standard. That means that 1,000 people would have had to die each year to justify OSHA's regulation. Taking into account discount rates, the picture becomes even more dismal. At a 3% discount rate, 200 people using the high estimate for life value or 2,000 people using the lower estimate would have had to die each year for OSHA to justify the costs. At a 10% discount rate, 700 people would have had to die using the former estimate and 7,000 using the lower estimate. Thus, the authors concluded, "using a 10 percent discount rate and the value of life estimated in the 1970s, it would be necessary to show that every worker in the industry, every year, would have died in the absence of the standard, in order to justify the regulation in cost-benefit terms."[82] Beyond their analysis, it turned out that the estimated cost of control was high as well.

REFERENCES

1. Butterworth H. The bird with a broken wing. In: George AH. *Up Through Childhood: A Study of Some Principles of Education in Relation to Faith and Conduct.* New York, NY: G.P. Putnam and Sons;1904:258.

2. Feinberg KR. What is a life worth? In: Feinberg, KR. *The Unprecedented Effort to Compensate the Victims of 9/11.* New York, NY: Public Affairs;2005.

3. Obama B. President Obama and Senate Republicans release job plans. In: Kerrigan H, ed. *Historic Documents of 2011.* Thousand Oaks, CA: CQ Press;2013:480–491.

4. O'Toole J, Hansot E, Herman W, et al. *Work in America: Report of a Special Task Force to the Secretary of Health, Education, and Welfare.* Cambridge, MA: MIT Press;1975.

5. Heilbroner R, Milberg W. *The Crisis of Vision in Modern Economic Thought.* New York, NY: Cambridge University Press;1995.

6. Lahart J. Rethinking health care and the GDP. *Wall Street Journal.* January 2007;25:C1.

7. Organisation for Economic Co-operation and Development. OECD health data 2012: how does the United States compare? Available at: http://www.oecd.org/unitedstates/BriefingNoteUSA2012.pdf. Accessed March 8, 2013.

8. Longest BB. *Health Policymaking in the United States.* Washington, DC: AUPHA Press;2007.

9. Gold MR, Siegel JE, Russell LB, Weinstein MC. *Cost-Effectiveness in Health and Medicine.* New York, NY: Oxford University Press;1996.

10. Leigh JP. Economic burden of occupational injury and illness in the United States. *Milbank Q.* 2011;89(4):728–772.

11. Leigh JP, Markowitz S, Fahs M, Landrigan P. *Costs of Occupational Safety and Health.* Ann Arbor, MI: University of Michigan Press;2000.

12. Go AS, Mozaffarian D, Roger VL, et al. Economic cost of cardiovascular disease. Heart disease and stroke statistics—2013 update: a report from the American Heart Association. *Circulation.* 2013;127:e234–e237. Available at: http://circ.ahajournals.org/content/127/1/e6.full.pdf+html. Accessed February 1, 2013.

13. Bureau of Labor Statistics. Inflation calculator. Available at: http://data.bls.gov/cgi-bin/cpicalc.pl. Accessed February 3, 2013.

14. Bureau of Labor Statistics. Consumer Price Index for all urban consumers: medical care. Available at: http://research.stlouisfed.org/fred2/data/CPIMEDSL.txt. Accessed February 3, 2013.

15. Bradley CJ, Yabroff KR, Dahman B, et al. Productivity costs of cancer mortality in the United States: 2000–2020. *J Natl Cancer Inst.* 2008;100(24):1763–1770.

16. Mariotto AB, Yabroff KR, Yongwu SY, et al. Projections of the cost of cancer care in the United States: 2010–2020. *J Natl Cancer Inst.* 2011;103(2):117–128.

17. United States Bone and Joint Initiative. Health care utilization and economic cost of musculoskeletal diseases. In: *The Burden of Musculoskeletal Diseases in the United States.* 2nd ed. Rosemont, IL: American Academy of Orthopaedic Surgeons;2011:219–252.

18. National Academy of Sciences. *Musculoskeletal Disorders and the Workplace: Low Back and Upper Extremities.* Washington, DC: The National Academies Press;2001.

19. Finkelstein EA, Corso PS, Miller TR, et al. *The Incidence and Burden of Injuries in the United States.* New York, NY: Oxford University Press;2006.

20. Alzheimer's Association. Changing the trajectory of Alzheimer's Disease: a national imperative. 2010. Available at: http://www.alz.org/documents_custom/final_trajectory_report_release-emb_5-11-10.pdf. Accessed February 1, 2013.

21. Riggs JL. *Engineering Economics.* New York, NY: McGraw-Hill;1977.

22. Mankiw NG. *Essentials of Economics*. Mason, OH: South-Western Cengage Learning;2009.

23. Feinman JM. *Un-Making Law: The Conservative Campaign to Roll Back the Common Law*. Boston, MA: Boston Press;2004.

24. Rodriguez P. *Why Economies Rise or Fall*. Chantilly, VA: The Teaching Company;2010.

25. Rogers DW. *Making Capitalism Safe: Work Safety and Health Regulation in America, 1880-1940*. Urbana, IL: University of Illinois Press;2009.

26. Ashford NA, Caldart CC. *Technology, Law, and the Working Environment*. Washington, DC: Island Press;1996.

27. Muller JZ. *Thinking About Capitalism*. Chantilly, VA: The Teaching Company; 2008.

28. De Soto H. *The Mystery of Capital: Why Capitalism Triumphs in the West and Fails Everywhere Else*. London, UK: Black Swan;2001.

29. O'Connor J. On the two contradictions of capitalism. *Capitalism Nature Socialism*. 1991;2(3):107–109.

30. Sengupta I, Reno V, Burton JF. *Workers' Compensation: Benefits, Coverage, and Costs, 2010*. Washington, DC: National Academy of Social Insurance;2012.

31. O'Leary P, Boden LI, Seabury SA, et al. Workplace injuries and the take-up of Social Security disability benefits. *Soc Secur Bull*. 2012;72(3):1–17.

32. Leigh PJ, Marcin JP. Workers' compensation benefits and shifting costs for occupational injury and illness. *J Occup Environ Med*. 2012;54(4):445–450.

33. Spieler EA. Perpetuating risk? Workers' compensation and the persistence of occupational injuries. *Houston Law Rev*. 1994;31(1):119–264.

34. U.S. Chamber of Commerce. *2004 Analysis of Workers' Compensation Laws*. Washington, DC: U.S. Chamber of Commerce;2004.

35. Office of Technology Assessment. *Preventing Illness and Injury in the Workplace*. Washington, DC: U.S. Congress;1985. OTA-H-256.

36. Little JW, Eaton TA, Smith GR. *Cases and Materials on Workers' Compensation*. St. Paul, MN: West Publishing Co.;1993.

37. Plumb JM, Cowell JWF. An overview of workers' compensation. *Occup Med*. 1998;13(2):241–272.

38. Guidotti TL. Workers' compensation: An introduction. Supercourse lecture. *Epidemiology, the Internet, and Global Health.* 2004. Available at: http://www.pitt.edu/~SUPER1/lecture/lec16661/index.htm. Accessed October 3, 2006.

39. Boden LI. Workers' compensation. In: Levy BS, Wegman DH, eds. *Occupational Health: Recognizing and Preventing Work-Related Disease.* Boston, MA: Little, Brown and Co.;1988:149–162.

40. Virta RL. *Worldwide Asbestos Supply and Consumption Trends From 1900 through 2003.* Washington, DC: U.S. Department of the Interior;2006. Circular 1298.

41. Carroll SJ, Hensler D, Gross J, et al. *Asbestos Litigation.* Santa Monica, CA: RAND Corporation;2005.

42. U.S. Department of Labor. *An Interim Report to Congress on Occupational Disease.* Washington, DC: U.S. Government Printing Office;1980.

43. Andersson BGJ, Cocchiarella L. *Guides to the Evaluation of Permanent Impairment.* Chicago, IL: American Medical Association;2004.

44. Sengupta I, Reno V. Recent trends in workers' compensation. *Soc Secur Bull.* 2007;67(1):17–26.

45. National Commission on State Workmen's Compensation Laws. *Report of the National Commission on State Workmen's Compensation Laws.* Washington, DC: U.S. Government Printing Office;1972.

46. Social Security Administration. Report of the National Commission on State Workmen's Compensation Laws. *Soc Secur Bull.* 1972;10:31–32, 56. Available at: http://www.ssa.gov/policy/docs/ssb/v35n10/v35n10p31.pdf, Accessed February 24, 2013.

47. George RP. What is law? A century of arguments. *First Things.* 2001;112(4):23–29.

48. *Hearing on Promoting Safe Workplaces through Voluntary Protection Programs, House Subcommittee on Workforce Protections* (June 28, 2012) (testimony of DI Levine, Randomized government safety inspections reduce worker injuries with no detectable job loss). Available at: http://edworkforce.house.gov/uploadedfiles/06.28.12_levine.pdf. Accessed February 28, 2013.

49. Smith RS. The impact of OSHA inspections on manufacturing incidence rates. *J Human Resources.* 1979;14(2):145–170.

50. Viscusi WK. The impact of occupational safety and health regulation. *Bell J Econ.* 1979;10(1):117–140.

51. Ruser JW, Smith RS. Reestimating OSHA's effects—Have the data changed? *J Human Resources.* 1991;26(2):212–235.

52. Haviland A, Burns R, Gray W, Ruder T, Mendeloff J. What kinds of injuries do OSHA inspections prevent? *J Safety Res.* 2010;41(4):339–345.

53. Haviland A, Burns R, Gray W, Ruder T, Mendeloff J. A new estimate of the impact of OSHA inspections on manufacturing injury rates, 1998-2005. *Am J Ind Med.* 2012;55(11):964–975.

54. Mendeloff J, Gray W. Inside the black box: How do OSHA inspections lead to reductions in workplace injuries? *Law Policy.* 2005;27(2):219–237.

55. Gray WB, Scholz JT. Does regulatory enforcement work? A panel analysis of OSHA enforcement. *Law Soc Rev.* 1993;27(1):177–214.

56. Baggs J, Silverstein B, Foley M. Workplace health and safety regulations: Impact of enforcement and consultation on workers' compensation claims rates in Washington State. *Am J Ind Med.* 2003;43(5):483–494.

57. Levine DI, Toffel MW, Johnson MS. Randomized government safety inspections reduce worker injuries with no detectable job loss. *Science.* 2012;336(6083):907–911.

58. Heaton P. *The Impact of Health Care Reform on Workers' Compensation Medical Care: Evidence From Massachusetts.* Santa Monica, CA: RAND Corporation;2012. Technical report.

59. U.S. Department of Justice, Civil Division. Radiation Exposure Compensation Program. November 5, 2007. Available at: http://www.justice.gov/civil/common/reca.html. Accessed January 25, 2013.

60. Wikipedia. Radiation Exposure Compensation Act. July 2013. Available at: http://en.wikipedia.org/wiki/Radiation_Exposure_Compensation_Act. Accessed January 25, 2013.

61. *Hearing Before House Subcommittee on National Security, Emerging Threats, and International Relations, Committee on Government Reform* (September 8, 2006) (testimony, John Howard, MD, MPH, Director, National Institute for Occupational Safety and Health, Centers for Disease Control and Prevention on progress since 9/11: protecting public health and safety of the responders and residents).

62. White MJ. Asbestos and the future of mass torts. *J Econ Perspect.* 2004;18(2):183–204.

63. Congressional Budget Office. The economics of U.S. tort liability: a primer. 2003. Available at: http://www.cbo.gov/sites/default/files/cbofiles/ftpdocs/46xx/doc4641/10-22-tortreform-study.pdf. Accessed January 31, 2013.

64. Geistfeld MA. *Principles of Product Liability.* New York, NY: Foundation Press; 2006.

65. Nicholson WJ, Perkel G, Selikoff IJ. Occupational exposure to asbestos: population at risk and projected mortality 1980–2030. *Am J Ind Med.* 1982;3(3):259–311.

66. Greenwald J. Lloyd's of London falling down. February 28, 2000. *Time* in partnership with CNN. Available at: http:www.time.com/time/printout/0,8816,996199,00.html. Accessed January 21, 2011.

67. *American Textile Manufacturers Institute v. Donovan,* 452 U.S. 490, 509 (1981).

68. Messonnier M, Meltzer M. Cost-benefit analysis. In: Haddix AC, Teutsch SM, Corso PS, eds. *Prevention Effectiveness: A Guide to Decision Analysis and Economic Evaluation.* New York, NY: Oxford University Press;2003:127–155.

69. Driesen D. Is cost-benefit analysis neutral? *Univ Colorado Law Rev.* 2006;77: 335–405.

70. Gift TL, Haddix AC, Corso PS. Cost-effectiveness analysis. In: Haddix AC, Teutsch SM, Corso PS, eds. *Prevention Effectiveness: A Guide to Decision Analysis and Economic Evaluation.* New York, NY: Oxford University Press;2003:156–177.

71. Dasbach EJ, Teutsch SM. Quality of life. In: Haddix AC, Teutsch SM, Corso PS, eds. *Prevention Effectiveness: A Guide to Decision Analysis and Economic Evaluation.* New York, NY: Oxford University Press;2003:77–91.

72. Max W, Rice DP, Sung H-Y, Michel M. Valuing human life: Estimating the present value of lifetime earnings, 2000. In: *Memio.* Center for Tobacco Control Research and Education, University of California, San Francisco. Available at: http://escholarship.org/uc/item/82d0550k#. Accessed June 13, 2014.

73. Corso PS, Haddix AC. Time effects. In: Haddix AC, Teutsch SM, Corso PS, eds. *Prevention Effectiveness: A Guide to Decision Analysis and Economic Evaluation.* New York, NY: Oxford University Press;2003:92–102.

74. Paxton J. *The Story of Medieval England: From King Arthur to the Tudor Conquest.* Chantilly, VA: The Teaching Company;2010.

75. Blincoe L, Seay A, Zaloshnja E, et al. The economic impact of motor vehicle crashes, 2000. Washington, DC: National Highway Traffic Safety Administration, U.S. Department of Transportation;2002. Report No. DOT HS 809 446.

76. Cullen L. The myth of workers' compensation. *Frontline*. 2000. Available at: http://www.pbs.org/wgbh/pages/frontline/shows/workplace/ect/fraud.html. Accessed March 7, 2014.

77. Michaels D. Fraud in the workers' compensation system: origin and magnitude. *Occup Med.* 1998;13(2):439–442.

78. Atkins WJ. Investigating fraud and insuring compliance in Georgia's workers' compensation system. *Journals.* 2000;12(71). Available at: http://www.deflaw.com/articles/investigating-fraud-and-insuring-compliance-in-georgias-workers-compensation-system. Accessed March 8, 2014.

78a. Gilbert DT, Malone PS. The correspondence bias. *Psychol Bull.* 1995;117(1): 21–38.

79. Kome P. *Wounded Workers: The Politics of Musculoskeletal Injuries.* Buffalo, NY: University of Toronto Press;1998.

80. Massin N, Moulin JJ, Wild P, et al. A study of the prevalence of acute respiratory disorders among workers in the textile industry. *Int Arch Occup Environ Health.* 1991;62(8):555–560.

81. Ringholz RC. *Uranium Frenzy: Saga of the Nuclear West.* Logan, UT: Utah State University Press;2002.

82. Ackerman F, Heinzerling L, Massey R. Applying cost-benefit to past decisions: was environmental protection ever a good idea? *Admin Law Rev.* 2005;57(1): 155–192.

14

Right-to-Know and Privacy

Asked recently whether he [Bill Moyers, Presidential press secretary] had to compromise his principles in his job, Moyers answered that he always followed a rule his father once gave him: "Tell the truth if you can. But don't tell a lie if you can't."

—Robert J. Longood[1]

THE SPERMICIDE NARRATIVE

In January 1976, the Oil, Chemical, and Atomic Workers union (OCAW) distributed a safety and health questionnaire to workers in Occidental Chemical's agricultural chemical department in a plant in Lathrop, California. The plant produced a nematicide called dibromochloropropane (DBCP). In March, the local union asked the national union's safety and health staff to conduct an industrial hygiene survey of the plant. The company's management refused this survey, while an uncomprehended epidemic lurked among the workers.[2] Meanwhile, wives sat on the stands watching their husbands, all of whom worked at a DBCP formulation plant, play baseball at a company ball game. The wives talked. None had been able to conceive babies in the last four years. Then in July, their concerns moved to their husbands, and the first complaints of being unable to father children emerged. Five of the husbands sought medical advice regarding their inability to father children. They were examined by a physician at the University of California and were found to have low sperm counts.[3] Then an examination of 36 of their coworkers indicated that 14 had reduced sperm counts, nine of whom had no sperm.[4] The union submitted a request for a health hazard evaluation (HHE) to the National Institute for Occupational Safety and Health (NIOSH). Of 114 workers exposed at the plant, NIOSH investigators found 38 men to be infertile.[5] At this point in 1977, the company moved to a position of full cooperation.[2] Low sperm counts were also found among DBCP workers at a Dow Chemical plant in Magnolia, Arkansas.[6] Of 86 tested there, 62 were found to be sterile or have very low sperm counts.[5] As a result, the Occupational Safety and Health Administration (OSHA) established a standard for DBCP in 1978.[7]

14.1. INTRODUCTION

Any standard promulgated under this subsection shall prescribe the use of labels or other appropriate forms of warning as are necessary to insure that employees are apprised of all hazards to which they are exposed, relevant symptoms and appropriate emergency treatment, and proper conditions and precautions of safe use or exposure.
    —Section 6(7), Occupational Safety and Health Act of 1970

Knowledge of exposure to hazards is a precondition to the elimination or control of these hazards. Right-to-know carries a dual meaning: an act of knowing and a source of rights. These rights have a social benefit by informing people of potential harm so that they can protect themselves from the harm, and they confer access to information from another party.[8] Right-to-know rules and laws have two purposes: (1) workers and other persons including employers are potentially enabled to act to avoid or limit exposures to toxic substances, and (2) creators, manufacturers, and users of these substances are encouraged to reduce or eliminate these toxic exposures.[9] This encouragement is consistent with the "precautionary principle" as defined and described in Chapter 6.

This chapter addresses the information aspects of the compensating differential argument that claims that workers will demand more compensation for increased exposure to hazards. It explains the rationale for right-to-know laws and rules and the role of warnings in the prevention of occupational injuries and diseases. It describes the evolution and the promulgation of the OSHA Hazard Communication (HazCom) Standard and how the standard grew to extend to all workers. It also describes how the Emergency Planning and Community Right to Know Act of 1986 is potentially helpful to workers and notes the recent integration of the HazCom Standard within the Globally Harmonized System. This chapter also describes the need for training workers about workplace hazards. It explains the information that is acquired through the discovery process prior to a trial, barriers to getting information about hazards and protective measures to workers, and issues regarding workers' privacy.

14.2. THE COMPENSATING DIFFERENTIAL ARGUMENT

The whole of the advantages and disadvantages of the different employments of labor and stock must, in the same neighborhood, be either perfectly equal or continually tending to equality. . . . The wages of labor vary with ease or hardship, the honorableness or dishonorableness of employment.

—Adam Smith[10]

Formulated by Adam Smith in his book *The Wealth of Nations* and advocated by many economists, the compensating differential argument claims that workers will demand more compensation for increased exposure to hazards. Economists that advocate this argument claim that "this wage mechanism leads to efficient levels of job safety and to optimal matchups of jobs and workers."[10] The essence of this argument is that employers will pay workers higher wages for more hazardous jobs in the labor market, which leads to an efficient balance between risk and the costs of control. However, the choices are not altogether financial. Other problems include workers' lack of information and understanding of the risks to life and limb, failings to adequately assign risk in the workers' compensation system, and the acceptance of risk by a worker that omits the social cost of acceptable risk (e.g., the welfare of the worker's family).

In a perfect market, the argument is founded on workers' awareness of the hazards that they face and that they have alternative job choices. The HazCom Standard addresses the first of these foundations, yet OSHA compliance officers routinely find noncompliance with the standard. As for the second foundation, high unemployment makes it difficult to find jobs, let alone switching to alternative jobs that may involve difficult if not impossible changes in location. Moreover, education levels contradict the argument in which higher pay for higher educated workers means that they are employed in safer workplaces than lower paid workers employed in more dangerous workplaces with a lower education.[2] In today's global market, Adam Smith's concept of neighborhood extends worldwide, and workers in thousands if not millions of jobs in developing countries work under extremely hazardous conditions with very low pay; these workers include children. Moreover, in the broader neighborhood of the nation or the world, mobility is a constraint for finding alternative jobs.

Workers typically are unable to "shop" for a safer workplace and must cope with conditions at their current workplace. The "perfect market" argument fails to account for many dimensions of modernity.

14.3. RIGHTS AND DUTIES

One cannot have a meaningful right to information unless someone else has a corresponding duty to provide that information.
—Charles C. Caldart[11]

In the 1980s, legislatures created laws, courts made decisions, and agencies issued rules to inform workers of potential exposures to chemicals that are often beyond detection by human senses. In 1974, NIOSH recommended a standard that employers should inform employees of potentially hazardous materials in the workplace.[12] Eight years later, OSHA promulgated the Haz-Com Standard, and in 1986, Congress passed the Emergency Planning and Community Right to Know Act, extending the right to communities.

Right-to-know is a mandatory sharing of information between management and labor and embodies workplace democracy. One person's right to information corresponds to a duty for someone else to provide the information, thus a worker's right-to-know requires manufacturers and employers to disclose information about hazardous chemicals.[11] The concept of information disclosure entails the provision of all information without request.[13] Caldart divided information transfer into three categories: (1) the duty to generate or retain information, (2) the right of access, and (3) the duty to inform.[11] The right of access depends upon a service in which a request is made for information, and the duty to inform depends upon an employer informing workers of any potential harm. The rights of one party depend upon duties from another party, as indicated in Figure 14-1.

Three conceptual rationales provide the foundation for right-to-know actions: moral, economic, and political.[11] These rationales follow the ethical principles laid out in the *Belmont Report,* written in 1979 by the National

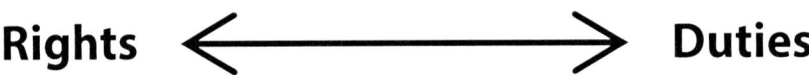

Figure 14-1. The social contract of rights and duties.

Commission for the Protection of Human Subjects of Biomedical and Behavioral Research.[14] Regarding the three conceptual rationales, the principles are respect for (human) persons, beneficence, and justice, which draw from the history of humans used as subjects in experiments.

14.3.1. Moral Rationale—The Autonomous Person

One rationale for right-to-know requirements is the moral perspective. This perspective is like the concept for informed consent in medicine. The principle of respect for persons follows two ethical convictions: first, individuals should be treated as autonomous agents, and second, persons with diminished autonomy are entitled to protection. Employees, as subordinate individuals, are among potentially vulnerable subjects, for they have limited autonomy and are unable to fully appreciate or participate in the consent process. Employees may perceive pressure of job loss, delayed promotion, or other influences by a superior. Vulnerability is more acute when children or pregnant women or decisionally impaired individuals are employed. Informed consent for these individuals involves (1) providing enough information so that a "reasonable" person can decide to participate (in a job with potential hazards) without deception; (2) providing the information in an organized, interactive, and timely way so that it is comprehended; and (3) accenting free of coercion (i.e., an overt threat of harm intentionally presented in order to gain compliance).[14]

14.3.2. Economic Rationale—Perfect Competition

The virtues of free enterprise are present when the checks and balances of perfect competition are complete. Adam Smith established perfect competition as the principle for the market economy in *The Wealth of Nations*, in which he described the principle of the "invisible hand." He claimed that

> every individual endeavors to employ his capital so that its produce may be of greatest value. He generally neither intends to promote the public interest, nor knows how much he is promoting it. He intends only his own security, only his own gain. And he is in this led by an "invisible hand" to promote an end, which was no part of his intention. By pursuing his own interest he frequently promotes that of society more effectively than when he really intends to promote it.[15]

Free market tenets provide the economic rationale for right-to-know, in which the provision of perfect information is a market-correcting mechanism. Right-to-know rules and laws seek to improve decision making in the marketplace. Classic economic theory, in which perfect competition exists, relies upon free access to "perfect" information regarding choices in the market. History has shown that workers lack perfect information about their job. Right-to-know initiatives seek to inform a worker about potential harm in the workplace, yet they also aim to create information about harm where that information was absent before. With this information, as the market theory goes, the worker will be better able to make a rational decision about whether to refuse to take a hazardous job or to change jobs. Nonetheless, the worker needs bargaining power to exercise these decisions.[11]

Ours is not an economy of perfect competition since it has a mix of government and private enterprise and a mixed system of competition and monopoly, and right-to-know regulation is needed to move toward perfect competition.[15] Consistent with the economic rationale is the concept of nudges, which is a regulatory approach that provides for freedom of choice without commanding people to do anything. Nudges include required disclosures that have a high potential benefit with a low cost and provide for high personal liberty.[16] Nevertheless, nudges are criticized as unethical since they may covertly manipulate an individual's behavior.

The principle of beneficence is applied to risk and benefits assessments. As a metaphor, the application of this principle to the workplace entails gathering systematic and comprehensive information about work. For the employer, it means assurance of an inherently safe job design. The term "risk" refers to a possibility that harm may occur both in probability and in severity. The term "benefit" refers to something of positive value related to health or welfare. Risks and benefits may affect individual persons, their families, or special groups in society.[14]

14.3.3. Political Rationale—Empowerment

The principle of justice relates to fairness in distribution. Under this principle, a benefit to which an individual is entitled should not be denied without good reason nor should a burden be imposed unduly.[14] The benefit of right-to-know is about empowerment and has the potential to become more effective at preventing harm as workers have more potential to exercise a right to act under right-to-know rules and laws.[11]

Workers have the right to refuse work under the Occupational Safety and Health Act (OSHAct, 1970) and the National Labor Relations Act (NLRA) of 1935. In establishing the right to refuse hazardous work, these statutes also protect the individual against reprisals through antidiscrimination remedies.[11] Organized workers have the right to strike under the NLRA rather than be exposed to abnormally dangerous conditions.[17]

14.3.4. Failure to Warn

The 1973 asbestos-related liability case, *Clarence Borel v. Fibreboard Paper Products Corporation, et al.*, was a jolt to the chemical manufacturing industry. In the ruling in this case, the 5th Circuit Court of Appeals (New Orleans) established liability for chemical producers for failure to warn workers of hazards. As a result, chemical manufacturers initiated voluntary labeling of their products, and they produced and distributed an early form of material safety data sheets (MSDSs). The court expressed the following points in its ruling, as paraphrased by Morse in 1998:[18]

1. If there is a failure to warn users of the hazards, then the product is unreasonably dangerous, even where there are benefits from the product.
2. The manufacturer is held to the knowledge and skill of an expert. The manufacturer has to keep up with current information and also has the duty to test the product.
3. The manufacturer may be liable to warn the ultimate consumer, unless an intermediary interferes (e.g., destroying the label).
4. Misuse by the consumer, such as not wearing a dust mask when told to do so, would result in no damages being awarded.
5. The warning must take into account the severity of the result. The court said, "The admonition that a worker should 'avoid breathing the dust' is black humor: there was no way for insulation workers to avoid breathing asbestos dust."[18]

14.4. WARNINGS

Contrary to common understanding, the history of warnings is perhaps most influenced by the needs of industry to maximize profit, not the desire to promote safety.

—David Egilman and Susanna Rankin Bohme[19]

Let us worry about the basics and not think about what we might do in the "Land of Oz."

—Richard Berman[18]

In the filming of the 1939 movie *The Wizard of Oz,* Margaret Hamilton played the Wicked Witch of the West, and as she left a scene in billows of smoke and fire, she suffered second- and third-degree burns. She endured pain as the film crew used alcohol to wipe away the green makeup of copper oxide from her face and hands so that her burns could be treated. Copper oxide is an explosive under certain conditions and toxic if inhaled or ingested. She was able to return to the set six weeks later; but that was not the only hazard in filming *The Wizard of Oz.* Buddy Ebsen was cast to play the Tin Man in the movie until he was coated with aluminum dust. He had an allergic reaction from inhaling the dust and nearly died. Another actor, Jack Haley, took his place, but this time, aluminum paste was painted onto him to avoid inhalation of the dust. Haley was not informed of Ebsen's reaction to the aluminum dust. Haley suffered an infection in one eye after the paste was applied, but doctors were able to intervene before serious eye damage occurred.[18]

In the hazard control hierarchy, the first priority is to design out or eliminate the hazard, the second priority is to guard against the hazard, and the third priority is to warn against the hazard.[20] The purpose of warnings is twofold. First, warnings are intended to reduce or prevent injuries, health problems, and property damage; the second purpose is to communicate safety-related information to a target audience so that they can influence their behavior with informed decisions for their safety (i.e., a right-to-know).[21] However, a litigious purpose may compromise these two purposes of warnings. Warnings may take on a legal defense position that can be used to counter liability suits with the argument that the victim was warned. Such warnings may proliferate on a machine with labels or clutter operator manuals with information that may not be readable or lack priority for safety.[22]

The New York State legislature required the first signal word of "poison" conspicuously displayed on containers of any substance or liquid known to be a poison in 1829.[23] Today, warning labels and signs based on American National Standards Institute (ANSI) Z535 standards have a precedence of signal words indicating a level of hazard: "danger," "warning," and "caution" (in all-capital letters). The implication of the associated description of the signal words is "shall" (meaning mandatory), "should" (meaning advisory), and "may" (meaning permissive), respectively. The first two signal words—"danger" and "warning"—should not be used for property damage, whereas "caution" can be used for property damage. The signal words are defined below.[24]

Danger: Indicates an imminently hazardous situation, which, if not avoided, will result in death or serious injury. This signal word is to be limited to the most extreme situations.

Warning: Indicates a potentially hazardous situation, which, if not avoided, could result in death or serious injury.

Caution: Indicates a potentially hazardous situation, which, if not avoided, may result in minor or moderate injury. It may also be used to alert against unsafe practices.

Warnings are important when attended to and comprehended by a worker at risk. However, there are technology-based warning devices that inherently demand the attention of a worker. These may be audible or visual devices that include backup alarms on off-road vehicles or proximity alarms on cranes to warn of electrical current. Technology can also be useful for informing workers of potential hazards to others, such as video cameras and proximity alarms on heavy equipment that warn of personnel or vehicles that are out of normal sight from an operator's station.

14.5. HAZARD COMMUNICATION

We've got young people here who don't have any family . . . everyone was having trouble having kids. No one was using contraceptives; none of the wives were on the pill. The sad thing is that we didn't get to it earlier. We just talked about it a lot. I guess that we knew we were sterile even before they took the tests.

—A worker at the Lathrop DBCP plant[25]

The HazCom Standard is the primary worker right-to-know rule promulgated under the OSH Act. After a recommended standard in 1974 by NIOSH, OSHA began developing the standard in 1977 and proposed a standard in January 1981 at the end of the Carter administration. However, President Ronald Reagan withdrew the proposal, but with chemical industry pressure his administration proposed its own rule in March 1982 and promulgated the final rule in November 1983. The standard required employers to inform employees of potentially hazardous materials in the workplace.[12] The standard emphasized providing information about risks, but it also provided instructions about how to avoid the risks. The standard came in two steps. The first step required manufacturers or importers of chemical materials to evaluate the safety of these materials and inform employers who purchased the material of the safety of the materials. The second step required employers to inform their employees of the hazards of chemicals with which they worked.[26]

14.5.1. A Recommended Standard

In 1972, NIOSH conducted a National Occupational Hazard Survey that found that chemical identification was nearly impossible when trade names were used, some of which were composed of products that were also identified with trade names. The institute followed this study with its criteria document and recommended a standard to OSHA for an Identification System for Occupationally Hazardous Materials in 1974.[18]

In response to the NIOSH recommended standard, OSHA convened a standards advisory committee to consider the NIOSH recommendation. The committee was composed of four employee representatives, four employer representatives, and three federal agency representatives: NIOSH, the U.S. Environmental Protection Agency (EPA), and the U.S. Department of Transportation (DoT). The employer representatives brought more resources to the table than the employee representatives. Of the employer representatives, C. Boyd Shaffer, representing American Cyanamid, shifted the consideration from the NIOSH recommendation to several working documents from chemical manufacturing companies. The employer-dominated proceedings led to the following arguments:[18]

1. The OSHAct does not sanction the requirement for MSDSs and, if they are provided, they should go to the employer and not the employees.
2. The U.S. Chamber of Commerce representative "bristled" at the suggestion that the label and MSDS should include the manufacturer's phone number as a contact in the event of an emergency, claiming that the OSHAct did not require this information.
3. There should be a performance-based system founded on hazards and symptoms and not a listing of maximum exposure levels, and it should be limited to the chemicals covered by the interim OSHA/NIOSH standards.
4. Laboratories and intermediate chemicals should not be covered by a standard.
5. Trade secrets should be protected.
6. Some plants would be forced to close.

In the meantime, the Manufacturers Chemists Association (now the Chemical Manufacturers Association) proposed and was able to establish the basis of a voluntary standard through ANSI. At congressional hearings in 1978, the Manufacturers Chemists Association claimed that there were no negative votes for the standard based upon 26 entities contacted, most of which were industry parties. Two unions that were approached rejected the approval of the ANSI standard. NIOSH was contacted and did not vote for it, which the association counted as an abstention.[18] The NIOSH policy from its beginning was to depend upon the science and not on a vote for consensus. Indeed, such misrepresentations led later to NIOSH declining to participate in consensus standards organizations.

In 1977, OSHA issued an Advance Notice of Rulemaking. Of the 49 responses to this notice, 59% were from chemical manufacturers, 24% were from chemical users, and 14% were from companies that claimed exemption because they were covered by DoT rules. Chemical manufacturers claimed that the proposed rule was impractical or not legally justified. They also claimed economic hardships such as increased workers' compensation claims, companies going out of business, and a lack of a cost-benefit analysis. Conversely, one company claimed a need for the standard since it was already warning its customers of hazards so that its competitors would be required to do likewise. However, chemical users differed from the producers, for they had a need-to-know about the chemical constituents from a manufacturing perspective. While only 43% of chemical producers favored the standard, 82% of chemical users supported the standard.[18]

The Public Citizen (a consumer advocacy organization begun by Ralph Nader, i.e., the people's voice) response countered arguments that chemical names would confuse workers with the argument that unions needed to know the chemicals so as to protect their members and the workers needed to know the chemical to which they were exposed so as to be able to request intervention by OSHA or NIOSH. The interventions included requesting a standard, an OSHA inspection, or an HHE from NIOSH.[18]

In January 1981, OSHA issued its "Proposed Labeling Standard" as President Jimmy Carter was leaving office. The first act of President Reagan's incoming Secretary of Labor, Raymond Donovan, was to withdraw the proposed standard.[18]

14.5.2. The Imperative

As early as the 1950s, industry-sponsored studies had found reproductive toxicity from DBCP in laboratory animals.[2] "The findings remained confidential until they were published in a scientific journal in 1961, and then were largely ignored until the furor broke out sixteen years later."[2] A National Cancer Institute study published in 1973 reported that DBCP was carcinogenic.[27]

On August 5, 1977, the OCAW union requested that NIOSH conduct an HHE at the Occidental Chemical company plant in Lathrop to investigate abnormally low sperm counts in a number of workers. Four days later, NIOSH conducted a walk-through at the plant and met with the physician, Dr. M. Donald Whorton at the University of California, Berkeley, who had examined the workers. The NIOSH investigators and Whorton conducted examinations of several other workers from the plant, at which 38 of 114 exposed workers were found to be affected. Occidental terminated production of DBCP at its plant. As investigations expanded, one-third of 432 exposed workers in Arkansas, California, and Colorado were found to be infertile.[5]

On August 12, 1977, OSHA informed approximately 80 manufacturers and formulators via telegram of the potential reproductive hazard of DBCP, and NIOSH requested information from DBCP manufacturers and formulators on August 19 so as to fully evaluate the extent of the hazard of exposure to DBCP. On August 23, OSHA issued guidelines that detailed work practices to these companies, and on the same day OCAW asked OSHA to issue an emergency temporary standard, which it issued on September 19, 1978, at a press conference that included EPA and the U.S. Food and Drug Administration. On November 1, OSHA proposed a permanent standard, and NIOSH issued a recommended standard with supporting criteria to OSHA in January 1978. The permanent standard went into effect in April 1978. No company sued OSHA over the standard, which is unique in OSHA's regulatory history.[4]

The DBCP experience spawned the right-to-know movement. In 1981, the city of Philadelphia passed the first community right-to-know ordinance. From 1981 to mid-1983, between 2,000 and 3,000 requests were received in Philadelphia under this ordinance, about half of them relating to air emissions. By mid-1983, 15 states or communities had passed right-to know statutes.[28] Industry opposed these laws because of inconsistency in their information requirements. Industry supported an OSHA HazCom standard so as to preempt conflicting state and local laws. This industry support for the HazCom standard explains the standard's success in promulgation during the antiregulatory years of the Reagan administration. Industry also opposed community right-to-know laws, which were part of many of the state and local worker right-to-know laws.

14.5.3. Expansion Beyond the Chemical Industry

The original standard was limited to employers in the chemical manufacturing sector. However, in 1985, the United Steelworkers of America[29] brought suit against the administrator of OSHA, contending that the standard should not be limited to this sector, and the judge for the 3rd Circuit Court of Appeals (Philadelphia) found that OSHA must extend the standard to all workers potentially exposed to hazardous chemicals. As a result, OSHA revised the standard in 1987 to cover all workers within its jurisdiction.[12]

14.5.4. Labeling and Material Safety Data Sheets

The use of labels can be traced back to the 9th century BC, when container seals in South Asia indicated the contents of the containers.[28] As referred to earlier, New York State required the signal word "poison" in all-capital letters on containers in 1829.[22] In 1906, Upton Sinclair's novel *The Jungle* described unsanitary working conditions in Chicago's meatpacking plants, which led to Congress passing the Meat Inspection Act and the Pure Food and Drug Act of 1906. The latter act was the first national labeling law in the United States. It did not require labeling, but if labels were used, they needed to include ingredients, proportions, and quantity. The Insecticides Act was passed in 1910 with labeling requirements, which defined the crimes of adulteration and mislabeling. In 1927, Congress passed the Federal Caustic Poison Act, which required the labeling of 12 substances with the word "poison" in all-capital letters. The Federal Hazardous Substances Labeling Act of 1960 moved from regulating specific substances to requiring labels on categories of substances.[28]

In order to ensure chemical safety in the workplace, information must be available about the identities and hazards of the chemicals. The OSHAct provided for labeling in each of its promulgated permanent standards and, under the HazCom standard, labeling had to bring together scientific information with communication theory.[26]

Manufacturers and importers are required to assess potential exposures, understand the possible effects of complex mixtures, and explain the risks for which precautionary information is to be printed. The HazCom standard requires chemical manufacturers and importers to evaluate the hazards of the chemicals and prepare not only labels but also MSDSs to convey the hazard information to their downstream customers. All employers with hazardous chemicals in their workplaces must have labels and MSDSs for their exposed workers and train them to handle the chemicals appropriately.

14.6. COMMUNITY RIGHT-TO-KNOW

The sad fact is that when our government is faced with a choice between public health and private gain, it almost invariably sides with private gain unless it's forced to do otherwise. And that just reflects the enormous power that these vested interests have over our legislators and politicians. And I think that the only way this changes is if people get educated enough, aroused enough and start a movement that changes the balance of power.

—Dr. Andrew Weil[30]

Many state and local right-to-know laws preceded federal right-to-know laws. Occupational health advocates such as OCAW and committees on occupational safety and health led the drive for passage of the Emergency Planning and Community Right-to-Know Act (EPCRA) of 1986 and the establishment therein of the Toxics Release Inventory (TRI).[31] These advocates had influenced the passage of 25 worker right-to-know and 18 community right-to-know laws in 29 states in addition to some municipal laws. These were the first laws that provided workers and citizens with the right to be informed of toxic chemicals to which they were potentially exposed. The variety of requirements across the nation led chemical manufacturers to support a national standard by OSHA so as to preempt the various state and local laws. In 1983, OSHA stated its intent that the HazCom Standard should preempt state and local workplace laws so as to "reduce the regulatory burden posed by multiple state laws."[12]

In 1985, the New Jersey State Chamber of Commerce brought suit to establish preemption of New Jersey's stringent law in its entirety, including its community right-to-know sections.[32] The court found that the OSHA rule did not preempt the New Jersey environmental hazard warning system.[33] A similar case in Pennsylvania brought by the Manufacturer's Association of Tri-County came to the same result.[34]

Two chemical incidents, one in Bhopal, India, in 1984, and another in Institute, West Virginia, in 1985, drove Congress to go beyond OSHA's action and pass EPCRA. The incident in Bhopal involved a release of methyl isocyanate at Union Carbide's pesticide manufacturing facility that immediately killed 4,000 people and another 4,000 in the weeks that followed. Then, eight months later a similar but much less tragic incident occurred in West Virginia that injured 100 Kanawah Valley residents. As a result, OSHA initiated a special emphasis program aimed at inspections of large chemical manufacturing facilities on November 4, 1985, followed by the EPA announcing its Chemical Emergency Preparedness Program two weeks later. Following these releases, the U.S. public demanded the protection of communities from similar incidents. States and localities followed suit with a plethora of pollution disclosure rules. Congress capitalized on the fervor in 1986 by enacting EPCRA, modeled on the HazCom Standard.[35,36]

Congress included EPCRA as Title III in its amendments to the Superfund Amendment and Reauthorization Act of 1986. It is a comprehensive federal community right-to-know law that, though not aimed at worker protection, workers can nonetheless use to gain access to chemical information reported locally by their employer or to evaluate the presence of chemicals at potential worksites. Four major requirements are embodied in EPCRA:[12]

1. All facilities that manufacture, use, or store certain extremely hazardous substances above a certain quantity must report a suspected leak of the substance to state and local commissions established under EPCRA that are responsible for emergency response.
2. Facilities covered by the OSHA HazCom Standard must provide MSDSs to the local county and city commissions and fire departments.
3. Many facilities are required to submit an inventory and the location of hazardous chemicals on the premises.
4. Manufacturers of these chemicals are required to submit an annual report to the EPA of routine releases of the substances.

The Pollution Prevention Act of 1990 amended EPCRA. This amendment requires facilities that submit the annual report of toxics substance releases to also report their source reduction and waste management practices as part of the report.[9] This requirement also has the potential to protect workers through a policy of toxics reduction.

14.7. GLOBALLY HARMONIZED SYSTEM OF CLASSIFICATION AND LABELING OF CHEMICALS

A globally harmonized hazard classification and compatible labeling system, including material safety data sheets and easily understandable symbols, should be available, if feasible, by the year 2000.

—United Nations[37]

In May 2012, OSHA promulgated regulations that require all hazardous substances to be labeled according to new international standards, called the Globally Harmonized System (GHS). The United Nations adopted GHS in 2002. This system established standards for three groupings that determine health, physical, and environmental hazards associated with chemical exposure. The system includes requirements for labeling and (material) safety data sheets (SDSs).[38]

The labeling requirements include standardized pictograms such as that shown in Figure 14-2, the "skull and crossbones" label that states: "Fatal if inhaled, swallowed, or in contact with skin." The requirements also include signal words such as "danger" or "warning," and harmonized label elements for each class within each group and category within each class. An example of a class within the health hazard group is "acute toxicity."

The SDS standard provides a uniform format for presenting a sequence of safety information in 16 sections, consistent with ANSI Z400.1 and related

Note: Border is red.

Figure 14-2. Occupational Safety and Health Administration skull-and-crossbones pictogram based on the Globally Harmonized System.

International Organization for Standardization (ISO) standards. International companies were already adopting the ISO standards.[38] The 16 sections of the SDS as adopted by OSHA are shown in Table 14-1 over a transition period from December 2013 and to 2015.

14.8. TRAINING

We have learned that safety and health training efforts must convey complex information on toxicity, safe work practices, and control measures in a way that is useful and understandable.

—Joseph Hughes[39]

If ignorance of specific job hazards and of proper work practices is even partly to blame for higher injury rates, then training is an important part of the HazCom Standard and right-to-know rationales. Furthermore, training workers is an important adjunct to other protective measures for occupational safety and health. This importance of training is amplified since OSHA is unable to inspect but a comparatively small number of millions of workplaces. Some workplaces are dynamic in time and location, such as construction, farm work, and transportation. Accordingly, OSHA follows a strategy of encouraging training as an essential part of every employer's safety and health program for protecting workers from injuries and illnesses.[10] The agency's policy is that employee training must be presented in a manner that employees can understand.

14.8.1. Occupational Safety and Health

Many standards require the employer to train employees in the safety and health aspects of their jobs, while other standards hold employers responsible for limiting certain jobs to employees who are "certified," "competent," or "qualified" based on special previous training. The term "designated" personnel means being qualified to perform specific duties. The HazCom Standard requires that employers train their workers about the potential exposure to hazardous chemicals, precautions to take, how to avoid the exposure, and how to respond to an incident.

Regardless of the regulatory language, the terms "train" and "instruct" mean that employees receiving information are capable of understanding so that they can perform work in a safe and healthful manner in compliance with the OSHA standards. Employers need to provide safety and health training to

Table 14-1. Globally Harmonized System (Material) Safety Data Sheet as Adopted by the Occupational Safety and Health Administration

SDS Headings	Content
1. Identification of the substance or mixture and of the supplier	GHS product identifier, other means of identification, recommended use of the chemical and restrictions on use, supplier's details, and emergency phone number
2. Hazards identification	Classification and label elements and other hazards that do not result in classification (e.g., dust explosion hazard)
3. Composition/information on ingredients	Substance: Chemical identity, common name, synonyms, etc., CAS number, EC number, etc., and impurities and stabilizing additives Mixture: The chemical identity and concentration or concentration ranges of all ingredients that are hazardous
4. First aid measures	Description of necessary measures (i.e., inhalation, skin and eye contact, and ingestion), most important acute and delayed symptoms or effects, immediate medical attention and special treatment needed
5. Firefighting measures	Suitable and unsuitable extinguishing media, specific hazards arising from the chemical, special protective equipment, and precautions
6. Accidental release measures	Protective equipment and emergency procedures, environmental precautions, methods and materials for containment and cleaning up
7. Handling and storage	Precautions for safe handling, safe storage conditions
8. Exposure controls/personal protection	Control parameters (e.g., PELs), engineering controls, individual protection measures (e.g., PPE)
9. Physical and chemical properties	Appearance, odor and odor threshold, pH, melting and freezing point, initial boiling point and boiling range, flash point, evaporation rate, flammability, upper/lower flammability or explosive limits, vapor pressure and density, relative density, solubility, partition coefficient, autoignition and/or decomposition temperature
10. Stability and reactivity	Chemical stability, possibility of hazardous reactions, conditions to avoid, incompatible materials, hazardous decomposition products
11. Toxicological information	Description of the toxicological effects and the available data used to identify those effects
12. Ecological information	Ecotoxicity, persistence and degradability, bioaccumulative potential, mobility in soil,* other adverse effects
13. Disposal considerations	Description of waste residues and information on their safe handling and methods of disposal
14. Transport information	Precautions that a user needs to be aware of or needs to comply with in connection with transport or conveyance either within or outside the premises
15. Regulatory information	Regulations specific to the product in question
16. Other information	Information on the preparation and revision of the SDS

Note: SDS = Safety Data Sheet; GHS = Globally Harmonizing System; CAS = Chemical Abstracts Service; EC = European Community; PELs = permissible exposure limits; PPE = personal protective equipment.

Source: Monroe et al.[38]

*May also be a source of occupational exposure such as carbon monoxide migration from blasting through the soil into tunnels or up into buildings.

the employees at the same vocabulary level or in a language other than English in the same manner as they communicate work instructions or other information to them. Employers may also teach English to non-English-speaking employees. Some standards require verification of "acquired" knowledge and skills from the training.

OSHA compliance officer investigations focus on training as a part of the HazCom Standard.[26] OSHA's training guidelines follow a model that even small employers can use.[40] The model consists of the following:

1. Determine if training is needed: Problems can arise from lack of knowledge of a work process, unfamiliarity with equipment, or incorrect execution of a task.
2. Identify training needs:
   - Use company records to identify how injuries occur and how to prevent them.
   - Request employees to provide their descriptions of jobs in their own words.
   - Observe employees as they perform tasks, ask about the work, and record their answers.
   - Examine similar training programs offered by other companies or from other sources.
3. Identify goals and objectives: Determine unnecessary training and set learning objectives.
4. Develop learning activities: Be able to demonstrate the learned knowledge and skills on the job.
5. Conduct the training: Train in a clear, unambiguous manner; motivate the employees to pay attention; have employees demonstrate their knowledge and skills.
6. Evaluate program effectiveness: Evaluate training through student feedback, instructor observations, and workplace improvements.
7. Improve the program: Drop what is known and unnecessary, correct what was confusing or distracting, and add what was missing from the program and what was learned or failed to be learned.

The agency offers training courses and educational programs to broaden worker and employer knowledge on the recognition, avoidance, and prevention of safety and health hazards in their workplaces. It also offers training and educational materials for businesses to train their workers: Through the

Outreach Training Program and the OSHA Training Institute, OSHA offers classes that include 10-hour and 30-hour courses and provides training materials for workers and employers. The OSHA Training Institute provides training and education for federal and state compliance officers, state consultants, other federal agency personnel, and the private sector. The agency's Susan Harwood Training Grant Program (formerly the New Directions Program) awards grants to nonprofit organizations to develop training and educational programs and train and educate workers and employers.

14.8.2. Mine Safety and Health

The Mine Safety and Health Administration (MSHA) delivers training through the National Mine Health and Safety Academy in Beckley, West Virginia; its Educational Field Services program; and its Small Mine Office. The agency also administers a state grants program to supplement mining health and safety programs at the state level and other competitive grants that target studies of specific mine safety and health problems. In addition, a unit evaluates qualifications and issues regarding certifications for instructors and miners.[41]

The mission of the academy is to reduce injuries and fatalities and improve health conditions in the mining industry through education and training. The academy conducts education and training programs and provides for hands-on training for MSHA inspectors and mining industry personnel.

In response to requests from the mining industry, MSHA created the Educational Field Services in 1998 to assist in developing mine safety and health programs. This service is located in 24 states, and its staff travel extensively to mines and training centers to assist in developing mine health and safety programs. The service also works closely with MSHA district enforcement offices to identify industry needs and assist individual mines with safety and health issues.

Mines employing five or fewer employees represent about 50% of all U.S. mining operations. From 2000 to 2002, the incidence of fatalities at these mines was about two and a half times greater than at larger mines.[42] These operations typically are unable to employ full-time safety and health professionals. Consequently, in October 2002, MSHA created the Small Mine Office to help small operations develop and improve safety and health programs tailored specifically to the needs of the miners in the operations.

In 1916, The Joseph A. Holmes Safety Association was formed and named after the first director of the Bureau of Mines. The association has a national council, state councils, district councils, and local chapters. Its aim is to prevent fatalities and injuries and to improve health and safety among officials and workers in all phases of mining, and consistent with this aim, it publishes a periodical bulletin. The MSHA is also a participant in association activities.

14.8.3. Hazardous Waste Work

The Superfund Amendments and Reauthorization Act of 1986 gave the National Institute of Environmental Health Sciences (NIEHS) the responsibility for initiating the Worker Education and Training Program through a grants process. The aim of this program is to fund nonprofit organizations that have a record of delivering quality occupational safety and health training to workers involved in handling hazardous substances or responding to emergency releases of hazardous materials.[42] These awards are made under the following program areas:

1. Hazardous Waste Worker Training Program
2. HazMat Disaster Preparedness Training Program
3. Minority Worker Training Program
4. Nuclear Weapons Cleanup Training Program (a U.S. Department of Energy program)

The Worker Education and Training Program has awarded grants to 20 organizations that support the training and education of workers engaged in activities related to hazardous materials and waste generation, removal, containment, transportation, and emergency response. The U.S. Department of Health and Human Services (DHHS), which includes the National Institutes of Health and its NIEHS, is a signatory to the National Response Plan, a single and comprehensive framework for the management of domestic incidents under the U.S. Department of Homeland Security. It provides for the coordination of federal support to state, local, and tribal incident managers and for the exercise of direct federal authorities and responsibilities. Under the plan's Worker Safety and Health Annex, OSHA may activate NIEHS to provide:

- Technical training for instructional staff, curriculum development experts, subject-matter experts, and professional staff.
- Safety training to worker target populations with respect to the nature and location of the incident and the particular hazards.

- Assistance and support in the development and delivery of site-specific health and safety training through appropriately qualified Worker Education and Training Program awardee instructional staff.
- Assistance such as respirator fit-testing and distribution of PPE.

14.9. DISCOVERY

If you once forfeit the confidence of your fellow citizens, you can never regain their respect and esteem. It is true that you may fool all of the people some of the time; you can even fool some of the people all of the time; but you can't fool all of the people all of the time.

—President Abraham Lincoln, 1865

The judicial system offers the last line of defense in protecting a worker's safety and health by way of seeking restitution for an injury. To resolve civil disputes in tort law, discovery is a right-to-know step that follows a plaintiff's complaint and defendant's response to assure that the case is decided on its merits rather than the rhetorical skills of the attorneys. The judge establishes a period of time in which the parties engage in the discovery of evidence that is pertinent to the case. The process helps level the field between rich and poor contenders in the case, since the expense is not exorbitant. Serious penalties can result from the lack of compliance with discovery procedures. The Federal Rules of Civil Procedure—and similar state rules—allow parties to obtain discovery regarding any matter relevant to the subject of the impending action.[43] Privileged material is not subject to discovery and includes the work products of the attorneys and information protected by attorney-client, doctor-patient, and priest-penitent privilege. The tools used in discovery include depositions, interrogatories, requests for production of documents and objects, physical and mental examinations, and requests for admission. These tools are described below:

- A deposition is testimony by a person who is examined under oath out of court by a party to the court. Most depositions are oral, but they can be written. Depositions are typically recorded by a certified court reporter, can also be video-recorded, and can be shown before a jury.
- Interrogatories are written questions issued by one party to be answered in writing by another party under oath. Interrogatories may be used to gain names of witnesses and the location of documents that may be used as evidence.

- A request for production is a request for documents and things for either specific materials or physical inspection of the documents.
- If the physical or mental condition of a party is at issue, the judge can order an examination of that person.
- A request of admission is the final discovery tool, which is a written request to admit certain facts or opinions, which avoids the necessity of proving the matter at trial.

14.10. LEGAL RESTRICTIONS ON INFORMATION DISCLOSURE

The corporate notion of "freedom" means a "freedom to" act without constraint even though it may cause serious harm to others. By the terms of the corporate "freedom to" model, all that matters is the unbridled freedom of the acting party. The freedom that a potential victim prizes, however, is of another sort entirely. Victims care most about "freedom from" harm; it is a defensive freedom. They seek to preserve certain elemental rights such as personal safety, good health, and the right to make informed decisions in the marketplace.

—David Bollier and Joan Claybrook[7]

Trade secrets are one form of restricting the disclosure of information, which regulatory agencies must address in rule making and enforcement. However, the judicial system also restricts a lot of information from disclosure through secret settlements. Moreover, in the process of litigation, the judge may deny an expert the opportunity of presenting testimony before a jury because of a *Daubert* challenge (explicated in 14.10.3 below), which may be either justified or ill informed.

14.10.1. Trade Secrets

The NLRA provides that unions can negotiate "wages, hours, and other terms and conditions of employment." The National Labor Relations Board, established by this act, and the federal courts addressed whether employers were required to disclose toxic-related information under the act but left unresolved two important issues: (1) if and how employers are required to substantiate their claims of trade secret protection, and (2) and what degree of disclosure is required if the claim is substantiated.

A trade secret is information that includes a formula, pattern, compilation, program device, method, technique, or process that derives independent economic value from not being generally known or readily ascertainable to other persons who can obtain economic value from its disclosure or use. Federal laws regarding trade secrets depend on state laws and establish criminal liability for federal agents who expose these secrets. While patents and trademarks are open to the public, trade secrets are protected by not disclosing the secret to the public.[12]

Soon after the OSHAct was passed, employers were required to inform workers of overexposure to the substances for which interim standards were established under § 6(a) of that act. However, employers had difficulty in complying with this provision of the standards since they were uninformed of the ingredients in the materials that they were using, knowing only their trade names. Without knowledge of the chemical constituents of these materials, the employers, indeed OSHA compliance officers, were ill informed as to what to sample for at workplaces. Many materials were shielded behind a veil of trade names, which many manufacturers claimed were trade secrets. In its 1972 National Occupational Hazard Survey, NIOSH was able to identify chemical constituents in only 5% of 200,000 trade name products. In the NIOSH request for information regarding trade name chemicals, it received 8,970 responses, and of these responses 35% claimed trade secret protection; of the 1,440 chemicals named in these claims, 46% contained substances covered by OSHA regulations.[18]

OSHA addressed the trade secret issue in the HazCom Standard, recognizing a balance between disclosure and a trade secret claim, but with a policy that workers' health takes primacy in the decision regarding disclosure.[44] An employer can claim a trade secret when it can support the claim. However, chemical ingredients of general knowledge in an industry or if disclosed by the goods one markets cannot be claimed as a trade secret. Indeed, if someone can reverse-engineer a trade secret through the trade literature, the claim for a trade secret fails. Even when a hazardous chemical is claimed as a trade secret, the PEL, threshold limit value, or other designated exposure limits, as well as properties and effects of the hazardous ingredients, must be included on an MSDS.[12] The EPCRA provides for trade secret protection if the following four factors are satisfied:[36]

1. The information has not been disclosed to any persons other than pertinent federal, state, and local individuals, and reasonable measures continue to be taken to protect its confidentiality.

2. The information is not required to be disclosed or otherwise available.
3. The disclosure of the information is not likely to cause substantial harm to the competitive position of the claimant.
4. If the information is chemical identity information, the chemical identity is not readily discoverable through reverse engineering.

A less recognized challenge to a trade secret is that no legitimate need exists to protect a product or service that hurts people. If the secret represents a dangerous product, then no one else will emulate it since it is defective, and thus there is no trade secret to protect. This recognition is based on the interest of public safety and health, not any privacy interests regarding trade secrets.[45]

14.10.2. Secret Settlements

About 97% of litigation in this country terminates in settlements negotiated by contesting parties, and there is a long-standing practice of sealing court records in these cases. Sealed court records include evidence obtained through pre-settlement agreements. The practice has become the focus of increasing controversy—and scrutiny—at local, state, and federal levels because it can limit access to information about harmful products. It is a practice that limits accountability to the public, and, in the view of some, it erodes public justice. Judges approve the terms of the settlement on behalf of the public, but the terms of those agreements can be withheld from the public, including the public interest for safety and health.[46]

Since 1938, federal rules have allowed judges to deny a request to seal a record, but the vast majority of judges agree to settlements given the demands on their time, the cost of a trial, and the litigants' agreement to settle. Moreover, judges may also encourage settlements between the litigants. Thus, the majority of judges regularly approve secret settlements and grant protective orders without an inquiry into the public's interest. Even though dockets are trimmed, justice may not be done.[46]

Settlement is the civil analogue of plea bargaining in criminal cases. While courts sometimes reserve the right to publicize a sealed record or settlement if the need arises, sealed records and settlements normally remain permanently sequestered from all nonparties. During litigation, parties frequently ask courts to seal records that contain potentially damaging or embarrassing information. A plaintiff may not want to expose medical records, a plaintiff's attorney may want a certain return on litigation cost with a settlement rather than an uncertain result from a jury, and a defendant may agree to settle on the condition that the court seal the records, which may include embarrassing documents exposed during discovery or through deposition, criminal culpability, or cause for additional and broader liability.[46] Moreover, a plaintiff may benefit from a settlement when faced with a long and litigious process before going to trial.

Advocates for settlements claim that secrecy is vital to the fluidity and viability of the courts, emphasizing that secrecy as an incentive to settle and the lack of secrecy can lead to public disclosure of embarrassing or financially injurious information with no bearing on public health and safety. A counterargument claims a presumption of universal access to all judicial records, which are the result of a public judicial process. A more limited counterargument is that settlements affecting public safety and health should be prohibited from sealing based upon a right of access to information with implications for public safety and health. In support of the argument for public safety and health is a long list of settlements that include the infamous Johns-Manville asbestos settlement, the Agent Orange settlement, and the Firestone/Ford Explorer settlement. Proponents of open information argue that if these and other settlements had been subject to the sunshine of universal access, they would have revealed significant dangers to the public and saved countless lives. Asbestos exposures led to the deaths of thousands per year, and more recently, the Ford Explorer and Firestone tires settlement, in which records were sealed for years and was followed by the death of 271 people and serious injury to an additional 800 victims.[46]

The need for legislative reform mandating the judiciary to take an active role in the creation and approval of secret settlement agreements and protective orders led to the failed Sunshine in Litigation Act of 2009 that aimed to "prohibit courts from shielding important health and safety information from the public as part of legal settlement agreements." The Sunshine in Litigation Act stood to address this problem and would have helped restore the public's right of access to information exchanged during discovery.[45] In another attempt, yet unsuccessful, Senator Herb Kohl (D) of Wisconsin and Representative Jerrold Nadler (D) of New York reintroduced the Sunshine in Litigation Act again in 2011. More recently, the bill was introduced in 2014 by the following senators: Richard Blumenthal (D) of Connecticut, Lindsay Graham (R) of South Carolina, Patrick Leahy (D) of Vermont, Sheldon Whitehouse (D) of

Rhode Island, and Ed Markey (D) of Massachusetts, as well as Representative Nadler in the House.

Opponents to this bill successfully denied that a problem exists and stated that empirical evidence is lacking that shows sealed settlements or protective orders are a problem. Even though information exchanged during pretrial discovery is presumptively public, proponents of restricted access to discovery materials assume that discovery is inherently private. They argue that the number of cases with any bearing on public health or safety is minuscule. Furthermore, so the argument goes, courts have neither the time nor inclination to review information for potential public safety and health impact before agreeing to secret settlement agreements, and the debate continues.[45]

14.10.3. Trial by Judge

A 1923 federal case, *Frye v. United States*,[47] set the precedent that admissibility of expert testimony should be based on a consensus (i.e., general acceptance) of the underlying theory in the relevant field. Some federal courts use the "Frye test" primarily in criminal cases, and it is still used in some states, such as California, Illinois, and New York. The Frye test is criticized on a number of grounds: (1) it fails to explain how to determine what the relevant field is, (2) it counts the number of experts rather than examining the validity of their opinions, and (3) it leads to self-validating experts who claim that their particular subspecialty is the relevant field. Trial judges have preferred to leave interpretation of expert testimony to the jury, particularly when the expert proof relates to complex scientific principles with which the judge is unfamiliar or uncomfortable.[48]

Empirical research has shown that juries understand the adversarial process and are not reluctant to be critical of expert testimony. Moreover, this research indicates that decisions reached by juries are as reliable as those of judges; indeed, juries bring the wisdom of several people to decide an issue rather than one judge.[49]

Nonetheless, a judge can restrict information as not probative in a case before a jury.[49] The pejorative term "junk science" is attributed to a witness presenting grossly fallacious interpretations of scientific data or opinions not supported by scientific evidence. However, the empirical basis supporting this term has not been made. Another pejorative term routinely used by business defendants in toxic tort liability cases is "frivolous lawsuits."[50] In 1993, regarding such a challenge to a witness, the Supreme Court ruled in *Daubert v. Merrell Dow Pharmaceuticals* that experts need to provide for legal reliability based upon scientific reliability.[51] An expert can be challenged on two conditions:

- First, an expert's testimony must be reliable, and knowledge must be more than subjective belief or speculation. The court opined that the expert must derived his or her conclusion by the scientific method, which can be defined as hypothesis testing, peer review and publication, known or potential rates of error, and the existence of standards controlling the methodology. General acceptance of the methodology in the relevant discipline is as an additional factor to be considered.[48] However, the test for reliability is problematic when the evidence is descriptive, which can be submitted not only by scientists but is also routinely submitted by forensic engineers, historians, literary scholars, and witnesses from the trades such as plumbers.[52]
- Second, the testimony of an expert must be relevant to the facts of the case. The regulatory perspective of relevance is a matter of policy that depends upon the weight of evidence. Even without a clear understanding of the cause of a disease, the weight of evidence is the best that can be done.[51] The classic example of the weight of evidence for public health is John Snow's removal of the pump handle in 1854 to control the outbreak of cholera in London.[53] Snow determined that a cholera outbreak was associated with drinking water from a single pump. Based upon the weight of the evidence, he had the pump handle removed, which resulted in the end of the epidemic, and this despite not knowing what in the water was the causative agent for cholera (the germ theory was yet to be discovered). Under the *Daubert* ruling, only after the judge decides which expertise and evidence will be admitted will the body of evidence be presented to the jury, and once admitted, the jury decides on the weight of evidence.[51]

The weight of evidence refers to a method in which all relevant scientific evidence regarding a causal hypothesis is considered. The scale of justice is appropriate as a symbol for understanding the instructions to a jury and the weight of evidence approach as a legal process. For criminal trials, the jury is instructed to consider the weight of evidence that will move the scale strongly in the direction of guilt "beyond reasonable doubt" so as to avoid convicting an innocent defendant. However, the weight of evidence for civil trials requires less in determining liability by taking measure of the preponderance of the evidence in which the scale tips one way or the other even slightly in favor of the plaintiff or the defendant.[54]

The challenge for the party seeking consideration of expert testimony is to convince the judge that the testimony fits into a larger and coherent framework so as to be admitted.[51] The *Daubert* ruling interferes with a case going to trial in two ways: first, the judge can determine whether experts are qualified and their testimony shows causation, and second, the judge can decide a case in a pre-trial *Daubert* hearing by denying an expert and evidence, leading to a summary judgment for the defendant and thus denying the plaintiff a jury trial.[55]

The *Daubert* ruling has provided an opportunity for defendants to exclude incriminating witness testimony. Indeed, judges have excluded information from jury consideration that at first may not appear relevant in which additional evidence presents background levels of an exposure to a known carcinogen (e.g., in drinking water) that an expert opines shortens the time for an occupational cancer to be manifest. Another factor leading to exclusion is the healthy worker effect, in which adjustments are made for those missing since they left the workforce because of the subject's illness.[56]

The *Daubert* ruling and subsequent rulings have moved from giving deference to science to questioning science that is proffered by plaintiffs and potentially denying evidence for a jury's consideration. The traditional authority of a judge is limited to points of law and proper trial procedure, and if a judge's prejudice enters into a ruling, an appeal to a higher court is warranted. A ruling in 1997 in *General Electric Co. v. Joiner* effectively negated an appeal of a *Daubert* ruling, and a 1999 ruling in *Kumho Tire Co. v. Carmichael* extended the judge's authority to deny any expert for trial.[55,57,58] In this trilogy of cases, several concerns have been raised about court decisions related to experts and evidence. Regarding the *Daubert* decision, there are no criteria to assess the validity of scientific evidence. The *Joiner* decision encourages judges to evaluate separate elements of scientific evidence rather the totality of the evidence, as in the weight of evidence approach. Challenges to witnesses raise the cost to the plaintiff's attorney, which is an incentive to not pursue a case.[59]

14.11. PRIVACY

Privacy involves the notion that a person can make a decision without outside interference, which includes the legal recognition of private property.

However, there is no explicit provision in the Constitution recognizing the right to privacy, and statutory protections of privacy are a recent phenomenon even though privacy has been a cherished value of citizens from the inception of the United States.

In 1965, in *Griswold v. Connecticut,* the general right of privacy was recognized for the first time between an individual and the government, whereas previously laws only protected privacy indirectly and under certain circumstances.[60] In *Griswold v. Connecticut,* the executive director of Planned Parenthood in Connecticut was arrested for giving information, instruction, and medical advice to married couples regarding contraception, which was a crime in that state at the time. The case made its way to the Supreme Court with the defense that the law violated the constitutional right to privacy. With a 7 to 2 decision, the court declared the Connecticut law unconstitutional. In that decision, Justice William Douglas wrote the majority opinion that articulated the constitutional right to privacy. He justified a zone of privacy for people based upon the "penumbras" of the following amendments from the Bill of Rights.[61]

- The First Amendment protects the freedom of religion and association without governmental interference.
- The Third Amendment protects against the mandatory billeting of soldiers in a person's home.
- The Fourth Amendment protects persons from governmental searches and seizures without due process of law.
- The Fifth Amendment protects people from self-incrimination.
- The Ninth Amendment states, "The enumeration in the Constitution, of certain rights, shall not be construed to deny or disparage others retained by the people."

The next case that built on the *Griswold* opinion was the 1972 *Eisenstadt v. Baird* case.[62] In Massachusetts, state law treated contraceptives as a prescription drug available only to married people. William Baird gave a lecture at Boston University on birth control and distributed free samples of contraceptives, whereupon deputies to Sheriff Thomas Eisenstadt arrested Baird. The sheriff charged Baird for exhibiting and giving contraceptives in violation of the law. Baird was convicted, but the State Supreme Court found that Baird had a right to free speech. Nonetheless, the justices upheld his conviction for distributing contraceptives. Baird appealed the case to the Supreme Court with a challenge under the equal protection clause of the Constitution regarding married versus unmarried people. Recognizing that unmarried women were being punished with pregnancy for premarital sex, the court found the state law discriminatory against unmarried people.

Also in 1972, the Supreme Court heard the Texas case of *Roe v. Wade*.[63] The court found that the "zones of privacy" (patient-physician privilege) protected under the Constitution include the right of a woman to terminate her pregnancy, but held that this right was not absolute. Two valid purposes existed for denying this right, according to the court. One was protecting the mother from a dangerous risk to her health after the first trimester of pregnancy, and the other was protecting viable prenatal life after the second trimester to protect the fetus. In a companion case from Georgia, *Doe v. Bolton*,[64] the court found that an abortion cannot be treated any differently than any other medical procedure.

Congress then passed the Privacy Act of 1974. This act gives private citizens access to federal government agency documents that pertain to themselves so as to correct inaccurate information about themselves in governmental records and limit a government agency's disclosure of personal information.[12] Other areas dealing with employee record confidentiality are the Americans with Disabilities Act of 1990 and the Family and Medical Leave Act of 1993. Preserving confidentiality of employee records in these areas is important because of the potential for defamation, invasion of privacy, or emotional distress claims by employees if information such as past medical problems is improperly released. Under these regulations, any information relating to the medical condition or history of an applicant or employee must be kept in separate medical files from general personnel information and treated as confidential. However, at the time these acts were established, no comprehensive protection existed at the federal level to guarantee the confidentiality and integrity of medical information, and existing state laws were incomplete and inadequate.

With the passage of the Health Insurance Portability and Accountability Act of 1996 (HIPAA), new federal regulations required physicians to ensure the protection of the privacy and security of patients' medical information. This act also ensures that a standard format be used when submitting electronic transactions, such as claims to payers. The DHHS issued the Privacy Rule in 2005 to implement provisions of HIPAA. The Privacy Rule applies to an entity that is a healthcare provider or business involved in the disclosure of protected health information (PHI). This information can be electronic, paper, or oral communications and does not need an individual's approval for disclosure under some circumstances, such as to protect the public health. Electronic storage or transmission of PHI also must meet additional conditions to secure the data.[65]

A RIGHT-TO-ACT NARRATIVE

Whirlpool Corporation suspended a horizontal steel mesh screen from the roof structure in its appliance factory in Marion, Ohio, to protect employees from falling objects that were carried in overhead conveyers. Maintenance workers routinely walked on the screen and angle iron frames for the screen to collect objects that fell from the conveyers and to spread paper on the screen to catch dripping grease. Several workers had fallen partially through the screen, and one worker had survived a fall through the screen onto the floor below. In 1973, many of the maintenance workers brought the unsafe condition of the screen to the attention of their supervisor, but the company reply was that the workers should step only on the angle iron frames. In 1974, a worker fell through the screen to his death. The company changed the procedure for removing the objects by requiring workers to use a powered mobile platform to hook the fallen objects. However, this was an inadequate procedure, and two maintenance workers raised the safety problem regarding the screen with the superintendent. The superintendent inspected the screen but nevertheless disagreed with the workers' concern.[66]

Two workers reported the hazard to OSHA. When the workers reported to work the next day, their foreman walked on the angle iron to show them how to maneuver around the screens and directed them to clean the screens. The men refused, claiming that it was unsafe. Then they were ordered to clock out, and they were reprimanded the next day. The Secretary of Labor brought suit against Whirlpool a month later claiming discrimination against the workers under § 11(c)(1) of the OSHAct and ordered Whirlpool to expunge the reprimands from the personnel files and to pay compensation to the two workers for the six hours for which they were ordered off the job for refusing to work in unsafe conditions. The district court agreed that the OSHA regulation justified the workers' refusal to work because of a genuine fear of death or serious bodily harm but denied relief, finding that the OSHA regulation was inconsistent with the intent of the OSHAct. The 6th Circuit Court of Appeals

(Cincinnati) reversed the lower court's finding and supported the OSHA regulation as consistent with the OSHAct.[66]

Six years after the incident, the case (*Whirlpool Corporation v. Marshall*) found its way to the Supreme Court in 1980, which found that the regulation clearly conformed to the law based upon the OSHAct's purpose and legislative history. Thereupon, the district court ordered Whirlpool to expunge the written reprimands from the workers' personnel files and to pay them for the time they were absent from work. Today, OSHA responds to complaints by whistle-blowers against their employers under 23 federal laws that include environmental, transportation, and financial institution statutes.[67]

REFERENCES

1. Longood RJ. Radiation accidents—the public's right to know. *Am J Public Health*. 1966;56(10):1751–1755.

2. Robinson JC. *Toil and Toxics: Workplace Struggles and Political Strategies for Occupational Health*. Los Angeles, CA: University of California Press;1991.

3. Siegel CS, Siegel DS. The history of DBCP from a judicial perspective. *Int J Occup Environ Health*. 1999;5:127–135.

4. McCaffrey DP. *OSHA and the Politics of Health Regulation*. New York, NY: Plenum Publishing Co.;1982.

5. Regenstein L. *America the Poisoned: How Deadly Chemicals Are Destroying Our Environment, Our Wildlife, Ourselves and—How We Can Survive!* Washington, DC: Acropolis Books;1982.

6. Bingham E, Monforton C. The pesticide DBCP and male infertility. In: *Late Lessons From Early Warnings: Science, Precaution, Innovation*. Copenhagen, Denmark: European Environmental Agency;2013:235–271. EEA Report No. 1/2013.

7. Bollier D, Claybrook J. *Freedom From Harm: The Civilizing Influence of Health, Safety, and Environmental Regulation*. Washington, DC: Public Citizen;1986.

8. O'Reilly JT. Worker "right to know" in 30-year retrospect: did we get it right, with what we know today? *Pitt J Environ Public Health Law*. 2007;2(1):3–26.

9. Ashford NA, Caldart CC. *Environmental Law, Policy, and Economics: Reclaiming the Environmental Agenda*. Cambridge, MA: MIT Press;2008.

10. Viscusi WK. *Risk by Choice: Regulating Health and Safety in the Workplace*. Cambridge, MA: Harvard University Press;1983.

11. Caldart C. Promises and pitfalls of workplace right to know. *Seminars in Occupational Medicine*. New York, NY: Thieme Medical Publishers, Inc.;1986.

12. Ashford NA, Caldart CC. *Technology, Law, and the Working Environment*. Washington, DC: Island Press;1996.

13. Millar JD, Myers ML. Occupational safety and health: Progress toward the 1990 objectives for the nation. *Public Health Rep*. 1983;98(4):324–335.

14. Dunn CM, Chadwick G. *Protecting Study Volunteers in Research: A Manual for Investigative Sites*. Boston, MA: CenterWatch, Inc.;2002.

15. Samuelson PA. *Economics*. 8th ed. New York, NY: McGraw-Hill Book Company;1970.

16. Sunstein CR. *Simpler: The Future of Government*. New York, NY: Simon & Schuster;2013.

17. Ashford N, Katz J. Unsafe working conditions: employee rights under the Labor Management Relations Act and the Occupational Safety and Health Act. *Notre Dame Lawyer*. 1977;52(2):802–837.

18. Morse T. Dying to know: A historical analysis of the right-to-know movement. *New Solut*. 1998;8(1):117–145.

19. Egilman D, Bohme SR. A brief history of warnings. In: Wogalter MS, ed. *Handbook of Warnings*. Mahwah, NJ: Lawrence Erlbaum Associates;2006:11–20.

20. Wogalter MS. Purposes and scope of warnings In: Wogalter MS, ed. *Handbook of Warnings*. Mahwah, NJ: Lawrence Erlbaum Associates;2006:3–9.

21. Laughery KR. Foreword. In: Wogalter MS, ed. *Handbook of Warnings*. Mahwah, NJ: Lawrence Erlbaum Associates;2006:xiii.

22. Tebeaux E. Improving tractor safety warnings: readability is missing. *J Agric Saf Health*. 2010;16(3):181–205.

23. Jones MM, Benrubi ID. Poison politics: a contentious history of consumer protection against dangerous household chemicals in the United States. *Am J Public Health*. 2013;103(5):801–812.

24. Peckham GM. An overview of the ANSI Z535 standards for safety signs, labels, and tags. In: Wogalter MS, ed. *Handbook of Warnings*. Mahwah, NJ: Lawrence Erlbaum Associates;2006:437–443.

25. Peterson B, Shinoff P. Firms had sterility data on pesticide. *Washington Post*. August 23, 1977:A1.

26. Fagotto E, Fung A. Improving workplace hazard communication. *Issues Sci Technol.* 2002;19(2):63–68.

27. Hathaway GJ, Proctor NH. *Proctor and Hughes' Chemical Hazards of the Workplace.* Hoboken, NJ: Wiley-Interscience;2004.

28. Hadden SG. *Read the Label: Reducing Risk by Providing Information.* Boulder, CO: Westview Press;1986.

29. *United Steelworkers of America, AFL-CIO-CLC v. Auchter,* 763 F.2d 728 (3rd Cir. 1985).

30. Weil A. EcoSense for living: environmental body makeover. Episode 5. Georgia Public Broadcasting. April 24, 2013. Available at: http://vimeo.com/81110107. Accessed June 9, 2014.

31. Gottlieb R, Smith M, Roque J, Yates P. New approaches to toxics: production design, right-to-know, and definition debates. In: Gottlieb R, ed. *Reducing Toxics: A New Approach to Policy and Industrial Decisionmaking.* Washington, DC: Island Press;1995:124–169.

32. *New Jersey State Chamber of Commerce v. Hughey,* 774 F.2d 587 (3rd Cir. 1985).

33. Horowitz CA. OSH Act Hazard Communication Standard preemption of state right to know laws under *New Jersey Chamber of Commerce v. Hughey,* 868F.2d 621. *Wash Univ J Urb Contemp Law.* 1990;38:243–258. Available at: http://digitalcommons.law.wustl.edu/urbanlaw/vol38/iss1/10. Accessed April 26, 2013.

34. *Manufacturers' Association of Tri-County v. Knepper,* 801 F.2 130 (3rd Cir. 1986).

35. Jasanoff S. The Bhopal disaster and the right to know. *Soc Sci Med.* 1988;27(10): 1113–1123.

36. Gray PL. *EPCRA: Emergency Planning and Community Right-to-Know Act.* Chicago, IL: American Bar Association;2002.

37. United Nations. Agenda 21. Presented at: United Nations Conference on Environment and Development; June 3–14, 1992; Rio de Janeiro, Brazil. Available at: http://sustainabledevelopment.un.org/content/documents/Agenda21.pdf. Accessed June 9, 2014.

38. Monroe KA, Orr G. Warnings and the U.S. Occupational Safety and Health Administration. In: Wogalter MS, ed. *Handbook of Warnings.* Mahwah, NJ: Lawrence Erlbaum Associates;2006:537–551.

39. Hughes J. The critical role of training in protecting workers. *New Solut.* 2012;22(3):253–254.

40. Occupational Safety and Health Administration. Training requirements in OSHA standards and training guidelines. OSHA 2254 [revised]. 1998. Available at: http://www.osha.gov/Publications/osha2254.pdf. Accessed March 4, 2013.

41. Mine Safety and Health Administration. Educational policy and development's programs and services. Available at: http://www.msha.gov/PROGRAMS/EPDPS.asp. Accessed April 19, 2013.

42. National Institute of Environmental Health Sciences. Hazmat safety and training: worker education and training program. Available at: http://www.niehs.nih.gov/careers/hazmat/index.cfm. Accessed April 19, 2013.

43. National Paralegal College. Discovery and Federal Rule of Civil Procedure 11. National Juris College. 2014. Available at: http://nationalparalegal.edu/public_documents/courseware_asp_files/researchLitigation/PreTrialPractice/Discovery.asp. Accessed August 16, 2014.

44. Gevertz JN. Workplace exposure to toxic chemicals: Information disclosure versus trade secret protection. *Rev Law Soc Change*. 1984-1985;8:149-172. Available at: http://www.law.nyu.edu/ecm_dlv4/groups/public/@nyu_law_website__journals__review_of_law_and_social_change/documents/documents/ecm_pro_070403.pdf. Accessed March 12, 2013.

45. Keaney ME. Don't steal my sunshine: deconstructing the flawed presumption of privacy for unfiled documents exchanged during discovery. *Hastings Law J*. 2011;62(3):795-820.

46. Sanson DS. The pervasive problem of court-sanctioned secrecy and the exigency of national reform. *Duke Law J*. 2003;53(2):807-832.

47. *Frye v. United States*, 130 S. Ct. 307, 175 Legal Ed. 2d 204 2009 U.S.

48. Berger MA. What has a decade of *Daubert* wrought? *Am J Public Health*. 2005;95(S1):S59-S65.

49. Vidmar N. Expert evidence, the adversary system, and the jury. *Am J Public Health*. 2005;95(S1):S137-S143.

50. McGarity TO. *Daubert* and the proper role for the courts in health, safety, and environmental regulation. *Am J Public Health*. 2005;95(S1):S92-S98.

51. Foster KR, Huber PW. *Judging Science: Scientific Knowledge and the Federal Courts*. Cambridge, MA: MIT Press;1999.

52. Haack S. Trial and error: the Supreme Court's philosophy of science. *Am J Public Health*. 2005;95(S1):S66-S73.

53. Johnson S. *The Ghost Map: The Story of London's Most Terrifying Epidemic—and How It Changed Science, Cities, and the Modern World*. New York, NY: Riverhead Books; 2006.

54. Krimsky S. The weight of scientific evidence in policy and law. *Am J Public Health*. 2005;95(S1):S129–S136.

55. Lakoff GP. A cognitive scientist looks at *Daubert*. *Am J Public Health*. 2005;95(S1):S114–S120.

56. Melnick RL. A *Daubert* motion: a legal strategy to exclude essential scientific evidence in toxic tort litigation. *Am J Public Health*. 2005;95:S30–S34.

57. *General Electric Co. v. Joiner*, 522 U.S. 136 (1997).

58. *Kumho Tire Co. v. Carmichael*, 526 U.S. 137 (1999).

59. Michaels D. Scientific evidence and public policy. *Am J Public Health*. 2005;95(S1):S5–S7.

60. *Griswold v. Connecticut*, 381 U.S. 479, 85 S. Ct. 1678, 14 Legal Ed. 2d 510, 1965 U.S.

61. Wing KR. *The Law and the Public's Health*. Ann Arbor, MI: Health Administration Press;1985.

62. *Eisenstadt v. Baird*, 405 U.S. 438 (1972).

63. *Roe v. Wade*, 410 U.S. 113 (1973).

64. *Doe v. Bolton*, 410 U.S. 179 (1973).

65. Karasz HN, Elden A, Bogan S. Text messaging to communicate with public health audiences: How the HIPAA security rule affects practice. *Am J Public Health*. 2013;103(4):617–622.

66. *Whirlpool Corporation v. Marshall*, 445 U.S. 1 (1980).

67. Occupational Safety and Health Administration. OSHA fact sheet: your rights as a whistleblower. Available at: http://www.osha.gov/OshDoc/data_General_Facts/whistleblower_rights.pdf. Accessed April 17, 2013.

15

Leadership and Ethics

Most of our experience, whatever it is going to be, is still ahead of us.
—Dr. Irving John Selikoff[1]

THE LUCIFER EFFECT NARRATIVE

In 1959, when U.S. workers in vinyl chloride monomer (VCM) plants were exposed to 500 ppm of VCM routinely when more than five billion pounds of VCM were produced annually, a worker complained to the company doctor of a pain in his hands.[2,3] Then on April 30, 1969, members of the industry's trade association met in Washington, DC, to consider a report from a group of medical researchers that recommended a reduction of exposure to VCM to 50 ppm. Most participants were medical doctors representing the companies and discounted the danger of VCM by their vote. A record of the meeting described the following: "The association between reactor cleaning and the occurrence of acroosteolysis is sufficiently clear-cut.... The severity of exposure of reactor cleaner to vinyl chloride should be kept at a minimum...." A motion to accept the report as submitted was defeated by a vote of 7 to 3. The participants agreed to a change in the report as follows: "Eliminate the last sentence 'Sufficient ventilation should be provided to reduce the vinyl chloride concentration below 50 parts per million.'"

Richard Lemen, former deputy director at the National Institute for Occupational Safety and Health (NIOSH), told Bill Moyers in a 2003 PBS documentary,

> I think that that reflects who the medical doctor's patient really was. Was their patient the workers in the plant—or were they representing their employer? This is a fundamental problem that we've had in public health

for a long time—and that is, who is more important? Is it the chemical being produced or is it the human being producing the chemical?[3]

In 1967, Dan Ross began working at a new Conoco VCM plant in Louisiana. Vinyl chloride monomer (VCM) is the raw material for the manufacture of polyvinyl chloride (PVC) plastic. Ross worked there for 23 years and was exposed to VCM every workday. When Ross contracted brain cancer, he engaged attorney William Baggett Jr. to sue his employers, including a charge of conspiracy, which resulted in more than a million pages of documents during discovery. These documents, all previously confidential, were the sources for Moyers's story.[3]

As described by VCM manufacturing company officials in Table 15-1, VCM exposure from hairspray was recognized as early as 1959, but the problem was kept a secret. In 1969, the industry took the hairspray problem seriously and quietly removed VCM from its hairspray products, without warning hairdressers or their customers of any potential hazard, thus avoiding future liability suits.

Columbia University historian David Rosner told Moyers,

> Vinyl chloride is a gas, and it is used as a propellant in hairsprays, in deodorants at that time, in a whole slew of pesticides and other cans that are propelling chemicals out into the environment. So, if it turns out that this relatively low threshold limit is poisoning workers, what is the potential danger if it ends up poisoning consumers? The problem that they're identifying is the giant elephant in the corner. It's the issue of what happens when workers' comp isn't there to shield them from suits in court, what happens if people who are not covered by workers' comp suddenly get exposed to vinyl chloride and begin to sue them for damages to their health.

In 1970, Dr. Publio L. Viola, medical director of the Italian PVC manufacturing firm Solvay et Cie, reported at an international cancer conference his discovery of cancer in laboratory rats that were exposed to VCM. Viola et al. published their results in May 1971, discounting the effect on workers. Four European PVC producers commissioned Italian researcher Dr. Cesare Maltoni to verify Viola's results.[1] In 1972, Maltoni found evidence of a rare liver cancer—angiosarcoma—at exposures of 250 ppm. U.S. and European industry representatives signed a confidential agreement to keep the results secret. Quotations from industry documents regarding a cover-up of these findings are shown in Table 15-1.

Table 15-1. Quotations Used in "Trade Secrets: A Moyers Report"

Hairspray Exposure, 1959, 1969	Workplace Inhalation Exposure, 1959, 1971-1973
"We have been investigating vinyl chloride a bit.... We feel quite confident that 500 parts per million is going to produce rather appreciable injury when inhaled 7 hours a day, five days a week for an extended period." (memo, Director, B.F. Goodrich Department of Industrial Hygiene, May 1959)	"An off-the record phone call from VK Rowe gives me incomplete data on their current repeated inhalation study.... Vinyl chloride monomer is more toxic than has been believed." (Union Carbide intercompany correspondence, November 24, 1959)
"Calculations have been made to show the concentration of propellant in a typical small hairdresser's room.... All of this suggests that beauty operators may be exposed to concentrations of vinyl chloride monomer equal to or greater than the level in our polys." (B.F. Goodrich document, March 24, 1969)	"Publishing of Dr. Viola's work in the United States could lead to serious problems with regard to the vinyl chloride monomer industry.... The present political climate in the United States is such that a campaign by Mr. R. Nader and others could force an industrial upheaval via new laws or strict interpretation of pollution and occupational health laws." (record from meeting of 20 VCM-producing companies, Washington, DC, November 16, 1971)
"If vinyl chloride proves to be hazardous to health, a producing company's liability to its employees is limited by various Workmen's Compensation laws. A company selling vinyl chloride ..." (Union Carbide confidential internal correspondence)	"The need to be able to assure the employees of the industry that management was concerned for, and diligent in seeking the information necessary to protect their health. The need to develop data useful in defense of the industry against invalid claims for injury for alleged occupational or community exposure." (industry ad hoc planning group for VCM research, December 14, 1971)
"Dow ... is questioning the aspect of making sales of vinyl chloride monomer when the known end use is as an aerosol propellant since market is small but potential liability is great." (Ethyl Corporation)	"Dow Chemical Company reviewed the work on the European study. They report the results on rats are probably undeniable" (confidential internal correspondence, Union Carbide, February 13, 1973). An Ethyl Corporation interoffice memo regarding VCM stated, "All agreed the results certainly indicate a positive carcinogenic effect above or at 250 parts per million" (interoffice memo, Ethyl Corporation).
"Concerning use of vinyl chloride monomer as aerosol propellant, serious consideration should be given to withdrawal from this market." (memo, Allied Chemical Corporation)	"We should not volunteer reference to the European project, but in response to direct inquiry, we could not deny awareness of the project and knowledge concerning certain preliminary results." (minutes, Manufacturing Chemists Association meeting, May 21, 1973)
	"[It] could be construed as evidence of an illegal conspiracy by industry ... if the information were not made public or at least made available to the government." (Union Carbide, May 31, 1973)

Note: VCM = vinyl chloride monomer.

Rosner said to Moyers,

> You kind of avoid as a historian the idea that there are conspiracies or that there are people planning the world in a certain way. You just try to avoid that because it's—it seems too—too unreal and too frightening in its implications. Yet when you look at these documents, you say yes, there are people who understood what was going on, people who thought about the crisis that was engulfing them or about to engulf them and tried in every which way to get out of that crisis and actually to, in some sense, to suppress an issue.

In January 1973, NIOSH published a request for safety and health information regarding VCM. In 1974, B.F. Goodrich broke ranks with the rest of the industry and informed NIOSH that four workers at its VCM plant in Louisville, Kentucky, had died from angiosarcoma. OSHA then issued an emergency temporary standard followed by a permanent standard for the control of VCM as a carcinogen.

In 1989, Dan Ross was told he had a rare form of brain cancer. He and his wife found a record that showed that he was exposed to an amount of VCM that exceeded short-term exposure limits on which was written, "Do not include on wire to Houston," where the company headquarters was located. Wanting answers, the Rosses sought out attorney Baggett, who brought charges that included conspiracy against the companies producing VCM. While most of the companies had settled, on October 9, 1990, Dan Ross died at age 46.

Historian Gerald Markowitz of John Jay College said to Moyers,

> Historians don't like to use broad political terms like "cover-up," but there is really no other term you can use for this because the industry had the information. They knew the significance of the information they had, and they refused to tell the government because they were afraid the government would take action to protect the workforce.

15.1. INTRODUCTION

How can a defensible compromise be reached between the protection of health and counteracting factors such as economic, technological, or political feasibility?
—Sven Ove Hansson[4]

This chapter addresses the dual issues of leadership and ethics. The opening narrative discusses the Lucifer effect and how it relates to situational attribution. A section then describes the ethics of leadership, followed by a discussion of the issue of blaming the victim. Next, a section addresses morality related to messaging, and the penultimate section addresses the irony surrounding the harm principle as related to human actions. Finally, a section describes how OSHA resolves the problem of situational attribution by changing the situation, with a discussion of situational leadership theory.

15.2. THE SITUATION

Corporations have neither bodies to be punished, nor souls to be condemned; they therefore do as they like.

—Lord Edward Thurlow[5]

The opening narrative shows how doctors and other men of good standing move away from what is good for the public interest by denying or obfuscating what is harmful to workers in corporate cultures. The doctors no longer abide by "first do no harm" for workers under their care, and management ignores the second part of their libertarian mantra, "free to act as long as it does not harm others." Moreover, conspiracy emerged in this industrial culture, defined as taking "place when two or more people meet or confer in secret to commit an illegal, treacherous, or evil act against a third party without the third party's knowledge or approval."[6]

While economics has dominated this field of industrial relations, another psychological theory is at work in the actions described in the narrative from the "Trade Secrets" documentary. This theory—situational attribution—is woven into this chapter to explain corporate behavior and the political economy of capitalism. This theory has much to do with efforts and barriers to reform occupational safety and health policy.

The doctors and managers referred to in the opening narrative were arguably captive to their situations according to situational attribution theory, which explains behavior based upon an external attribute: the situation. According to this theory, the situation can cause good people to engage in terrible behaviors. Evidence for this theory comes from three dramatic psychological experiments.

1. In a 1961 experiment, Stanley Milgram of Yale University recruited and paid 40 student subjects to apply electricity under a supervisor's direction to victims strapped to a chair in the next room. The victims were

actors, out of sight from the subject administering the shocks. Despite the sound of tape-recorded screams and the actor banging a chair against a wall, the subjects continued to administer shocks even when the victim fell silent after lethal shocks that reached 450 volts. Only one subject refused to administer the shock above 300 volts.[7]

2. In 1970, John Darley and Daniel Batson of Princeton University conducted an experiment using 67 seminary student volunteers. These students drew lots to be placed in one of four cohorts. Two cohorts were instructed individually to walk to the other side of the campus and deliver a sermon about the Biblical Good Samaritan, half of whom had to hurry to give their sermon while the other half could take their time. The other two cohorts were instructed in the same way, but their sermon was about job opportunities for the seminary students. On each student's path to the lecture site, a person (an actor) was slumped over in an alleyway in obvious need of help. The students assigned the Good Samaritan story stopped in no higher proportion than all the subjects; those in a hurry, less so. Overall, only 10% of the subjects stopped to render aid to the person in the alleyway.[8]

3. In 1971, Philip Zimbardo of Stanford University recruited subjects to participate in a prison experiment in the basement of a university building. Twenty-one subjects, tested to be psychologically stable students, were divided by lot into roles as either prison guards or prisoners. The subjects as guards were given uniforms, mirrored glasses, and a baton; and the subjects as prisoners were arrested at their homes and taken to the mock prison by real police officers, registered, assigned numbers, and outfitted with prisoner smocks and caps. All knew this was an experiment. All of the guards became domineering, and by the end of the experiment, one-third of them exhibited sadistic tendencies. The prisoners formed into a group and rioted on the second day. Zimbardo and his colleagues believed that this experiment revealed that people are creatures of context even when the situation is temporary or implausible. He called this the Lucifer effect.[9]

These three studies demonstrate that there is a broader field of social science than just economics that can apply to occupational safety and health policy. Evident from situational attribution theory discussed above, we have much to learn regarding ethical leadership.

15.3. THE ETHICS OF LEADERSHIP

Why do they believe as they do? Why do they act as they do? Is there something to their position that I don't understand or that I've been wrong about? The most disturbing thing now is the rigidity of some you know: "We are right, we are 100 percent right, and if you don't agree with us, you're not just wrong, you are not an American!"

—George Mitchell[10]

While Chapter 6 addressed analytical approaches to critical thinking and advocacy, leadership may be necessary for occupational safety and health professionals who are employed or engaged by corporate or government entities, or for advocacy organizations to improve occupational safety and health. This section addresses leadership as an instrument for advocacy, the art of persuasion, and ethics.

15.3.1. Leadership

Advocacy within institutions involves influencing decision making. This type of advocacy is important within organizations where it is known as "persuasive influence" on an issue or "leadership" regarding change.

Leadership is intertwined with followership, for without followers there is no leader. Public health leadership competency has been defined by four core categories: (1) transformation, (2) legislation and politics, (3) transorganization, and (4) team and group dynamics. Characteristics of these categories are described in Table 15-2.[11]

While transformational leaders appeal to moral values of their followers to mobilize them for major policy change in society, a contrasting style, transactional leaders, motivate followers by appealing to their self-interest with incentives in exchange for their contribution.[12] Servant leadership is another type that leads with the motivation to serve others; since followers trust this leader, they freely follow.[13] An example of a servant leader is the late César Chávez of the United Farm Workers.[14] Section 15.3.4 below discusses these leadership types in further detail.

Another aspect of leadership is based upon contingency theory, in which a leader's course of action depends upon the situation. This theory suggests a sliding scale of moving from task direction to empowerment and delegation to followers based upon their capacity to do the work, which is discussed further

Table 15-2. Leadership Competency Categories, Characteristics, and Examples for Public Health Professionals

Category	Characteristics	Examples
Transformation	Systems thinking, analytical and critical thinking processes, visioning potential futures, strategic and tactical assessment, communication, change dynamics	Apply critical thinking through argument "to assure so far as possible every working man and woman in the Nation safe and healthful working conditions"*
Legislation and politics	Facilitate, negotiate, and collaborate in an increasingly competitive and contentious political environment	Build policy networks to inform protective standards at the state level
Transorganization	Move beyond scope and boundaries of single stakeholder groups, communities, professions, disciplines, organizations, agencies	Cooperate with consumer groups in building coalitions
Team and group dynamics	Communications, team building, capacity and capability building	Use informal leadership to move to precautionary policies

Source: Wright et al.[11]
*From the purpose of the Occupational Safety and Health Act.

in the last section of this chapter. All leaders engage in some kind of process, act, or influence that finds ways to get people to do something.[13]

Leaders need to establish credibility through expertise as well as trust among peers and subordinates; and with audiences find common ground, provide evidence beyond data through stories and examples, and connect emotionally. Most occupational safety and health professionals employed by an organization may be in a position as a staff member. Thus, they must lead as an informal leader. The following strategies can be used by informal leaders to persuade others to improve safety and health policies:[12]

- Understand the audience and how they think and learn.
- Examine the history of prior attempts regarding the issue (make no enemies in the process).
- Build a coalition of allies (find common ground).
- Connect with gatekeepers who have access to those in authority.
- Do not engage; use divergent thinking to get potential opponents to think in a different way about an issue.
- Present solutions to problems (do not be "the" problem, be part of the solution).

15.3.2. Persuasion

Leaders need to learn to persuade others. The following persuasion tools may be helpful to the advocate:[12,15]

- Authority is important, and for the professional this may be expert power, which is respect based on knowledge and the ability to communicate that knowledge.
- Consistency and commitments are important, observed by prior actions. They may take some time. Gaining commitment to a course of action by others once established may be hard to stop, which is a good thing as long as that course does not require significant change.
- Reciprocity is a profound tool. Once resources have been given to another, that person feels an obligation to reciprocate. Sometimes, concessions work when one party caves in on an issue, and the other person is motivated to reciprocate (e.g., compromise). The opposite is true too: When a politician asks for a vote, and if given, will likely result in a commitment by the voter to support the politician (e.g., confirmation bias).
- Social proof is important. People look to others to determine what is appropriate. Recall the narrative about Wag Dodge in Chapter 6. His subordinates saw their respected peers running away from the "black," which was an example of social proof as they followed their peers up the hill. Wag Dodge initially showed no concern about the Mann Gulch Fire, so the firefighters assumed no concern. A leader must provide social proof by establishing respect and be an example to be emulated. Social proof seeking by others is augmented by uncertainty, ambiguity, or complexity regarding the situation.
- The liking principle is a phenomenon that motivates others to be persuaded by someone they like, which depends upon physical attractiveness, similarity (but diversity in appearance or beliefs may be critical), extending compliments, familiarity that engenders comfort, and association with positive results. Small incremental gains are important.
- The scarcity principle suggests that if something is not widely available, it is seen as more attractive. Framing something as a scarcity can persuade. Constant scarcity is more acceptable than moving from abundance to scarcity. Once freedoms or choices are given, hatred can emerge when they are taken away, such as the removal of personal autonomy.

15.3.3. Public Health Ethics

At the core of public health ethics in the United States is the "Belmont Report," published in the *Federal Register* in 1979, that addressed the ethics of working with human subjects in research.[16] This report was in response to a 1974 statute that created the National Commission for the Protection of Human Subjects of Biomedical and Behavioral Research. The report addressed three basic principles similar to the three rationales regarding rights and duties described in the previous chapter. First was the principle of "Respect for Persons," which acknowledges the autonomy of a person free from both controlling interferences by others and personal limitations that prevent meaningful choice. This principle also acknowledges the requirement to protect those with diminished autonomy, including employees as subordinate individuals who could be at risk of coercive tactics such as fear of job loss, delayed promotion, or other influences of a superior. Autonomous individuals act intentionally, with understanding, and without controlling influences.

Second is the principle of beneficence: action (research) involving a subject but for the benefit of others. Beneficent actions can be taken to help prevent or remove harms or to simply improve the situation of others. Expressions of beneficent actions are to (1) do not harm and (2) maximize possible benefits and minimize possible harms.

Third is the principle of justice that depends upon fairness of distribution. The "Belmont Report" expressed the converse of justice: "An injustice occurs when some benefit to which a person is entitled is denied without good reason or when some burden is imposed unduly...."[16] Regarding justice, the perils of the workplace inflict death, illness, and disability on a minority of our society at any given time. The dominant model of justice in the United States has been market justice, which emphasizes individual responsibility, minimal collective action, and freedom of action while respecting one another's rights. Even though society recognizes collective action to protect a person from harm from another or when vast populations are endangered, the traditional social norm is that individuals are on their own in fighting death, illness, and disability. The issue for the polity is whether a majority or powerful minority should help bear the burden of death, illness, and disability systematically placed upon a minority.

The challenge to the polity is the acceptance that death, illness, and disability are a collective problem and that all persons are entitled to health protection.[17]

The Western liberal tradition of social justice in society is a high-quality ethic of caring for each other in sharing the burdens and benefits of protection against death, illness, and disability (e.g., protecting against workplace hazards). This public health ethic is a social justice in which all persons are entitled to equal protection from death, illness, and disability based on the following three principles:[18]

- Identification and control of hazards rather than blaming individual defects.
- Prevent damaging exposures and mitigate the effects of exposures when they cannot be prevented.
- Take collective action to control hazards that cannot be achieved through voluntary methods.

15.3.4. Business Ethics

The transformational type of leadership may serve as a model for ethical leadership, as shown in contrast with transactional leadership in Table 15-3. Servant leadership may be another model for ethical leadership. It elevates people, passing a test that those served grow as persons; while being served, they become healthier, wiser, freer, more autonomous, and more likely themselves to become servants and have a positive effect on the least privileged in society.[13]

Table 15-3. Values for Three Leadership Types and Ethical Test Criteria

Leadership Type	Criteria	
	Modal-values (means)	End-values
Transforming	Responsibility, fairness, honesty, promise-keeping	Liberty, justice, equality
Transaction	Supply lower-level wants and needs so that they can move to higher-level needs	Raise followers up through various stages of morality and need
Servant	Motivated to serve others, elevate people	Trust, freely follow, followers become servants

Source: Ciulla.[13]

Table 15-4. Comparison of Public Health and Business (Transforming) Leadership Principles

Principle	Public Health Ethics	Business Ethics
Respect for persons	Free from both controlling interferences by others and from personal limitations that prevent meaningful choice; protect those with diminished autonomy	Respect: treat people as human beings not just a means to an end; treat each stakeholder group as people would like to be treated if they were on the other side of the exchange
Justice	Fairness of distribution: equals ought to be treated equally—each an equal share; each according to individual need, effort, societal contribution, merit	Fairness (distributive justice): each according to merit, each according to free market exchanges (libertarian ethic); but must honor each according to their rights

Source: Public Health Ethics, Dunn et al.;[16] Business Ethics, Ciulla.[13]

The ethical test for transforming leadership includes the following criteria: (1) honor, integrity, equality, advancing standards of good conduct for humankind regarding modal values; (2) justice for end-values; and (3) impact on well-being of people touched.[13] Leadership principles are similar between public health ethics and transformational business ethics as shown in Table 15-4. In this comparison, the public health ethics are drawn from the "Belmont Report"[16] and an analysis of applied ethics to business.[18,19]

Leadership ethics must also address effectiveness, which is in conflict many times with ethics. To be effective, a leader follows three processes: (1) establish a compelling direction with a vision for the future and strategies for means and ends for reaching the vision; (2) get buy-in by aligning followers, communicating the direction, building shared understanding, engendering belief in the vision, and persuading them to follow the vision; and (3) motivate followers to enact the articulated changes and vision.[12] Moral assessment of leadership comes down to three criteria:[18]

1. The ethics of the leader, including both intentions and personal ethics, which are conditioned by internalized beliefs.
2. The ethics of the means that the leader uses (the leadership process), which is the way challenges or opportunities are addressed.
3. The ethics regarding the leader's effectiveness, which are the results of leadership behavior.

15.4. BLAMING THE VICTIM

So you've come to Pittsburgh to study accidents, have you? Well, I've been in business fifteen years, and I can tell you one thing right now—95 percent of our accidents are due to carelessness of the man who gets hurt.

—Crystal Eastman[20]

Another barrier for a prevention ethic is placing fault upon individuals to control their own victimization (i.e., blaming the victim).[17] A historical social phenomenon places the blame for an injury upon the victim or the blame for a disease upon fate. It has become ingrained in the way Americans think.[21] Indeed, in product liability cases, the defense can argue that the injury is the victim's fault. Looking back after the period of slavery in the United States, the tenet of social Darwinism justified industrial titans' control over the workforce; the idea of survival of the fittest placed blame on workers for their own injuries.

This blaming-the-victim phenomenon is known as a fundamental attribution error, which is an inclination to attribute others' behavior to their internal failings in the situation or environment.[12] It is not only a thing of the past. It resides in the United States today. In the hearings for the proposed Occupational Safety and Health Act (OSHAct; see Appendix), many industry witnesses blamed worker fault for their injuries and diseases. One piece of testimony to the House Committee on Education and Labor included the following claim: "Safety authorities have estimated that three quarters of accidents on the job result from unsafe acts rather than unsafe conditions."[22]

Market justice feeds off of an understanding of social problems, with a focus on an individual's behavior and associated failures as perceived rather than on organizational design and the situation at hand. Remedies for these unusual events or circumstances are in the hands of the individual.[21] Blaming the victim justifies inequality by finding defects in the victim and depends upon remedial or reactionary action rather than preventive or progressive action. This exceptionalist ideology views the problems as unusual, unique exceptions to the rule that result from a defect in the individual or by "accident."

A contrasting ideology depends upon a universalist viewpoint in which problems are public, legislated, general, and inclusive. It views problems as social arrangements that are predictable and preventable through public action. They are not unique to the individual, and the individual is not defective or abnormal.[23]

The more recent view raised by W. Edward Deming in the Total Quality Management (TQM) movement in the 1980s and 1990s described most problems regarding workers as systemic in the management structure, representing 95% of such problems; workers were the victims of these systems. The remaining 5% of problems were unique and required special attention to understand the causes. He placed blame on the managerial system, not the victim.[24] However, in occupational safety and health settings, TQM morphed into behavior-based safety procedures, which placed the obligation on workers to identify and change to safe behavior over unsafe behavior. While worker training is important, true to TQM, managerial behavior is where the ultimate control of safety and health lies.

In product liability cases, the defense may attempt to place blame on the victim. Figure 15-1 shows that a potentially injurious product can be controlled most easily by its upstream source, at its design and manufacturing steps, rather than by passing warnings—such as "be careful"—down the line to the potential victim. On a related note, the designer and manufacturer are the first line of defense in establishing safe processes and products, for they are the most knowledgeable of the potential hazards and their elimination or control. It is their experience that precedes protective consensus standards, which follow in time, and government standards that follow even later. The front-line defense lies with the creator of the problem (i.e., the precautionary principle).

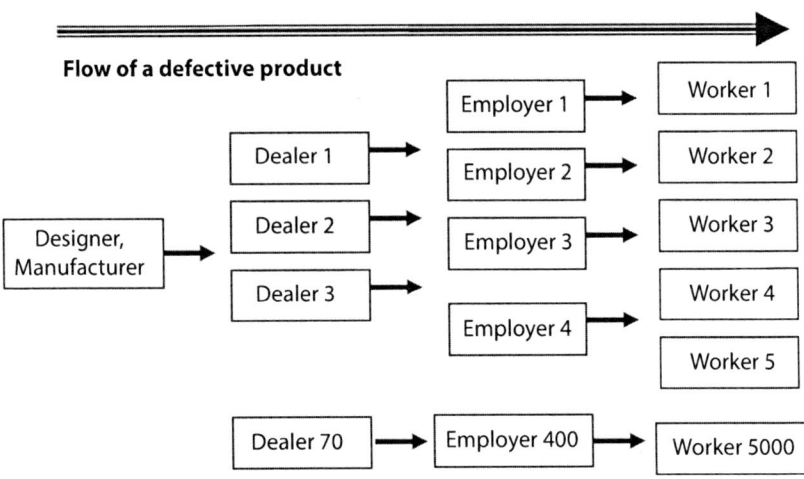

Figure 15-1. Flow of a product that is reasonably dangerous to the worker and has the potential to cause a significant injury, and for which a safer alternative exists.

15.5. MORALITY FOUNDATIONS

Good and evil are always at war. Good men must choose.

—Nelson Mandela[25]

Conceptual frames place messages into existing concepts that give order and meaning. Advocates can generate messages from different levels ranging from values to issues to policy, as shown in Table 15-5. Messages have more influence if they first address values before issues, and issues before minutia-laden policy.[26] The advantage lies with the advocate who sets the frame around values. The message can then progress down this hierarchy to policy.

Regarding moral foundations, social psychologists have looked to morality as a bridge between individualism and society. Paradigms have shifted from moral reasoning to include moral emotion and intuition. On this path, morality has centered on the two concepts of not harming and not cheating other people. Three principles have generated a synthesis for morality in public discourse: (1) intuitive primacy, (2) moral thinking for doing, and (3) morality that binds and builds.[27]

As shown by the opening narrative in Chapter 6 regarding the wildfire at Mann Gulch, the intuitive primacy principle (intuition precedes reason) rests on the sudden arousal of a feeling that goes to a polar opposite, such as "good or bad," "right or wrong," or "fight or flee." This spontaneous evaluation precedes reasoning and immediately leads to confirmation bias. The average citizen uses virtually no reason in decision making. A search for evidence to confirm the feeling is sought, and when found, the search stops. Intuition happens more quickly and frequently than moral reasoning. Conversely, reasoning involves multiple steps—also affected by intuition—and can win the day in discussion when confirmation bias is challenged with evidence. This may take time, however, which Wag Dodge did not have at Mann Gulch.[27]

Table 15-5. Levels for Messaging Against Conceptual Frames

Message Level	Examples	Explanation
1. Overarching values (moral foundations)	Harm/care, fairness/reciprocity, ingroup/loyalty, authority/respect, purity/sanctity	Core values that motivate people to change the world or not change it
2. The issue	Environment, health, safety	The problem to be solved
3. Policy details	Strategy and tactics for change	What needs change and how the change should occur

Politicians are intuitively sensitive to their instincts and the desires of their audiences, responding rapidly but not necessarily logically. Intuitive politicians are thus swayed by their perception of audience desires. Politicians engage in moral hypocrisy, for it is easy for them (or anyone) to justify their bad behavior through hypocrisy, finding excuses for their own selfishness. Conscience can counter hypocrisy when people are facing a quandary, motivating them to try to do the right thing, especially if they believe they are being watched, which argues for transparency and publicity.[27]

The "moral thinking for doing" principle (population-based values drive policy) addresses evolutionary thinking for going beyond the survival of the fittest to working together in endeavors of agriculture, trade, infrastructure, and governance. What evolves is the building of reputation among individuals who have elicited future cooperation in these endeavors. Over time, word-of-mouth evolves in the form of gossip to identify those of good reputation versus selfish exploiters and free riders (e.g., nonunion workers who benefit from rules pioneered by unions). Indeed, gossip is critical as a catalyst for cooperation as a way to investigate the actions of others against norms of behavior and cheating. Much gossip occurs today through social media.[28]

The "morality binds and builds" principle (ever more inclusive communities) focuses on building communities for cooperation, which individuals

Table 15-6. Moral Foundations as Overarching Issues Mapped Against Message Levels of Conceptual Frames as Related to the Legislative History of the Occupational Safety and Health Act

Overarching values (moral foundations)	→ The Issue	→ Policy Details
Harm/care	Prevent causes of injuries and diseases	Enact legislation to protect workers
Fairness/reciprocity	State versus federal control	The DoL will establish standards, but states can enforce them
Ingroup/loyalty	Antilabor proclivity of opposition	Establish an appeals board outside of the DoL
Authority/respect	Public involvement	Appeals to circuit courts
Purity/sanctity	Compassion for injured and sick people	Provide workers' compensation insurance

Note: DoL = U.S. Department of Labor.

alone cannot accomplish. The villains in this principle include the free riders, the norm-violators, and the cheaters: those who gain without contributing to the group's success. These communities historically were tribes with norms of behavior and cohesion. So-called inside-the-head psychological mechanisms and outside-the-head cultural inventions interlock to suppress selfishness and build social life.[27]

The synthesis derived from these principles extends morality foundations beyond the two traditional overarching values of "harming versus helping" and "fairness/justice/rights" to three more. All five values are quoted below:[27,28]

1. Harm/care: Concerns for the suffering of others, including the virtues of caring and compassion.
2. Fairness/reciprocity: Concerns about unfair treatment and cheating, and more abstract notions of justice and rights.
3. Ingroup/loyalty: Concerns related to obligation of group membership, such as loyalty, self-sacrifice, and rights.
4. Authority/respect: Concerns related to social order and the obligations of hierarchical obedience, respect, and the fulfillment of role-based duties.
5. Purity/sanctity: Concerns about physical and spiritual contagion, including virtues of chastity, wholesomeness, and control of desires.

Traditional public health approaches have derived from the first two values listed above, which are considered "liberal." Harm/care is at the foundation of doing no harm, prevention, and precaution. Fairness/reciprocity provides a focus on public justice in which harmed minorities (e.g., small or dispersed worker populations) need protection.[17] The conservative viewpoint on harm/care as well as "reciprocity" can, respectively, extend to law-and-order issues and can generate blame-the-victim claims. It is important for the public health advocate to understand conservative viewpoints so as to broaden public support or argue effectively to protect the safety and health of workers and other members of the public. Table 15-6 applies these five values to the message levels described above in Table 15-5.

15.6. THE HARM PRINCIPLE

I see in the near future a crisis approaching that unnerves me and causes me to tremble for the safety of my country . . . corporations have been enthroned and an

era of corruption in high places will follow, and the money power of the country will endeavor to prolong its reign by working upon the prejudices of the people until all wealth is aggregated in a few hands and the Republic is destroyed.
—President Abraham Lincoln. Letter to Colonel William F. Elkins; November 21, 1864

President Lincoln foresaw many potential horrors that were to emerge. This penultimate section presents examples of antiscience arguments that stand in the way of prevention, which an advocate must overcome. These arguments are a significant shift from attacks upon the rule-making process to attacks on the underlying science behind regulation or against the scientist who reports discomfiting scientific findings (ad hominem fallacy). Regulation is always seen as a constraint on the free market. The challenge is to overcome beliefs in individualism when shared responsibility is needed.[17]

The oath from the *Hippocratic Corpus*, "first do no harm," is well known in medical and public health circles. This moral principle is also part of the libertarian mantra: John Stuart Mill's harm principle states that the only reason to restrict the action of another individual is to prevent harm to others. However, according to this ethic, in market justice a business has a minimal obligation to protect the common good; it is rooted in the belief that an unfettered marketplace is the best way to serve the desires of people.[17] At issue is who has the burden to identify the harm. Institutions contribute to absolution for harmful acts by blaming or dehumanizing victims, diffusing responsibility, or minimizing negative consequences.[29,30]

Many books have documented the safety and health horrors perpetuated by deliberate industrial ignorance. David Michaels, appointed by President Barack Obama as OSHA administrator in 2009, published a book in 2008 entitled *Doubt Is Their Product*.[31] The subtitle of this book is *How Industry's Assault on Science Threatens Your Health*. Michaels shows how powerful interests cloud the issue of the public's health with profits as the trade-off. A number of other books address the challenge to science from industry, including *The Merchants of Doubt*,[32] *The Hockey Stick and the Climate Wars*,[33] *Deceit and Denial*,[34] and *Bending Science*.[35]

A united corporate community strongly opposed the creation of OSHA as both a possible precedent for enlarging government regulation and a potential stronghold for unions. By the 1980s, the corporate community had turned the agency into a "political prisoner" through delays in providing information, legislative amendments limiting its power, legal victories that further reduced its power, and budget cuts that made inspections fewer and more superficial. These changes occurred despite strong public sentiment in favor of enforcing workplace safety laws.[36,37] Several examples are described below that show a callousness toward the harm principle.

15.6.1. Beryllium

The original standard for occupational exposure to beryllium was set in 1949 by the U.S. Atomic Energy Commission at 2 µg/m³, which was established in a taxicab conversation.[31] By the 1970s, evidence was clear that damaging health effects were occurring below the standard. OSHA and the U.S. Department of Energy moved to lower the standard. The leading producer of beryllium products contended that the science was unsound. Hundreds of workers in the weapons industry and some engaged in ore grinding had come down with chronic beryllium disease. The industry argued that the standard was not at fault but that at some time in the past these sick people must have been exposed to levels above the standard. During the period 1975–1979, three studies by NIOSH of exposure to beryllium and its association to lung cancer were published in the peer-reviewed literature. However, with industry reconstruction of the scientific data and political influence, OSHA terminated rule making.[38] The politics surrounding this issue was addressed in more detail in Chapter 9, regarding research and the OSHAct.

15.6.2. Asbestos

Investigators had identified a serious asbestosis problem among workers associated with asbestos exposure in the early 1930s, and asbestosis was correlated with lung cancer in the 1940s. After World War II, Johns-Manville funded research with mice that did not address cancer and falsely concluded that asbestosis was a nonprogressive disease. In 1957, the industry-created Asbestos Textile Institute wrote that evidence of cancer or asbestosis was lacking to warrant more research. By 1964, the asbestos industry's decade long cover-up of the problem of asbestosis and cancer fell apart with a conference on the biological effects of asbestos. The industry tried to silence Dr. Irving Selikoff, the organizer of the conference. In 1967, the Asbestos Information Association defended the industry by claiming the lack of "unequivocal" scientific evidence of the hazard. In a 1968 study of asbestos installers, Selikoff found an "unequivocal" lung cancer rate seven times higher than expected.[31] By one calculation, 2.1 million workers in the United States were expected to die over several decades from asbestos-related diseases.[39]

As revelations of the asbestos hazard led to crippling lawsuits for the industry in the United States,[33] the battle shifted to international science organizations. The first drafts of the World Health Organization's (WHO) International Program on Chemical Safety (IPCS) criteria document on chrysotile asbestos were prepared by scientists associated with the asbestos industry in 1996 (see Chapter 12 regarding international policy). The scientific community and the U.S. Department of State intervened to bring balance among the writers of the final criteria document, which was published in 1998.

In another incident, the International Fibre Safety Group was an industry front that worked with the International Labour Organization (ILO) to sponsor a 1997 draft monograph, which was written by industry confederates including those involved with the early draft of the IPCS criteria document. Scientists from several nations railed against industry involvement, leading the ILO to withdraw publication of the monograph. Likewise, two industry-friendly WHO reports emerged out of its European office in Copenhagen (Denmark) regarding asbestos that the scientific community challenged as inaccurate.[40] This controversy was described in more detail in Chapter 12.

15.6.3. White Lead

Alice Hamilton, the first U.S. physician to dedicate her career to occupational medicine, as described in Chapter 5, said in 1908 that lead poisoning had endangered workers' health for nearly two millennia. In 1910, she said that lead enters the body through inhalation and ingestion and not just through the skin, and in 1913 she said that white lead paint should not be used for interior work, where painters were at particular risk. In the 1920s, children were also found to be poisoned by lead paint where it was used on toys and within households. The industry countered with advertisements using the Dutch Boy brand and promoting the sanitizing effect of painted walls. By the 1930s, substitutes for lead as a pigment in paint were known, but the lead industry was effective at controlling information regarding the hazard of lead poisoning through its sponsored research, challenges to research results by others, and at times outright intimidation. In the 1940s and 1950s, the industry framed its argument as a "prejudice against lead," countering arguments of the public health problem of lead poisoning as absurd.[41]

The battles between lead promotion and scientific findings of its hazards continued. In 1971, President Richard Nixon signed the Lead Based Paint Poisoning Prevention Act, which stopped paint use inside of houses when federal funds were used.[34] It was not until 1978 that the U.S. Environmental Protection Agency's (EPA) lead abatement requirements became effective to protect children from exposure in housing and when OSHA promulgated a standard to protect workers from lead exposures. In 1993, OSHA promulgated another standard to protect construction workers exposed to lead paint—80 years after Alice Hamilton's 1913 claim.

15.6.4. Leaded Gasoline

Tetraethyl lead became an important antiknocking compound in gasoline in the mid-1920s. Deaths in the tetraethyl lead formulation plants were a sentinel event of a new hazard, and the U.S. Surgeon General convened a conference to elicit voluntary industry controls of exposures to lead formulation and fumes from leaded gasoline. The industry agreed to maintain standards to prevent further deaths among workers. The Ethyl Corporation and the automobile industry funded grants to Robert Kehoe of the Kettering Laboratories in the 1950s, which resulted in claims that leaded gasoline posed no hazard to the public. Kehoe conducted experiments on 16 of his employees, exposing them to lead, and contended that their high blood lead levels did not indicate symptoms of poisoning. Another argument regarding the safety of lead exposure was an existing threshold level value, which Harriet Hardy disputed.[41a] Hardy, described in Chapter 5, was a pioneering occupational health toxicologist and colleague of Alice Hamilton. She claimed that threshold levels are meaningless when developing children are at risk from a known toxin.

When the lead industry paradigm of safe levels was challenged effectively, the industry shifted its argument in 1968 to claiming that the lead problem resulted from the old use of white lead in paint and not its new use in gasoline. The industry also funded efforts to discredit Dr. Herbert Needleman for his work on lead toxicity by paying two scientists to bring scientific misconduct charges against him. He was cleared of these charges after 10 years of intimidation.[35] Control came first indirectly in the early 1970s, when leaded gasoline was banned from new automobiles to avert damage to a pollution-controlling device, the catalytic converter. During the 1970s, occupational and environmental policies coalesced further to eliminate leaded gasoline exposures.

15.6.5. Tractor Overturns

A John Deere engineer reported in 1970 that 30,000 farmers had been killed as a result of tractor overturns. During the period when he made the report, an average of 500 farmers were killed annually in the United States as a result of overturns. Rollover protective structures (ROPS) had been found to be effective in preventing 98% of these deaths in Sweden, which had implemented mandatory ROPS on new tractors in 1959. John Deere made its Roll-Guard design patent available to all manufacturers in 1967. However, the industry did not make ROPS mandatory on tractors until 18 years and an estimated 7,200 deaths later in 1985.[42]

15.6.6. Short-Handled Hoe

California companies and contractors hired farmworkers to weed and thin their crops with the use of a short-handled hoe. Growers claimed that workers did a better job with the short hoe rather than the long-handled hoe. Doctors claimed that the stooped position workers had to use with the short hoe was associated with degeneration and herniation of the discs in the spine and that three out of four farmworkers had permanent disabling back injury after age 40. In 1970, César Chávez of the United Farm Workers led a campaign to eradicate the use of the short hoe based on a state law that banned unsafe hand tools. University of California students conducted a survey comparing farmworker use of the short hoe and the long hoe with results of 15.6 and 3.7% permanent disabling back injuries, respectively. Governor Ronald Reagan (R) had appointed the members of the California Industrial Safety Board, which dismissed a petition to ban the use of the short hoe. The board ruled that the short hoe was not unsafe and that the cost of discarding the short hoe outweighed its harm. Lawyers for the farmworkers then took the case to the state court of appeals in 1973, where it was denied, and then to the California Supreme Court in 1974, where the petition was granted in 1975. As a result, a new board under newly elected Governor Jerry Brown (D) reconsidered the petition. The new board banned the short hoe, and ironically, growers found that the use of the long-handled hoe improved "stamina" among the workers and thus improved productivity.[14]

15.6.7. Hexavalent Chromium

Thomas F. Mancuso and Wilhelm C. Hueper published results of a study of hexavalent chromium exposed workers in 1951 that found an excess of lung cancer among that cohort. Several study results followed with the same conclusion. After the passage of the OSHAct, the hexavalent chromium industry mounted a campaign to delay OSHA hexavalent chromium rule making. The industry argued that there was no effect from exposure at low levels. The EPA published a study in 2000 of 2,300 workers exposed to hexavalent chromium from 1950 to 1974. A significant elevated risk of lung cancer was found. Industry investigators acquired the raw data from the study, conducted their own analysis, and challenged the EPA conclusions, which OSHA rejected when responding to a court order to issue a standard. The agency published its proposed rule in 2004. The industry responded by funding a study to support its position, reporting results of a statistically underpowered part of that study that showed negative results. In another paper, they combined data from two exposed populations that diluted the reported health effect. When their complete study report was uncovered as a result of a separate bankruptcy case, it became available to the public. That report confirmed elevated lung cancer at low exposure levels.[38] Under court order, OSHA promulgated a hexavalent chromium standard in 2006.

15.6.8. Synthetic Dyes

In the early 1900s, European investigators found that exposure to two chemicals (beta-naphthylamine and benzidine) used in the production of dyes were associated with bladder cancer. The ILO published a monograph on occupational bladder cancer in 1921. By 1925, the Swiss government recognized benzidine as an occupational carcinogen. Hueper, a physician employed by DuPont, published his first article on bladder cancer in 1934, but the company disallowed his publication of additional findings and dismissed him. DuPont contended that benzidine was not a human carcinogen. Nonetheless, bladder cancer cases continued to be identified across the synthetic dye industry into the 1950s and 1960s. Workers exposed to benzidine were later found to have a bladder cancer rate 10 times higher than the population as a whole, and hundreds of workers had died from exposure to synthetic dye-related chemicals. Voluntary action to protect workers failed because of managerial ignorance or recalcitrance. Indeed, the industry for many years took no responsibility for taking note of the scientific literature regarding chemical hazards.[43] It was OSHA that intervened when it promulgated standards for these two chemicals in 1974.

There are other stories of the lack of ethical behavior for protecting workers' safety and health from exposures to occupational hazards. These hazards include silica,[44,45] cotton dust,[46] pesticides,[47] coal workers' pneumoconiosis (miners' asthma, or black lung),[48] secondhand tobacco smoke,[31] and ergonomic challenges.[49,50] Advocating for occupational safety and health presents a quandary: "Why do so many powerful and intelligent people distort the scientific truth about the negative effects of hazardous exposures?"[31]

Market justice hearkens back to earlier pioneer American individualism that extolled the value of self-reliance and personal independence. In the new individualism, monetary gain has become the goal built on the modern machine age.[51,52] We live in an age of pecuniary gain that undercuts the autonomy and health of the individual worker. Industrial leaders, those who are not transformational, are enslaved by avarice and greed in the corporation. In 1930, John Dewey argued that science along with social reform would be a new and countervailing path to new and improved truths and values.[51,52] The public health advocate is challenged to defend the science and examine the enslavement of powerful and influential leaders of industry to the enemies of prevention as described in Chapter 6: time, distance, and ignorance, but most of all, greed.

15.7. SITUATIONAL LEADERSHIP THEORY

The place to improve the world is first in one's own heart and head and hands.
—Robert M. Pirsig[53]

This chapter began by examining a situation as governing the behavior of leaders within organizations, and that situation is a profit-first rather than a safety-first doctrine. Situational leadership theory posits that a leader's styles should adapt in different ways to the situation presented by the majority of followers.[54] Flipping this theory on its head from the viewpoint of management-labor relations, the problem regarding occupational safety and health is the situation of

Table 15-7. Adaptation of Situational Leadership Theory to Occupational Safety and Health Administration Leadership Orientation (Support Versus Direction) Contingent on Employer Readiness at Different Levels of Development, With Examples

Supportive Behavior	Directive Behavior	
	Low	High
High support	Level 3. Consultation Program (supporting style): OSHA is collaborative with employers; includes consultation and consensus.	Level 2. Training and inspection programs (coaching style): OSHA provides considerable input about task accomplishment and intervenes to protect worker safety and health.*
Low Support	Level 4. Voluntary Protection Program (delegating style): OSHA delegates responsibility for worker safety and health to an employer and is kept informed of progress.	Level 1. Severe Violator Enforcement Program (directing style): OSHA produces a lot of direction.

(Supportive Behavior axis: (Low) → (High))

(Low) → Directive (task) Behavior → (High)

Employer Readiness to Protect Workers From Hazards			
	High	Moderate	Low
Follower Maturity	Competent and committed	High competence and variable commitment	Some competence but low commitment	Committed but low competence

Employer-Directed   OSHA-Directed
Developed ← ← ← Development Progression → → → Developing

Note: OSHA = Occupational Safety and Health Administration.
*In many situations, this orientation produces the best result.[53]

viewing OSHA as the leader and employers as the followers. The agency can change the situation that employers experience regarding safety and health.

Consistent with this theory, which is shown in Table 15-7, the leader (i.e., OSHA) has four styles to address different levels of development: level 1—directing, level 2—coaching, level 3—supporting, and level 4—delegating. The concept of development under this theory is defined as a continuum (e.g., from OSHA-directed to employer-directed) based on the competence and commitment to accomplish a specific task (e.g., provide a workplace free of recognized hazards). From the occupational safety and health policy perspective, employer competence is the mastery of knowledge, experience, and skills to provide a safe workplace, and employer commitment is the extent to which confidence and a positive attitude exist to provide a safe workplace.

In level 1, the "directing" style (guiding, telling) addresses the situation in which an employer is unable and unwilling to provide a safe workplace, which is represented by the OSHA Severe Violator Enforcement Program. The "coaching" style (persuading, explaining) under this theory can address the low to moderate transition of development; and the "supporting" style (participating, encouraging problem solving) can address the moderate to high transition of development. These two styles are represented by, first, OSHA's outreach training program and inspection programs[55] (e.g., planned or scheduled investigations) and, second, by the OSHA Consultation Program, respectively, in levels 2 and 3. Finally, the "delegating" style (observing, monitoring) in level 4 can address the situation in which an employer has both the competence and the commitment to provide a safe workplace. This latter style is represented by the OSHA Voluntary Protection Program.

In the application of this theory, the most effective style depends on the development level of an employer. While it is intuitive, this theory is not a panacea. It depends upon choices and not principles. Nonetheless, it does address the situation that was identified earlier regarding situational attribution as to why good people act unethically.

The explosion on the Deepwater Horizon in the Gulf of Mexico on April 20, 2010, as described in Chapter 11 shows how a situation can control safety behavior (situational attribution theory). The president's National Commission on the BP Deepwater Horizon Oil Spill and Offshore Drilling found that the immediate causes of the well blowout and resulting explosion that killed 11 workers can be traced to a series of identifiable mistakes made by the management of three companies (BP, Halliburton, and Transocean) that were drilling on the day of the explosion, which "reveal such systematic failures in risk management that they place in doubt the safety culture of the entire industry." The commission identified the lack of technology, laws and regulations, and practices to prevent blowouts and explosions from large, high-pressure, and deep reservoirs of oil and gas. It recommended that "government must close the existing gap and industry must support rather than resist that effort." This investigation points out the need for the application of situational leadership theory in which government must change the situation and provide leadership in that change. Changes did happen at the U.S. Department of the Interior, which is responsible for regulating rig safety, and which is also described in Chapter 11.[56]

On a related note, NIOSH provided a starting point for moving employers along the development scale toward increased competence and commitment to provide a workplace free of recognized hazards. In the 1980s, it developed a curriculum to introduce occupational safety and health education to managers through a business school curriculum. This program was named Project MINERVA, and its curriculum comprised eight units. It did not take hold, partly because business schools were not ready to define management as a profession with a code of ethics similar to medicine or engineering. The ILO later suggested a study program for managers that covered the following units:[57]

1. The management of occupational health and safety,
2. Occupational health management,
3. Occupational hygiene,
4. Ergonomics,
5. Safety and health law,
6. Risk management,
7. Injury investigation,
8. Statistics and information systems.

PUSHING-THE-LUCK NARRATIVE

Seven workers' lives were at risk. The space shuttle Challenger sat on the pad on January 27, 1986, when the temperature was predicted to drop below freezing at launch time on the following morning. Engineers at Morton Thiokol in Utah—the designers of the rocket that would carry the shuttle into space—were concerned that the O-rings would be too stiff to seal at that low temperature, resulting in escaping hot gas that could cause the rocket to explode. Their evidence for this concern was a history of O-ring damage during previous launches, that resiliency of the rings was known to decline exponentially with cooling, and confirmation of this decline from experimental data. As a result of this concern, Thiokol managers faxed a recommendation to the National Aeronautics and Space Administration (NASA) that claimed that the launch should be delayed for warmer conditions, as evidenced by their engineering data. This was the first time that Thiokol had made a no-launch recommendation in 12 years, during which 24 launches had been successful. Even though early tests showed that the field joints that were sealed by O-rings expanded slightly during test firings rather than tightening as they were designed to do, aborting launches because of the O-ring problem had been waived routinely since 1982. The administration had an ambitious launch schedule to keep, and Thiokol wanted to please NASA.[58,59]

A lot of publicity surrounded this launch with a schoolteacher aboard and the president poised for comment. Managers at NASA questioned the reasoning behind the recommendation. An intense debate between Thiokol and NASA ensued in the afternoon and evening before the planned launch, which addressed the issue, "Will the rubber O-rings fail catastrophically tomorrow because of cold weather?" To support its recommendation, Thiokol faxed 13 charts as evidence to NASA at Cape Canaveral in Florida. In a rush to judgment, Thiokol used existing charts with handwritten notations added. Doubt was engendered when the charts used Thiokol identifiers rather than NASA terms. The key chart showed the history of O-ring damage from previous flights with handwritten dates of launches added. Six observed factors regarding O-ring damage were shown, which muddled the engineers' message. As for temperature, the coldest launch had been at 53°F, and this and one other launch at 75°F were the only two of the 24 earlier launches for which temperatures were shown on the charts, although other supporting experimental temperature data were shown. The chart of the 24 launches showed dates but not temperatures.

During a teleconference between Thiokol and NASA, a high official at NASA stated that he was "appalled" and suggested that Thiokol reconsider its recommendation so that the launch could go ahead, thus intimidating the Thiokol managers. This official claimed that damage was "true of every other flight we have had." He further stated, "My God, Thiokol, when do you expect me to launch, next April?" Another NASA official claimed he had no reason to believe that the O-rings would malfunction since blow-by had occurred at temperatures much higher than freezing at 53°F with no catastrophe, and thus there was no correlation between temperature and the likelihood of blow-by. During a caucus while the teleconference was on mute, Thiokol managers discussed their recommendation. Three of four managers voted to bow to NASA's desire. The fourth manager was an engineer and was reluctant to change the recommendation. Finally, when the holdout was challenged with the statement, "Take off your engineering hat, and put on your manager hat," he caved, and at midnight, Thiokol reversed its recommendation.[60]

The next morning, an on-site Thiokol manager expressed his opposition to the launch but was told it had been resolved. He stated, "I sure wouldn't want to be the person who had to stand in front of a board of inquiry to explain why we launched this outside of the qualification of the solid rocket motor on any shuttle system." His concern was not forwarded to higher levels at NASA.[59]

NASA launched the Challenger on January 28, the O-rings failed, and 73 seconds after liftoff the rocket exploded, killing all aboard.

A display of the causal relations is key to using numbers as evidence. The engineers were right in their conclusion, they were correct in their theory and causal thinking, but the persuasive argument failed in part because of the lack of a chart associating O-ring failure to temperature. Persuasive influence failed, but reason failed too, and fallacies abounded.[58]

REFERENCES

1. Northrup HR, Rowan RL, Perry CR. *The Impact of OSHA.* Philadelphia, PA: University of Pennsylvania;1978. Labor Relations and Public Policy Series, No. 17.

2. Zimbardo P. *The Lucifer Effect: Understanding How Good People Turn Evil.* New York, NY: Random House;2008.

3. Moyers B, Jones S. Trade secrets: a Moyers report [transcript]. PBS. 2001. Available at: http://www.pbs.org/tradesecrets/transcript.html. Accessed July 12, 2013.

4. Hansson SO. *Setting the Limit: Occupational Health Standards and the Limits of Science.* New York, NY: Oxford University Press;1988.

5. Chandler, DB, Werther, WB. *Strategic Corporate Social Responsibility: Stakeholders, Globalization, and Sustainable Value Creation.* Thousand Oaks, CA: Sage;2014:250.

6. Shermer M. *Skepticsm 101: How to Think Like a Scientist.* Chantilly, VA: The Great Courses;2013. Course Guidebook.

7. Milgram S. *Obedience to Authority.* New York, NY: Harper Touchbooks;1974.

8. Darley JM, Batson CD. "From Jerusalem to Jericho": A study of situational and dispositional variables in helping behavior. *J Pers Soc Psychol.* 1973;27(1):100–108.

9. Zimbardo PG. On the ethics of intervention in human psychological research: With special reference to the Stanford prison experiment. *Cognition.* 1973;2(2): 243–256.

10. Mitchell G. Q&A with George Mitchell. *Sunday Morning.* CBS News. September 2, 2012. Available at: http://www.cbsnews.com/news/qa-with-george-mitchell. Accessed June 10, 2014.

11. Wright K, Rowitz L, Merkle A, et al. Competency development in public health leadership. *Am J Public Health.* 2000;90(8):1202–1207.

12. Roberto MA. *Transformational Leadership: How Leaders Change Teams, Companies, and Organizations*. Chantilly, VA: The Teaching Company;2011.

13. Ciulla JB. Leadership ethics: mapping the territory. *Bus Ethics Q*. 1995;5(1):5–28.

14. Jourdane M. *The Struggle for the Health and Legal Protection of Farmworkers: El Cortito*. Houston, TX: Arte Público Press;2004.

15. Cialdini R. *Influence: The Psychology of Persuasion*. New York, NY: Harper; 2006.

16. Dunn CM, Chadwick GL. *Protecting Study Volunteers in Research: A Manual for Investigative Sites*. Boston, MA: Centerwatch;2002.

17. Beauchamp DE. Public health as social justice. *Inquiry*. 1976;13(1):3–14.

18. Ciulla JB. The state of leadership ethics and the work that lies before us. *Bus Ethics Europ Rev*. 2005;14(4):323–335.

19. Robin D. Toward an applied meaning for ethics in business. *J Bus Ethics*. 2009;89:139–150.

20. Eastman C. *Work Accidents and the Law*. New York, NY: Russell Sage Foundation; 1910.

21. Wallack L, Dorfman L, Jernigan D, Themba M. *Media Advocacy and Public Health: Power for Prevention*. London, UK: Sage Publications;1993.

22. Page JA, O'Brien M-W. *Bitter Wages*. New York, NY: Grossman Publishers;1973.

23. Ryan W. *Blaming the Victim*. New York, NY: Vintage Books;1976.

24. Deming WE. *Out of the Crisis*. Cambridge, MA: Massachusetts Institute of Technology;1986.

25. Natola S. Nelson Mandela's body left us today, but not his spirit. *Brave Gnu Whirled: Political and Social Commentary*. December 5, 2013. Available at: http://bravegnuwhirled.blogspot.com/2013/12/nelson-mandelas-body-left-us-today-but.html. Accessed June 10, 2014.

26. Dorfman L, Wallack L, Woodruff K. More than a message: framing public health advocacy to change corporate practices. *Health Educ Behav*. 2005;32(3): 320–336.

27. Haidt J, Kesebir S. Morality. In: Fiske S, Gilbert D, Lindzey G, eds. *Handbook of Social Psychology*. 5th ed. Hoboken, NJ: Wiley;2010:797–832.

28. Haidt J. The new synthesis in moral psychology. *Science*. 2007;316(5827): 998–1002.

29. Schapiro M. Chemical Revolution. In: *Exposed: The Toxic Chemistry of Everyday Products and What's at Stake for American Power.* White River Junction, VT: Chelsea Green Publishing;2007.

30. Tindale CW. *Fallacies and Argument Appraisal.* New York, NY: Cambridge University Press;2007.

31. Michaels D. *Doubt Is Their Product: How Industry's Assault on Science Threatens Your Health.* New York, NY: Oxford University Press;2008.

32. Oreskes N, Conway EM. *Merchants of Doubt: How a Handful of Scientists Obscured the Truth on Issues From Tobacco Smoke to Global Warming.* New York, NY: Bloomsbury Press;2010.

33. Mann ME. *The Hockey Stick and the Climate Wars.* New York, NY: Columbia University Press;2012.

34. Markowitz G, Rosner D. *Deceit and Denial.* Berkeley, CA: University of California Press;2002.

35. McGarity TO, Wagner WE. *Bending Science: How Special Interests Corrupt Public Health Research.* Cambridge, MA: Harvard University Press;2008.

36. Noble C. *Liberalism at Work: The Rise and Fall of OSHA.* Philadelphia, PA: Temple University Press;1986.

37. Szasz A. Industrial resistance to occupational safety and health legislation: 1971–1981. *Soc Probl.* 1984;32:103–116.

38. Michaels D, Monforton C, Lurie P. Selected science: an industry campaign to undermine an OSHA hexavalent chromium standard. *Environmental Health: A Global Access Science Source.* 2006;5(5). Available at: http://www.ehjournal.net/content/pdf/1476-069X-5-5.pdf. Accessed August 23, 2013.

39. O'Hare JA. Asbestos litigation: the dust is yet to settle. *Fordham Urb Law J.* 1978;7(1):55–91.

40. Castleman BI, Lemen RA. The manipulation of international scientific organizations. *Int J Occup Environ Health.* 1998;4(1):53–55.

41. Sicherman B. *Alice Hamliton. A Life of Letters.* Cambridge, Massachusetts: Harvard University Press;1984.

41a. Warren C. *Brush with Death: A Social History of Lead Poisoning.* Baltimore, MD: Johns Hopkins University Press;2001.

42. Myers ML. Prevention effectiveness of roll-over protective structures, part I: strategy evolution. *J Agric Saf Health.* 2000;6(1):29–40.

43. Michaels D. Waiting for the body count: Corporate decision making and bladder cancer in the U.S. dye industry. *Med Anthro Q.* 1988;2(3):215–232.

44. Rosen D, Markowitz G. *Deadly Dust: Silicosis and the Politics of Occupational Disease in Twentieth-Century America.* Princeton, NJ: Princeton University Press;1991.

45. Cherniak M. *The Hawk's Nest Incident: America's Worst Industrial Disaster.* New Haven, CT: Yale University Press;1986.

46. Levenstein C, DeLaurier GF, Dunn ML. *Cotton Dust Papers: Science, Politics, and Power in the "Discovery" of Byssinosis in the U.S.* Amityville, NY: Baywood Publishing Company;2001.

47. Regenstein L. *America the Poisoned: How Deadly Chemicals Are Destroying Our Environment, Our Wildlife, Ourselves, and How We Can Survive!* Washington, DC: Acropolis Books;1982.

48. Derickson A. *Black Lung: Anatomy of a Public Health Disaster.* Ithaca, NY: Cornell University Press;1998.

49. Kome P. *Wounded Workers: The Politics of Musculoskeletal Injuries.* Toronto, ON: University of Toronto Press;1998:177–189.

50. Maraniss D, Weisskopf M. *"Tell Newt to Shut Up!"* New York, NY: Simon and Schuster;1996:60–64.

51. Dewey J. *Individualism: Old and New.* Amherst, NY: Prometheus Books;1999.

52. Crosby P. Leading with soul: an uncommon journey of spirit. *J Coll Char.* 2004;5(4). Available at: http://journals.naspa.org/cgi/viewcontent.cgi?article=1383&context=jcc. Accessed November 13, 2012.

53. Pirsig RM. *Zen and the Art of Motorcycle Maintenance.* New York, NY: William Morrow;1974.

54. Blanchard KH, Zigarmi D, Nelson RB. Situational Leadership® after 25 years: a retrospective. *J Lead Org Stud.* 1993;1(1):21–36.

55. Levine DI, Toffel MW, Johnson MS. Randomized government safety inspections reduce worker injuries with no detectable job loss. *Science.* 2012;336(6083):907–911.

56. National Commission on the BP Deepwater Horizon Oil Spill and Offshore Drilling. Deep water: the gulf oil disaster and the future of offshore drilling. Final Report. 2011. Available at: http://cybercemetery.unt.edu/archive/oilspill/20121210200431/http:/www.oilspillcommission.gov/final-report. Accessed June 12, 2014.

57. Rudge J. Safety and health training of managers. In: Stellman SM et al., eds. *Encyclopaedia of Occupational Safety and Health*. Geneva, Switzerland: International Labour Office;1998:18.18–18.22.

58. Gouran DS. The failure of argument in decisions leading to the "Challenger Disaster": a two-level analysis. In: Schiappa E, ed. *Warranting Assent: Case Studies in Argument Evaluation*. Albany, NY: State University of New York Press;1995: 57–77.

59. Vaughan D. *The Challenger Launch Decision: Risky Technology, Culture, and Deviance at NASA*. Chicago, IL: University of Chicago Press;1996.

60. Tufte ER. *Visual Explanations: Images and Quantities, Evidence, and Narrative*. Cheshire, CT: Graphics Press;1997.

16

Occupational Safety and Health Policy Analysis

One should think of law as a first, rather than a last, step in the process of producing desired policy results.

—Denise Asheberle[1]

A PUBLIC HEALTH ACHIEVEMENT NARRATIVE

During the 20th century, life expectancy at birth among U.S. residents increased by 62%, from 47.3 years in 1900 to 76.8 years in 2000.[2] One aspect of this success is a century-long advocacy that resulted in one of the 20th century's "Ten Great Public Health Achievements" in the United States, in which occupational safety and health policies resulted in safer workplaces during the period 1900 to 1999 with a large impact on the reduction in death, illness, and disability. Safer workplaces helped reduce the rate of fatal occupational injuries by approximately 40%. Work-related diseases, such as coal workers' pneumoconiosis, silicosis, and lead poisoning, which were common early in the century, have come under better control. In the latter part of the century after the passage of the Occupational Safety and Health Act (OSHAct; see Appendix), severe injuries and deaths related to mining, manufacturing, construction, and transportation decreased.[2] In 1970, when President Richard Nixon signed the OSHAct, more than 10,000 people were dying of work-related injuries every year. The decline to half that number today reflects technological advancements as well as the imposition of Occupational Safety and Health Administration (OSHA) standards. But even considering that decline, workplace deaths still occur with disturbing frequency.

Jim Fall of the 3M Industrial Adhesives and Tapes Division spoke of government intervention at the Specialty Tools and Fasteners Distributors Association Conference on November 5, 2012. He stated that government regulations can provide opportunities for business. Specifically, he acknowledged the impact of OSHA on the market for personal protective equipment and fall protection and of the National Institute for Occupational Safety and Health (NIOSH) on respirator certifications. He also spoke of OSHA's impact on the reduction of thousands of occupational fatalities since 1970.[3]

16.1. REVIEW

A plan once made and visualized becomes a reality along with other realities—never to be destroyed but easily to be attacked.

—John Steinbeck[4]

The introduction to this book began with the promise quoted from the OSH Act: "to assure so far as possible every working man and woman in the Nation safe and healthful working conditions." This promise has been the thread woven into these chapters, with an emphasis on the prevention of irreversible morbidity and premature mortality. In review, Chapter 1 introduced the book and emphasized the occupational safety and health problem of work-related diseases and injuries. It also offered a definition of policy as "a definite course of action selected from among alternatives with regard to certain conditions to guide and determine present and future actions." The next five chapters addressed precepts for occupational safety and health policy, followed by six chapters that addressed the implementation of this policy, and the latter four chapters, including this chapter, address important instruments of policy.

Chapter 2 focused on the public health principle of prevention and the different models that are used in implementing prevention policies, and Chapter 3 addressed the connections between occupational and environmental health and the subsuming of occupational health as part of environmental health. This chapter also introduced injury control and prevention as part of occupational and environmental health. Chapter 4 addressed law as a necessary policy tool in the protection of occupational safety and health, and Chapter 5 described the history of occupational safety and health policy, which builds on the idea of precedence in law and is important as a foundation for continuing progress in more effective protection of workers. Since policy is nothing unless acted upon, Chapter 6 addressed the need for advocacy with the use of argument, persuasion, and ways to combat fallacies and denials regarding the problem. It incorporated the arguments for the creation of the OSHAct.

The following six chapters described the implementation of occupational safety and health policy. Chapters 7 through 9 covered the 34 sections of the OSHAct and its ramifications regarding ongoing controversies. Chapter 7 addressed the standards-setting process, Chapter 8 described the enforcement of these standards, and Chapter 9 considered the role of research and outreach to the public under the OSHAct. Chapter 10 described the history and controversies regarding mine safety and health policies, showing progress in injury prevention as driven by disasters and revealing how fixed paradigms of science can stymie progress in disease prevention. Chapter 11 described other prevention policies that lie outside of the jurisdictions of the OSHAct. Chapter 12 addressed global occupational safety and health policies, which present emerging challenges to national policies and are expanded upon later in this concluding chapter.

The latter four chapters addressed instruments of policy (in addition to the instruments of law discussed in Chapter 4 and advocacy discussed in Chapter 6) that are important to occupational safety and health policy. Chapter 13 described the economics of occupational safety and health, which provides support for as well as a bane to prevention efforts. Chapter 14 described the need for and power of information as a prevention tool, including the multifaceted impact of worker right-to-know strategies for the protection of workers from occupational injuries and diseases. Chapter 15 addressed issues closely related to the discussion of advocacy in Chapter 6 with a discussion of leadership and ethics related to occupational safety and health. This, the final chapter, addresses the role of policy analysis related to occupational safety and health, which shines a light on the dark past of our subject, reveals progress in advancing protective policies, and opens windows to see possible futures for occupational safety and health policies.

16.2. INTRODUCTION TO CHAPTER 16

By analysis we mean the process of deducing consequences from initial conditions, of attending scrupulously to chains of reasoning, and of guarding against the always present temptation to substitute demagoguery for intellectual exchange.
—Robert Heilbroner and William Milberg[5]

Policy analysis is founded on applying the social sciences to policy. Analysis as it is applied to policy leads to (1) inferring consequences from initial conditions, (2) attending to chains of reasoning, and (3) guarding against anything but intellectual exchange.[5] Policy analysis is client-oriented advice relevant to public decisions and informed by social values.[6] Indeed, policy analysis is defined as the act of helping clients to develop a response to public dilemmas.[7] Beyond rational determinations, political actions can have dramatic effects on occupational safety and health policy. Policy analysis must also extend to the polis as well and may need to change rather than buy into the existing system.

Policy analyses traditionally depended upon persuasion and objectivity. While admitting to the naivety of excluding ideology from analysis, Lawlor provided three principles for the profession of policy analysis:[8]

- First, policy analysis functions as a distinct form of applied social science. Lawlor accepted the argumentative school for examining alternative frames of discovery that may lead to change agent activism. However, his scope was limited to the social sciences, and the OSHAct, which is social legislation, depends upon the analysis of policy well beyond the disciplines of the social sciences such as the fields of toxicology and epidemiology.
- Second, policy analysis occurs in real time and in the context of real policy processes. This principle distinguishes analysis from both applied and basic science since policy analysis depends upon meeting a schedule and influencing a policy audience. Advice is required against a calendar and actions in motion.
- Third, policy analysis ultimately produces arguments about choice. These arguments involve distinctive formal structures and reasoning based upon external criteria. As discussed later in this chapter, there is another school of thought about policy analysis, which is analyzing and using narratives.

This chapter could easily be a precept of policy making and could have been placed earlier in this book, but policy analysis provides advantages as the concluding chapter by referring back to multiple chapters and thus serving a review function. The order of the sections in this chapter is consistent with a previous policy analysis of occupational safety and health by Mendeloff that followed a two-step process.[9] One step explored the rationale for governmental action. Accordingly, this chapter first addresses the argument for regulation as a way to address the promise of the OSHAct as stated above, and second, it explores the transitions of policy as it affects occupational safety and health over a century of change.

The other step considered alternative actions that governments may take. Consistent with this step, third, this chapter examines, by way of political economy, reform options of the OSHAct; fourth and fifth, it describes contrasting analytical approaches through examples of governmental action: narrative and paradigmatic analyses, respectively; and it sixth addresses the challenge of the global economy to occupational safety and health policy. Finally and seventh, this chapter offers some conclusions, using an analytical framework based upon economics and the polis.

16.3. THE ARGUMENT FOR REGULATION

Occupational safety and health regulation is probably the best-known and most controversial federal regulatory enterprise.

—Kenneth J. Meier[10]

As situational attribution theory explains, well-meaning people can engage in decisions that are harmful to workers. To control the context or situation within which these decisions are made, regulations as defined in Chapter 4 are any attempt by government to control the behavior of citizens, corporations, or subgovernments. Regulations are essential in modern society to govern behaviors between individuals and interests. As applied to occupational safety and health, regulations govern disparate behaviors between different employers by assuring fair competition so that one company does not have an unfair advantage over another company that invests in safety; and between employers and employed workers by assuring that workers' health is not compromised by their work or workplace. Consistent with the field of policy analysis, the study of regulations includes law, economics, history, organization theory, and political science.[10]

Using the method of diagramming arguments described in Chapter 6, Figure 16-1 shows the evidence supporting the promise of the OSHAct: the imperative to prevent work-related injuries and diseases, the failure of volunteerism as an effective prevention strategy, the inadequacy and inconsistency of state programs to protect workers, the importance of protecting workers

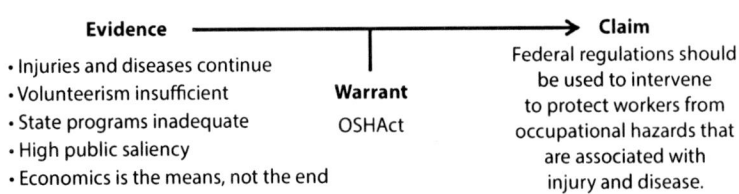

Figure 16-1. Diagram of the argument for occupational safety and health regulations.

from injury and disease exhibited by high public salience, and the recognition that health and not economics comes first.

Traditional occupational safety and health rationales for regulation are many, including problematic economic arguments. First, regarding fairness, bargaining between employers and employees is asymmetrical, with employers having more power and resources than employees. Second, regarding externalities, one party places a cost on one or more other parties regarding injury or disease that are not represented in the bargain. Third, regarding a market-based informational defect, a worker is uninformed about hazards, risks, and the consequences of an exposure. Fourth, workers underestimate the future effects of a potential injury or illness and its effect upon others. Fifth, regarding moral hazard, an employer may fail to provide a safe workplace since the cost of an injury will be diluted when the cost is shared through workers' compensation insurance.[11] Beyond economic perspectives, an additional rationale, indeed a norm that has emerged with high salience, is the protection of the public health, including occupational health.

Standards are the type of regulation used to protect occupational safety and health under the OSHAct. Regulation by OSHA is a governmental standard-setting method for both the goal (i.e., health protection) and the means (e.g., engineering controls) in its standards.[10] The method used is standards aimed at the purpose of the OSHAct. Administrative law guides the process, which is described in the OSHAct. One type of standard embedded in the law is the general duty clause in § 5 of the OSHAct, which is a standard of care as a duty of employers, including a duty to comply with standards set under the act. Section 6 specifies three types of standards: (1) temporary interim, (2) permanent, and (3) emergency temporary standards. The Mine Act has the same types of standards, and it also specifies standards as a matter of law that include limits on coal mine dust exposure. Following the collection of sufficient information to formulate a standard, the following questions are addressed prior to rule making:[11]

1. Should the standard aim directly at the evil targeted (e.g., lead poisoning) or should it aim at a surrogate (e.g., blood lead levels)?
2. What degree of specificity should the standard embody (e.g., 1 µg/m^3 or "avoid so far as practicable")?
3. Should there be a performance standard (e.g., 1 µg/m^3) or a design standard (e.g., guardrail height)?
4. Should a technology-based standard be used (e.g., best available technology)?
5. Should the agency develop a technology forcing the standard (e.g., coke oven emissions standard)?
6. Is regulatory screening (burden of proof at the origin of the potential hazard) an alternative to setting standards (burden of proof on the government)?

The Federal Coal Mine Health and Safety Act (1969) and Mine Act (1977) provide an example of the effectiveness of occupational safety and health regulations as shown in Figure 16-2,[11a] which shows a dramatic reduction in both

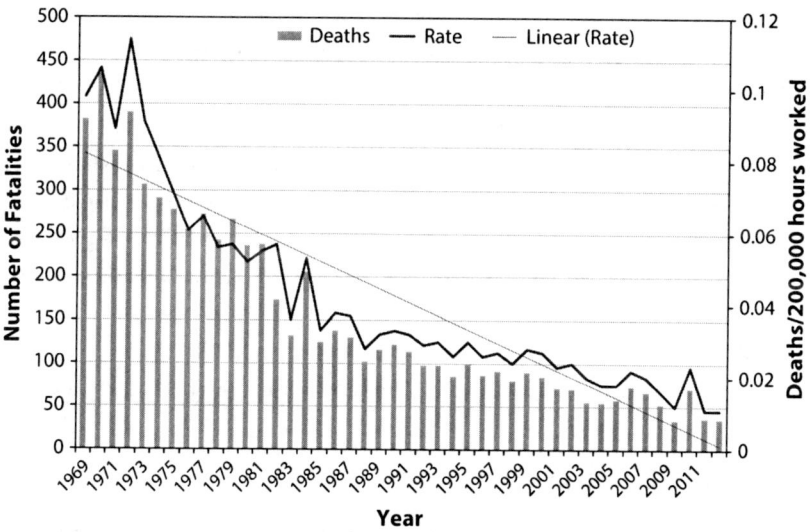

Figure 16-2. Annual frequency and rate of occupational fatalities among U.S. miners, 1969-2012.

the frequency and rate of occupational fatalities among U.S. miners after their establishment. Moreover, OSHA standards aimed at individual hazards have had a multiplier effect for greater overall safety and health awareness and capabilities at the workplace; promulgation of standards has often spurred industrial sectors affected by the standards to develop programs, hire professionals, and train workers and managers in safety and health.[12]

Coalitions of actors form in support and opposition regarding occupational safety and health, and they are partisans with links to political parties. Beyond attempts to influence the regulatory subsystem, these coalitions intervene at the macropolitical level, including through the president, Congress, and the judiciary.

The OSHA and NIOSH subsystem is straightforward and is part of the overall political system, but they are weak entities since they are not independent of top-down control as an independent board or commission. The OSHA administrator reports to the Secretary of the U.S. Department of Labor (DoL) who controls the priorities and the separate Solicitor's Office that provides legal input into the subsystem; in addition, the White House exercises much control over agency actions through the Office of Management and Budget (OMB). NIOSH is not immune to OMB interference, witnessed by its intervention to stop a study of the effects of working with video display terminals in 1987 and the Secretary of the U.S. Department of Health and Human Services (DHHS) intervening to replace three nominees on an ergonomics advisory committee in 2002. Moreover, the subsystem is further controlled by Congress, particularly through the appropriations process, within which riders are attached to limit agency discretion by restricting funding for certain statutory authorities, such as inspections at small farms with fewer than 11 employees, or delaying investigations and rules as was the case regarding the OSHA ergonomics standard, which is discussed later. Nonetheless, this subsystem is of high salience since its actions rarely escape controversy. Salience is used to describe the importance of an issue to the public, but more specifically salience means that actors in politics are motivated to intervene in the regulatory subsystem.

16.4. TRANSITIONS IN POLICY

The way history works: You don't get a lot of credit for what didn't happen. No, this is one of those kind[s] of situations. It's not so much what you achieved as [it] is what you prevented.

—Dick Cheney[13]

The irony and dissonance of former Vice-President Cheney's quote is that he would not use it to describe the concept of prevention in public health even while it rings true for public health. While disasters are newsworthy, successes in preventing problems are often obscured from public view. The issues that result in policy conflicts are typically contests between means and ends, which pits free trade issues against "quality of life" issues rather than considering alternative means to reach the ends, such as having no adverse health effects associated with work.

In many ways the evolution of occupational safety and health policy was incremental. Policies during the period of 1880 to the early 1900s, marked by President Theodore Roosevelt's Square Deal, addressed episodic problems of occupational injury such as at the railroads and in mines, and the disfiguring problem of phossy jaw. The Public Health Service Act was set up to help the states with a focus on infectious and occupational diseases, and it set the stage for a century of occupational health research. The Bureau of Mines initially addressed explosions that helped preserve mine operators' capital investment while saving lives, and workers' compensation systems replaced tort law as an insurance system.

The next period through the 1950s, marked by President Franklin Roosevelt's New Deal, saw a major change during the Great Depression through the Walsh-Healey Public Contracts Act of 1936 that started the process of setting safety standards, although limited to federal government contracts, and through grants to states to establish industrial hygiene programs. These programs led to the creation of the American Conference of Governmental Industrial Hygienists and its formulations of threshold limit values.

At the beginning of the 1960s, positive public policy became the norm that established rights across the full population including the workforce. This period was marked by President Lyndon Johnson's "Great Society." A positive right "specifies obligations of someone to provide whatever the entitlement is," whereas a negative right is "to be free of restraint; says no one can prevent you from doing something."[14] Positive public policy has been revolutionary, leading to the Coal Act of 1969, the OSHAct of 1970, and the Mine Act of 1976 on the wave of the environmental movement. Indeed, as positive public policy, the OSHAct extended its reach economy-wide.[10] The economy-wide laws were much different from sector specific laws of the past.

Then from 1980 to the end of the century, the issue of efficiency captured the occupational safety and health policy agenda, which argued against the negative economic effects of regulations. This antiregulatory agenda instituted obstructions to standard setting with several new administrative laws,

Table 16-1. Framework for understanding the regulatory politics of occupational safety and health policy

Regimes	Policy Goal	Policy Examples
Market: 1880–early 1900s	Create market-like results through administrative means	Safety Appliances Act of 1892, Organic Act of 1910 creating the BoM, White Phosphorus Matches Prohibition Act of 1912; Public Health Service Act of 1912, State Workmen's Compensation acts
Associative: late 1920s–1950s	Promote industrial stability and redistribute national income	Surgeon General's Agreements (e.g., tetra-ethyl lead), National Labor Relations Act of 1935, Title IV of the Social Security Act of 1936 (state industrial hygiene programs), Walsh-Healey Public Contracts Act of 1936, Fair Labor Standards Act of 1938
Societal: 1960s–1970s	Prevent hazards to health and the environment	Federal Metal and Nonmetallic Mine Safety Act of 1966, Federal Coal Mine Health and Safety Act of 1969, Occupational Safety and Health Act of 1970, Federal Mine Safety and Health Act of 1977
Efficiency: 1980–1990s	Eliminate policies that interfere with the market or impose high compliance costs	Negotiated Rulemaking Act of 1990, Paperwork Reduction Act of 1995, Congressional Review Act of 1996, Small Business Regulatory Enforcement Act of 1998, Information Quality Act of 2000
Global: 2000 forward	Manage the impact on domestic constituents, expand commerce, regulate transborder externalities	EU Registration, Evaluation, Authorization, and Restriction of Chemicals Program of 2003, UN Globally Harmonized System of Classification and Labeling of Chemicals of 2003, ILO Better Factories Cambodia Program of 2008

Source: Eisner.[15]
Note: BoM = Bureau of Mines; EU = European Union; UN = United Nations; ILO = International Labour Organization.

as shown in Table 16-1.[15] This period is marked by President Ronald Reagan's mantra, "Get Government Off Our Back."

With the new century, the great change is the globalization of the economy, which presents a dynamic challenge. Indeed, policy has yet to be marked by an effective slogan. Nonetheless, global health and health disparities are considerations that cannot be ignored. Perhaps the tattered adage, "Think Globally, Act Locally," may be a fitting mark for the future. Section 16.8 addresses globalization.

16.4.1. Before the OSHAct

They all die so slowly that none call it murder.

—Samuel Taylor Coleridge[16]

Following World War II, collective bargaining became salient as a wave of labor strikes surged. The strikes came as result of a combination of factors that included returning veterans who were on 52 weeks of unemployment at $20 per week and unions making up for wages and fringe benefits frozen during the war effort as inflation rose. In 1955, the American Federation of Labor (AFL) and the Congress of Industrial Organizations (CIO) merged into a single organization for labor. Older policies of supporting laissez-faire economics as formerly advocated by Samuel Gompers were abandoned; they were associated with a distrust of governments as an agent of employers. The president of the AFL-CIO, George Meany, focused on collective bargaining to reestablish wages that had been eroded by inflation, provide for benefits such as health care, and shift benefit payments to the employer. During the war, businesses had conceded to industrial union power, but after the war, employers bargained strongly to reverse some of the concessions they had made.[17]

Despite employer-labor conflict, collective bargaining worked well. Collective bargaining established the general principle that workers have an interest in their working conditions. Nonetheless, unions traded off safety issues for higher wages and benefits in the bargaining process. Some in the unions raised concerns for the safety and health of workers, including Dr. Lorin Kerr of the United Mine Workers of America, César Chávez of the United Farm Workers, and Tony Mazzocchi of the Oil, Chemical, and Atomic Workers union.[18-20] In addition, Jack Sheehan of the United Steelworkers of America lobbied for mine safety and health legislation, and George Taylor of the AFL-CIO was instrumental in writing the 1985 "Frye Report," *Protecting Eighty Million American Workers,* for the U.S. Public Health Service's (USPHS) Division of Occupational Health. Taylor was also instrumental in stopping USPHS plans to abolish the division—the predecessor agency for the Bureau of Occupational Safety and Health (BOSH), which later became NIOSH.[21,22]

In the 1960s, policies moved the center of debates from interest groups to a standards-based regulatory approach across society. Positive public policy established rights for its citizens and corresponding duties for many to honor these rights. These policies covered civil rights, pollution control, education, and unemployment.[17] As positive public policy, the OSHAct applied economy-wide. The spark that ignited interest in the OSHAct came in a 1965 speech by President Johnson, planted by Jack Hardesty of BOSH,[21] as the Johnson White House mounted a "Quality of Life" initiative that incorporated occupational safety and health. The USPHS, DoL, and AFL-CIO demurred, so the

White House took on the issue, and its Bureau of the Budget (the predecessor to OMB) composed an early draft of the legislation. Then, stimulated by a BOSH study of uranium miners and visits to the mines, Assistant Secretary of Labor Esther Peterson pressed for DoL action that led to a draft bill in 1967.[23]

Howard McQuiggen of the AFL-CIO Industrial Union Department joined the earlier advocates for developing a bill to protect workers from occupational hazards.[23] When Richard Nixon was elected president, he proposed a more business-friendly bill, which union leaders claimed as an "abomination" and mustered to back former President Johnson's version of the bill.[21] Sheehan of the United Steelworkers had worked on early versions of the Clean Air Act, which provided the framework for passage of the Coal Act in 1969, followed by the OSH Act in 1970 under President Nixon.[20]

16.4.2. The First Decade

Paul Weaver argues that the "vast" federal bureaucracy and its "allies" in the national press, professions (such as law and epidemiology), and research institutions were largely responsible for the creation of the new regulation.

—Alfred A. Marcus[24,25]

The new OSHA was quick to issue temporary interim standards under § 6(a) from 1971 to 1973. In that haste, many consensus standards were adopted such as the height of a toilet seat, which received much ridicule. Moreover, early standards and enforcement emphasized safety and not health (i.e., injuries not diseases). During the 1970s, NIOSH recommended many health standards in criteria documents regarding health protection that were submitted to the Secretary of Labor. When Mort Corn became the Assistant Secretary of Labor in President Gerald Ford's administration, he moved in the direction of promulgating health standards, but it was Eula Bingham under President Jimmy Carter who set OSHA on a course to terminate the temporary safety standards that were not associated with safety and health and issue several health standards.

Employers and/or unions have challenged the majority of health and safety standards and all health standards issued by OSHA except for the dibromochloropropane (DBCP) standard. Employers have generally challenged rules on the grounds that available evidence failed to demonstrate a significant risk or that required measures were too costly or infeasible. Union challenges have

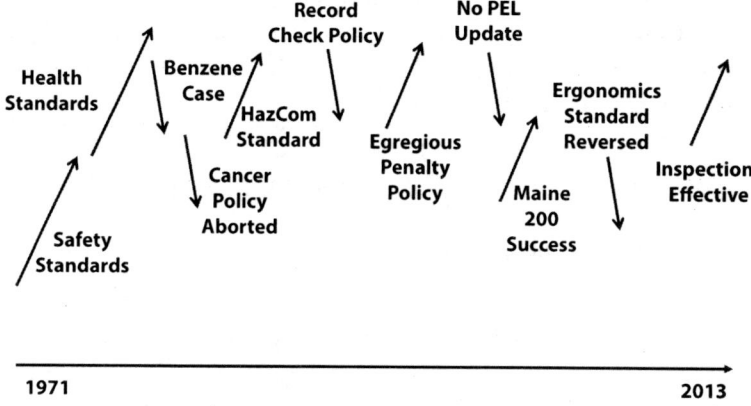

Note: PEL = permissible exposure limit; HazCom Standard = Hazard Communication Standard.

Figure 16-3. Jagged process of policy under the Occupational Safety and Health Act, 1971–2013.

sought to have rules strengthened on the grounds that evidence and the law supported a more protective rule. Of the more than 80 final § 6(b) safety and health standards issued by OSHA, two issued in OSHA's first decade were overturned by the courts—4,4'-Methylenebis(O-Chloroaniline), abbreviated as MOCA, and benzene. The agency's 1974 MOCA standard was overturned on procedural grounds, and the 1978 benzene standard was overturned when a court ruled that OSHA had failed to show that the requirement to reduce exposure to 1 ppm was reasonably necessary to protect workers from a significant risk of harm. Figure 16-3 depicts the uneven progress made under the OSHAct to protect workers' safety and health by showing the ups and downs of events affecting policy at OSHA over more than 40 years.

In 1987, OSHA issued a new benzene standard that reduced the permissible exposure level (PEL) to 1 ppm, the same level as the 1978 rule, which was vacated by the Supreme Court in 1980. The risk of regulatory delay in the benzene standard was calculated to be between 30 and 490 ultimate excess leukemia deaths as a result of nine extra years of occupational exposures to benzene greater than 1 ppm. Deaths from aplastic anemia and lymphoma likely added to this toll.[26] The courts also overturned the air contaminants standard that was issued in the second decade: Faced with dated interim standards set up in its first two years, OSHA had attempted to update the PELs for 428 substances in one rule making, which is described in Chapter 7. To accomplish this rule making, OSHA grouped the substances into 18 categories. The 11th Circuit Court of Atlanta (Georgia) ruled that OSHA must issue separate rules for each substance. The court vacated the air contaminants standard and remanded the rule for OSHA to make specific findings with respect to each substance.

16.4.3. What Is Good for Business Is Good for America

After all, the chief business of the American people is business.
—President Calvin Coolidge[27]

Johnson's positive public policy in the form of his "Quality of Life" initiative was countered in the early 1970s by Nixon in his cost-based "Quality of Life" review (see Chapter 4) that signaled a harbinger to come in the 1980s. From the challenge of positive public policy, there emerged at the beginning of the Reagan presidency in 1981 a new strategy by business interests to counter the revolution of regulations, including occupational safety and health standards. Prior to 1960, business was regulated more at an industry sector level, and interest groups were able to intervene at the subsystem level to represent their positions. This led over time to the potential of agency capture, where an interest group could control an agency. Positive public policy was different, because it raised the specter of regulation to the social level across the economy.

The positive public policy approach that extended economy-wide caught the business community "flat-footed." It took years for business to understand and develop a political response to this approach. Responses led to a number of reactions. Corporations hired legal staff, intermediaries such as Washington-based lawyers proliferated, corporate planning linked up with governmental affairs units, CEOs engaged in lobbying, and corporations developed political action committees.[24]

From the beginning, employers demanded relief from OSHA standards. However, fighting the positive public policy approach with negative attacks against public norms regarding the prevention of work-related injuries and diseases was a losing battle. Thus, the business community had to find a generalizable and positive message to advocate in this emergent megapolitical environment, and it found this message in the economy: efficiency to grow the economy. The employers' strategy was based on three arguments: (1) reduce the costs of regulation to firms to release capital for investments, (2) vet safety and health standards by economic analysis to weigh the benefits of the intervention to the cost of regulation to society, and (3) give managers discretion to organize work and provide the most efficient protective measures.[22]

16.4.4. Shift to Deregulation

In the early 1970s, it took about six months to two years for OSHA to develop and issue major rules such as those on asbestos and vinyl chloride monomer (VCM), even though these rules were controversial and contentious. In the early 1980s, the time for standards development and issuance became even longer as action was taken in response to congressional mandates or court orders. None of these time frames included the demand on time for litigation on final rules, which can take years to resolve. The delay in the issuance of rules meant that workers continued to be exposed to serious recognized safety and health hazards causing unnecessary injury disease and death.

Mendeloff developed an uncertainty principle regarding regulations.[28] The stricter the exposure standard, the more the pace of rule making is slowed, and the pace of OSHA's standard-setting process has slowed into oblivion. One way to generate more standards is to dedicate more staff to standards development. Another improvement is to reduce the procedural requirements including regulatory analysis, quantitative risk analysis, and public hearings. Furthermore, the burden of proof is on OSHA, and each standard requires significant involvement by the agency head and DoL attorneys.[28]

Today, much of OSHA's progress in implementing its policy under the OSHAct has been compromised by one roadblock after another. The agency must provide notice that it has undertaken an analysis calculating the most cost-effective means of accomplishing its regulatory objective in order to fully comply with the Unfunded Mandates Reform Act of 1995. This is required when any executive agency action imposes costs in excess of $100 million per year on the private sector.

The agency's standard-setting process has become more complex and burdensome as additional requirements have been imposed on the agency. The Paperwork Reduction Act, Regulatory Flexibility Act, Unfunded Mandates Reform Act, and Small Business Regulatory Enforcement Fairness Act have required additional analyses and reviews. Executive orders on regulatory reform and federalism impose further analytical and process requirements. All of these are on top of the additional justification and analyses that have been required as a result of court reviews. The impact of these requirements can be seen in both the increased time to develop and issue standards and the expansion of the preambles and analyses that accompany OSHA rules.

While OSHA standards have routinely and consistently been opposed by industry groups, in recent years opposition has increased. Similarly, political opposition to OSHA standards has also increased with more members of Congress seeking to block, delay, or weaken many OSHA rules through appropriations riders, legislation, or intense oversight of agency actions. Congressional efforts to block and ultimately overturn OSHA's ergonomics rule is the most notable. The irony of the focus on efficiency promoted by the regulated sector during this period has been an increase in governmental inefficiency at OSHA established by different administrations, Congress, and the courts.

16.5. REFORMS BY DIFFERENT NAMES

We are going to look at policy making as an extremely complex analytical and political process to which there is no beginning or end, and the boundaries of which are most uncertain. Somehow a complex set of forces that we call "policy making," all taken together, produces effects called "policies."

—Charles E. Lindblom[29]

Two major movements in Congress sought to dramatically reform the OSHAct in opposite directions and within the span of two years. These movements serve to explicate the role of politics in policy making. After the influence of politics on policy making is discussed below, this section notes that the first major movement occurred when Bill Clinton became president and the Democrats prepared to enact substantive amendments to the OSHAct to correct many aspects of the law that had been problematic in protecting workers. The second movement came at the next national election, when the Republicans took control of both houses of Congress and prepared amendments to the OSHAct that swung the pendulum to the extreme right. Finally, the impact of an interest group that mounted a fierce effort to stop OSHA from promulgating an ergonomics standard is described.

16.5.1. Politics and Policy Analysis

We know that genuine political reform is not only a matter of immediate pragmatic success, but also a process of political education by which citizens come to believe that other citizens have [brought] legitimate claims to their attention and legitimate grievances to be redressed.

—Robert D. Holsworth[30]

The market is conceived as an aggregation of individuals, each competing for scarce resources to satisfy their self-interest. There is no cooperation among competitors, whether producers or consumers. Conversely, in the polis, politics is defined as policies or expressions of the state will,[15] in which there is cooperation in achieving goals through alliances or organizations. Alliances are necessary whenever there are two or more sides to an issue or two or more people acting on the issue. Cooperation typically trumps coercion as a strategy.[14] Furthermore, markets are a social creation to advance communal progress.[31]

Figure 16-4 shows two triangles that represent the complexity of policy making within the polis. First, the iron triangle has been used to depict the problem of agency capture by interest groups.[32] It shows that interest groups support candidates for election with the implied expectation of friendly legislation and oversight in return. Congress provides funding and voice in support of agencies in return for actions consistent with its member's political agenda. Multiple iron triangles may exist for a member of Congress, which he or she must balance. The interaction between interest groups and agencies can result in the protection of members of those groups in return for lobbying support. President Nixon was intent on breaking this triangle by creating the OMB in 1970 from the Bureau of the Budget and thereby exerting administration control and coordination over agency actions. This triangle still exists today, but it may not always be positive for an agency; it can turn on an agency, as this section addresses later.

Nevertheless, Paul Weaver argued that a new "iron triangle" has emerged that is made up of public interest groups, the press, and the federal government

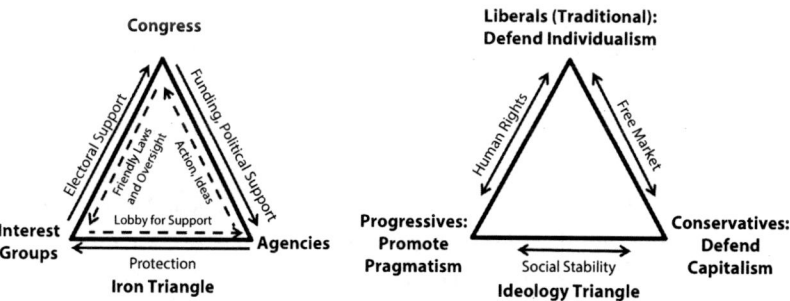

Figure 16-4. Triad depictions of political influences upon policy formulation.

as a whole (especially the courts and Congress).[25] His observation was consistent with the emergence of positive public policy, which was discussed earlier. Whereas the old iron triangle was responsive mainly to the concerns of business, the new iron triangle addresses concerns for health, safety, and the environment. However, since Weaver observed a new iron triangle in 1978, coalitions have reacted to positive public policy and have shifted back toward the old iron triangle, with business interests arguing for deregulation based on the concept of economic efficiency.

Second, the ideology triangle represents the current state of affairs in U.S. politics as a triad.[33] Liberals (i.e., neoliberals) focus on individual liberty and reflect Jeffersonian values of liberal democracy in the Declaration of Independence and strict interpretation of the Constitution, especially the Bill of Rights. While their position reflects the rugged individualism of the frontier of more than two centuries ago, the power of something absolute still has political influence, represented by libertarians. Conservatives are known as reactionaries wanting to protect institutions of property rights, free trade, and religion. They argue for the status quo or a return to a past before governmental interference. The conservative agenda of maintaining tradition moderates radical change. Progressives emerged during the Gilded Age, when abuses against citizens by zealous businesses and agencies suppressed personal freedom and damaged emerging individual rights. Progressives look to progress with an eye on what people learn from history and science. They promote change, at times radical, with the view that government is the solution, which is in opposition with the ossified values of neoliberals and conservatives guided by former President Reagan's view that "government is the problem." A genuine irony of this claim is that corporations are creatures of and gain their legitimacy from the government.

Business viewpoints are advocated by the Business Roundtable, the National Association of Manufacturers, and the U.S. Chamber of Commerce, which was created by the federal government in 1912.[34] These viewpoints are consistent with the idea of efficiency in economics and have had support from academic economists, particularly from business schools. Moreover, the business coalition is an effective interest group able to articulate its advocacy against regulations or to weaken occupational safety and health regulations. It has resources, prestige, status, and knowledge about the system.[10]

The other coalition, headed by the AFL-CIO, counters anti-OSHA lobbying.[10] Individual unions bring expertise to bear in defense and support of regulations. On particular issues, the coalition may broaden to include consumer groups or other interested parties (e.g., recently, the Sierra Club and the National Association for the Advancement of Colored People). This coalition typically includes occupational safety and health professionals, including the National Council for Occupational Safety and Health. The balance of power in the political system depends upon pluralism that is represented by engagement between these two interest groups, uneven as they are.[35]

As noted in Chapter 5, when neither interest group takes up the problem of work-related injuries and diseases, the "state" can take that mantle as a moral act to protect disadvantaged people. In the face of the resistance from DoL and Department of Health, Education, and Welfare, President Johnson directed the Bureau of the Budget to draft what later, through debate and into the Nixon administration, became the OSHAct. This action by President Johnson led to the first occupational safety and health legislation proposal even in the face of resistance from the departments that held that responsibility.

16.5.2. Reinventing Government

President Clinton launched a government reinvention initiative upon taking office in 1992, with the intention of promoting more efficiency and flexibility in agencies and policies.[16] One approach in this initiative was to reduce the layers in governmental agencies; thus, the USPHS was removed as a layer in the DHHS, becoming a staff entity headed by the Surgeon General. This action raised the Centers for Disease Control and Prevention up one layer, reporting directly to the Secretary of Health and Human Services and thereby raising NIOSH up one layer closer to par with OSHA.

Upon the Democratic Party gaining control of both Congress and the presidency in 1992, Congress acted with two bills to reform the OSHAct by correcting many barriers to efficient and flexible regulation of occupational safety and health. One bill, introduced by Senator Edward Kennedy (D) of Massachusetts, was cosponsored by 12 other senators (S 575), and a companion bill introduced by Representative William Ford (D) of Michigan was cosponsored by 83 other Representatives (HR 1280). The tables of contents of the two bills are shown in Table 16-2, which shows a remarkable similarity between the bills.

Furthermore, these bills provided a progressive agenda for the improvement of the OSHAct regarding worker safety and health. Both bills were

Table 16-2. Similarity between Occupational Safety and Health Administration Reform Bills in the Senate and the House, 1993: Comprehensive Occupational Safety and Health Reform Act

Senate Bill S 575 (1993) (Kennedy Bill)[a]	House Bill HR 1280 (1993) (Ford Bill)[b]
Title I—Safety and Health Programs	Title I—Safety and Health Programs
Sec. 101. Safety and health programs	Sec. 101. Safety and health programs
Title II—Safety and Health Committees And Employee Safety and Health Representatives	Title II—Safety and Health Committees And Employee Safety and Health Representatives
Sec. 201. Safety and health committees and employee safety and health representatives	Sec. 201. Safety and health committees and employee safety and health representatives
Title III—Coverage	Title III—Coverage
Sec. 301. Extension of coverage to public employees	Sec. 301. Extension of coverage to public employees
Sec. 302. Application of act	Sec. 302. Congressional coverage
Sec. 303. Application of OSHA to DoE nuclear facilities	Sec. 303. Application of OSHA to DoE nuclear facilities.
Sec. 304. Extension of employer duties to all employees working at a place of employment	Sec. 304. Extension of employer duties to all employees working at a place of employment
Title IV—Occupational Safety and Health Standards	Title IV—Occupational Safety and Health Standards
Sec. 401. Time frames for setting standards	Sec. 401. Time frames for setting standards
Sec. 402. Basis for standards	Sec. 402. Occupational safety and health standard
Sec. 403. Recording of work-related adverse medical conditions	Sec. 403. Recording of adverse medical conditions
Sec. 404. Public disclosure of all communications on standards	Sec. 404. Public disclosure of all communications on standards
Sec. 405. Revision of PELs	Sec. 405. Revision of PELs
Sec. 406. Exposure monitoring and health surveillance	Sec. 406. Exposure monitoring and health surveillance
Sec. 407. Standard on ergonomic hazards	Sec. 407. Standard on ergonomic hazards
Sec. 408. Emergency temporary standards	Sec. 408. Emergency temporary standard
Sec. 409. Air contaminants	Sec. 409. Air contaminants
Title V—Enforcement	Title V—Enforcement
Sec. 501. No loss of employee pay for inspections	Sec. 501. No loss of employee pay for inspections
Sec. 502. Time frame for response to complaints	Sec. 502. Time frame for response to complaints
Sec. 503. Complaints	Sec. 503. Complaints
Sec. 504. Mandatory special emphasis	Sec. 504. Mandatory special emphasis
Sec. 505. Investigations of deaths and serious incidents	Sec. 505. Investigations of deaths and serious incidents
Sec. 506. Abatement of serious hazards during employer contests to a citation	Sec. 506. Abatement of serious hazards during employer contests to a citation
Sec. 507. Right to contest citations and penalties	Sec. 507. Right to contest citations and penalties

Table 16-2. (Continued)

Senate Bill S 575 (1993) (Kennedy Bill)[a]	House Bill HR 1280 (1993) (Ford Bill)[b]
Sec. 508. Right of employee representatives to participate in other proceedings	Sec. 508. Right of employee representatives to participate in other proceedings
Sec. 509. Objections to modification of citations	Sec. 509. Objections to modification of citations
Sec. 510. Imminent danger inspections	Sec. 510. Imminent danger inspections
Sec. 511. Citations and penalties for violations of § 27, 28, and 31	Sec. 511. Citations and penalties for violations
Sec. 512. OSHA criminal penalties	Sec. 512. OSHA criminal penalties
Sec. 513. Commission members' terms	Sec. 513. Commission members' terms
Sec. 514. Inspections	Sec. 514. Inspections
Sec. 515. Employee accountability	Sec. 515. Employee accountability
	Sec. 516. Serious penalty
Title VI—Protection of Employees From Discrimination	**Title VI—Protection of Employees From Discrimination**
Sec. 601. Antidiscrimination provisions	Sec. 601. Antidiscrimination provisions
Sec. 602. Posting of employee rights	Sec. 602. Posting of employee rights
Title VII—Technical Assistance and Training	**Title VII—Technical Assistance and Training**
Sec. 701. Technical assistance to employers and employees	Sec. 701 Technical assistance to employers and employees.
Sec. 702. OSHA assistance fund	
Title VIII—Recordkeeping and Reporting	**Title VIII—Recordkeeping and Reporting**
Sec. 801. Data collected by Secretary of HHS	Sec. 801. Data collected by Secretary of HHS
Sec. 802. Employee-reported illnesses	Sec. 802. Employee-reported illnesses
Sec. 803. Employee access	Sec. 803. Employee access
Title IX—NIOSH	**Title IX—NIOSH**
Sec. 901. Hazard evaluation reports	Sec. 901. Hazard evaluation reports
Sec. 902. Safety research	Sec. 902. Safety research
Sec. 903. Contractor rights	Sec. 903. Contractor rights
Sec. 904. National surveillance program	Sec. 904. National surveillance program
Sec. 905. Establishment of NIOSH as a separate agency within USPHS	Sec. 905. Establishment of NIOSH as a separate agency within USPHS
Sec. 906. NIOSH training	Sec. 906. Conforming amendments changing references from HEW to HHS
	Sec. 907. NIOSH training
Title X—State Plans	**Title X—State Plans**
Sec. 1001. State plan committees and programs	Sec. 1001. State plan committees and programs
Sec. 1002. Access to information; employee rights	Sec. 1002. Access to information; employee rights
Sec. 1003. Application of federal standards	Sec. 1003. Application of federal standards
Sec. 1004. Complaints against a state plan	Sec. 1004. Complaints against a state plan
Sec. 1005. Action against a state plan	Sec. 1005. Action against state plan
Sec. 1006. State plan conforming amendments	Sec. 1006. State plan conforming amendments
Sec. 1007. Effect on state laws	Sec. 1007. Validity of state laws
Title XI—Victim's Rights	**Title XI—Victim's Rights**
Sec. 1101. Victim's rights	Sec. 1101. Victim's rights

(Continued)

Table 16-2. (Continued)

Senate Bill S 575 (1993) (Kennedy Bill)[a]	House Bill HR 1280 (1993) (Ford Bill)[b]
Title XII—Construction Safety	Title XII—Construction Safety
Sec. 1201. Short title	Sec. 1201. Definitions
Sec. 1202. Definitions	Sec. 1202. Office of Construction Safety, Health, and Education
Sec. 1203. Office of Construction Safety, Health, and Education	Sec. 1203. Construction safety and health plans and programs
Sec. 1204. Construction safety and health plans and programs	Sec. 1204. Inspections, investigations, reporting, and recordkeeping
Sec. 1205. Inspections, investigations, reporting, and recordkeeping	Sec. 1205. Advisory Committee on Construction Safety and Health
Sec. 1206. Advisory Committee on Construction Safety and Health	Sec. 1206. State construction safety and health plans
Sec. 1207. State construction safety and health plans	Sec. 1207. Construction Safety and Health Academy
Sec. 1208. Construction Safety and Health Academy	Sec. 1208. Enforcement
Sec. 1209. Enforcement	Sec. 1209. Reports to Congress
Sec. 1210. Reports to Congress	Sec. 1210. Federal construction contracts
Sec. 1211. Federal construction contracts	Sec. 1211. Relationship to existing law and regulations
Sec. 1212. Relationship to existing law and regulations	Sec. 1212. Timetable for regulations
Sec. 1213. Timetable for regulations	
	Title XIII—Workers' Compensation Study
	Sec. 1301. Commission
Title XIV—Administration	Title XIV—Administration
Sec. 1301. Administration	Sec. 1401. Administration
Title XV—Effective Date	Title XV—Effective Date
Sec. 1401. Effective date	Sec. 1501. Effective date

Note: OSHA = Occupational Safety and Health Administration; DoE = U.S. Department of Energy; HHS - U.S. Department of Health and Human Services; USPHS = U.S. Public Health Service; HEW = (the former) U.S. Department of Health, Education, and Welfare; NIOSH = National Institute for Occupational Safety and Health.

[a] Senate Bill S 575. Comprehensive Occupational Safety and Health Reform Act. Committee on Labor and Human Resources, 103rd Cong, 1st Sess, Mar 11, 1993.
[b] House Bill HR 1280. Comprehensive Occupational Safety and Health Reform Act. Committee on Education and Labor, 103rd Cong, 1st Sess, March 3, 1993.

structured under 15 titles, starting with the requirement that each employer establish a written occupational safety and health program (§ 101) and that each employer with more than 10 employees establish at least one health committee with employee representation (§ 201) and employee participation in OSHA inspections (§ 202). Sections 301–304 extended the coverage under the OSHAct to employees of state and local governments and federal nuclear facilities and on an employer's worksite even when employed by other employers. Sections 401–409 extended the emergency temporary standards from 6 months to 18 months, set time frames for setting standards, established exposure limits on a regular basis, and promulgated an exposure monitoring and medical surveillance standard, an ergonomics standard, and air contaminants standards for different industries. Sections 501–515 reformed enforcement, including the requirement that OSHA investigate work-related deaths or serious injuries to more than one employee from a single incident. These sections also addressed several employee rights, including the requirement that the Occupational Safety and Health Review Commission (OSHRC) inform affected employees of its actions and extending criminal penalties to officials and supervisors employed by the employer. Section 905 of both bills established NIOSH as a separate agency at the same level as OSHA.

Senator Kennedy's bill redefined a standard to nullify the Supreme Court interpretation under the benzene case (§ 402), and it included a provision for a revolving fund to pay for OSHA training and assistance that could be supplemented with fees (§ 702). An earlier version of a Construction Safety, Health, and Education Improvement Act proposal by Senator Kennedy was integrated into the Kennedy bill (§ 1201). Representative Ford's bill set the minimum penalty for serious violations at $1,000 (§ 515) and established a second Federal Worker's Compensation Commission to review the recommendations of the original National Commission on State Workmen's Compensation Laws, the relationship of workers' compensation to the prevention of occupational injuries and diseases, and the adequacy of the system to provide medical care and compensation associated with injuries (§ 1301). With a Democratic-controlled Congress and a Democratic president, this reform had a good chance of passage after the upcoming election.

16.5.3. Contract With America

What a difference a year makes. In the election of 1994, the Republicans took majority control of the House and Senate. Prior to the election, Republicans running for office in the House issued a one-page, 10-point "Contract With America: A Program for Accountability," on October 5, 1994. The eighth point stated, "Roll back government regulations: Let's slash regulations that strangle small business and let's make it easier for people to invest in order to create jobs and increase wages."[36]

One section in Representative Ford's bill (§ 302) found its way into the "Contract With America." A preamble to the contract stated, "Force Congress to live under the same laws as every American." Accordingly, the Congressional Accountability Act of 1995 made the civil rights and labor laws applicable to Congress. An applicable law was the OSHAct, which was administered by Congress and not the executive branch. However, OSHA provided technical assistance to Congress.

In 1995, the two houses of the new Congress created starkly different reform bills to amend the OSHAct. The tables of contents of the new bills, one in the Senate and the other in the House, are shown in Table 16-3. These two bills were remarkably different from the two Democratic-sponsored bills of 1993. First, they reversed the movement to make the OSHAct more effective, and second, while the two Democratic bills were nearly word-for-word similar, the two Republican bills were extremely different from one another with a few exceptions. This difference spelled doom for viable legislation, as did the potential veto by President Clinton that loomed if the bills were reconciled and passed.

The lead legislator on the House side was Representative Cass Ballenger (R) of North Carolina. Representative Ballenger had owned a plastic bag manufacturing company in Hickory, North Carolina. Reminiscent of a description in Chapter 15 of the blame-the-victim attitude, when someone would lose a finger in a machine at his factory, Representative Ballenger would say, "See what can happen? Put the guard back on and don't do that again. You learn not to do that anymore." Representative Ballenger explained that before OSHA, employers and workers relied on "simple common sense." After the passage of the OSHAct, his experience with the state OSHA was quarrelsome, and when he was elected in 1987 as Representative, he boasted that he was the only member who had ever been cited by OSHA. With the "Republican Revolution" in 1994 with a majority in the House, Ballenger chaired the Workplace Protection Subcommittee, for which he recruited members with an aim of dismantling OSHA. They produced a bill entitled the Safety and Health Improvement and Regulatory Reform Act of 1995 (the Ballenger bill), which organized labor tagged the "Death and Injury Enhancement (DIE) Act."[37]

The Ballenger bill (HR 1834), cosponsored by 66 other representatives, had extensive and regressive proposals for reforming occupational safety and health

Table 16-3. Dissimilarity Between Occupational Safety and Health Administration Reform Bills in the Senate and the House, 1995

Senate Bill S. 1423, Occupational Safety and Health Reform and Reinvention Act	House Bill HR 1834, Safety and Health Improvement and Regulatory Reform Act of 1995
Gregg Bill[a]	Ballenger Bill[b]
Sec. 1. Short title; reference	Sec. 1. Short title: table of contents; reference
Sec. 2. Employee participation	Sec. 2. Standards
Sec. 3. Inspections	Sec. 3. Notice of violation
Sec. 4. Worksite-based initiatives	Sec. 4. Consultation, incentives for voluntary action, and technical assistance
Sec. 5. Employer defenses	Sec. 5. Removal of barriers to voluntary safety and health activities
Sec. 6. Inspection quotas	Sec. 6. Inspections
Sec. 7. Warnings in lieu of citations	Sec. 7. Employer defenses
Sec. 8. Penalties	Sec. 8. Penalties
Sec. 9. Consultation services	Sec. 9. Review by the (Occupational Safety and Health Review) Commission
Sec. 10. Voluntary protection programs	Sec. 10. NIOSH repealed
	Sec. 11. State Workmen's Compensation Commission repealed
	Sec. 12. State programs
	Sec. 13. Discrimination
	Sec. 14. Coverage of federal agencies
	Sec. 15. Federal agency safety programs
	Sec. 16. Prevention of alcohol and substance abuse
	Sec. 17. Mine safety and health
	Sec. 18. Recordkeeping and reporting
	Sec. 19. Definitions
	Sec. 20. Miscellaneous technical amendments
	Sec. 21. Effective date

Note: NIOSH = National Institute for Occupational Safety and Health.
[a] Senate Bill S.1423. Occupational Safety and Health Reform and Reinvention Act. Committee on Labor and Human Resources, 104th Cong, 1st Sess, November 17, 1995.
[b] House Bill H.R. 1834, Safety and Health Improvement and Regulatory Reform Act of 1995. Committee on Economic and Educational Opportunities, 104th Cong, 1st Sess, June 14, 1995.

regulations. It would abolish OSHAct § 20–22 regarding research, education, and training and thus eliminate NIOSH, and it would abolish the Mine Act and the Mine Safety and Health Administration (MSHA), subsuming its standards as OSHA standards. As for OSHA, the Ballenger bill set down specific requirements for risk assessment, cost-benefit analysis (CBA), determination of significant risk, and feasibility. It also specified a regulatory impact analysis, a process for applying these requirements to existing standards, and the role of an external panel to review the scientific and economic basis of a standard prior to promulgation. Regarding inspections, an employee would have to first bring violations to the attention of the employer prior to requesting an OSHA inspection, and certain farming and small business operations would be excluded from inspections. An innovative insertion was made in the bill for training of any federal or state inspectors under federal law in identifying fire hazards in workplaces and referring identified hazards to OSHA; this came on the heels of the chicken processing plant fire in Hamlet, North Carolina, as described in Chapter 8. As for penalties, willful and repeated violations would be redefined as serious violations, the OSHRC would establish the penalty, and no penalties would be assigned unless a standard existed, thus terminating general duty clause penalties. The bill sanctioned alcohol and substance abuse testing programs when there was a potential for harm to workers from the abuse.

The Ballenger bill and the more modest Senate bill (S 1423) proposed by Senator Judd Gregg (R) of New Hampshire and cosponsored by four other senators overlapped in four areas: work-based incentives, inspections, employer defenses, and penalties. Both bills provided for work-based incentives ("reinvention initiatives" in the Gregg bill, consistent with the president's reinvention initiative) that would provide for consultation services that would exempt firms from OSHA inspections for a multimonth period. Regarding inspections, the two bills differed markedly, for the Gregg bill did not require employees to report violations to employers prior to reporting violations to OSHA as did the Ballenger bill. While the Ballenger bill exempted small businesses with fewer than 50 employees from inspections, the Gregg bill placed that number at 10 employees. Employer defenses were similar in both bills, which included employee negligence and proof of the employer's knowledge or that the employer should have known of the violation. Concerning penalties, the Senate bill was strident, reducing the maximum penalty per violation from $7,000 to $100.

With the challenge of the "Contract With America," there developed a widening gap between OSHA's mission and resources provided by Congress for protecting American workers. While the number of workplaces and workers had increased substantially since the passage of the OSH Act, OSHA's resources had dropped. Between 1980 and 1994, the number of employees at OSHA dropped by 15%, and from 1988 to 1994, the number of inspections dropped by 40%. As a result, OSHA's strategy moved toward targeting resources to protect the greatest number of workers who were at the greatest risk.[15]

President Clinton's reinvention initiative took hold at OSHA in 1995 in response to the "Contract With America" and a hostile Republican-led Congress. The AFL-CIO instituted an active lobbying campaign funded through an assessment of $1.80 per union member to counter the threat of a weakened OSHAct.[15]

A series of acts were introduced in the following years that provided for employer relief from OSHA inspections.[38] These acts carried the acronym "SAFE" and included the Safety Advancement for Employees Acts of 1997 (S 1237 and HR 2579) and the SAFE Act of 1999 (HR 1427). These bills passed neither the Senate nor the House.

16.5.4. National Coalition on Ergonomics

No one ever died of ergonomics.

—Representative Cass Ballenger[39]

Congress enacted the Contract With America Advancement Act of 1996 that included as § 251 the Congressional Review Act (CRA). The CRA allows Congress to review new regulations and eliminate those it deems too burdensome or inconsistent with congressional intent. The act requires agencies to report new regulations to Congress, which has 60 legislative days to strike down by a simple resolution of disapproval, which the president can veto. The only time that such a resolution was passed by both houses and acted on by the president was for the disapproval of the OSHA ergonomics standard. The rise and fall of the ergonomics standard was described in Section 7-12 in Chapter 7.

Behind this action was a massive political battle in the United States, which entailed the political interaction shown earlier in Figure 16-4. Regarding the iron triangle, an antiregulatory interest group exercised persistent influence on congressional members to defeat the proposed standard. Another interest group, the AFL-CIO, supported the standard and OSHA and exerted influence within the triangle. Regarding the ideology triangle, progressives who supported the standard were pitted against an alliance of conservatives and neoliberals opposing the standard.

As far back as 1978, a report from a President Carter task force had recommended that OSHA develop ergonomic standards to eliminate musculoskeletal hazards through equipment design.[40] In 1983, NIOSH identified musculoskeletal injuries as a leading work-related disease and injury (see Chapter 9).[41] In 1985, the Office of Technology Assessment (OTA) devoted a chapter to ergonomics and human factors in the report *Preventing Illness and Injury in the Workplace*.[42] A year later, NIOSH published *A Proposed National Strategy for the Prevention of Musculoskeletal Injuries*.[43] In 1990, in the George H.W. Bush administration, Secretary of Labor Elizabeth Dole announced that OSHA would begin working on an ergonomics standard.[39] Dorothy Strunk was the acting OSHA administrator when the ergonomics standard was proposed.[44]

Court cases regarding the general duty clause and ergonomics in the meatpacking industry had led to OSHA considering a regulation. Proposing a regulation released OSHA from the authority to identify ergonomic shortcomings and prove that feasible remedies exist. The agency moved to shift this burden for identifying ergonomic risks and remedies to employers. In the OSHA draft proposal, companies would identify situations with a high risk of injury from strains that built over time or came from lifting heavy objects. While OSHA lacked the capacity to inspect many worksites that would be affected by the standard, employers would be forced to educate themselves and workers to the importance of ergonomics.[44]

In 1994, in response to the OSHA proposal, the National Association of Manufacturers formed a coalition on ergonomics. The association asked each member company to contribute $5,000 to help build a $600,000 fund, and soon, 185 companies had signed up.[44] Not long thereafter, the Chamber of Commerce renamed the coalition the National Coalition on Ergonomics (NCE), which allied with the association and the National Federation of Independent Business, the Small Business Survival Committee with 40,000 members, and the Labor Policy Association. In June 1994, NCE announced its opposition to the ergonomics standard, boasting of an alliance of 300 corporations and trade organizations with a budget of $600,000.[39] Former Acting OSHA Administrator Dorothy Strunk was also a lobbyist for the United Parcel Service and led the coalition against the ergonomics standard.[44]

The Heritage Foundation stated in 1995 that when faced with reducing unnecessary and expensive laws not justified on public health grounds, Congress should use appropriation riders to stop regulations. In that year, stopping work on the ergonomics standard became a target for such a rider. One claim was that there had been too little scientific research on ergonomic disorders to provide adequate guidance for such a broad standard.[45] Thus, the

Republican-controlled Congress used appropriation riders to keep OSHA from developing and issuing an ergonomics standard in 1995.

On June 12, 1995, the NCE issued a statement that read, "Experimental ergonomic regulation would have assumed that every workplace in every job is a potential disorder waiting to happen." In the face of congressional action against OSHA in reducing the budget related to the ergonomics standard, OSHA abandoned plans for the regulation.[46] This setback for OSHA was short-lived.

The "ergo-rider" came off the proposed standard in 1996 when the House approved an amendment to strip the rider from the 1997 appropriations bill (H.R. 3755) sponsored by Representative Nancy Pelosi (D) of California, but the rider returned again in 1997 for 1998 appropriations. The rider prohibited OSHA from promulgating an ergonomics standard or guidelines, but with the compromise that the restriction would last for only one year.[47] Following a series of attacks by the NCE against the science of ergonomics as presented by NIOSH and at OSHA hearings, Congress asked the National Academy of Sciences to conduct reviews of ergonomics at two different times as a delay tactic that further stretched a two-year rule-making time frame into a six-year ordeal for OSHA and NIOSH. Finally, in November 2000, in the waning days of Bill Clinton's presidency, OSHA issued the final standard.[39] The NCE immediately filed a suit with the U.S. Court of Appeals in Washington, DC, to overturn the ergonomics regulation.[48]

Then in 2001 under the CRA, the regulation was reversed when Congress passed a resolution to eliminate the ergonomics standard, and the newly elected President George W Bush signed the bill that terminated the regulation. In 2005, the NCE was still active when it appealed ergonomic guidelines issued by OSHA for poultry processing, retail grocery stores, and nursing homes under the Information Quality Act. The plague of musculoskeletal disorders continues with 387,820 cases in 2011 that accounted for 33% of all occupational injury and illness cases in that year.[49]

16.6. NARRATIVE ANALYSIS

Stories reassert a kind of conventional wisdom about what can be expected, even (or especially) what can be expected to go wrong and what might be done to restore or cope with the situation.

—Jerome Bruner[50]

The perspective of reason is one worldview, but there are other worldviews such as those revealed by politics. Moreover, the economic model of the market is based upon preferences and not on how people get these preferences within a community—which guides politics. And claims based upon objectivity need to be defended in the milieu of a political economy. This is why narrative and its analysis are important.[15]

This section is based upon a distinction made by Bruner between narrative and paradigmatic thought, much like the different functions of the right and left hemispheres of the brain. The narrative approach is context-free and universal, and if it is successful, it means more than what is said. Truth is in the interpretation of the text and is open and not literal. A story can have a compelling believability.[51]

Stories describe change over time. When stories are rearranged to group incidents by their significance, the narrative becomes analysis.[7] What follows are five approaches that can apply narratives in analysis. The first one, narrative analysis, aims to resolve intractable policy issues. An example of amendments to the OSHAct shows how narrative analysis can work. The second approach examines change theory with a focus on how reading narratives can reveal stark differences in strategies between winners and losers and how these positions can be reversed. The example of policy change here is the rise and demise of the ergonomics standard. The third approach is the use of policy analytics to influence the adoption of policy advice. Policy analytics is demonstrated by the narratives used throughout this book—which suggest more than they say. The fourth and fifth approaches relate to precautionary analyses: one describes the approach used in Europe, and in a similar vein, the other one explains how to make the shift a precautionary assessment.

16.6.1. Narrative Analysis and Metanarratives

The key step in this methodology is the creation of a "metanarrative" story that is built upon both the dominant conception of the policy problem as well as other latent and often unarticulated stories.

—Edward F. Lawlor[8]

Policy narratives are the drivers for this analysis: stories that include scenarios and arguments that endorse and advocate a proposed governmental action (i.e., a policy). Narrative analysis reformulates highly complex, polarized, and uncertain policy problems into tractable problems for paradigmatic analysis. It is a process that accepts complexity, polarization, and uncertainty as input into the analysis by examining stories that expose the sources of this triad. Complexity results from the internal intricacy of an issue and its interdependences with other issues. Polarization is exhibited by groups taking extreme and polar positions on an issue or issues. Both complexity and polarization can drive uncertainty, which is an analyst's lack of knowledge about an issue that may also include risk and ignorance. Uncertainty may add further to the complexity of the issue.[52] Narrative analysis follows four steps: (1) identify stories and argument, (2) identify nonstories and counterstories, (3) create metanarratives, and (4) recast the policy narrative to resolve polarity.

The first step identifies stories or arguments that describe the context of the issue and have high complexity and uncertainty regarding the issue. A story has a beginning, middle, and ending, and arguments have claims with supporting evidence as was described in Chapter 6. In the second step, nonstories and counterstories are identified. This type of narrative lacks context and may represent fallacies such as circular arguments. The third step compares the set of stories and arguments and nonstories and counterarguments so as to generate a metanarrative. The metanarrative is constructed by writing about what the issue is not. A controversy may not have a metanarrative, or it may have more than one metanarrative. The last step of narrative analysis evaluates the metanarrative so as to recast the policy narrative to assimilate assumptions, so that one can escape the paralysis of decision making caused by the complexity, uncertainty, and polarization generated by the initial policy narrative.[52]

As an example, Representative Ballenger's 1995 bill to reform OSHA failed to go forward. While it attained high salience within his committee in the House, it mustered little attention and was quite dissimilar to Gregg's companion bill in the Senate. Moreover, it did not move forward in Congress since President Clinton claimed he would veto it even before it came out of committee.[53]

Representative Ballenger later sought alliances with the Senate and concordance with President Clinton's reinvention agenda. He referred to President Clinton's comments about a "new OSHA" and the need to move to prevention rather than punishment.[54] Representative Ballenger did not have to look far to find nonnarratives, for they were listed in the "Contract With America." Moreover, the title of Senator Gregg's 1995 bill, the Occupational Safety and Health Reform and Reinvention Act, adopted President Clinton's terminology for reinvention. Representative Ballenger was able to construct a metanarrative in a new bill (HR 3234) that a congressional staffer said "literally takes the words out of the administration's mouth and puts them on paper."[55]

On April 15, 1996, Representative Ballenger introduced his revised bill as the "Small Business OSHA Relief Act."[53] This bill had five provisions: (1) balancing costs and benefits with reference to Secretary of Labor Robert Reich's comments regarding commonsense regulations (e.g., clear priorities, focusing rules on problems, reforming out-of-date and confusing standards, and working together with businesses and workers to develop rules), (2) a penalty waiver for small businesses based on a directive issued by the president, (3) a reduction in employer paperwork for which OSHA had issued citations, (4) setting the OSHA state consultation program into law, and (5) the elimination of quotas as performance measures for compliance officers (which was in Senator Gregg's 1995 bill). The multisectioned bill was broken down into five separate bills in the Senate, the latter two provisions were enacted, and the president signed the two amendments to the OSHAct into law in 1998: first, there would be no quotas regarding citations issued by compliance officers, in § 8(h), and second, a consultation program that would buffer participating firms from OSHA inspections for a specified time period, in § 21c(2) and (d) (Public L. 105-197 and 105-198). The intractable problem of Representative Ballenger's 1995 bill that was rendered dead before it came out of committee was resolved by his 1996 bill being winnowed down to five separate bills in the Senate, leading to the ultimate passage of two bills as amendments to the OSHAct. Congress provided funding for the consultation program.

16.6.2. Policy Change Theories

Ergonomics is an overly ambitious, burdensome, and possibly the most expensive and far-reaching and intrusive regulation ever written by the federal government.

—Representative Henry Bonilla[56]

Chapter 6 addressed some policy change theories that included prospect theory, agenda setting, and incrementalism. Based on policy change theories, McBeth et al. conducted a study in 2007 that indicated that interest groups use narrative strategies in turbulent policy environments. Their findings are instructive regarding policy change in occupational safety and health, especially when examining the ergonomics standard as an example. Their study looked at five political strategies based upon content analysis of narratives: (1) identifying winners and losers, (2) construction of benefits and costs, (3) the use of condensation symbols (e.g., words that stir a person's passions to act), (4) the policy surrogate, and (5) scientific certainty and disagreement.[57] In the example of the ergonomics standard controversy herein, OSHA is the presumed winner, which can be validated with a content analysis of narratives regarding ergonomics rule making.

Here is why: The standard was initiated under a Republican administration, and it had administration support through the Clinton years but with some important compromises. The rule-making process, while cumbersome, keeps moving toward a final standard. The strategy of a winning actor is to maintain this status quo as reflected in narratives. Conversely, as identified by an analysis of narratives, the losing actor will implement a strategy early on of growing a wide coalition of potential losers and attacking the status quo[57]—thus, in the ergonomics narrative, the creation of the NCE.

The winner expresses diffusion of the benefits to a wide worker population in its argument, while the loser's voice narrows the scope of the benefits to empowering federal OSHA inspectors and a new cadre of ergonomists. As for cost, the strategies are the converse, with losers diffusing the cost to a broadening number of affected parties. Meanwhile, OSHA has concentrated its cost estimates to the affected industries, aggregations of the affected parties.

According to McBeth et al., losing narratives are more than three times as likely as winning narratives to use policy surrogates in their political narratives. Surrogates are used to expand the scope of the debate for competitive advantage and are typically larger and more controversial problems (e.g., a "straw man" fallacy, as described in Chapter 6).[57] One issue raised by Eugene Scalia, an organizer of NCE, claimed back pain to be a much broader issue than a relationship to the workplace. In addition, he raised the *Daubert* case as an issue that questioned the reliability of evidence as found in tort law (see Chapter 14), which is associated with the tag line "junk science."[58] Furthermore, rhetoric like that in Representative Bonilla's quote from above indicates the wide-ranging surrogates of "far-reaching and intrusive regulation" that were used to challenge the ergonomics standard.

In the McBeth et al. study, no significant difference was found in how science was used in the winning-losing frames. In that study, both sides used science to support their camp with scientific certainty. OSHA and the pro-ergonomics interest parties used science to bolster their core beliefs in the policy. However, the anti-ergonomic standard interests attacked the certainty of the science as a major issue. Indeed, they attacked the science so as to delay the issuance of the standard, which led to ultimate success for the NCE and defeat for the standard.[57]

The agency entered this rule making as a policy monopoly with the support of both Presidents George H.W. Bush and Bill Clinton. In cases like this, the winner narrative expresses belief in controversy containment and winning with a perception of a slow march to victory. As OSHA expected, it was victorious in issuing the standard in November 2000, but unexpectedly for OSHA, this victory was short-lived. The new Congress convened in 2001, passed a resolution to stop the standard, and antiregulation President George W. Bush signed the congressional resolution that terminated the ergonomics standard. Throughout the ergonomics controversy, the losing narrative interest groups became more confrontational over time, expanded the scope of the conflict, and drew in ever more interested parties; thus, the issue became increasingly intractable. In spite of marshalling a substantial coalition against what seemed like unsurmountable odds of regulatory power, OSHA's hard-won victory was quickly reversed.[57]

16.6.3. Analytic Narratives

Stories are surely not innocent: they always have a message, most often so well concealed that even the teller knows not what ax he may be grinding.

—Jerome Bruner[50]

Stories are persuasive and deal with complex happenings by explaining why they happened, which is the essence of analytic narratives. A story can explain a current dilemma and policies to address the dilemma, and give complex advice about the future. It may achieve more change than a formal process of defined external criteria and a proposal based upon the criteria.[7]

Using policy analysis as a tool for policy advocacy is abhorrent to the classical field of policy analysis, which stresses objectivity. However, bias in policy analysis is inherently present given the support by a client. Analytical narratives are advocacy-in-motion founded on strategic planning principles such as attending to stakeholder values and to the elements of the traditional "SWOT analysis": perceived internal strengths and weaknesses and external opportunities and threats.[7]

Resolution of policy dilemmas may not depend upon a priori criteria, especially when criteria are unavailable to parties to explain why a course of action should be taken. Resolution may depend upon narrative analytics that are proactive stories. External criteria for a rational policy analysis may be problematic when parties are trying to maximize multiple objectives and deal with disagreements. Solutions to a problem may depend upon iterations between observed facts and ideas to improve the coherence of criteria (an abductive logic process, as explained in Chapter 6), which time and resources may constrain. Clear criteria may fail to incorporate both the means to accomplish an objective and the objective itself.[7]

Narrative analytics depends on stories that are true, such as the narratives that have served as bookends for each chapter in this book. Opponents may counter with different stories, which may also be true. Analytic narrative stories must be rich by encompassing how they are relevant to the problem that is addressed and how other stories are not relevant to the problem or are false (e.g., a story may include a counternarrative for this purpose). An actor can enrich a story further by conveying the many possible stories and selecting the one that is most appropriate. Good analytic stories are personal with actors and settings and impose a natural order into a complex world.

Similar to the craft of fiction writing, tests of consistency, congruency, and unity need to be met. Regarding consistency, stories are temporal, following actions through time; regarding congruency, any conflict must be explained, especially the arc in the story where expectations are jolted; regarding unity, all parts of the story must be related. The obscure must have meaning.[7]

Related to stories based on narrative analytics, "scenario" writing goes beyond the known. It posits possible stories with actions leading to consequences that lead to more actions and to additional consequences. Scenarios may imagine a slippery slope, or they may provide an enlightened and convincing future consequence of one or more actions.

16.6.4. Precautionary Principle Analysis in Europe

When an activity raises threats of harm to human health or the environment, precautionary measures should be taken even if some cause and effect relationships are not fully established scientifically.

—Wingspread Statement on the Precautionary Principle[59]

In the 1970s, concerns regarding the limitations of science and policy structures to address complexity and uncertainty in risks to health and the environment led to the precautionary principle. The essence of this principle, quoted from the above Wingspread Statement, is the prevention of damage to health founded upon the *Hippocratic Corpus*, "first do no harm." Central components of the principle follow:[59]

1. Take preventive action in the face of uncertainty.
2. Shift burdens onto proponents of potentially harmful activities.
3. Explore a wide range of alternatives to possible harmful actions.
4. Increase public participation in decision making.

However, the precautionary principle turns the harm principle on its head by starting with protecting health as opposed to first attacking the harm, which may be possible but unknown. As positive law, European Union (EU) law speaks to the "high level" of health and environmental protection, in contrast with negative law such as the avoidance of significant risk. Moreover, health protection is seen as the end goal on policy, whereas economics is relevant as a means for protection regarding the most feasible intervention to use. The EU focus is on a high level of health protection, whereas the U.S. position is to rely on cost-benefit and market-oriented values. EU is the leader in implementing the precautionary principle, which has become the international norm as customary law for the protection of public health and the environment.[60]

The precautionary principle is a narrative analysis approach to occupational safety and health that precedes the determination of risk from which risk assessment would follow. Science becomes one consideration in the precautionary principle, for it depends on assumptions and intuition where data are unavailable and is biased in favor of avoiding false positives as a trade-off for avoiding false negatives.[60]

People are generally risk averse, and thus regulatory agencies pursue policies to avoid risk. The elimination of risk can be accomplished by eliminating the hazard, and a zero risk strategy has been used as a policy before. This was the case regarding the 1958 Delaney Clause in the United States. Named after Representative James Delaney (D) of New York, the amendment to the Food, Drugs, and Cosmetic Act of 1938 required the U.S. Food and Drug Administration to not approve any chemical additive for use in food found to induce cancer in humans or animals. It has also been the case in the banning of many pesticides including the use of DBCP in the United States and many nations banning asbestos sales and use (see Chapter 12). These examples followed after failures to take precautions that resulted in occupational illnesses and injuries.

People's perception of risk may be a minor issue in policy making, but it has everything to do with acceptable risk that can be accomplished. Some perceptual factors include familiarity with risk, catastrophic potential, irreversibility of harm, voluntary exposure, threat to posterity, individual control of the risk, possibility for risk control, and benefit to society. Transparency and public dialogue with people is important to determine acceptable risk for both risk management and the precautionary principle.[60]

In Europe, products, substances, and processes are presumed dangerous until the originator demonstrates its safety or lack of harm. The burden of proof is on the manufacturer.

burden of proof = burden of producing evidence + burden of persuasion

When the precautionary principle does not apply, such as on existing chemicals, the burden of proof falls onto the public and its representatives. However, when scientific uncertainty enters this argument, regulatory authorities intervene to place the burden on the manufacturer.[60] When the burden of proof is placed upon manufacturers, this responsibility likely leads them to adopt analysis techniques such as risk assessment.

16.6.5. Precautionary Assessment

Pursuing meaningful, positive goals leads us to necessary collaborations among biological and social sciences, engineering, and political courage.

—Mary O'Brien[61]

While Chapter 6 discussed the precautionary principle, the problem is how to make it operational in the United States. This problem is grounded in the lack of a quantification approach, but a qualitative process is available: precautionary assessment, which is also called a qualitative Bayesian approach. The precautionary assessment is a positive, goal-driven approach that changes the argument to one of public health rather than an initial focus on hazard control.[62]

The OSHAct states positive goals, one of which is in its purpose, "to assure so far as possible every working man and woman in the Nation safe and healthful working conditions," and another regarding protection from toxic materials and harmful physical agents: "that no employee will suffer material

Table 16-4. Changes Needed in Decision-Making Processes for Precautionary Assessment

Changes	From	To
Redirect questions	How safe is safe?	What safer options may achieve the goal?
Alter basic assumptions	Substances are safe until proven dangerous	Those undertaking the activities are responsible for ensuring safety
Modify decision making	Rapid implementation of new technologies and activities	Slow the process for safety evidence when impacts are not understood
Expand participation	Policy maker deliberations	Citizen participation
Reconfigure science framework	Science for scientists	Science to inform prevention policy

impairment of health or functional capacity even if such employee has regular exposure to the hazard dealt with by such standard for the period of his working life." The Mine Act sets out the following goal: "the first priority and concern of all in the coal or other mining industry must be the health and safety of its most precious resource—the miner." Clearly, these are positive goal statements founded on public health protection.

The positive goals are there, and that is where the deliberations need to start. A shift from a harm-driven process to the goal-driven process requires asking different questions and approaches, as indicated in Table 16-4.[62]

Precautionary assessment proceeds through several steps consistent with business textbook approaches. While the steps are sequential, they are also iterative, whereby one step may feed back to previous steps. In this process, every decision is different, and qualitative analysis is important so as to deal with uncertainty and complexity and not narrow analysis or the use of yes-no algorithms. The first step is to define and scope out the problem, identifying needs and potential impacts. The second step is to analyze participation by determining who should be involved and defining trigger mechanisms for adding participants. Third is an analysis of the allocation of burden and responsibility for resources for the assessment.[62]

A fourth step is an analysis of the health impact and, more broadly, the environmental impact of the activity. This step includes a hazard and exposure analysis. It also examines the magnitude and severity of potential impacts considering spatial and temporal dimensions and effects on subpopulations, and the reversibility of impacts. It considers uncertainty and ways to decrease uncertainty, and it considers the weight of evidence of the threat to health and the environment.[62] The fifth step is an identification and comparison of alternatives, the selection of the best alternative, and acting on its implementation. Finally, the sixth step is to determine the level of precaution based upon the threat and establish feedback for continuous improvement.

This process is not meant to be rigid but to provide an approach for considering precaution. It is not unlike the OSHA rule-making process, to consider the weight of the evidence absent a narrowing of focus on the numbers, and it typically needs to be broad enough to address environmental and consumer concerns.[62]

16.7. PARADIGMATIC ANALYSIS

Policymakers often have to act, even though we may not fully understand the full range of possible outcomes, let alone each possible outcome's likelihood. As a result, risk management often involves significant judgment as we evaluate the risks of different events and that our actions will alter those risks.

—Alan Greenspan[63]

This section now turns to the language of numbers. Paradigmatic analysis depends upon formal verification procedures and empirical proof. It also seeks explanations that are sensitive to context and are particular. In this type of analysis, the analyst attempts to be explicit and mean what he or she says.[51] Quantification appears neutral and has provided refuge for regulatory agency officials.[64]

While policy analysis is a term typically applied to the social sciences of economics, organization theory, and political science, in occupational safety and health the multidisciplinary teams are much broader and more diverse. The following subsections address this diversity by first describing risk assessment, then prospective assessment and economic analysis.

16.7.1. Risk Assessment

The right to life and health is the most fundamental of all human rights, and no restriction should be placed on it without proper consideration.

—Theofanis Christoforou[60]

In 1994, the National Research Council codified the four elements of risk assessment: hazard identification, exposure assessment, dose/response assessment, and risk characterization.[65] Risk assessment is traditionally a linear process that follows these elements stepwise. OSHA's approach to risk assessment is guided by Supreme Court interpretations of the OSH Act, namely decisions involving benzene (*Industrial Union Department, AFL-CIO v. American Petroleum Institute,* 1980) and cotton dust (*American Textile Manufacturers Institute v. Donovan,* 1981).[66,67] The court ruled in these cases that OSHA may not promulgate a standard unless it has determined, based on substantial evidence in the record considered as a whole, that there is a significant risk of health impairment at existing permissible exposure levels and that a new standard is necessary to achieve a significant reduction of that risk. The court defined a significant risk as one case in 1,000, whereas an insignificant risk is one in a billion. Even though this spread is large, regulators have been focused more on the court's definition of significant risk since there is little argument against acting at that level. Risk assessment is structured to feed into risk management, as depicted in Figure 16-5. The steps of traditional risk assessment follow:[68]

- Hazard assessment: the determination of whether a particular agent (e.g., chemical) is or is not causally linked to particular health effects.
- Exposure assessment: the determination of the extent of human exposure.
- Dose/response assessment: the determination of the relationship between exposure and the health effects in question.
- Risk characterization: the description of the nature and often the magnitude of human risk.

Although in the cotton dust case the Supreme Court rejected the use of CBA in setting OSHA standards, it reaffirmed its earlier holding in the benzene case that a risk assessment relating to worker health is not only appropriate but is required in order to identify a significant worker health risk and to determine whether a proposed standard will achieve a reduction in that risk. Although the court did not require OSHA to perform a quantitative risk

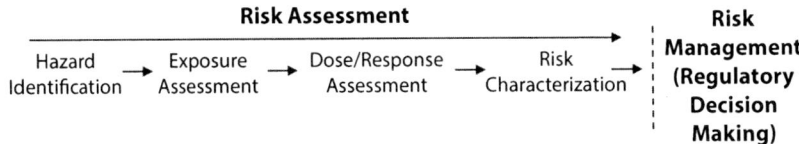

Figure 16-5. Risk assessment and risk management logic diagram.

assessment in every case, the court implied, and OSHA as a policy matter has agreed, that such assessments should be put in quantitative terms to the extent possible.

For example, several approaches can be used to estimate cancer risk from exposure to toxic agents. A standard approach uses mathematical models to describe the relationship between dose (such as airborne concentration) and response (e.g., cancer). In all cases it is assumed that the mathematical curves are reflective of biological processes that control the biological fate and action of the toxic compound. To date, many health-related factors have not been quantitatively linked to mathematical models.[65]

Major risk assessments for some chemicals take more than 10 years. Decision making based on risk assessment is also bogged down. Uncertainty, an inherent property of scientific data, continues to lead to multiple interpretations and contribute to decision-making gridlock. Stakeholders—including community groups, environmental organizations, industry, and consumers—are often disengaged from the risk assessment process at a time when risk assessment is increasingly intertwined with societal concerns. Disconnects between the available scientific data and the information needs of decision makers hinder the use of risk assessment as a decision-making tool.[69]

Risk assessment should continue to capture and accurately describe what various research findings do and do not publicize about threats to human health and to the environment. It should address risk management questions that need to be clearly posed with careful evaluation of the options available to manage risk or potential risk.[69]

Safety standards from OSHA have always been based upon § 3(8) of the OSHAct, which states that companies should adopt safety and health policies that are "reasonably necessary or appropriate to provide safe or healthful employment and places of employment" regarding the avoidance of injuries and not the § 6(2)(b) language regarding toxic materials or harmful physical agents stating that "no employee will suffer material impairment of health or functional capacity even if such employee has regular exposure to the hazard dealt with by such standard for the period of his working life." To assess the significance of many workplace-related fatality rates, a NIOSH study that estimated risk accumulated over a working lifetime found that the risk of work-related fatal injuries in 50 industries and in 50 occupations with the highest risks was "significant." Researchers found that the risks of certain work-related fatal injuries in some occupations (e.g., loggers being struck by falling objects) were of the same magnitude as risks previously identified for specific occupational illness exposures (e.g., lung cancer among uranium miners exposed to radon progeny). Over a 45-year working lifetime, fatal injury risks were found to range from a minimum of 1 death per 1,000 lifetime workers to 36.4 deaths per 1,000 lifetime workers, which by the Supreme Court ruling on the benzene case are significant risks justifying rule making. Much attention has been given to protecting populations experiencing health effects that are considered significant, but conversely, workers exposed to significant risk from fatal injury at more than one death per 1,000 lifetime workers has escaped serious attention. Pointing out this double standard between safety and health standards, the authors suggested that risk assessment for traumatic causes of occupational death should be considered equally with risk assessments for health exposures, such as potential carcinogens.[70]

16.7.2. Prospective Analysis

Whereas risk assessment becomes locked into a lengthy and stepwise process, prospective analysis is a streamlined risk assessment model that provides a foundation for an analysis of emerging technologies and an examination of their risks and benefits to occupational safety and health. This approach is different because it analyzes technologies rather than evaluating the risks of individual agents. Modifications to risk assessment using this approach include the consideration of benefits and injuries and informed research through continuous iterations of current and accrued knowledge. Iterations break the mold of moving through a stepwise process without reflecting on previous steps that become ossified as a finished product. Prospective assessment builds on risk assessment, incorporates these modifications, and aims to forecast potential consequences of the technology by systematically asking the question, "What if?" A companion element in prospective analysis is seeking inherently safer designs. The elements in a prospective analysis in sequence are described below.[71,72]

- Hazard or benefit identification: Qualitatively describe emerging technologies, the potential applications of these technologies, the full range of information available about one or more of these applications, and the implications of that information for occupational health.
- Exposure or contact assessment: Evaluate the probability of workers' exposure to or contact with an identified new technology.

- Dose/contact response assessment: Quantitatively determine the nature and magnitude of the adverse or beneficial effects to worker safety and health that would be potentially associated with exposure to or contact with an emerging technology.
- Risk and benefit characterization: Separate significant risks or benefits from those that are trivial, address uncertainties, and identify principal knowledge gaps.
- Prospective assessment: Extrapolate beyond what is known about an emerging technology and attempt to forecast future risks and benefits and embed this element into the rest of the other elements.
- Inherently safer design: Avoid and not just control occupational hazards.

16.7.3. The Political Economy of Economic Analysis

Using cost-benefit analysis will not necessarily result in greater benefits to citizens, but it will result in the termination of many regulatory programs.
—Kenneth J. Meier[73]

From a public health perspective, economic analysis is important for evaluating the cost-effectiveness of alternative interventions when resources are limited. Nonetheless, the public health professional must be informed about the broader economic analysis techniques in use that are applied in policy analyses.

Economics has outpaced other social science disciplines as a source of ideas and methodologies for public policy.[74] In theory, economic analysis is meant to be a neutral and objective method of evaluating policies and offering transparent judgments on the merits of a proposal. Moreover, economic analysis of proposed regulations aims to avoid adopting inefficient rules that would impose ruinous economic costs on the targeted industry.[75] While Chapter 13 described the advantages and limitations of cost analyses, the stalking horse for regulatory relief is the analysis of the cost and benefit of rules on the regulated parties.

Chapter 13 described a 1995 OTA analysis of the cost and feasibility of OSHA's standards. The OTA found that the actual costs of control were far lower than those predicted by industry.[76]

The chapter also introduced two types of economic analyses: Cost-benefit analysis (CBA) and cost-effectiveness analysis (CEA). These analyses have efficiency as a goal and emerged as a policy analysis procedure during the 1980s and 1990s, as previously shown in Table 16-2. Below is a critique of their appropriateness for evaluating prevention efforts in occupational safety and health.

CBA is an economic analysis in which all costs and benefits are converted into monetary values, and results are used to compare dollars expended to dollars of benefit. CEA is another economic tool that calculates the incremental cost per health outcome averted by an intervention. It is used to choose the most cost-effective intervention in public health for the reduction of an adverse health effect. Meanwhile, CBA is a policy-making tool by which the costs of a regulation are weighed against the potential benefits of harm reduction. It systematically organizes the impacts of policy proposals and forces the explicit assignment of values to the impacts and judgments into the open.

There is an inherent bias away from prevention when efficiency is the goal. As an example, OSHA determined through years of hearings and stakeholder involvement that the ergonomics standard would cost industry $4.7 billion per year but that it would lead to approximately $10.4 billion in cost savings from avoided workplace injuries and improved productivity, for a net savings to society of about $5.7 billion. This was the kind of analysis called for in the name of efficiency. However, the bastion of economists who ignore protection for public health is large.[77] Dudley and DeLong opened an issue of the *Journal of Labor Research* based upon an earlier symposium with a description of the OSHA ergonomics standard in some detail and delivered a message that was not about prevention but claimed the lack of the preventability for nearly all musculoskeletal disorders (MSDs). They also posed a number of open-ended questions regarding the rule-making process and referred to iatrogenic-related (induced by treatment or diagnostic procedures) symptoms suggested by Scalia, the originator of the NCE.[77]

While agreeing with the cost to industry in another article, Berkman and David took issue with the portion of benefits in the proposed OSHA ergonomics standard that related to improved productivity and the presumed failure of the market to intervene to reduce costs.[78] While the authors addressed the "at-risk" industries, they did not address the "at-risk" workers as part of the savings to society, which is the point of the standard. In another article, Cochran criticized OSHA's use of a study by Liberty Mutual Insurance Company regarding workers' compensation claims to support the standard and OSHA's translation of cumulative trauma disorder data from that study into MSD data, but they did not address the plight of workers with MSD.[79] Dudley was critical of a Government Accountability Office study result that OSHA used in formulating the standard while at the same time applauding the value of volunteerism as addressed in the same study.[80] Moreover, she was critical of the cost-benefit methodology that was used and denied that the standard had merit, and she concluded that the standard would impose a significant cost on employers, workers, and society without acknowledging another cost metric, the prevalence of MSDs.

Johnson, Gramm, and Viscusi concluded that workers' preferences would lead to trade-offs between wages and safety and that the standard would be "extremely" expensive for some high-risk industries.[81] They appealed to the tired compensating differential argument, which was shown to be a failed concept in practice (see Chapter 14). Lambert stated that OSHA's primary task is to correct market failures and to respond to these failures efficiently, and not to use command-and-control approaches but rather provide information. This is a misreading of the purpose of the OSH Act. He advised that employees should be informed of the risk and that employers should provide information to protect workers against the risk.[82]

While CBA is considered a neutral tool in policy making, legal scholars have found that CBA is inherently political and even at times supports positions taken against public health protection. The following discussion of the neutrality of CBA and CEA is drawn from three articles. First, among these is an analysis of three case studies that Ackerman, Heinzerling, and Massey compiled, one regarding the OSHA VCM standard of 1974.[75] They found that if a CBA had been conducted at that time, the standard would not have been justified by its economic efficiency based upon the data offered at the time. The same would have been true of the other two case studies that included the removal of lead from gasoline in the 1970s and 1980s by U.S. Environmental Protection Agency (EPA) rules. Regarding the OSHA VCM standard, a 1978 study of the rule found that the cost to industry was one-tenth of its claim at the time that the rule was issued. The authors concluded that CBA would have stood as an obstacle to early regulatory successes regarding the case studies evaluated.

Second, Driesen addressed the neutrality of CBA and showed that OMB reviews of regulations during the George W Bush administration produced numerous antienvironmental, health, and safety changes and no pro-protection changes in the rules.[83] More specifically, cost-benefit criteria applied to the Toxic Substances Control Act (TSCA) of 1976 and the Federal Insecticide, Fungicide, and Rodenticide Act of 1972 have halted regulation under key provisions of these two statutes. In addition, the EPA has not banned a single chemical under TSCA since the U.S. Court of Appeals for the Fifth Circuit ruled in *Corrosion Proof Fittings v. EPA* (1991) that bans must pass a cost-benefit test, rejecting an EPA ban on asbestos.[84] Driesen argued that CBA as a form of analysis should be limited to when costs govern a decision and that it is not a "principle" to be blindly followed. He also concluded that an objective, value-neutral CBA is a theoretical impossibility because of choices of methods for quantifying benefits. His finding was that CBA does not have a neutral effect.[83]

Third, Parker addressed the control of regulations by OMB, stating that PhD statisticians do not render "OMB economists more expert in risk assessment than the entire scientific staff of EPA and OSHA."[85] He criticized analyses by John H. Morrall and Robert W. Hahn, both of whom had altered OSHA benefit estimates. According to Parker, Morrall considered only deaths and not morbidity (a significant cost factor), and Hahn addressed only studies that quantified health effect costs and ignored additional qualitative information on health effects where cost data were not quantified. Parker specifically addressed OMB's Morrall, who gave OSHA's formaldehyde rule a cost of $72 billion per life saved. This analysis used a methodological limitation of CEA to generate this estimate in which there was only one outcome measure, and Morrall chose death as the measure. Parker acknowledged that although the formaldehyde rule may only save one life a year, Morrall's calculation omitted many other benefits, including "reduced or avoided burning eyes or noses, sore or burning throats, asthma attacks, chronic bronchitis, allergic reactions, dermatitis and skin sensitization." Parker noted that OSHA estimated that more than 500,000 U.S. "workers were regularly exposed to formaldehyde at concentrations that have been found to cause one or more of these illnesses or discomforts." According to Parker, Morrall's calculations missed the broader harm that a regulation is actually averting by using simplistic calculations and limiting the analysis to only lives saved.[85]

In Parker's critique of an analysis conducted by Hahn et al., (posted on the AEI-Brookings Joint Center for Regulatory Studies website; Hahn founded the center in 2008) he found a remarkable distortion. Out of 106 rules analyzed, Hahn placed a zero benefit in 32 of them because the benefits were not quantified but were expressed in narrative form. Hahn claimed he used government numbers, and since the rules used narrative and not numbers to describe the benefit, he gave them a zero value. Parker found that neither in theory nor in application are CEA and CBA neutral analytical tools.[85] The efficiency agenda from the regulated community has effected CBA as a precondition for governmental regulation promulgation—which is an indirect form of agency capture to counter the positive public policy movement.

16.8. GLOBAL POLICY

Only this time the beneficiaries of legal creativity "should" not be U.S. citizens alone, tenaciously "protecting" the safety of their own backyards against encroachment by dirty, unsafe industries. This time U.S. legal ingenuity should be put in service of a global ethic of precaution, corresponding to the global spread of environmental (and occupational) hazards and corporate capital.
—Sheila Jasanoff[64]

This section brings closure to the discussion of transitions in policy over time and to modernity and its global regime as shown in Table 16-1. Globalization as seen today happens in the context of receding government, deregulation, and reduced social obligations within national economies.[31] Global economic policy is designed for a monetary and trade system with occupational safety and health only a footnote at best, as demonstrated by the experience with the North American Free Trade Agreement (NAFTA; see Chapter 12). As this global monetary and trade integration has emerged, every nation is vulnerable to decisions made elsewhere across the globe. Transnational corporations have become stateless corporations in which the nation-state is losing its capacity to protect its citizens, and more specifically its workers. Indeed, positive public policy is compromised, and the nation-state is increasingly irrelevant as political leaders lack coherent answers to questions of the impact of the global economy on citizens. In this milieu, OSHA has a more difficult time addressing the national norm of a commitment by corporations to take on responsibility for their workers' welfare.[16]

Discordant as it is, Systematic Occupational Health and Safety Management (SOHSM) models are gaining legitimacy around the world. This model is discussed next, followed by discussions of four major problems regarding the global economy that confront domestic policies: goal diversity, externalities (the cost of doing business), institutions and sanctions, and participation and accountability.[16]

16.8.1. Systematic Occupational Health and Safety Management

Globalization and labor standards are not mortal enemies but complementary ways—Siamese twins, in our analogy—to make modern economic growth work better for all.

—Kimberly Ann Elliott and Richard B Freeman[86]

Incentives are important. The manufacturers of machines are liable for the safety of the machines that they make and, as a result, responsible to think and act proactively no matter the specific hazard. An international network regarding food safety is emerging: systems for tracing food-borne hazards back to their source are being built, thereby providing an incentive for producers to think and act proactively no matter the specific hazard. More difficult challenges emerge regarding precaution when the possible hazard is of long latency or when it is a condition of work. Part of the SOHSM approach is to provide incentives to induce employers to take responsibility for comprehensive, systematic, and precautionary approaches for occupational safety and health. These approaches are in contrast with just prescribing specific solutions as a regulatory strategy. Moreover, SOHSM has been voluntarily adopted by a number of large organizations.

The need for precaution on a global scale is represented by international norms present in trade today. The precautionary principle is codified in the EU 1989 Framework Directive, within which a strategy for SOHSM is embedded. This strategy aims to prevent work-related injuries and illnesses as "a permanent and enduring improvement and optimization of the work environment by involving all the key actors and key processes in companies."[87]

In recent years, SOHSM has become a common approach for occupational safety and health protection in developed countries. Furthermore, developing and transitional countries have started to adopt elements of this approach as well.

A problem regarding SOHSM is that it considers management as the agent of rationality and workers as a source of irrationality. However, SOHSM lacks defined management approaches. After a series of rational management theories developed over the years, starting with Taylorism in the early 1900s, a current viewpoint held by management is contingency theory. This theory claims that an organization is contingent upon its environment (circumstances and history), which shapes its strategy, technology, size, and innovations. However, caution needs to be exercised, as demonstrated by the opening narrative of Chapter 15 regarding situation attribution theory.

Rational theories focus on management as the rational agent that protects the worker from hazards or hazardous behavior, which can be easily exaggerated as being overly paternalistic.[88] Nonrational theories look to human relations and a sociotechnical tradition that focuses on social rather than rational characteristics of organizations. The nonrational characteristics take political and labor perspectives that include social organizations, power relations, conflict and consent, and how goals and interest are invented.[88]

The SOHSM model takes on two perspectives. One is the regulated system, and the other is the voluntary system, which remains as a work in progress.[89] Chapter 9 noted that NIOSH has adopted a research focus on the "total health" of workers, and OSHA is using a hybrid regulatory-voluntary approach in its programs as described in Chapter 15. The regulatory approach is a legal mandate for OSHA through the enforcement of standards, and its voluntary approach includes the Voluntary Protection Program (VPP) and its state consultation services, each with the threat of the regulatory approach as a backup system.

16.8.2. Goal Diversity

Contrary to what many economists believe, we lack a full understanding of how globalization works.

—Dani Rodrik[31]

The antagonistic ideologies of the Cold War have been replaced by proponents of the global economy versus proponents of global standards to protect labor and the environment.[86] The challenge is to evolve a synthesis of these two contenders in a world that has extreme differences in cultures. The SOHSM model deals with the tensions of two sets of goals regarding occupational safety and health—one is prevention through regulation versus voluntarism, and the other is rational-based versus nonrational-based theories. Another set of goals in developing countries involves conflict between employment as a path out of extreme poverty and safe work, despite arguments for both. A fundamental dilemma for developing nations is the prevalence of poverty in one-third of the world's population, with incomes at less than US$1 or $2 per day per person versus the unsafe jobs that they take to live. Thus, unfortunately, nations in poverty promote economic growth no matter the human cost.

Moreover, as discussed in Chapter 12, even when science and the actions of many nations have united to ban the use of asbestos, the economic powers in other developed as well as developing countries have advocated for the use of asbestos as a matter of policy despite overwhelming scientific evidence of the danger of a multinational pandemic of cancer. Another example of diverse goals and a source of tension between the global market and social stability (e.g., low unemployment) is asymmetry between groups that can easily cross international borders, such as capital, and those that cannot, such as labor.[31]

A major international influence on occupational safety and health is the effect of changes in the structure and organization of work. These changes are driven by emerging networks of production driven by global movement of capital, technological change, and deregulation in the developed countries. This is in the midst of vast differences in work life between developed, transitional, and developing countries.[90]

The publicity of the employment of children or of catastrophic events, such as those described in Chapter 12, are a repeat of the early history of occupational safety and health protection in the United States that was most vividly expressed in Chapters 5 and 10. Proponents of the international enforcement of labor standards present two perspectives.[91]

- Organized labor and social activists in the industrialized countries argue that "unfair" labor practices and conditions exist in many developing country trading partners and need to be offset by appropriate trade policy measures in order to "level the playing field."
- Many social activists argue that workers in developing countries are subject to exploitative and abusive working conditions, and that their wages are suppressed.

Conflicts within and between nations arise over domestic norms within and among countries and social institutions (e.g., domestic society versus international trade). Globalization engenders conflicts over social norms and the institutions that embody them. Trade becomes contentious when it unleashes forces that undermine these norms.[31]

One approach to evolve concordance of norms across cultures is to consider the spectrum of prevention that was described in Chapter 2 from an international perspective. This spectrum—inform individuals → launch media campaigns → educate advocates → engender coalitions → change practices → influence policies—can serve as a model for improving global occupational safety and health. Social media technology is in place to intervene with the first two steps. Moreover, as discussed in Chapter 13, the metric for longevity of the average life span in each nation can be used as a gauge for where geographically and where on the occupational safety and health spectrum intervention should focus.

16.8.3. The Cost of Doing Business

Despite enormous costs (of work-related injuries and diseases), it was not until OSHA began focusing its enforcement efforts on these job hazards that most industries began paying attention to them.
        —Deborah Berkowitz, United Food and Commercial Workers[56]

Elliott and Freeman[86] referred to Joseph Heller's novel, *Catch-22*, in which the catch results from rules, regulations, or procedures that an individual is subject to but has no control over. Specifically, they contrasted the international mobility of capital and the international immobility of labor in response to dynamic changes in comparative economic advantage across nations. One has an exit option, and the other does not, which presents a paradox for the worker in which there is no escape from a "race to the bottom."

As a social norm, the cost of business in the United States includes the cost of compliance with occupational safety and health standards. As production is outsourced to nations that lack these protections, a product may not incorporate these costs. Tensions arise between markets and societal norms across borders, which can lead to conflict.[90] A commonplace tension is that transnational companies obscure the protection of workers' safety and health through offshore operations and outsourcing of jobs, and they escape having to provide that protection as a cost of doing business, which is one of capitalism's contradictions as described in Chapter 13. The absence of these safeguards places a negative externality upon the workers, their families, and society for the cost of injuries and illnesses. Moreover, the importing countries experience indirect externalities if they provide these safeguards domestically but are unable to compete globally because of the expressed cost of these safeguards. Thus, unemployment or underemployment may be a result, which is another contradiction of capitalism as described earlier in Chapter 13.

Driven by the lower cost of production and the "magic" of comparative advantage, globalization makes the labor of large segments of the working population more easily substituted for the labor of other working populations across borders.[31] Mogensen contended that neoliberal policies and globalization operate with their own rules. On the one hand, they focus on opening, deregulating, and privatizing to make an economy more competitive and attractive to foreign investment. On the other hand, they dismantle the decades-old, grassroots-built regulatory safety nets, setting workplace safety back by a century to a legal doctrine whereby the worker, rather than the employer, assumes the risks and costs of injury, illness, and death.[92]

The past has shown that transnational corporations outsource their jobs to companies in developing countries where worker protections are tenuous and where the cost of the product fails to account for the cost of an occupational injury or illness. Indeed, "competitiveness" is code for reducing labor costs, including the cost of compliance with occupational safety and health regulations.[31]

The incentive to reduce costs is a strong motivation to shift costs to the public. Even companies that cannot export jobs from the service economy in the United States claim that they can ill afford to protect their workers in a global, free market economy. These externalities threaten the sustainability of occupational safety and health policies by accentuating the differences between the limited-mobility workers and the greater mobility of other factors of production including capital, highly skilled workers, and professionals.[39] Traditional occupational safety and health rationales for regulation apply to the problems inherent in globalization as described in Section 16-3, and how this is done remains an open question.

16.8.4. Institutions and Sanctions

Institutions are durable systems of established and embedded social rules that structure social interactions. In short, institutions are social rule systems.
—Geoffrey M. Hodgson[93]

Two institutional approaches are available for regulating occupational safety and health globally. One approach is working within the existing trade structure of the World Trade Organization (WTO). The other approach is to use separate structures that address the problem directly, perhaps through the International Labour Organization (ILO) or the Organisation for Economic Co-operation and Development (OECD).

Markets are social institutions, and their legitimacy needs to be affirmed in both their processes and outcomes. Since international markets are not controlled by overarching governance, their legitimacy is most at question in national governments (e.g., the case in France as described in Chapter 12 regarding the ban on asbestos). When legitimacy is lost, institutions can no longer function. Legitimacy is driven by the resolution of conflicts through national debate and deliberation.[31]

In the United States, the U.S. Department of Commerce is the national judge regarding in-country claims. Thus, an important issue is the staffing of the organizations that have sanction authority, which bring expertise regarding economics to the table but not necessarily regarding public health. Despite the strong emphases of protecting worker safety and health by the World Health Organization (WHO) and ILO, the trade organizations win out.[18] An argument can be made that it is a lack of policy space—and not a lack of market access—that may become the binding constraint on a prosperous global economy.[94]

A major international issue is how nation-states will join together for the protection of occupational safety and health. The EU is demonstrating how nation-states can come together on this issue (see Chapter 12).[90] Conflicts regarding multilateral institutions come down to two issues. One is how to reduce tensions that arise out of domestic practices when multilateral institutions encourage the convergence of policies and standards between nations. The other issue is how nations can selectively safeguard domestic policies that are in conflict with multinational trade policies.[31] Table 16-5 describes the options available regarding the regulatory realms available to nation-states to protect their citizens.[16]

Rules are needed regarding how a nation can depart from multilateral rules. The WTO escape clause, the Agreement on Safeguards from the 1994 General Agreement on Tariffs and Trade (GATT), was designed for this purpose, except that it has a bias for promoting importers through antidumping procedures. The safeguards do not address nontrade norms at the domestic level. One way to address this problem is to recast the "serious injury" test regarding safeguards to address public health safeguards such as occupational safety and health. Article X of the GATT states the following:

> This investigation [by the nation introducing the safeguard measure] shall include public hearings or other appropriate means in which importers, exporters, and other interested parties could present evidence and their

views, including the opportunity to respond to the presentations of other parties and to submit their views, inter alia, as to whether or not the application of a safeguard measure would be in the public interest.[95]

The problem with the interpretation of this clause is that groups other than those raising the claim are consistently excluded from testimony. Regarding the inherent conflicts between the market and society at the country level, Rodrik argued that these safeguard hearings should include all relevant parties to determine if broad support exists for the safeguards.[31] Imagine this scenario: if an importer's goods were manufactured by slave labor, would testimony be offered to defend slave labor in response to claims lodged by opposing testimony? The advantage of this approach is establishing the legitimacy, within international forums and of national norms, of what is considered free trade.[31]

There are few international institutions that impose sanctions for violating international regulations, and international regulations are lacking for protecting occupational safety and health. International organizations that

Table 16-5. Options regarding international regulatory institutions

Type	Description	Examples
Cooperation	Recognize the legitimacy of policies of one nation that are incompatible with policies of another nation	NAFTA
Harmonization	Harmonize domestic policies for international compatibility	UN Globally Harmonized System of Classification and Labeling of Chemicals
International regulatory accords	Create international bodies of executive, legislative, and judicial functions	EU regulation of occupational safety and health
International recommendations	Adopt domestic policies recommended by international bodies	ILO recommendations, OECD codes
Governmental international standards	Treaty policies developed by international organizations	ILO standards
NGO international standards	Self-regulation by regulated entities	ISO standards

Source: Eisner.[15]
Note: NAFTA = North American Free Trade Agreement; UN = United Nations; EU = European Union; ILO = International Labour Organization; OECD = Organisation for Economic Co-operation and Development; ISO = International Organization for Standardization.

impose sanctions include the International Monetary Fund, the WTO, and the OECD. Regional regulatory organizations include NAFTA and the EU. There are many other international agreements that contribute to fragmented policies. Many of these organizations lack strong sanctions, including NAFTA (see Chapter 12).

The Safeguards Agreement could be broadened to a wider set of circumstances. Accordingly, any interested party could pursue an exemption or opt-out based on a compelling case that the international economic transactions in question are in conflict with a widely shared social norm within a country, which could include a ban on imports of certain goods from a country because of safety concerns as an unacceptable economic transaction. A well-designed set of procedures would help bring out the relevant considerations on all sides.[94]

The preceding would be open for review in a multilateral setting. The scheme forces deliberation and debate at the national level on the nature of the international economy, the economic gains it generates, and the circumstances in which domestic practices and needs come into conflict.[94]

From a perspective of employers, labor standards such as workplace safety rules are seen as a tax on employment.[31] Regarding tax policy, nations have combined to thwart tax evasion policies by nations outside of a norm of fair behavior. The OECD has been successful at tightening controls over financial centers that permit tax evasion, including money laundering, by threatening reprisals from members of the organization that included economic sanctions, a ban on banking transactions, and a cutoff of development aid. Consistent with this action, the Paris-based Financial Action Task Force was ready to publish a "blacklist of countries that permitted tax evasion in 2008.[96] Outsourcing to nations where workplace safety standards do not measure up to international norms such as those recommended by the ILO or proposed by the OECD could be an argument for international sanctions (see Chapters 4 and 12).

A critical rethinking of strategy among occupational safety and health activists in the labor movement is needed to protect workers who form unions or complain about safety violations.[97] An example of U.S. labor coordinating with labor movements in other countries is the World Summit on Sustainable Development of 2002, as identified in Chapter 12 along with WHO activities. Workplace safety is clearly intertwined with protection of the environment, as illustrated by the Bhopal (India) disaster.

Global economy advocates have argued that rather than adding a social clause to the WTO's mandate, another agency should contend with the issue of labor standards.[86] The ILO is such an agency—with connections to WHO and the UN Environment Programme (UNEP) regarding occupational safety and health. The ILO sets international labor standards, but it also publicizes country ratifications and performances regarding these standards. Moreover, it provides technical assistance to developing countries regarding occupational safety and health (e.g., the Better Factories Cambodia Program).

Nevertheless, the ILO also has international enforcement powers.[86] Through Article 24 and 26 of the ILO Charter, respectively, any worker or employer around the world can file a complaint against a member government regarding violation of an ILO convention, and if the complaint goes unresolved, a government can raise it against another country. This power is compromised by the U.S. government, since it has only ratified a measly 13 conventions and two of the four core conventions. However, given the tripartite structure of the ILO, U.S. representatives to the ILO—the U.S. Council for International Business, for employers, or the AFL-CIO, for labor—can bring a complaint regardless of U.S. ratification. The complaint can be appealed to the International Court of Justice. Nonetheless, the ILO has sanction authority in Article 33 of its charter that does not exclude economic sanctions.[86] The ILO allied with OECD may build a policy regarding sanctions for the violation of norms for the protection of occupational safety and health.

16.8.5. Participation and Accountability

The whole debate pertaining to free trade [NAFTA] assumed working people have no families, but are autonomous economic selves in a natural relationship of subjugation and subordination. They experience obedience because of fear of being made unemployed, since unemployment is an injury just as sure as one loses a finger in a punch press.

—Robert Sass[98]

The concept of participation is necessary for addressing the anticipation, identification, evaluation, and control of work-related hazards. Accountability is a related concept for assuring that participation takes place. Participation involves three important actors: two are management and labor, and the other is scientists. As for science, it brings reason and objectivity as a political resource for setting international norms and accords. Indeed, international accords cannot escape the consideration of science. A challenge for scientists is to bring together its different fields, especially social science and physical or biological sciences. An important aspect of science is the development of international standards, which involves a process of stabilizing policy-relevant knowledge across a mix of social interests. Standardization may include risk assessment and economic analysis, but quantification may "strip away" complex perspectives of problems and prematurely level these differences against domestic agendas. The challenge is to build the conditions in which participants recognize the need to standardize protections within their own domains as part of a global belief system. Mismatches of perception can lead to failures in compliance with international accords, even when agreements have been held in accord by various nations.[89]

Regarding management, self-interest has led corporations to voluntarily adopt the ISO 14000 standard regarding environmental protection, and as a matter of corporate policy, many trade only with other corporations that comply with ISO 14000, which provides for a system of accountability. Compliance with ISO 14000, which came about because of advocacy by UNEP, has become common with large companies worldwide, and by association, with smaller companies that are vendors.[16] Transnational companies are a potential resource within developing countries for introducing occupational safety and health norms, which are easily lost in the pyramid of contractors and subcontractors.

The most crucial issue regarding SOHSM is the level of worker participation, including co-determination (i.e., allows workers to elect half of the members of the board of directors in the company in which they are employed, which is common in Germany). Workers are the most aware of many hazards since they see them firsthand, which is an aspect of contingency theory that offers continuous grassroots feedback. The SOHSM model can be informed by the continuous improvement doctrine of worker participation as a pillar of Total Quality Management.

Likewise, the OECD could advocate for its corporate code of conduct in support of labor participation and occupational safety and health as described in Chapter 4. Another pathway to broader labor participation regarding working conditions is based on Germany's co-determination laws that state that union leaders or employee representatives must receive as many as half of the seats on the supervisory boards that control an automaker's major investments and hire or fire executives. Special work councils handle decisions on issues like working conditions. In the United States, the United Automobile Workers sees co-determination as an important avenue for increasing participation within the corporate structure.[99]

Despite the ILO being periodically starved of financial contributions by member nations, notably by the United States, its power lies in a policy of transparency regarding violations of conventions and the availability of protective standards. The Internet can instill inducements for improved attention to occupational safety and health by posting violations. It also provides an avenue for mass distribution of information, interaction in service-related activities, and training by way of webinars over the Internet and social media, and thus offers an avenue for circumventing budgetary barriers.[86]

16.9. CONCLUSION

This chapter returns now to the "problem": work-related injuries and diseases. Evident in the debates regarding passage of the OSHAct as described in Chapter 6, the anchor point for occupational safety and health advocacy is the threat to human life and its quality. The opportunity is positive public policy (establishment of a duty of one to another versus a freedom from this duty) to rid the world of perceived hazards that affect individual workers but also their families and the broader network of society. As referred to earlier, the adage "think globally, act locally" may be useful for coping within the global economy with the challenges to national norms including occupational safety and health.

As this book concludes, a discussion of Jacobson and Weiss provides a framework for the analysis of the implementation of, compliance with, and effectiveness of laws based upon factors present in the economy and the polis.[100] A brief analysis of the results of the U.S. mandate and norms for occupational safety and health follows.

16.9.1. Implementation

Implementation refers to the measures that the United States or other countries use to effect the goal of preventing work-related injuries and illnesses. The United States has enacted and implemented several laws that protect occupational safety, including the OSHAct, the Mine Act, and several specific laws such as protecting the safety of commercial fishers. However, standards promulgation was nearly halted because of the administrative barriers constructed to slow down rule making as part of deregulation policies. These barriers include riders on appropriation bills, the resolution to terminate the ergonomics standard, executive orders, OMB reviews, administrative laws, and court challenges and rulings; these barriers have been called "paralysis by analysis." However, several safety standards are in place and a number of health standards have been promulgated with few court cases that have denied the rules. Omitted from protection are state and local government employees unless covered by a state OSHA plan and self-employed workers. Nevertheless, self-employed workers are indirectly protected by the changes in social norms that occur through regulations and safer products that arise from regulations or tort claims. Workers' compensation laws have been established in all jurisdictions in the United States.

16.9.2. Compliance

Compliance goes beyond implementation and refers to whether the United States or other countries adhere to the goal to prevent work-related injuries and illnesses. Compliance may entail procedural or substantive obligations and behavior regarding the spirit of the law. In the United States, the cost estimated by the regulated community regarding standards has been consistently exaggerated. OSHA's compliance with the law for standard setting has slowed dramatically. More than 100 recommended standards have been issued by NIOSH, and OSHA has been able to promulgate less than a quarter of these recommendations. As for the OSHA-NIOSH standards completion project, now dated, in which more than 300 chemicals were identified for future rule making, only a fraction of these chemicals has been acted on. While OSHA complied with the OSHAct regarding ergonomics to address the major cause of lost-time injuries and the largest contribution to workers' compensation cost, Congress and President George W. Bush reversed that standard in 2001 for reasons other than the prevention of disabilities. This effort diverted staff from developing other standards for nearly a decade.

The OSHA cancer policy would have expedited the control of carcinogens, which was rendered dormant by the benzene court ruling. A standard to update the air contamination PELs was reversed by a court ruling. The Hazard Communication (HazCom) Standard was a major success that has reached virtually every workplace in the United States, augmented by EPA enforcement of the Community Planning and Right-to-Know Act, which the OSHA Haz-Com standard influenced greatly. In addition, OSHA acted on issuing standards referred to it by the EPA under the TSCA (e.g., formaldehyde). Moreover, NIOSH addressed with public health principles many worker populations including farmers and firefighters that were excluded from enforcement under the OSHAct or by congressional riders. The institute's research results have been a positive externality for occupational safety and health programs worldwide. While there is broad compliance with workers' compensation laws, there are holes in this safety net. Some sectors may be excluded (e.g., agriculture) from OSHA oversight, and the workers' compensation system's no-fault foundation is compromised when insurance companies challenge claims (e.g., back pain).

The overarching standard in the OSHAct, the general duty clause, places the responsibility for compliance with the act on employers. For compliance in the workplace, one looks at employer behavior. Both OSHA and MSHA do not need to look far to find workplaces out of compliance, including egregious cases. Citations are regularly issued when compliance officers visit workplaces. Indeed, mine disasters are preceded by citations for violations that could have prevented the disasters. OSHA issues large penalties for egregious violations of standards. However, taken as a whole after the passage of the OSHAct, workplaces are much cleaner and safer, suggesting that U.S. employers have largely adopted the norm of protection of the safety and health of their workers.

A consistent and troubling acceptance by society is a double standard in which a death through negligence is a felony when it occurs outside the workplace but is a misdemeanor when it occurs on the job. Worldwide, legal punishment of employers is rare and typically less severe than legal punishment for violations of environmental or financial rules. Negligent employers escape criminal prosecution, even when major workplace disasters arouse public outrage.[101]

16.9.3. Effectiveness

While the United States or other countries may be in compliance with the law, the law may be ineffective in addressing the goal to prevent work-related injuries and illnesses. In the United States, although the number of fatalities has dropped by more than half since the OSHAct went into effect in 1971, studies have been hard pressed to associate that reduction completely with the act.

Confounding factors included changes in technology (e.g., robotics) and demographic shifts to jobs in the service sector. A high proportion of the occupational deaths that have occurred since 1971 are outside of the jurisdiction of OSHA, principally in transportation. Nonetheless, much of the reduction can be related to safer working conditions, and the ultimate responsibility lies with employers.

A study has found that OSHA inspections do influence the reduction in reportable injuries and an associated reduction in workers' compensation costs.[102] Moreover, where OSHA has promulgated standards, the effect has been positive. Asbestos and DBCP are gone, cancer from coke oven fume exposure is undetectable, and byssinosis has been substantially reduced. Under the HazCom Standard, workers are not the only people informed of hazards—employers now know of the hazards and available interventions to control them. Furthermore, when a standard is promulgated there is a multiplier effect, for an investment in resources such as professional staff or consultants leads to expansion of their expertise more broadly at worksites.

While workers' compensation is a help in secondary (cure) and tertiary (care) prevention, its effectiveness is in question as an incentive for primary prevention (protection). Small- or high-hazard companies are typically placed into insurance pools where their injury experience is averaged into that of other employers. The exception is in those larger companies who have unique control over the adjustment of their injury experience rating.

Mine-related deaths have fallen dramatically, as was shown in Figure 16-2. The Mine Act has been very effective in preventing disasters, injuries, and dust-related diseases. Overall, the effectiveness of the OSHAct and the Mine Act has been effective for reducing injuries and diseases, improving knowledge and awareness of these problems and relevant controls, and creating a professional workforce that is knowledgeable and skilled at preventing occupational injuries and diseases.

THE CASE FARMS NARRATIVE

On March 26, 2013, Case Farms received a Worker Safety Recognition Award from the American Meat Institute at its Goldsboro, North Carolina, poultry plant. A news report referred to the plant adopting standards developed by OSHA's VPP that covered the company's four complexes. Case Farms was recognized for meeting or exceeding industry standards, increasing awareness about worker safety, and making efforts to reduce occupational injuries and illnesses.[103] Missing from the news release was a key indicator of success under the VPP program, which is a reduction in the incidence of injuries and illnesses. Moreover, Case Farms did not appear on the OSHA list of participating VPP companies.[104] Relatedly, an OSHA press release addressed the ergonomics guidelines for the poultry processing industry that was issued in 2004, which was built on a 1986 poultry processing industry guideline that advocated training, ergonomics, and medical intervention as a means to reduce the occurrence of MSDs and their associated costs.[105]

One of the Case Farms complexes is located in Morganton, North Carolina, and it has a history. In 1995, this complex was located in Representative Cass Ballenger's congressional district; Ballenger was out to change OSHA into a consultation agency, as described in Section 16.5 of this chapter.

Mary Williams (a pseudonym used at the time) worked on the chicken processing line at Case Farms in Morganton for more than 10 years, and she liked her job. She started with cutting oil sacs from the bird carcasses, then over the years she moved to different tasks that included gutting, deboning, and chopping the dead chickens. When she started, the required speed on the line was 45 birds per minute, then it was 70, then 80, and by 1995 it was 90 birds per minute. Workers had to buy their own personal protective equipment and sanitary apparel that included metal mesh gloves, rubber boots, hairnets, earplugs, and aprons, at a cost of more than $70. The company refused to post injury records as required by OSHA.

By the late 1980s, Williams began feeling the results of exposure to the "traumatogens" (a term coined by Vernon Putz Anderson at NIOSH in the mid-1980s to describe those conditions that result in cumulative trauma disorders and MSDs such as those from twisting, bending, and lifting). Her affliction started with a dull pain in the middle of her palms to her elbows. Her arms began to swell and feel numb. She could no longer wear her wedding ring because of the swelling. This was the early onset of a repetitive strain injury known as carpal tunnel syndrome (CTS). Every day, 15 to 20 of 450 workers at the plant visited the company nurse about pain in their arms; the nurse treated the conditions with wrist bandages and ibuprofen. When Williams asked to see a doctor about her pain, company management threatened to fire her. As the pain got worse, she told management that she aimed to see a lawyer, and only then did they let her see a doctor. The doctor diagnosed the condition as work-related CTS, but the workers' compensation carrier refused to honor the claim, contending that it was unrelated to work. She sought opinions from other doctors, and they agreed with the initial diagnosis. These doctors insisted that she see a specialist for an operation to relieve the pain (a typical cost was $20,000). She could not sleep at night because of the pain, and she had to drive with her palms on the steering wheel, unable to grip the wheel because of pain. The doctors also told Case Farms to give her work that would not aggravate the injury, but to no avail. Finally, after four years she got the operation, and the surgeon required that she be given light-duty work: no gripping, pulling, or overhead lifting (all traumatogens with repetitive or awkward and heavy loading of the body).[56]

At first, Williams was given paperwork and inspection jobs, but then Case Farms returned her to the line. The CTS was still present, and the crushing pain was driving Williams to tears. While she was earning less than $7 per hour, afflicted by CTS, and unable to grip, pull, or lift, the company fired her. Williams—unemployed, disabled, and unable to do many household chores—struggled to keep her marriage together. She saw other Case Farms workers with bandages around their wrists and said, "I know where they're headed, and there's nothing I can do about it."[56]

While Williams was employed at Case Farms, she witnessed a shift in employment from the local population to immigrants from Guatemala and Mexico. A local Catholic priest attested that they were guided to the company and employed because they were seen as putting up with anything including abuse, standing in chicken guts all day, and a minimum wage. Their voice was muted by language barriers and fear of deportation.[56]

Then in 1995, three workers requested to speak to management about the dangers of the accelerated speed on the line. Management had them arrested and hauled off in handcuffs for trespassing. A strike by 300 workers ensued, and one month later the workers voted to join the Laborers International Union. With a sense of community as part of their culture and religion, these Latino workers collectively joined with a voice: "An injury to one is an injury to all."[56]

After 1995, no OSHA inspections occurred at Case Farms in North Carolina until 2004, which was based on a complaint. By that time, Case Farms had become a nonunion employer again. The agency investigated two injuries in 2005, a foot amputation and an electrical shock. In 2004 and since then, OSHA reported that 20 inspections had been conducted at North Carolina Case Farm workplaces. Eight inspections were based upon complaints, four of which occurred in 2012. As of 2013, Williams's fate is unknown, since her name was protected with a pseudonym.

REFERENCES

1. Asheberle D. *Federalism and Environmental Policy.* Washington, DC: George Washington University Press;2004.
2. Centers for Disease Control and Prevention. Ten great public health achievements—United States, 1900–1999. *MMWR Morb Mortal Wkly Rep.* 1999;48(12):241–243.
3. Fall J. Megatrends for STAFDA distributors: Finding advantage in megatrends for businesses of any size. Presented at: Specialty Tools and Fasteners Distributors Association Conference; November 5, 2012; Orlando, FL.
4. Steinbeck J. *The Pearl.* New York, NY: Penguin;1947.
5. Heilbroner R, Milberg W. *The Crisis of Vision in Modern Economic Thought.* New York, NY: Cambridge University Press;1995.
6. Weimer DL, Vining AR. *Policy Analysis: Concepts and Practice.* Upper Saddle River, NJ: Prentice Hall;1999.
7. Kaplan JT. The narrative structure of policy analysis. *J Policy Anal Manage.* 1986;5(4):761–778.
8. Lawlor EF. Book reviews. *J Policy Anal Manage.* 1996;15(1):110–146.
9. Mendeloff J. *Regulating Safety: An Economic and Political Analysis of Occupational Safety and Health Policy.* Cambridge, MA: MIT Press;1979.
10. Meier KJ. *Regulation: Politics, Bureaucracy, and Economics.* New York, NY: St. Martin's Press;1985.
11. Breyer S. *Regulation and Its Reform.* Cambridge, MA: Harvard University Press;1982.
11a. U.S. Department of Labor. Celebrating 40 years of mine safety and health. Mine Safety and Health Administration. Available at: http://www.msha.gov/FocusOn/40thAnniversary/40thAnniversary.asp. Accessed January 30, 2015.
12. *Hearing Before the House Committee on Employment and Education, Subcommittee on Workforce Protection* (June 14, 2001) (testimony, M Seminario, OSHA's standard-setting process). Available at: http://archives.republicans.edlabor.house.gov/archive/hearings/107th/wp/osha61401/seminario.htm. Accessed September 17, 2013.

13. Cheney D. Documentary. In: Cutler RJ. The world according to Dick Cheney. *Showtime.* 2013. Available at: http://www.sho.com/sho/reality-docs/titles/3370771/the-world-according-to-dick-cheney#/index. Accessed March 18, 2013.

14. Stone D. *Policy Paradox: The Art of Political Decision Making.* New York, NY: W.W. Norton & Company;2002.

15. Eisner MA. *Regulatory Politics in Transition.* Baltimore, MD: John Hopkins University Press;2000.

16. Coleridge ST. A desultory poem, written on the Christmas Eve 1794. In: Keach W, ed. *The Complete Poems of Samuel Taylor Coleridge.* New York, NY: Penquin Books;2004.

17. Morris RB, ed. *The U.S. Department of Labor History of the American Worker.* Washington, DC: U.S. Government Printing Office;1977.

18. Kerr L. Black lung: The struggle to help its victims. In: *Protecting People at Work: A Reader in Occupational Safety and Health.* Washington, DC: U.S. Government Printing Office;1980:281–295.

19. Ganz M. *Why David Sometimes Wins: Leadership, Organization, and Strategy in the California Farm Worker Movement.* New York, NY: Oxford University Press;2009.

20. Leopold L. *The Man Who Hated Work and Loved Labor: The Life and Times of Tony Mazzocchi.* White River Junction, VT: Chelsea Green Publishing Company;2007.

21. Page JA, O'Brien M-W. *Bitter Wages.* New York, NY: Grossman Publishers;1973.

22. Noble C. *Liberalism at Work: The Rise and Fall of OSHA.* Philadelphia, PA: Temple University Press;1986.

23. Kelman S. Occupational Safety and Health Administration. In: Wilson JG, ed. *The Politics of Regulation.* New York, NY: Basic Books;1980.

24. Marcus AA. Whatever happened to the "New Class"? In: Stone A, Harpham EJ, eds. *The Political Economy of Public Policy.* Thousand Oaks, CA: Sage;1982:93–114.

25. Weaver PH. Regulation, social policy, and class conflict. *Public Int.* 1978;50(4):45–63.

26. Nicholson WJ, Landrigan PJ. Quantitative assessment of lives lost due to delay in the regulation of occupational exposure to benzene. *Environ Health Perspect.* 1989;82(7):185–188.

27. Coolidge C. Address to the American Society of Newspaper Editors, Washington, DC. January 17, 1925. The American Presidency Project. Available at: http://www.presidency.ucsb.edu/ws/?pid=24180. Accessed June 11, 2014.

28. Mendeloff JM. *The Dilemma of Toxic Substance Regulation: How Overregulation Causes Underregulation at OSHA.* Cambridge, MA: MIT Press;1988.

29. Lindblom CE. *The Policy-Making Process.* Englewood Cliffs, NJ: Prentice-Hall, Inc.;1968.

30. Holsworth RD. Why liberalism failed. In: Stone A, Harpham EJ, eds. *The Political Economy of Public Policy.* Thousand Oaks, CA: Sage;1982:29–47.

31. Rodrik D. *Has Globalization Gone Too Far?* Washington, DC: Institute for International Economics;1997.

32. Peterson MA. Political influence in the 1990s: From iron triangles to policy networks. *J Health Polit Policy Law.* 1993;18(2):395–438.

33. Ferris T. *The Science of Liberty: Democracy, Reason, and the Laws of Nature.* New York, NY: HarperCollins Publishers;2010.

34. Werking RH. Bureaucrats, businessmen, and foreign trade: The origins of the United States Chamber of Commerce. *Bus Hist Rev.* 1978;52(3):321–341.

35. McCaffrey DP. *OSHA and the Politics of Health Legislation.* New York, NY: Plenum Press;1982.

36. Balz DJ, Brownstein R. *Storming the Gates: Protest Politics and the Republican Revival.* Boston, MA: Little, Brown;1996.

37. Maraniss D, Weisskopf M. *"Tell Newt to Shut Up."* New York, NY: Touchstone Books;1996.

38. McQuiston TH, Zakocs RC, Loomis D. The case for stronger OSHA enforcement—evidence from evaluation research. *Am J Public Health.* 1998;88(7):1022–1024.

39. Mogensen V. State or society? The rise and repeal of OSHA's ergonomics standard. In: Mogensen V, ed. *Worker Safety Under Siege: Labor, Capital, and the Politics of Workplace Safety in a Deregulated World.* Armonk, NY: M.E. Sharpe;2006:108–139.

40. Interagency Task Force on Workplace Safety and Health. *Making Prevention Pay: Final Report of the Interagency Task Force on Workplace Safety and Health.* Washington, DC: U.S. Department of Commerce;1979.

41. Centers for Disease Control and Prevention. Leading work-related diseases and injuries—United States. *MMWR Morb Mortal Wkly Rep.* 1983;32(14):189–191.

42. Office of Technology Assessment. *Preventing Illness and Injury in the Workplace.* Washington, DC: U.S. Government Printing Office;1985.

43. National Institute for Occupational Safety and Health. *A Proposed National Strategy for the Prevention of Musculoskeletal Injuries.* Cincinnati, OH: NIOSH;1986. U.S. Department of Health and Human Services (NIOSH) Publication No. 89-129.

44. Swoboda F. OSHA targets repetitive motion injuries: safety rules would hit most workplaces. *Washington Post.* November 4, 1994. Available at: http://www.highbeam.com/doc/1P2-917486.html. Accessed June 11, 2014.

45. Shanahan J, Wilson M. *Using Appropriations Riders to Curb Regulatory Excess.* Washington, DC: The Heritage Foundation;1995. Issue Bulletin No. 218.

46. Skrzycki C. OSHA abandons rules effort on repetitive injury opposition by GOP, business cited. *Washington Post.* June 13, 1995. Available at: http://www.highbeam.com/doc/1P2-839065.html. Accessed June 11, 2014.

47. International Brotherhood of Teamsters. Chronology of OSHA's ergonomics standard. Stop the pain, start the healing: hands off the ergo standard. 2001. Available at: http://old1.teamster.org/sh/pdf/Ergo%20Chronology%20-%20Feb%2001%20-%20Teamster.pdf. Accessed June 11, 2014.

48. EHS Today Staff. Coalition files lawsuit to stop ergonomics regulation. November 22, 2000. Available at: http://ehstoday.com/print/news/ehs_imp_33888. Accessed September 9, 2013.

49. Johnson R. Letter to Keith L. Goddard, OSHA, re: Appeal of information quality correction request No. 123 (April 1, 2005) ergonomics guidelines for poultry processing, retail grocery stores, and nursing Homes; October 27, 2005.

50. Bruner J. *Making Stories: Law, Literature, Life.* Cambridge, MA: Harvard University Press;2002.

51. Bruner J. Narrative and paradigmatic modes of thought. In: Bruner JS. *In Search of Pedagogy, Volume II: The Selected Works of Jerome S. Bruner.* New York, NY: Routledge;1985:116–128.

52. Roe E. *Narrative Policy Analysis: Theory and Practice.* Durham, NC: Duke University Press;1994.

53. Introduction of Small Business OSHA Relief Act. *Congressional Record.* April 15, 1996: E528. 104th Cong, 2nd Sess. H.R. 3234, Small Business OSHA Relief Act.

54. Ballenger C. Commemorating a 25th anniversary—and creating a new OSHA. *Congressional Record.* May 1, 1996: E91. 104th Cong, 2nd Sess. Statement from the record.

55. Bureau of National Affairs. New Ballenger bill seizes on key concepts of administration's reinvention agenda; April 17, 1996.

56. Anderson S. OSHA under siege. *The Progressive.* 1995;59(12):26–28.

57. McBeth MK, Shanahan EA, Arnell RJ, Hathaway PL. The intersection of narrative policy analysis and policy change theory. *Policy Studies J.* 2007;35(1):87–108.

58. Scalia E. OSHA's ergonomics litigation record: three strikes and it's out. *J Safety Res.* 2001;22(1):55–74.

59. Tickner JA. Introduction. In: Tickner JA, ed. *Precaution: Environmental Science and Preventive Public Health Policy.* Washington, DC: Island Press;2003:xiii–xix.

60. Christoforou T. The precautionary principle in European Community law and science. In: Tickner JA, ed. *Precaution: Environmental Science and Preventive Public Health Policy.* Washington, DC: Island Press;2003:241–264.

61. O'Brien M. Science in the service of good: The precautionary principle and positive goals. In: Tickner JA, ed. *Precaution: Environmental Science and Preventive Public Health Policy.* Washington, DC: Island Press;2003:279–295.

62. Tickner JA. Precautionary assessment: A framework for integrating science, uncertainty, and preventive public policy. In: Tickner JA, ed. *Precaution: Environmental Science and Preventive Public Health Policy.* Washington, DC: Island Press;2003:265–278.

63. Greenspan A. Risk and uncertainty in monetary policy. Remarks at: Meetings of the American Economic Association; January 3, 2004; San Diego, CA. Available at: http://www.federalreserve.gov/boarddocs/speeches/2004/20040103. Accessed September 16, 2013.

64. Jasanoff S. A living legacy: The precautionary ideal in American law. In: Tickner JA, ed. *Precaution: Environmental Science and Preventive Public Health Policy.* Washington, DC: Island Press;2003:227–240.

65. National Research Council. *Science and Judgment in Risk Assessment.* Washington, DC: National Academy Press;1994.

66. *Industrial Union Department, AFL-CIO v. American Petroleum Institute et al.,* 448 U.S. 607 (1980). 100 S. Ct. 2844, 65 Legal Ed. 2d 1010.

67. *American Textile Manufacturers Institute v. Donovan,* 452 U.S. 490 (1981). 101 S. Ct. 2478, 69 Legal Ed. 2d 185.

68. U.S. Environmental Protection Agency. Guidelines for carcinogenic risk assessment. EPA/630/P-03/001B. 2005. Available at: http://www.epa.gov/ttnatw01/cancer_guidelines_final_3-25-05.pdf. Accessed September 16, 2013.

69. National Research Council. Science and decisions: advancing risk assessment. 2008. Available at: http://www.nap.edu/catalog/12209.html. Accessed August 3, 2013.

70. Fosbroke DE, Fisner SM, Myers JR, et al. Working lifetime risk of occupational fatal injury. *Am J Indust Med.* 1997;31(4):459–461.

71. Myers ML. Emerging technologies: inherently safer designs. *Prof Saf.* 2006;51(10):20–26.

72. National Institute for Occupational Safety and Health. *Emerging Technologies and the Safety and Health of Working People.* Cincinnati, OH: NIOSH;2006. U.S. Department of Health and Human Services (NIOSH) Publication No. 2006-13.

73. Meier KJ. Political economy and cost-benefit analysis: problems of bias. In: Stone A, Harpham EJ, eds. *The Political Economy of Public Policy.* Thousand Oaks, CA: Sage;1982:143–162.

74. Heineman RA, Bluhm WT, Peterson SA, Kearny EN. *The World of the Policy Analyst: Rationality, Values, and Politics.* New York, NY: Chatham House Publishers;2002.

75. Ackerman F, Heinzerling L, Massey R. Applying cost-benefit to past decisions: was environmental protection ever a good idea? *Admin Law Rev.* 2005;57(1):155–192.

76. Office of Technology Assessment. *Gauging Control Technology and Regulatory Impacts in Occupational Safety and Health.* Washington, DC: U.S. Government Printing Office;1995.

77. Dudley SE, Delong WB. OSHA's ergonomics program standard and musculoskeletal disorders: an introduction. *J Labor Res.* 2001;22(1):1–14.

78. Berkman MP, David J. Where is the market failure? A review of OSHA's economic analysis for its proposed ergonomics standard. *J Labor Res.* 2001;22(1):75–94.

79. Cochran J. The robustness of OSHA ergonomics benefits: A note. *J Labor Res.* 2001;22(1):111–115.

80. Dudley SE. The benefits and costs of OSHA's proposed ergonomics program standard. *J Labor Res.* 2001;22(1):95–109.

81. Johnson JM, Gramm WL, Viscusi WK. Do workers want OSHA's ergonomics regulations? *J Labor Res.* 2001;22(1):137–143.

82. Lambert TA. Avoiding "regulatory mismatch" in regulating workplace ergonomics: the case for an informational approach. *J Labor Res.* 2001;22(1):117–135.

83. Driesen D. Is cost-benefit analysis neutral? *Univ Colorado Law Rev.* 2006;77: 335–405.
84. *Corrosion Proof Fittings v. EPA*, 947 F2d 1201 (5th Cir 1991).
85. Parker RW. Is government regulation irrational? A reply to Morrall and Hahn. 2004. Available at: http://lsr.nellco.org/uconn_wps/31. Accessed August 3, 2013.
86. Elliott KA, Freeman RB. *Can Labor Standards Improve Under Globalization?* Washington, DC: Institute for International Economics;2003.
87. Ohlsson I. Foreword. In: Frick K, Jensen PL, Quinlan M, Wilthagen T, eds. *Systematic Occupational Health and Safety Management: Perspectives on an International Development.* Bingley, UK: JAI Press;2008:vii.
88. Nielsen KT. Organizational theories implicit in various approaches to OHS management. In: Frick K, Jensen PL, Quinlan M, Wilthagen T, eds. *Systematic Occupational Health and Safety Management: Perspectives on an International Development.* Bingley, UK: JAI Press;2007:99–125.
89. Jasanoff S. Contingent knowledge: Importance for implementation and compliance. In: Weiss EB, Jacobson HK, eds. *Engaging Countries: Strengthening Compliance With International Environmental Accords.* Cambridge, MA: Massachusetts Institute of Technology;2000:61–87.
90. Walters D. International developments and their influence on occupational health and safety in advanced market economies. In: Peterson CL, Mayhew C, eds. *Occupational Health and Safety: International Influences and the "New" Epidemics.* Amityville, NY: Baywood Publishing Company, Inc.;2005:13–30.
91. Stern RM, Terrell K. *Labor Standards and the World Trade Organization: A Position Paper.* Ann Arbor, MI: University of Michigan;2003.
92. Mogensen V. Introduction. In: Mogensen V, ed. *Worker Safety Under Siege: Labor, Capital, and the Politics of Workplace Safety in a Deregulated World.* Armonk, NY: M.E. Sharpe;2006:xiii–xxix.
93. Hodgson GM. *The Evolution of Institutional Economics: Agency, Structure, and Darwinism in American Institutionalism.* New York, NY: Routledge;2004.
94. Rodrik D. How to save globalization from its cheerleaders. *J Int Trade Dipl.* 2007;1(2):1–33.
95. World Trade Organization. Uruguay Round agreement: agreement on safeguards. 1994. Available at: http://www.wto.org/english/docs_e/legal_e/25-safeg_e.htm. Accessed June 11, 2014.

96. James B. Tax havens face OECD threat of sanctions. *New York Times.* June 14, 2000. Available at: http://www.nytimes.com/2000/06/14/news/14iht-launder.2.t.html. Accessed September 9, 2013.

97. Storey R, Tucker E. All that is solid melts into air: worker protection and occupational health and safety regulation in Ontario, 1970–2000. In: Mogensen V, ed. *Worker Safety Under Siege: Labor, Capital, and the Politics of Workplace Safety in a Deregulated World.* Armonk, NY: M.E. Sharpe;2006:157–186.

98. Sass R. A conversation about the work environment. *Int J Health Serv.* 1995;25(1):117–128.

99. Nelson G, Wilson A. German labor model wins support from UAW's King: U.S. union boss has first-hand experience with system as Opel board member. *Automotive News Europe.* June 20, 2013. Available at: http://europe.autonews.com/apps/pbcs.dll/article?AID=/20130620/ANE/306209944/german-labor-model-wins-strong-support-from-uaws-king#axzz2Wqt6oQCI. Accessed September 15, 2013.

100. Jacobson HK, Weiss EB. A framework for analysis. In: Weiss EB, Jacobson HK, eds. *Engaging Countries: Strengthening Compliance With International Environmental Accords.* Cambridge, MA: Massachusetts Institute of Technology; 2000:1–18.

101. O'Neill R. Criminal neglect: How dangerous employers stay safe from prosecution. In: Mogensen V, ed. *Worker Safety Under Siege: Labor, Capital, and the Politics of Workplace Safety in a Deregulated World.* Armonk, NY: M.E. Sharpe;2006:17–33.

102. Levine DI, Toffel MW, Johnson MS. Randomized government safety inspections reduce worker injuries with no detectable job loss. *Science.* 2012;336(6083):907–911.

103. Martinat M. Case Farms Chickens [press release]. March 26, 2013. Available at: http://www.casefarms.com/uploads/news/CaseFarms_AMI_WorkerSafetyAward.pdf. Accessed August 31, 2013.

104. Occupational Safety and Health Administration. Current federal and state-plan sites. June 30, 2013. Available at: https://www.osha.gov/dcsp/vpp/sitebystate.html. Accessed August 31, 2013.

105. Occupational Safety and Health Administration. Guidelines for poultry processing: ergonomics for the prevention of musculoskeletal disorders. OSHA 3213-09N. 2004. Available at: https://www.osha.gov/ergonomics/guidelines/poultryprocessing/poultryprocessing.html. Accessed August 31, 2013.

Appendix
Occupational Safety and Health Act of 1970

84 STAT. 1590

Public Law 91-596
84 STAT. 1590
91st Congress, S.2193
December 29, 1970,
as amended through January 1, 2004. (1)

An Act

To assure safe and healthful working conditions for working men and women; by authorizing enforcement of the standards developed under the Act; by assisting and encouraging the States in their efforts to assure safe and healthful working conditions; by providing for research, information, education, and training in the field of occupational safety and health; and for other purposes. *Be it enacted by the Senate and House of Representatives of the United States of America in Congress assembled*, That this Act may be cited as the "Occupational Safety and Health Act of 1970."

2. Congressional Findings and Purpose

(a) The Congress finds that personal injuries and illnesses arising out of work situations impose a substantial burden upon, and are a hindrance to, interstate commerce in terms of lost production, wage loss, medical expenses, and disability compensation payments.

29 USC 651.

(b) The Congress declares it to be its purpose and policy, through the exercise of its powers to regulate commerce among the several States and with foreign nations and to provide for the general welfare, to assure so far as possible every working man and woman in the Nation safe and healthful working conditions and to preserve our human resources --

(1) by encouraging employers and employees in their efforts to reduce the number of occupational safety and health hazards at their places of employment, and to stimulate employers and employees to institute new and to perfect existing programs for providing safe and healthful working conditions;

(2) by providing that employers and employees have separate but dependent responsibilities and rights with respect to achieving safe and healthful working conditions;

(3) by authorizing the Secretary of Labor to set mandatory occupational safety and health standards applicable to businesses affecting interstate commerce, and by creating an Occupational Safety and Health Review Commission for carrying out adjudicatory functions under the Act;

(4) by building upon advances already made through employer and employee initiative for providing safe and healthful working conditions;

(5) by providing for research in the field of occupational safety and health, including the psychological factors involved, and by developing innovative methods, techniques, and approaches for dealing with occupational safety and health problems;

(6) by exploring ways to discover latent diseases, establishing causal connections between diseases and work in environmental conditions, and conducting other research relating to health problems, in recognition of the fact that

occupational health standards present problems often different from those involved in occupational safety;

(7) by providing medical criteria which will assure insofar as practicable that no employee will suffer diminished health, functional capacity, or life expectancy as a result of his work experience;

(8) by providing for training programs to increase the number and competence of personnel engaged in the field of occupational safety and health;

(9) by providing for the development and promulgation of occupational safety and health standards;

84 STAT. 1591

(10) by providing an effective enforcement program which shall include a prohibition against giving advance notice of any inspection and sanctions for any individual violating this prohibition;

(11) by encouraging the States to assume the fullest responsibility for the administration and enforcement of their occupational safety and health laws by providing grants to the States to assist in identifying their needs and responsibilities in the area of occupational safety and health, to develop plans in accordance with the provisions of this Act, to improve the administration and enforcement of State occupational safety and health laws, and to conduct experimental and demonstration projects in connection therewith;

(12) by providing for appropriate reporting procedures with respect to occupational safety and health which procedures will help achieve the objectives of this Act and accurately describe the nature of the occupational safety and health problem;

(13) by encouraging joint labor-management efforts to reduce injuries and disease arising out of employment.

3. Definitions

For the purposes of this Act --   29 USC 652.

(1) The term "Secretary" means the Secretary of Labor.

(2) The term "Commission" means the Occupational Safety and Health Review Commission established under this Act.

(3) The term "commerce" means trade, traffic, commerce, transportation, or communication among the several States, or between a State and any place outside thereof, or within the District of Columbia, or a possession of the United States (other than the Trust Territory of the Pacific Islands), or between points in the same State but through a point outside thereof.

For Trust Territory coverage, including the Northern Mariana Islands, *see Historical and Statutory Notes, infra.*

(4) The term "person" means one or more individuals, partnerships, associations, corporations, business trusts, legal representatives, or any organized group of persons.

(5) The term "employer" means a person engaged in a business affecting commerce who has employees, but does not include the United States (not including the United States Postal Service) or any State or political subdivision of a State.

(6) The term "employee" means an employee of an employer who is employed in a business of his employer which affects commerce.

(7) The term "State" includes a State of the United States, the District of Columbia, Puerto Rico, the Virgin Islands, American Samoa, Guam, and the Trust Territory of the Pacific Islands.

(8) The term "occupational safety and health standard" means a standard which requires conditions, or the adoption or use of one or more practices, means, methods, operations, or processes, reasonably necessary or appropriate to provide safe or healthful employment and places of employment.

(9) The term "national consensus standard" means any occupational safety and health standard or modification thereof which (1), has been adopted and promulgated by a nationally recognized standards-producing organization under procedures whereby it can be determined by the Secretary that persons interested and affected by the scope or provisions of the standard have reached substantial agreement on its adoption, (2) was formulated in a manner which afforded an opportunity for diverse views to be considered and (3) has been designated as such a standard by the Secretary, after consultation with other appropriate Federal agencies.

(10) The term "established Federal standard" means any operative occupational safety and health standard established by any agency of the United States and presently in effect, or contained in any Act of Congress in force on the date of enactment of this Act.

(11) The term "Committee" means the National Advisory Committee on Occupational Safety and Health established under this Act.

(12) The term "Director" means the Director of the National Institute for Occupational Safety and Health.

(13) The term "Institute" means the National Institute for Occupational Safety and Health established under this Act.

(14) The term "Workmen's Compensation Commission" means the National Commission on State Workmen's Compensation Laws established under this Act.

4. Applicability of This Act

(a) This Act shall apply with respect to employment performed in a workplace in a State, the District of Columbia, the Commonwealth of Puerto Rico, the Virgin Islands, American Samoa, Guam, the Trust Territory of the Pacific Islands, Wake Island, Outer Continental Shelf Lands defined in the Outer

84 STAT. 1592

December 29, 1970

29 USC 653. For Canal Zone and Trust Territory coverage, including the Northern Mariana

Continental Shelf Lands Act, Johnston Island, and the Canal Zone. The Secretary of the Interior shall, by regulation, provide for judicial enforcement of this Act by the courts established for areas in which there are no United States district courts having jurisdiction.

(b)(1) Nothing in this Act shall apply to working conditions of employees with respect to which other Federal agencies, and State agencies acting under section 274 of the Atomic Energy Act of 1954, as amended (42 U.S.C. 2021), exercise statutory authority to prescribe or enforce standards or regulations affecting occupational safety or health.

(2) The safety and health standards promulgated under the Act of June 30, 1936, commonly known as the Walsh-Healey Act (41 U.S.C. 35 et seq.), the Service Contract Act of 1965 (41 U.S.C. 351 et seq.), Public Law 91-54, Act of August 9, 1969 (40 U.S.C. 333), Public Law 85-742, Act of August 23, 1958 (33 U.S.C. 941), and the National Foundation on Arts and Humanities Act (20 U.S.C. 951 et seq.) are superseded on the effective date of corresponding standards, promulgated under this Act, which are determined by the Secretary to be more effective. Standards issued under the laws listed in this paragraph and in effect on or after the effective date of this Act shall be deemed to be occupational safety and health standards issued under this Act, as well as under such other Acts.

(3) The Secretary shall, within three years after the effective date of this Act, report to the Congress his recommendations for legislation to avoid unnecessary duplication and to achieve coordination between this Act and other Federal laws.

(4) Nothing in this Act shall be construed to supersede or in any manner affect any workmen's compensation law or to enlarge or diminish or affect in any other manner the common law or statutory rights, duties, or

Islands, see Historical and Statutory Notes, infra.
67 Stat. 462.
43 USC 1311 note.

73 Stat. 688.

49 Stat. 2036
79 Stat. 1034.
83 Stat. 96.
72 Stat. 835.
79 Stat. 845;
Ante, p. 443.

Report to Congress.

84 STAT. 1593

liabilities of employers and employees under any law with respect to injuries, diseases, or death of employees arising out of, or in the course of, employment.

5. Duties

(a) Each employer --   29 USC 654.
   (1) shall furnish to each of his employees employment and a place of employment which are free from recognized hazards that are causing or are likely to cause death or serious physical harm to his employees;
   (2) shall comply with occupational safety and health standards promulgated under this Act.

(b) Each employee shall comply with occupational safety and health standards and all rules, regulations, and orders issued pursuant to this Act which are applicable to his own actions and conduct.

6. Occupational Safety and Health Standards

(a) Without regard to chapter 5 of title 5, United States Code, or to the other subsections of this section, the Secretary shall, as soon as practicable during the period beginning with the effective date of this Act and ending two years after such date, by rule promulgate as an occupational safety or health standard any national consensus standard, and any established Federal standard, unless he determines that the promulgation of such a standard would not result in improved safety or health for specifically designated employees. In the event of conflict among any such standards, the Secretary shall promulgate the standard which assures the greatest protection of the safety or health of the affected employees.

29 USC 655.
80 Stat. 381;
81 Stat. 195.
5 USC 500.

(b) The Secretary may by rule promulgate, modify, or revoke any occupational safety or health standard in the following manner:

(1) Whenever the Secretary, upon the basis of information submitted to him in writing by an interested person, a representative of any organization of

employers or employees, a nationally recognized standards-producing organization, the Secretary of Health and Human Services, the National Institute for Occupational Safety and Health, or a State or political subdivision, or on the basis of information developed by the Secretary or otherwise available to him, determines that a rule should be promulgated in order to serve the objectives of this Act, the Secretary may request the recommendations of an advisory committee appointed under section 7 of this Act. The Secretary shall provide such an advisory committee with any proposals of his own or of the Secretary of Health and Human Services, together with all pertinent factual information developed by the Secretary or the Secretary of Health and Human Services, or otherwise available, including the results of research, demonstrations, and experiments. An advisory committee shall submit to the Secretary its recommendations regarding the rule to be promulgated within ninety days from the date of its appointment or within such longer or shorter period as may be prescribed by the Secretary, but in no event for a period which is longer than two hundred and seventy days. **Advisory committee, recommendations**

(2) The Secretary shall publish a proposed rule promulgating, modifying, or revoking an occupational safety or health standard in the Federal Register and shall afford interested persons a period of thirty days after publication to submit written data or comments. Where an advisory committee is appointed and the Secretary determines that a rule should be issued, he shall publish the proposed rule within sixty days after the submission of the advisory committee's recommendations or the expiration of the period prescribed by the Secretary for such submission. **84 STAT. 1594 Publication in Federal Register.**

(3) On or before the last day of the period provided for the submission of written data or comments under paragraph (2), any interested person may file with the **Hearing Notice.**

Secretary written objections to the proposed rule, stating the grounds therefor and requesting a public hearing on such objections. Within thirty days after the last day for filing such objections, the Secretary shall publish in the Federal Register a notice specifying the occupational safety or health standard to which objections have been filed and a hearing requested, and specifying a time and place for such hearing.

Publication in Federal Register.

(4) Within sixty days after the expiration of the period provided for the submission of written data or comments under paragraph (2), or within sixty days after the completion of any hearing held under paragraph (3), the Secretary shall issue a rule promulgating, modifying, or revoking an occupational safety or health standard or make a determination that a rule should not be issued. Such a rule may contain a provision delaying its effective date for such period (not in excess of ninety days) as the Secretary determines may be necessary to insure that affected employers and employees will be informed of the existence of the standard and of its terms and that employers affected are given an opportunity to familiarize themselves and their employees with the existence of the requirements of the standard.

(5) The Secretary, in promulgating standards dealing with toxic materials or harmful physical agents under this subsection, shall set the standard which most adequately assures, to the extent feasible, on the basis of the best available evidence, that no employee will suffer material impairment of health or functional capacity even if such employee has regular exposure to the hazard dealt with by such standard for the period of his working life. Development of standards under this subsection shall be based upon research, demonstrations, experiments, and such other information as may be appropriate. In addition to the attainment of

Toxic Materials.

the highest degree of health and safety protection for the employee, other considerations shall be the latest available scientific data in the field, the feasibility of the standards, and experience gained under this and other health and safety laws. Whenever practicable, the standard promulgated shall be expressed in terms of objective criteria and of the performance desired.

(6)(A) Any employer may apply to the Secretary for a temporary order granting a variance from a standard or any provision thereof promulgated under this section. Such temporary order shall be granted only if the employer files an application which meets the requirements of clause (B) and establishes that (i) he is unable to comply with a standard by its effective date because of unavailability of professional or technical personnel or of materials and equipment needed to come into compliance with the standard or because necessary construction or alteration of facilities cannot be completed by the effective date, (ii) he is taking all available steps to safeguard his employees against the hazards covered by the standard, and (iii) he has an effective program for coming into compliance with the standard as quickly as practicable. Any temporary order issued under this paragraph shall prescribe the practices, means, methods, operations, and processes which the employer must adopt and use while the order is in effect and state in detail his program for coming into compliance with the standard. Such a temporary order may be granted only after notice to employees and an opportunity for a hearing: *Provided*, That the Secretary may issue one interim order to be effective until a decision is made on the basis of the hearing. No temporary order may be in effect for longer than the period needed by the employer to achieve compliance with the standard or one year, whichever is shorter, except that such an order may be renewed not more than twice (I) so long

Temporary variance order.

84 STAT. 1595

Notice, hearing.

Renewal.

as the requirements of this paragraph are met and (II) if an application for renewal is filed at least 90 days prior to the expiration date of the order. No interim renewal of an order may remain in effect for longer than 180 days.

Time limitation.

(B) An application for temporary order under this paragraph (6) shall contain:

(i) a specification of the standard or portion thereof from which the employer seeks a variance,

(ii) a representation by the employer, supported by representations from qualified persons having firsthand knowledge of the facts represented, that he is unable to comply with the standard or portion thereof and a detailed statement of the reasons therefor,

(iii) a statement of the steps he has taken and will take (with specific dates) to protect employees against the hazard covered by the standard,

(iv) a statement of when he expects to be able to comply with the standard and what steps he has taken and what steps he will take (with dates specified) to come into compliance with the standard, and

(v) a certification that he has informed his employees of the application by giving a copy thereof to their authorized representative, posting a statement giving a summary of the application and specifying where a copy may be examined at the place or places where notices to employees are normally posted, and by other appropriate means.

A description of how employees have been informed shall be contained in the certification. The information to employees shall also inform them of their right to petition the Secretary for a hearing.

(C) The Secretary is authorized to grant a variance from any standard or portion thereof whenever he determines, or the Secretary of Health and Human

Services certifies, that such variance is necessary to permit an employer to participate in an experiment approved by him or the Secretary of Health and Human Services designed to demonstrate or validate new and improved techniques to safeguard the health or safety of workers.

(7) Any standard promulgated under this subsection shall prescribe the use of labels or other appropriate forms of warning as are necessary to insure that employees are apprised of all hazards to which they are exposed, relevant symptoms and appropriate emergency treatment, and proper conditions and precautions of safe use or exposure. Where appropriate, such standard shall also prescribe suitable protective equipment and control or technological procedures to be used in connection with such hazards and shall provide for monitoring or measuring employee exposure at such locations and intervals, and in such manner as may be necessary for the protection of employees. In addition, where appropriate, any such standard shall prescribe the type and frequency of medical examinations or other tests which shall be made available, by the employer or at his cost, to employees exposed to such hazards in order to most effectively determine whether the health of such employees is adversely affected by such exposure. In the event such medical examinations are in the nature of research, as determined by the Secretary of Health and Human Services, such examinations may be furnished at the expense of the Secretary of Health and Human Services. The results of such examinations or tests shall be furnished only to the Secretary or the Secretary of Health and Human Services, and, at the request of the employee, to his physician. The Secretary, in consultation with the Secretary of Health and Human Services, may by rule promulgated pursuant to section 553 of title 5, United States Code,

Labels, etc.

Protective equipment, etc.

84 STAT. 1596
Medical examinations.

make appropriate modifications in the foregoing requirements relating to the use of labels or other forms of warning, monitoring or measuring, and medical examinations, as may be warranted by experience, information, or medical or technological developments acquired subsequent to the promulgation of the relevant standard.

(8) Whenever a rule promulgated by the Secretary differs substantially from an existing national consensus standard, the Secretary shall, at the same time, publish in the Federal Register a statement of the reasons why the rule as adopted will better effectuate the purposes of this Act than the national consensus standard.

80 Stat. 383.
Publication in Federal Register.

(c)(1) The Secretary shall provide, without regard to the requirements of chapter 5, title 5, Unites States Code, for an emergency temporary standard to take immediate effect upon publication in the Federal Register if he determines (A) that employees are exposed to grave danger from exposure to substances or agents determined to be toxic or physically harmful or from new hazards, and (B) that such emergency standard is necessary to protect employees from such danger.

Temporary standard.
Publication in Federal Register.
80 Stat. 381;
81 Stat. 195.
5 USC 500.

(2) Such standard shall be effective until superseded by a standard promulgated in accordance with the procedures prescribed in paragraph (3) of this subsection.

Time limitation.

(3) Upon publication of such standard in the Federal Register the Secretary shall commence a proceeding in accordance with section 6(b) of this Act, and the standard as published shall also serve as a proposed rule for the proceeding. The Secretary shall promulgate a standard under this paragraph no later than six months after publication of the emergency standard as provided in paragraph (2) of this subsection.

(d) Any affected employer may apply to the Secretary for a rule or order for a variance from a standard promulgated under this section. Affected employees shall be given notice of each such application and an opportunity to participate in a hearing. The Secretary shall issue such rule or order if he determines on the record, after opportunity for an inspection where appropriate and a hearing, that the proponent of the variance has demonstrated by a preponderance of the evidence that the conditions, practices, means, methods, operations, or processes used or proposed to be used by an employer will provide employment and places of employment to his employees which are as safe and healthful as those which would prevail if he complied with the standard. The rule or order so issued shall prescribe the conditions the employer must maintain, and the practices, means, methods, operations, and processes which he must adopt and utilize to the extent they differ from the standard in question. Such a rule or order may be modified or revoked upon application by an employer, employees, or by the Secretary on his own motion, in the manner prescribed for its issuance under this subsection at any time after six months from its issuance.

Variance rule.

(e) Whenever the Secretary promulgates any standard, makes any rule, order, or decision, grants any exemption or extension of time, or compromises, mitigates, or settles any penalty assessed under this Act, he shall include a statement of the reasons for such action, which shall be published in the Federal Register.

84 STAT. 1597
Publication in Federal Register.

(f) Any person who may be adversely affected by a standard issued under this section may at any time prior to the sixtieth day after such standard is promulgated file a petition challenging the validity of such standard with the United States court of appeals for the circuit wherein such person resides or has his principal place of business, for a judicial review of such

Petition for judicial review.

standard. A copy of the petition shall be forthwith transmitted by the clerk of the court to the Secretary. The filing of such petition shall not, unless otherwise ordered by the court, operate as a stay of the standard. The determinations of the Secretary shall be conclusive if supported by substantial evidence in the record considered as a whole.

(g) In determining the priority for establishing standards under this section, the Secretary shall give due regard to the urgency of the need for mandatory safety and health standards for particular industries, trades, crafts, occupations, businesses, workplaces or work environments. The Secretary shall also give due regard to the recommendations of the Secretary of Health and Human Services regarding the need for mandatory standards in determining the priority for establishing such standards.

7. Advisory Committees; Administration

(a)(1) There is hereby established a National Advisory Committee on Occupational Safety and Health consisting of twelve members appointed by the Secretary, four of whom are to be designated by the Secretary of Health and Human Services, without regard to the provisions of title 5, United States Code, governing appointments in the competitive service, and composed of representatives of management, labor, occupational safety and occupational health professions, and of the public. The Secretary shall designate one of the public members as Chairman. The members shall be selected upon the basis of their experience and competence in the field of occupational safety and health.

(2) The Committee shall advise, consult with, and make recommendations to the Secretary and the Secretary of Health and Human Services on matters relating to the administration of the Act. The Committee shall hold no fewer than two meetings during

29 USC 656. Establishment; membership.

80 Stat. 378
5 USC 101.

each calendar year. All meetings of the Committee shall be open to the public and a transcript shall be kept and made available for public inspection.

(3) The members of the Committee shall be compensated in accordance with the provisions of section 3109 of title 5, United States Code.

(4) The Secretary shall furnish to the Committee an executive secretary and such secretarial, clerical, and other services as are deemed necessary to the conduct of its business.

(b) An advisory committee may be appointed by the Secretary to assist him in his standard-setting functions under section 6 of this Act. Each such committee shall consist of not more than fifteen members and shall include as a member one of more designees of the Secretary of Health and Human Services, and shall include among its members an equal number of persons qualified by experience and affiliation to present the viewpoint of the employers involved, and of persons similarly qualified to present the viewpoint of the workers involved, as well as one or more representatives of health and safety agencies of the States. An advisory committee may also include such other persons as the Secretary may appoint who are qualified by knowledge and experience to make a useful contribution to the work of such committee, including one or more representatives of professional organizations of technicians or professionals specializing in occupational safety or health, and one or more representatives of nationally recognized standards-producing organizations, but the number of persons so appointed to any such advisory committee shall not exceed the number appointed to such committee as representatives of Federal and State agencies. Persons appointed to advisory committees from private life shall be compensated in the same manner as consultants or experts under section 3109 of title 5, United States Code. The

Public transcript.

60 Stat. 416.

84 STAT. 1598

Secretary shall pay to any State which is the employer of a member of such a committee who is a representative of the health or safety agency of that State, reimbursement sufficient to cover the actual cost to the State resulting from such representative's membership on such committee. Any meeting of such committee shall be open to the public and an accurate record shall be kept and made available to the public. No member of such committee (other than representatives of employers and employees) shall have an economic interest in any proposed rule.

80 Stat. 416.

Recordkeeping.

(c) In carrying out his responsibilities under this Act, the Secretary is authorized to --

(1) use, with the consent of any Federal agency, the services, facilities, and personnel of such agency, with or without reimbursement, and with the consent of any State or political subdivision thereof, accept and use the services, facilities, and personnel of any agency of such State or subdivision with reimbursement; and

(2) employ experts and consultants or organizations thereof as authorized by section 3109 of title 5, United States Code, except that contracts for such employment may be renewed annually; compensate individuals so employed at rates not in excess of the rate specified at the time of service for grade GS-18 under section 5332 of title 5, United States Code, including travel time, and allow them while away from their homes or regular places of business, travel expenses (including per diem in lieu of subsistence) as authorized by section 5703 of title 5, United States Code, for persons in the Government service employed intermittently, while so employed.

Ante, p. 198-1.

8. Inspections, Investigations, and Recordkeeping

(a) In order to carry out the purposes of this Act, the Secretary, upon presenting appropriate credentials to the owner, operator, or agent in charge, is authorized --

80 Stat. 499;
83 Stat. 190.

(1) to enter without delay and at reasonable times any factory, plant, establishment, construction site, or other area, workplace or environment where work is performed by an employee of an employer; and

(2) to inspect and investigate during regular working hours and at other reasonable times, and within reasonable limits and in a reasonable manner, any such place of employment and all pertinent conditions, structures, machines, apparatus, devices, equipment, and materials therein, and to question privately any such employer, owner, operator, agent or employee.

(b) In making his inspections and investigations under this Act the Secretary may require the attendance and testimony of witnesses and the production of evidence under oath. Witnesses shall be paid the same fees and mileage that are paid witnesses in the courts of the United States. In case of a contumacy, failure, or refusal of any person to obey such an order, any district court of the United States or the United States courts of any territory or possession, within the jurisdiction of which such person is found, or resides or transacts business, upon the application by the Secretary, shall have jurisdiction to issue to such person an order requiring such person to appear to produce evidence if, as, and when so ordered, and to give testimony relating to the matter under investigation or in question, and any failure to obey such order of the court may be punished by said court as a contempt thereof.

(c)(1) Each employer shall make, keep and preserve, and make available to the Secretary or the Secretary of Health and Human Services, such records regarding his activities relating to this Act as the Secretary, in cooperation with the Secretary of Health and Human Services, may prescribe by regulation as necessary or appropriate for the enforcement of this Act or for developing information regarding the causes and prevention of occupational accidents and illnesses. In order to carry out the provisions of this paragraph such regulations may include provisions requiring employers to conduct periodic inspections. The Secretary shall also issue regulations requiring that employers, through posting of notices or other appropriate means, keep their employees informed of their protections and obligations under this Act, including the provisions of applicable standards.

(2) The Secretary, in cooperation with the Secretary of Health and Human Services, shall prescribe regulations requiring employers to maintain accurate records of, and to make periodic reports on, work-related deaths, injuries and illnesses other than minor injuries requiring only first aid treatment and which do not involve medical treatment, loss of consciousness, restriction of work or motion, or transfer to another job.

(3) The Secretary, in cooperation with the Secretary of Health and Human Services, shall issue regulations requiring employers to maintain accurate records of employee exposures to potentially toxic materials or harmful physical agents which are required to be monitored or measured under section 6. Such regulations shall provide employees or their representatives with an opportunity to observe such monitoring or measuring, and to have access to the records thereof. Such regulations shall also make appropriate provision for each employee or former employee to have access to such records as will indicate his own exposure to toxic materials or harmful physical agents. Each employer shall promptly notify any employee who has been or is being exposed to toxic materials or harmful physical agents in concentrations or at levels which exceed those prescribed by an applicable occupational

safety and health standard promulgated under section 6, and shall inform any employee who is being thus exposed of the corrective action being taken.

(d) Any information obtained by the Secretary, the Secretary of Health and Human Services, or a State agency under this Act shall be obtained with a minimum burden upon employers, especially those operating small businesses. Unnecessary duplication of efforts in obtaining information shall be reduced to the maximum extent feasible.

(e) Subject to regulations issued by the Secretary, a representative of the employer and a representative authorized by his employees shall be given an opportunity to accompany the Secretary or his authorized representative during the physical inspection of any workplace under subsection (a) for the purpose of aiding such inspection. Where there is no authorized employee representative, the Secretary or his authorized representative shall consult with a reasonable number of employees concerning matters of health and safety in the workplace.

(f)(1) Any employees or representative of employees who believe that a violation of a safety or health standard exists that threatens physical harm, or that an imminent danger exists, may request an inspection by giving notice to the Secretary or his authorized representative of such violation or danger. Any such notice shall be reduced to writing, shall set forth with reasonable particularity the grounds for the notice, and shall be signed by the employees or representative of employees, and a copy shall be provided the employer or his agent no later than at the time of inspection, except that, upon the request of the person giving such notice, his name and the names of individual employees referred to therein shall not appear in such copy or on any record published, released, or made available pursuant to subsection (g) of this section. If upon receipt of such notification the Secretary determines there are reasonable grounds to believe that such violation or danger exists, he shall make a special inspection in accordance with the provisions of this section as soon as practicable, to determine if such violation or danger exists. If the Secretary determines there are no reasonable grounds to believe that a violation or danger exists he shall notify the employees or representative of the employees in writing of such determination.

(2) Prior to or during any inspection of a workplace, any employees or representative of employees employed in such workplace may notify the Secretary or any representative of the Secretary responsible for conducting the inspection, in writing, of any violation of this Act which they have reason to believe exists in such workplace. The Secretary shall, by regulation, establish procedures for informal review of any refusal by a representative of the Secretary to issue a citation with respect to any such alleged violation and shall furnish the employees or representative of employees requesting such review a written statement of the reasons for the Secretary's final disposition of the case.

(g)(1) The Secretary and Secretary of Health and Human Services are authorized to compile, analyze, and publish, either in summary or detailed form, all reports or information obtained under this section.

(2) The Secretary and the Secretary of Health and Human Services shall each prescribe such rules and regulations as he may deem necessary to carry out their responsibilities under this Act, including rules and regulations dealing with the inspection of an employer's establishment.

(h) The Secretary shall not use the results of enforcement activities, such as the number of citations issued or penalties assessed, to evaluate employees directly involved in enforcement activities under this Act or to impose quotas or goals with regard to the results of such activities.

9. Citations

(a) If, upon inspection or investigation, the Secretary or his authorized representative believes that an employer has violated a requirement of section 5 of this Act, of any standard, rule or order promulgated pursuant to section 6 of this Act, or of any regulations prescribed pursuant to this Act, he shall with reasonable promptness issue a citation to the employer. Each citation shall be in writing and shall describe with particularity the nature of the violation, including a reference to the provision of the Act, standard, rule, regulation, or order alleged to have been violated. In addition, the citation shall fix a reasonable time for the abatement of the violation. The Secretary may prescribe procedures for the issuance of a notice in lieu of a citation with respect to de minimis violations which have no direct or immediate relationship to safety or health.

(b) Each citation issued under this section, or a copy or copies thereof, shall be prominently posted, as prescribed in regulations issued by the Secretary, at or near each place a violation referred to in the citation occurred.

(c) No citation may be issued under this section after the expiration of six months following the occurrence of any violation.

84 STAT. 1601
29 USC 658.

Limitation.

10. Procedure for Enforcement

(a) If, after an inspection or investigation, the Secretary issues a citation under section 9(a), he shall, within a reasonable time after the termination of such inspection or investigation, notify the employer by certified mail of the penalty, if any, proposed to be assessed under section 17 and that the employer has fifteen working days within which to notify the Secretary that he wishes to contest the citation or

29 USC 659.

proposed assessment of penalty. If, within fifteen working days from the receipt of the notice issued by the Secretary the employer fails to notify the Secretary that he intends to contest the citation or proposed assessment of penalty, and no notice is filed by any employees or representative of employees under subsection (c) within such time, the citation and the assessment, as proposed, shall be deemed a final order of the Commission and not subject to review by any court or agency.

(b) If the Secretary has reason to believe that an employer has failed to correct a violation for which a citation has been issued within the period permitted for its correction (which period shall not begin to run until the entry of a final order by the Commission in the case of any review proceedings under this section initiated by the employer in good faith and not solely for delay or avoidance of penalties), the Secretary shall notify the employer by certified mail of such failure and of the penalty proposed to be assessed under section 17 by reason of such failure, and that the employer has fifteen working days within which to notify the Secretary that he wishes to contest the Secretary's notification or the proposed assessment of penalty. If, within fifteen working days from the receipt of notification issued by the Secretary, the employer fails to notify the Secretary that he intends to contest the notification or proposed assessment of penalty, the notification and assessment, as proposed, shall be deemed a final order of the Commission and not subject to review by any court or agency.

(c) If an employer notifies the Secretary that he intends to contest a citation issued under section 9(a) or notification issued under subsection (a) or (b) of this section, or if, within fifteen working days of the issuance of a citation under section 9(a), any employee or representative of employees files a notice with the

84 STAT. 1602

Secretary alleging that the period of time fixed in the citation for the abatement of the violation is unreasonable, the Secretary shall immediately advise the Commission of such notification, and the Commission shall afford an opportunity for a hearing (in accordance with section 554 of title 5, United States Code, but without regard to subsection (a)(3) of such section). The Commission shall thereafter issue an order, based on findings of fact, affirming, modifying, or vacating the Secretary's citation or proposed penalty, or directing other appropriate relief, and such order shall become final thirty days after its issuance. Upon a showing by an employer of a good faith effort to comply with the abatement requirements of a citation, and that abatement has not been completed because of factors beyond his reasonable control, the Secretary, after an opportunity for a hearing as provided in this subsection, shall issue an order affirming or modifying the abatement requirements in such citation. The rules of procedure prescribed by the Commission shall provide affected employees or representatives of affected employees an opportunity to participate as parties to hearings under this subsection.

80 Stat. 384.

11. Judicial Review

(a) Any person adversely affected or aggrieved by an order of the Commission issued under subsection (c) of section 10 may obtain a review of such order in any United States court of appeals for the circuit in which the violation is alleged to have occurred or where the employer has its principal office, or in the Court of Appeals for the District of Columbia Circuit, by filing in such court within sixty days following the issuance of such order a written petition praying that the order be modified or set aside. A copy of such petition shall be forthwith transmitted by the clerk of the court to the Commission and to the other parties, and

29 USC 660.

thereupon the Commission shall file in the court the record in the proceeding as provided in section 2112 of title 28, United States Code. Upon such filing, the court shall have jurisdiction of the proceeding and of the question determined therein, and shall have power to grant such temporary relief or restraining order as it deems just and proper, and to make and enter upon the pleadings, testimony, and proceedings set forth in such record a decree affirming, modifying, or setting aside in whole or in part, the order of the Commission and enforcing the same to the extent that such order is affirmed or modified. The commencement of proceedings under this subsection shall not, unless ordered by the court, operate as a stay of the order of the Commission. No objection that has not been urged before the Commission shall be considered by the court, unless the failure or neglect to urge such objection shall be excused because of extraordinary circumstances. The findings of the Commission with respect to questions of fact, if supported by substantial evidence on the record considered as a whole, shall be conclusive. If any party shall apply to the court for leave to adduce additional evidence and shall show to the satisfaction of the court that such additional evidence is material and that there were reasonable grounds for the failure to adduce such evidence in the hearing before the Commission, the court may order such additional evidence to be taken before the Commission and to be made a part of the record. The Commission may modify its findings as to the facts, or make new findings, by reason of additional evidence so taken and filed, and it shall file such modified or new findings, which findings with respect to questions of fact, if supported by substantial evidence on the record considered as a whole, shall be conclusive, and its recommendations, if any, for the modification or setting aside of its original order. Upon the filing of

72 Stat. 941;
80 Stat. 1323.

the record with it, the jurisdiction of the court shall be exclusive and its judgment and decree shall be final, except that the same shall be subject to review by the Supreme Court of the United States, as provided in section 1254 of title 28, United States Code.

84 STAT. 1603

62 Stat. 928.

(b) The Secretary may also obtain review or enforcement of any final order of the Commission by filing a petition for such relief in the United States court of appeals for the circuit in which the alleged violation occurred or in which the employer has its principal office, and the provisions of subsection (a) shall govern such proceedings to the extent applicable. If no petition for review, as provided in subsection (a), is filed within sixty days after service of the Commission's order, the Commission's findings of fact and order shall be conclusive in connection with any petition for enforcement which is filed by the Secretary after the expiration of such sixty-day period. In any such case, as well as in the case of a noncontested citation or notification by the Secretary which has become a final order of the Commission under subsection (a) or (b) of section 10, the clerk of the court, unless otherwise ordered by the court, shall forthwith enter a decree enforcing the order and shall transmit a copy of such decree to the Secretary and the employer named in the petition. In any contempt proceeding brought to enforce a decree of a court of appeals entered pursuant to this subsection or subsection (a), the court of appeals may assess the penalties provided in section 17, in addition to invoking any other available remedies.

(c)(1) No person shall discharge or in any manner discriminate against any employee because such employee has filed any complaint or instituted or caused to be instituted any proceeding under or related to this Act or has testified or is about to testify in any such proceeding or because of the exercise by such employee on behalf of himself or others of any right afforded by this Act.

(2) Any employee who believes that he has been discharged or otherwise discriminated against by any person in violation of this subsection may, within thirty days after such violation occurs, file a complaint with the Secretary alleging such discrimination. Upon receipt of such complaint, the Secretary shall cause such investigation to be made as he deems appropriate. If upon such investigation, the Secretary determines that the provisions of this subsection have been violated, he shall bring an action in any appropriate United States district court against such person. In any such action the United States district courts shall have jurisdiction, for cause shown to restrain violations of paragraph (1) of this subsection and order all appropriate relief including rehiring or reinstatement of the employee to his former position with back pay.

(3) Within 90 days of the receipt of a complaint filed under this subsection the Secretary shall notify the complainant of his determination under paragraph 2 of this subsection.

12. The Occupational Safety and Health Review Commission

29 USC 661. Establishment; membership.

(a) The Occupational Safety and Health Review Commission is hereby established. The Commission shall be composed of three members who shall be appointed by the President, by and with the advice and consent of the Senate, from among persons who by reason of training, education, or experience are qualified to carry out the functions of the Commission under this Act. The President shall designate one of the members of the Commission to serve as Chairman.

(b) The terms of members of the Commission shall be six years except that (1) the members of the Commission first taking office shall serve, as designated by the

84 STAT. 1604
Terms.

President at the time of appointment, one for a term of two years, one for a term of four years, and one for a term of six years, and (2) a vacancy caused by the death, resignation, or removal of a member prior to the expiration of the term for which he was appointed shall be filled only for the remainder of such unexpired term. A member of the Commission may be removed by the President for inefficiency, neglect of duty, or malfeasance in office.

(c)(1) Section 5314 of title 5, United States Code, is amended by adding at the end thereof the following new paragraph: 80 Stat. 460.

> "(57) Chairman, Occupational Safety and Health Review Commission."

(2) Section 5315 of title 5, United States Code, is amended by adding at the end thereof the following new paragraph: Ante, p. 776.

> "(94) Members, Occupational Safety and Health Review Commission."

(d) The principal office of the Commission shall be in the District of Columbia. Whenever the Commission deems that the convenience of the public or of the parties may be promoted, or delay or expense may be minimized, it may hold hearings or conduct other proceedings at any other place. Location.

(e) The Chairman shall be responsible on behalf of the Commission for the administrative operations of the Commission and shall appoint such administrative law judges and other employees as he deems necessary to assist in the performance of the Commission's functions and to fix their compensation in accordance with the provisions of chapter 51 and subchapter III of chapter 53 of title 5, United States Code, relating to classification and General Schedule pay rates: Provided, That assignment, removal and compensation of administrative law judges shall be in accordance with sections 3105, 3344, 5372, and 7521 of title 5, United States Code. 5 USC 5101, 5331. Ante, p. 198-1.

(f) For the purpose of carrying out its functions under this Act, two members of the Commission shall constitute a quorum and official action can be taken only on the affirmative vote of at least two members.

Quorum.

(g) Every official act of the Commission shall be entered of record, and its hearings and records shall be open to the public. The Commission is authorized to make such rules as are necessary for the orderly transaction of its proceedings. Unless the Commission has adopted a different rule, its proceedings shall be in accordance with the Federal Rules of Civil Procedure.

Public Records.

(h) The Commission may order testimony to be taken by deposition in any proceedings pending before it at any state of such proceeding. Any person may be compelled to appear and depose, and to produce books, papers, or documents, in the same manner as witnesses may be compelled to appear and testify and produce like documentary evidence before the Commission. Witnesses whose depositions are taken under this subsection, and the persons taking such depositions, shall be entitled to the same fees as are paid for like services in the courts of the United States.

28 USC app.

(i) For the purpose of any proceeding before the Commission, the provisions of section 11 of the National Labor Relations Act (29 U.S.C. 161) are hereby made applicable to the jurisdiction and powers of the Commission.

61 Stat. 150;
Ante, p. 930.

(j) A administrative law judge appointed by the Commission shall hear, and make a determination upon, any proceeding instituted before the Commission and any motion in connection therewith, assigned to such administrative law judge by the Chairman of the Commission, and shall make a report of any such determination which constitutes his final disposition of the proceedings. The report of the administrative law judge shall become the final order of the Commission within thirty days after such report by the

84 STAT. 1605
Report

administrative law judge, unless within such period any Commission member has directed that such report shall be reviewed by the Commission.

(k) Except as otherwise provided in this Act, the administrative law judges shall be subject to the laws governing employees in the classified civil service, except that appointments shall be made without regard to section 5108 of title 5, United States Code. Each administrative law judge shall receive compensation at a rate not less than that prescribed for GS-16 under section 5332 of title 5, United States Code.

80 Stat. 453.

Ante, p. 930.

13. Procedures to Counteract Imminent Dangers

(a) The United States district courts shall have jurisdiction, upon petition of the Secretary, to restrain any conditions or practices in any place of employment which are such that a danger exists which could reasonably be expected to cause death or serious physical harm immediately or before the imminence of such danger can be eliminated through the enforcement procedures otherwise provided by this Act. Any order issued under this section may require such steps to be taken as may be necessary to avoid, correct, or remove such imminent danger and prohibit the employment or presence of any individual in locations or under conditions where such imminent danger exists, except individuals whose presence is necessary to avoid, correct, or remove such imminent danger or to maintain the capacity of a continuous process operation to resume normal operations without a complete cessation of operations, or where a cessation of operations is necessary, to permit such to be accomplished in a safe and orderly manner.

29 USC 662.

(b) Upon the filing of any such petition the district court shall have jurisdiction to grant such injunctive relief or temporary restraining order pending the outcome of an enforcement proceeding pursuant to this Act. The proceeding shall be as provided by Rule

28 USC app.

65 of the Federal Rules, Civil Procedure, except that no temporary restraining order issued without notice shall be effective for a period longer than five days.

(c) Whenever and as soon as an inspector concludes that conditions or practices described in subsection (a) exist in any place of employment, he shall inform the affected employees and employers of the danger and that he is recommending to the Secretary that relief be sought.

(d) If the Secretary arbitrarily or capriciously fails to seek relief under this section, any employee who may be injured by reason of such failure, or the representative of such employees, might bring an action against the Secretary in the United States district court for the district in which the imminent danger is alleged to exist or the employer has its principal office, or for the District of Columbia, for a writ of mandamus to compel the Secretary to seek such an order and for such further relief as may be appropriate.

14. Representation in Civil Litigation

Except as provided in section 518(a) of title 28, United States Code, relating to litigation before the Supreme Court, the Solicitor of Labor may appear for and represent the Secretary in any civil litigation brought under this Act but all such litigation shall be subject to the direction and control of the Attorney General.

84 STAT. 1606
29 USC 663.
80 Stat. 613.

15. Confidentiality of Trade Secrets

All information reported to or otherwise obtained by the Secretary or his representative in connection with any inspection or proceeding under this Act which contains or which might reveal a trade secret referred to in section 1905 of title 18 of the United States Code shall be considered confidential for the purpose of that section, except that such information may be disclosed to other officers or employees concerned with carrying out this Act or when relevant in any proceeding under this Act. In any such proceeding the Secretary, the

29 USC 664.

62 Stat. 791.

Commission, or the court shall issue such orders as may be appropriate to protect the confidentiality of trade secrets.

16. Variations, Tolerances, and Exemptions

29 USC 655.

The Secretary, on the record, after notice and opportunity for a hearing may provide such reasonable limitations and may make such rules and regulations allowing reasonable variations, tolerances, and exemptions to and from any or all provisions of this Act as he may find necessary and proper to avoid serious impairment of the national defense. Such action shall not be in effect for more than six months without notification to affected employees and an opportunity being afforded for a hearing.

17. Penalties

(a) Any employer who willfully or repeatedly violates the requirements of section 5 of this Act, any standard, rule, or order promulgated pursuant to section 6 of this Act, or regulations prescribed pursuant to this Act, may be assessed a civil penalty of not more than $70,000 for each violation, but not less than $5,000 for each willful violation.

29 USC 666. Maximum allowed criminal fines under this subsection have been increased by the Sentencing Reform Act of 1984, 18 USC § 3551 et seq., see *Historical and Statutory Notes,* *infra.*

(b) Any employer who has received a citation for a serious violation of the requirements of section 5 of this Act, of any standard, rule, or order promulgated pursuant to section 6 of this Act, or of any regulations prescribed pursuant to this Act, shall be assessed a civil penalty of up to $7,000 for each such violation.

(c) Any employer who has received a citation for a violation of the requirements of section 5 of this Act, of any standard, rule, or order promulgated pursuant to section 6 of this Act, or of regulations prescribed pursuant to this Act, and such violation is specifically determined not to be of a serious nature, may be assessed a civil penalty of up to $7,000 for each violation.

(d) Any employer who fails to correct a violation for which a citation has been issued under section 9(a) within the period permitted for its correction (which period shall not begin to run until the date of the final order of the Commission in the case of any review proceeding under section 10 initiated by the employer in good faith and not solely for delay or avoidance of penalties), may be assessed a civil penalty of not more than $7,000 for each day during which such failure or violation continues.

(e) Any employer who willfully violates any standard, rule, or order promulgated pursuant to section 6 of this Act, or of any regulations prescribed pursuant to this Act, and that violation caused death to any employee, shall, upon conviction, be punished by a fine of not more than $10,000 or by imprisonment for not more than six months, or by both; except that if the conviction is for a violation committed after a first conviction of such person, punishment shall be by a fine of not more than $20,000 or by imprisonment for not more than one year, or by both.

84 STAT. 1607

(f) Any person who gives advance notice of any inspection to be conducted under this Act, without authority from the Secretary or his designees, shall, upon conviction, be punished by a fine of not more than $1,000 or by imprisonment for not more than six months, or by both.

(g) Whoever knowingly makes any false statement, representation, or certification in any application, record, report, plan, or other document filed or required to be maintained pursuant to this Act shall, upon conviction, be punished by a fine of not more than $10,000, or by imprisonment for not more than six months, or by both.

(h)(1) Section 1114 of title 18, United States Code, is hereby amended by striking out "designated by the Secretary of Health and Human Services to conduct investigations, or inspections under the Federal Food, Drug, and Cosmetic Act" and inserting in lieu thereof "or of the Department of Labor assigned to perform investigative, inspection, or law enforcement functions".   65 Stat. 721; 79 Stat. 234.

(2) Notwithstanding the provisions of sections 1111 and 1114 of title 18, United States Code, whoever, in violation of the provisions of section 1114 of such title, kills a person while engaged in or on account of the performance of investigative, inspection, or law enforcement functions added to such section 1114 by paragraph (1) of this subsection, and who would otherwise be subject to the penalty provisions of such section 1111, shall be punished by imprisonment for any term of years or for life.   62 Stat. 756.

(i) Any employer who violates any of the posting requirements, as prescribed under the provisions of this Act, shall be assessed a civil penalty of up to $7,000 for each violation.

(j) The Commission shall have authority to assess all civil penalties provided in this section, giving due consideration to the appropriateness of the penalty with respect to the size of the business of the employer being charged, the gravity of the violation, the good faith of the employer, and the history of previous violations.

(k) For purposes of this section, a serious violation shall be deemed to exist in a place of employment if there is a substantial probability that death or serious physical harm could result from a condition which exists, or from one or more practices, means, methods, operations, or processes which have been adopted or are in use, in such place of employment unless the employer did not, and could not with the exercise of reasonable diligence, know of the presence of the violation.

(l) Civil penalties owed under this Act shall be paid to the Secretary for deposit into the Treasury of the United States and shall accrue to the United States and may be recovered in a civil action in the name of the United States brought in the United States district court for the district where the violation is alleged to have occurred or where the employer has its principal office.

18. State Jurisdiction and State Plans

(a) Nothing in this Act shall prevent any State agency or court from asserting jurisdiction under State law over any occupational safety or health issue with respect to which no standard is in effect under section 6.

(b) Any State which, at any time, desires to assume responsibility for development and enforcement therein of occupational safety and health standards relating to any occupational safety or health issue with respect to which a Federal standard has been promulgated under section 6 shall submit a State plan for the development of such standards and their enforcement.

(c) The Secretary shall approve the plan submitted by a State under subsection (b), or any modification thereof, if such plan in his judgement --

(1) designates a State agency or agencies as the agency or agencies responsible for administering the plan throughout the State,

(2) provides for the development and enforcement of safety and health standards relating to one or more safety or health issues, which standards (and the enforcement of which standards) are or will be at least as effective in providing safe and healthful employment and places of employment as the standards promulgated under section 6 which relate

84 STAT. 1608
29 USC 667.

to the same issues, and which standards, when applicable to products which are distributed or used in interstate commerce, are required by compelling local conditions and do not unduly burden interstate commerce,

(3) provides for a right of entry and inspection of all workplaces subject to the Act which is at least as effective as that provided in section 8, and includes a prohibition on advance notice of inspections,

(4) contains satisfactory assurances that such agency or agencies have or will have the legal authority and qualified personnel necessary for the enforcement of such standards,

(5) gives satisfactory assurances that such State will devote adequate funds to the administration and enforcement of such standards,

(6) contains satisfactory assurances that such State will, to the extent permitted by its law, establish and maintain an effective and comprehensive occupational safety and health program applicable to all employees of public agencies of the State and its political subdivisions, which program is as effective as the standards contained in an approved plan,

(7) requires employers in the State to make reports to the Secretary in the same manner and to the same extent as if the plan were not in effect, and

(8) provides that the State agency will make such reports to the Secretary in such form and containing such information, as the Secretary shall from time to time require.

(d) If the Secretary rejects a plan submitted under subsection (b), he shall afford the State submitting the plan due notice and opportunity for a hearing before so doing. **Notice of Hearing.**

(e) After the Secretary approves a State plan submitted under subsection (b), he may, but shall not be required to, exercise his authority under sections 8, 9, 10, 13, and 17 with respect to comparable standards promulgated under section 6, for the period specified in the next sentence. The Secretary may exercise the authority referred to above until he determines, on the basis of actual operations under the State plan, that the criteria set forth in subsection (c) are being applied, but he shall not make such determination for at least three years after the plan's approval under subsection (c). Upon making the determination referred to in the preceding sentence, the provisions of sections 5(a)(2), 8 (except for the purpose of carrying out subsection (f) of this section), 9, 10, 13, and 17, and standards promulgated under section 6 of this Act, shall not apply with respect to any occupational safety or health issues covered under the plan, but the Secretary may retain jurisdiction under the above provisions in any proceeding commenced under section 9 or 10 before the date of determination.

84 STAT. 1609

(f) The Secretary shall, on the basis of reports submitted by the State agency and his own inspections make a continuing evaluation of the manner in which each State having a plan approved under this section is carrying out such plan. Whenever the Secretary finds, after affording due notice and opportunity for a hearing, that in the administration of the State plan there is a failure to comply substantially with any provision of the State plan (or any assurance contained therein), he shall notify the State agency of his withdrawal of approval of such plan and upon receipt of such notice such plan shall cease to be in effect, but the State may retain jurisdiction in any case commenced before the withdrawal of the plan in order to enforce standards under the plan whenever the issues involved do not relate to the reasons for the withdrawal of the plan.

Continuing evaluation.

Plan rejection, review.

(g) The State may obtain a review of a decision of the Secretary withdrawing approval of or rejecting its plan by the United States court of appeals for the circuit in which the State is located by filing in such court within thirty days following receipt of notice of such decision a petition to modify or set aside in whole or in part the action of the Secretary. A copy of such petition shall forthwith be served upon the Secretary, and thereupon the Secretary shall certify and file in the court the record upon which the decision complained of was issued as provided in section 2112 of title 28, United States Code. Unless the court finds that the Secretary's decision in rejecting a proposed State plan or withdrawing his approval of such a plan is not supported by substantial evidence the court shall affirm the Secretary's decision. The judgment of the court shall be subject to review by the Supreme Court of the United States upon certiorari or certification as provided in section 1254 of title 28, United States Code.

72 Stat. 941;
80 Stat. 1323.

(h) The Secretary may enter into an agreement with a State under which the State will be permitted to continue to enforce one or more occupational health and safety standards in effect in such State until final action is taken by the Secretary with respect to a plan submitted by a State under subsection (b) of this section, or two years from the date of enactment of this Act, whichever is earlier.

62 Stat. 928.

December 29, 1970

19. Federal Agency Safety Programs and Responsibilities

29 USC 668.

(a) It shall be the responsibility of the head of each Federal agency (not including the United States Postal Service) to establish and maintain an effective and comprehensive occupational safety and health program which is consistent with the standards promulgated under section 6. The head of each agency shall (after consultation with representatives of the employees thereof) --

(1) provide safe and healthful places and conditions of employment, consistent with the standards set under section 6;

(2) acquire, maintain, and require the use of safety equipment, personal protective equipment, and devices reasonably necessary to protect employees;

(3) keep adequate records of all occupational accidents and illnesses for proper evaluation and necessary corrective action;

84 STAT. 1610
Recordkeeping.

(4) consult with the Secretary with regard to the adequacy as to form and content of records kept pursuant to subsection (a)(3) of this section; and

(5) make an annual report to the Secretary with respect to occupational accidents and injuries and the agency's program under this section. Such report shall include any report submitted under section 7902(e)(2) of title 5, United States Code.

Annual Report.

(b) The Secretary shall report to the President a summary or digest of reports submitted to him under subsection (a)(5) of this section, together with his evaluations of and recommendations derived from such reports.

80 Stat. 530.
Report to President.

(c) Section 7902(c)(1) of title 5, United States Code, is amended by inserting after "agencies" the following: "and of labor organizations representing employees".

(d) The Secretary shall have access to records and reports kept and filed by Federal agencies pursuant to subsections (a)(3) and (5) of this section unless those records and reports are specifically required by Executive order to be kept secret in the interest of the national defense or foreign policy, in which case the Secretary shall have access to such information as will not jeopardize national defense or foreign policy.

Records, etc.; availability.

20. Research and Related Activities

(a)(1) The Secretary of Health and Human Services, after consultation with the Secretary and with other

29 USC 669.

appropriate Federal departments or agencies, shall conduct (directly or by grants or contracts) research, experiments, and demonstrations relating to occupational safety and health, including studies of psychological factors involved, and relating to innovative methods, techniques, and approaches for dealing with occupational safety and health problems.

(2) The Secretary of Health and Human Services shall from time to time consult with the Secretary in order to develop specific plans for such research, demonstrations, and experiments as are necessary to produce criteria, including criteria identifying toxic substances, enabling the Secretary to meet his responsibility for the formulation of safety and health standards under this Act; and the Secretary of Health and Human Services, on the basis of such research, demonstrations, and experiments and any other information available to him, shall develop and publish at least annually such criteria as will effectuate the purposes of this Act.

(3) The Secretary of Health and Human Services, on the basis of such research, demonstrations, and experiments, and any other information available to him, shall develop criteria dealing with toxic materials and harmful physical agents and substances which will describe exposure levels that are safe for various periods of employment, including but not limited to the exposure levels at which no employee will suffer impaired health or functional capacities or diminished life expectancy as a result of his work experience.

(4) The Secretary of Health and Human Services shall also conduct special research, experiments, and demonstrations relating to occupational safety and health as are necessary to explore new problems, including those created by new technology in occupational safety and health, which may require ameliorative action beyond that which is otherwise provided

84 STAT. 1611.

for in the operating provisions of this Act. The Secretary of Health and Human Services shall also conduct research into the motivational and behavioral factors relating to the field of occupational safety and health.

(5) The Secretary of Health and Human Services, in order to comply with his responsibilities under paragraph (2), and in order to develop needed information regarding potentially toxic substances or harmful physical agents, may prescribe regulations requiring employers to measure, record, and make reports on the exposure of employees to substances or physical agents which the Secretary of Health and Human Services reasonably believes may endanger the health or safety of employees. The Secretary of Health and Human Services also is authorized to establish such programs of medical examinations and tests as may be necessary for determining the incidence of occupational illnesses and the susceptibility of employees to such illnesses. Nothing in this or any other provision of this Act shall be deemed to authorize or require medical examination, immunization, or treatment for those who object thereto on religious grounds, except where such is necessary for the protection of the health or safety of others. Upon the request of any employer who is required to measure and record exposure of employees to substances or physical agents as provided under this subsection, the Secretary of Health and Human Services shall furnish full financial or other assistance to such employer for the purpose of defraying any additional expense incurred by him in carrying out the measuring and recording as provided in this subsection.

Toxic substances, records.

Medical examinations.

(6) The Secretary of Health and Human Services shall publish within six months of enactment of this Act and thereafter as needed but at least annually a list of all known toxic substances by generic family or other

Toxic substances, publication.
December 29, 1970

useful grouping, and the concentrations at which such toxicity is known to occur. He shall determine following a written request by any employer or authorized representative of employees, specifying with reasonable particularity the grounds on which the request is made, whether any substance normally found in the place of employment has potentially toxic effects in such concentrations as used or found; and shall submit such determination both to employers and affected employees as soon as possible. If the Secretary of Health and Human Services determines that any substance is potentially toxic at the concentrations in which it is used or found in a place of employment, and such substance is not covered by an occupational safety or health standard promulgated under section 6, the Secretary of Health and Human Services shall immediately submit such determination to the Secretary, together with all pertinent criteria.

(7) Within two years of enactment of the Act, and annually thereafter the Secretary of Health and Human Services shall conduct and publish industry wide studies of the effect of chronic or low-level exposure to industrial materials, processes, and stresses on the potential for illness, disease, or loss of functional capacity in aging adults. **Annual studies.**

(b) The Secretary of Health and Human Services is authorized to make inspections and question employers and employees as provided in section 8 of this Act in order to carry out his functions and responsibilities under this section. **Inspections.**

(c) The Secretary is authorized to enter into contracts, agreements, or other arrangements with appropriate public agencies or private organizations for the purpose of conducting studies relating to his responsibilities under this Act. In carrying out his responsibilities under this subsection, the Secretary shall cooperate with the Secretary of Health and Human **Contract authority.**

84 STAT. 1612

Services in order to avoid any duplication of efforts under this section.

(d) Information obtained by the Secretary and the Secretary of Health and Human Services under this section shall be disseminated by the Secretary to employers and employees and organizations thereof.

(e) The functions of the Secretary of Health and Human Services under this Act shall, to the extent feasible, be delegated to the Director of the National Institute for Occupational Safety and Health established by section 22 of this Act. **Delegation of functions.**

21. Training and Employee Education

(a) The Secretary of Health and Human Services, after consultation with the Secretary and with other appropriate Federal departments and agencies, shall conduct, directly or by grants or contracts (1) education programs to provide an adequate supply of qualified personnel to carry out the purposes of this Act, and (2) informational programs on the importance of and proper use of adequate safety and health equipment. **29 USC 670.**

(b) The Secretary is also authorized to conduct, directly or by grants or contracts, short-term training of personnel engaged in work related to his responsibilities under this Act.

(c) The Secretary, in consultation with the Secretary of Health and Human Services, shall (1) provide for the establishment and supervision of programs for the education and training of employers and employees in the recognition, avoidance, and prevention of unsafe or unhealthful working conditions in employments covered by this Act, and (2) consult with and advise employers and employees, and organizations representing employers and employees as to effective means of preventing occupational injuries and illnesses.

(d)(1) The Secretary shall establish and support cooperative agreements with the States under which employers subject to this Act may consult with State personnel with respect to --

(A) the application of occupational safety and health requirements under this Act or under State plans approved under section 18; and

(B) voluntary efforts that employers may undertake to establish and maintain safe and healthful employment and places of employment. Such agreements may provide, as a condition of receiving funds under such agreements, for contributions by States towards meeting the costs of such agreements.

(2) Pursuant to such agreements the State shall provide on-site consultation at the employer's worksite to employers who request such assistance. The State may also provide other education and training programs for employers and employees in the State. The State shall ensure that on-site consultations conducted pursuant to such agreements include provision for the participation by employees.

(3) Activities under this subsection shall be conducted independently of any enforcement activity. If an employer fails to take immediate action to eliminate employee exposure to an imminent danger identified in a consultation or fails to correct a serious hazard so identified within a reasonable time, a report shall be made to the appropriate enforcement authority for such action as is appropriate.

(4) The Secretary shall, by regulation after notice and opportunity for comment, establish rules under which an employer --

(A) which requests and undergoes an on-site consultative visit provided under this subsection;

(B) which corrects the hazards that have been identified during the visit within the time frames established by the State and agrees to request a subsequent consultative visit if major changes in

working conditions or work processes occur which introduce new hazards in the workplace; and
(C) which is implementing procedures for regularly identifying and preventing hazards regulated under this Act and maintains appropriate involvement of, and training for, management and non-management employees in achieving safe and healthful working conditions, may be exempt from an inspection (except an inspection requested under section 8(f) or an inspection to determine the cause of a workplace accident which resulted in the death of one or more employees or hospitalization for three or more employees) for a period of 1 year from the closing of the consultative visit.

(5) A State shall provide worksite consultations under paragraph (2) at the request of an employer. Priority in scheduling such consultations shall be assigned to requests from small businesses which are in higher hazard industries or have the most hazardous conditions at issue in the request.

22. National Institute for Occupational Safety and Health

(a) It is the purpose of this section to establish a National Institute for Occupational Safety and Health in the Department of Health and Human Services in order to carry out the policy set forth in section 2 of this Act and to perform the functions of the Secretary of Health and Human Services under sections 20 and 21 of this Act.

29 USC 671. Establishment.

(b) There is hereby established in the Department of Health and Human Services a National Institute for Occupational Safety and Health. The Institute shall be headed by a Director who shall be appointed by the Secretary of Health and Human Services, and who shall serve for a term of six years unless previously removed by the Secretary of Health and Human Services.

Director, appointment, term.

(c) The Institute is authorized to --
   (1) develop and establish recommended occupational safety and health standards; and
   (2) perform all functions of the Secretary of Health and Human Services under sections 20 and 21 of this Act.

(d) Upon his own initiative, or upon the request of the Secretary of Health and Human Services, the Director is authorized (1) to conduct such research and experimental programs as he determines are necessary for the development of criteria for new and improved occupational safety and health standards, and (2) after consideration of the results of such research and experimental programs make recommendations concerning new or improved occupational safety and health standards. Any occupational safety and health standard recommended pursuant to this section shall immediately be forwarded to the Secretary of Labor, and to the Secretary of Health and Human Services. **84 STAT.1613**

(e) In addition to any authority vested in the Institute by other provisions of this section, the Director, in carrying out the functions of the Institute, is authorized --
   (1) prescribe such regulations as he deems necessary governing the manner in which its functions shall be carried out;
   (2) receive money and other property donated, bequeathed, or devised, without condition or restriction other than that it be used for the purposes of the Institute and to use, sell, or otherwise dispose of such property for the purpose of carrying out its functions;
   (3) receive (and use, sell, or otherwise dispose of, in accordance with paragraph (2)), money and other property donated, bequeathed, or devised to the Institute with a condition or restriction, including a

condition that the Institute use other funds of the Institute for the purposes of the gift;

(4) in accordance with the civil service laws, appoint and fix the compensation of such personnel as may be necessary to carry out the provisions of this section;

(5) obtain the services of experts and consultants in accordance with the provisions of section 3109 of title 5, United States Code; **80 Stat. 416.**

(6) accept and utilize the services of voluntary and noncompensated personnel and reimburse them for travel expenses, including per diem, as authorized by section 5703 of title 5, United States Code; **83 Stat. 190.**

(7) enter into contracts, grants or other arrangements, or modifications thereof to carry out the provisions of this section, and such contracts or modifications thereof may be entered into without performance or other bonds, and without regard to section 3709 of the Revised Statutes, as amended (41 U.S.C. 5), or any other provision of law relating to competitive bidding;

(8) make advance, progress, and other payments which the Director deems necessary under this title without regard to the provisions of section 3324 (a) and (b) of Title 31; and

(9) make other necessary expenditures.

(f) The Director shall submit to the Secretary of Health and Human Services, to the President, and to the Congress an annual report of the operations of the Institute under this Act, which shall include a detailed statement of all private and public funds received and expended by it, and such recommendations as he deems appropriate. **Annual report to HHS, President, and Congress.**

(g) LEAD-BASED PAINT ACTIVITIES.

(1) Training Grant Program. --

(A) The Institute, in conjunction with the Administrator of the Environmental Protection Agency, may make grants for the training and education of workers and supervisors who are or may be directly engaged in lead-based paint activities.

(B) Grants referred to in subparagraph (A) shall be awarded to nonprofit organizations (including colleges and universities, joint labor-management trust funds, States, and nonprofit government employee organizations) --

> (i) which are engaged in the training and education of workers and supervisors who are or who may be directly engaged in lead-based paint activities (as defined in Title IV of the Toxic Substances Control Act),
>
> (ii) which have demonstrated experience in implementing and operating health and safety training and education programs, and
>
> (iii) with a demonstrated ability to reach, and involve in lead-based paint training programs, target populations of individuals who are or will be engaged in lead-based paint activities.

15 USC 2681 et. seq.

Grants under this subsection shall be awarded only to those organizations that fund at least 30 percent of their lead-based paint activities training programs from non-Federal sources, excluding in-kind contributions. Grants may also be made to local governments to carry out such training and education for their employees.

(C) There are authorized to be appropriated, a minimum, $10,000,000 to the Institute for each of the fiscal years 1994 through 1997 to make grants under this paragraph.

(2) Evaluation of Programs. -- The Institute shall conduct periodic and comprehensive assessments of the efficacy of the worker and supervisor training programs developed and offered by those receiving grants under this section. The Director shall prepare reports on the results of these assessments addressed to the Administrator of the Environmental Protection Agency to include recommendations as may be appropriate for the revision of these programs. The sum of $500,000 is authorized to be appropriated to the Institute for each of the fiscal years 1994 through 1997 to carry out this paragraph.

23. Grants to the States

(a) The Secretary is authorized, during the fiscal year ending June 30, 1971, and the two succeeding fiscal years, to make grants to the States which have designated a State agency under section 18 to assist them -- 29 USC 672.

 (1) in identifying their needs and responsibilities in the area of occupational safety and health,

 (2) in developing State plans under section 18, or

 (3) in developing plans for -- **84 STAT. 1614**

  (A) establishing systems for the collection of information concerning the nature and frequency of occupational injuries and diseases;

  (B) increasing the expertise and enforcement capabilities of their personnel engaged in occupational safety and health programs; or

  (C) otherwise improving the administration and enforcement of State occupational safety and health laws, including standards thereunder, consistent with the objectives of this Act.

(b) The Secretary is authorized, during the fiscal year ending June 30, 1971, and the two succeeding fiscal years, to make grants to the States for experimental and demonstration projects consistent with the objectives set forth in subsection (a) of this section.

(c) The Governor of the State shall designate the appropriate State agency for receipt of any grant made by the Secretary under this section.

(d) Any State agency designated by the Governor of the State desiring a grant under this section shall submit an application therefor to the Secretary.

(e) The Secretary shall review the application, and shall, after consultation with the Secretary of Health and Human Services, approve or reject such application.

(f) The Federal share for each State grant under subsection (a) or (b) of this section may not exceed 90 per centum of the total cost of the application. In the event the Federal share for all States under either such subsection is not the same, the differences among the States shall be established on the basis of objective criteria.

(g) The Secretary is authorized to make grants to the States to assist them in administering and enforcing programs for occupational safety and health contained in State plans approved by the Secretary pursuant to section 18 of this Act. The Federal share for each State grant under this subsection may not exceed 50 per centum of the total cost to the State of such a program. The last sentence of subsection (f) shall be applicable in determining the Federal share under this subsection.

(h) Prior to June 30, 1973, the Secretary shall, after consultation with the Secretary of Health and Human Services, transmit a report to the President and to the Congress, describing the experience under the grant programs authorized by this section and making any recommendations he may deem appropriate.

24. Statistics   29 USC 673.

(a) In order to further the purposes of this Act, the Secretary, in consultation with the Secretary of Health and Human Services, shall develop and maintain an effective program of collection, compilation, and analysis of occupational safety and health statistics. Such program may cover all employments whether or not subject to any other provisions of this Act but shall not cover employments excluded by section 4 of the Act. The

Secretary shall compile accurate statistics on work injuries and illnesses which shall include all disabling, serious, or significant injuries and illnesses, whether or not involving loss of time from work, other than minor injuries requiring only first aid treatment and which do not involve medical treatment, loss of consciousness, restriction of work or motion, or transfer to another job.

(b) To carry out his duties under subsection (a) of this section, the Secretary may -- **84 STAT. 1615**

(1) promote, encourage, or directly engage in programs of studies, information and communication concerning occupational safety and health statistics;

(2) make grants to States or political subdivisions thereof in order to assist them in developing and administering programs dealing with occupational safety and health statistics; and

(3) arrange, through grants or contracts, for the conduct of such research and investigations as give promise of furthering the objectives of this section.

(c) The Federal share for each grant under subsection (b) of this section may be up to 50 per centum of the State's total cost.

(d) The Secretary may, with the consent of any State or political subdivision thereof, accept and use the services, facilities, and employees of the agencies of such State or political subdivision, with or without reimbursement, in order to assist him in carrying out his functions under this section.

(e) On the basis of the records made and kept pursuant to section 8(c) of this Act, employers shall file such reports with the Secretary as he shall prescribe by regulation, as necessary to carry out his functions under this Act. **Reports.**

(f) Agreements between the Department of Labor and States pertaining to the collection of occupational safety and health statistics already in effect on the effective date of this Act shall remain in effect until superseded by grants or contracts made under this Act.

25. Audits

(a) Each recipient of a grant under this Act shall keep such records as the Secretary or the Secretary of Health and Human Services shall prescribe, including records which fully disclose the amount and disposition by such recipient of the proceeds of such grant, the total cost of the project or undertaking in connection with which such grant is made or used, and the amount of that portion of the cost of the project or undertaking supplied by other sources, and such other records as will facilitate an effective audit.

29 USC 674.

(b) The Secretary or the Secretary of Health and Human Services, and the Comptroller General of the United States, or any of their duly authorized representatives, shall have access for the purpose of audit and examination to any books, documents, papers, and records of the recipients of any grant under this Act that are pertinent to any such grant.

26. Annual Report

Within one hundred and twenty days following the convening of each regular session of each Congress, the Secretary and the Secretary of Health and Human Services shall each prepare and submit to the President for transmittal to the Congress a report upon the subject matter of this Act, the progress toward achievement of the purpose of this Act, the needs and requirements in the field of occupational safety and health, and any other relevant information. Such reports shall include information regarding occupational safety and health standards, and criteria for such standards, developed during the preceding year; evaluation of standards and criteria previously developed under this Act, defining areas of emphasis

29 USC 675.

for new criteria and standards; an evaluation of the degree of observance of applicable occupational safety and health standards, and a summary of inspection and enforcement activity undertaken; analysis and evaluation of research activities for which results have been obtained under governmental and nongovernmental sponsorship; an analysis of major occupational diseases; evaluation of available control and measurement technology for hazards for which standards or criteria have been developed during the preceding year; description of cooperative efforts undertaken between Government agencies and other interested parties in the implementation of this Act during the preceding year; a progress report on the development of an adequate supply of trained manpower in the field of occupational safety and health, including estimates of future needs and the efforts being made by Government and others to meet those needs; listing of all toxic substances in industrial usage for which labeling requirements, criteria, or standards have not yet been established; and such recommendations for additional legislation as are deemed necessary to protect the safety and health of the worker and improve the administration of this Act.

84 STAT. 1616

27. National Commission on State Workmen's Compensation Laws

(a)(1) The Congress hereby finds and declares that --

29 USC 676.

(A) the vast majority of American workers, and their families, are dependent on workmen's compensation for their basic economic security in the event such workers suffer disabling injury or death in the course of their employment; and that the full protection of American workers from job-related injury or death requires an adequate, prompt, and equitable system of workmen's compensation as well as an effective program of occupational health and safety regulation; and

(B) in recent years serious questions have been raised concerning the fairness and adequacy of present workmen's compensation laws in the light of the growth of the economy, the changing nature of the labor force, increases in medical knowledge, changes in the hazards associated with various types of employment, new technology creating new risks to health and safety, and increases in the general level of wages and the cost of living.

(2) The purpose of this section is to authorize an effective study and objective evaluation of State workmen's compensation laws in order to determine if such laws provide an adequate, prompt, and equitable system of compensation for injury or death arising out of or in the course of employment.

28. Economic Assistance to Small Businesses

(a) Section 7(b) of the Small Business Act, as amended, is amended --   72 Stat. 387; 83 Stat. 802. 15 USC 636.

(1) by striking out the period at the end of "paragraph (5)" and inserting in lieu thereof "; and"; and;

(2) by adding after paragraph (5) a new paragraph as follows:

"(6) to make such loans (either directly or in cooperation with banks or other lending institutions through agreements to participate on an immediate or deferred basis) as the Administration may determine to be necessary or appropriate to assist any small business concern in effecting additions to or alterations in the equipment, facilities, or methods of operation of such business in order to comply with the applicable standards promulgated pursuant to section 6 of the Occupational Safety and Health Act of 1970 or standards adopted by a State pursuant to a plan approved under section 18 of the Occupational Safety and

Health Act of 1970, if the Administration determines that such concern is likely to suffer substantial economic injury without assistance under this paragraph."

(b) The third sentence of section 7(b) of the Small Business Act, as amended, is amended by striking out "or (5)" after "paragraph (3)" and inserting a comma followed by "(5) or (6)".

80 Stat. 132.
15 USC 633.

(c) Section 4(c)(1) of the Small Business Act, as amended, is amended by inserting "7(b)(6)," after "7(b)(5),".

79 Stat. 556.
42 USC 3142.

(d) Loans may also be made or guaranteed for the purposes set forth in section 7(b)(5) of the Small Business Act, as amended, pursuant to the provisions of section 202 of the Public Works and Economic Development Act of 1965, as amended.

29. Additional Assistant Secretary of Labor

(a) Section 2 of the Act of April 17, 1946 (60 Stat. 91) as amended (29 U.S.C. 553) is amended by --

75 Stat. 338.

(1) striking out "four" in the first sentence of such section and inserting in lieu thereof "five"; and

84 STAT. 1619

(2) adding at the end thereof the following new sentence, "One of such Assistant Secretaries shall be an Assistant Secretary of Labor for Occupational Safety and Health."

(b) Paragraph (20) of section 5315 of title 5, United States Code, is amended by striking out "(4)" and inserting in lieu thereof "(5)".

80 Stat. 462.

30. Additional Positions

Section 5108(c) of title 5, United States Code, is amended by --

5 USC 5108(c).

(1) striking out the word "and" at the end of paragraph (8);

(2) striking out the period at the end of paragraph (9) and inserting in lieu thereof a semicolon and the word "and"; and

(3) by adding immediately after paragraph (9) the following new paragraph:

> (10)(A) the Secretary of Labor, subject to the standards and procedures prescribed by this chapter, may place an additional twenty-five positions in the Department of Labor in GS-16, 17, and 18 for the purposes of carrying out his responsibilities under the Occupational Safety and Health Act of 1970;
> (B) the Occupational Safety and Health Review Commission, subject to the standards and procedures prescribed by this chapter, may place ten positions in GS-16, 17, and 18 in carrying out its functions under the Occupational Safety and Health Act of 1970."

32. Separability

If any provision of this Act, or the application of such provision to any person or circumstance, shall be held invalid, the remainder of this Act, or the application of such provision to persons or circumstances other than those as to which it is held invalid, shall not be affected thereby.

29 USC 677.

33. Appropriations

There are authorized to be appropriated to carry out this Act for each fiscal year such sums as the Congress shall deem necessary.

84 STAT. 1620
29 USC 678.

34. Effective Date

This Act shall take effect one hundred and twenty days after the date of its enactment.

Approved December 29, 1970.

Source: Occupational Safety and Health Act, 29 U.S.C. § 651–678 (1970). Available at: https://www.osha.gov/pls/oshaweb/owasrch.search_form?p_doc_type=OSHACT&p_toc_level=0. Accessed July 22, 2014.

Index

A

abductive reasoning, 127, 149–151
Abel, Iorwith Wilber, 113–114
abortion, 557
"accidents" on event scale, 413–414
accountability, 654–656
ACCSH. *See* Advisory Committee for Construction Safety and Health
ACGIH. *See* American Conference of Governmental Industrial Hygienists
acroosteolysis, 159
Act for the Protection of Lives of Miners (1891), 314–315
ad hominem fallacy, 157, 582
administrative law. *See also* Administrative Procedures Act
   administrative court of OSHRC, 217
   administrative law judges (ALJs), 67, 216, 217, 218, 243, 330, 485
   established by statute, 65–66
   examples of, 67–73
   in law hierarchy, 52
   separation of powers, 194
   workers' compensation administration, 485
Administrative Procedures Act (APA; 1946)
   administrative court of OSHRC, 217
   challenging OSHA standards, 214–215
   established by statute, 65
   formal and informal rule making, 66–67, 178
   Negotiated Rulemaking Act, 68, 69–70, 182
   OSHAct conference committee, 147
   OSHAct over APA, 66, 177
   regulatory procedure versus, 66, 67
   substantial evidence test, 178
admissibility of expert testimony, 553–555
Advisory Committee for Construction Safety and Health (ACCSH), 181, 182, 205
advisory committees

ad hoc advisory committees, 69
Advisory Committee for Construction Safety and Health, 181, 182, 205
Advisory Committee on Safety and Health at Work, 434
Board of Scientific Councilors, 288
Commercial Fishing Industry Vessel Safety Advisory Committee, 370, 391
Cranes and Derricks Negotiated Rulemaking Advisory Committee, 70, 182
Federal Advisory Committee Act, 68, 69, 182
Federal Advisory Council on Occupational Safety and Health, 227
Federal Radiation Council, 161, 371
Medical Advisory Committee on Beryllium, 275
Mine Act (1977), 323, 325
National Advisory Committee for Occupational Safety and Health, 180–181
National Advisory Committee on Ergonomics, 231
National Advisory Environmental Health Committee, 277
OSHAct (Section 7), 180–182
Standards Advisory Committee on Agriculture, 181–182
advisory standards "should," 177, 413, 534
advocacy
   advocates of public health, 127–137
   agenda setting, 152–155
   argument advancing policy, 126–127, 129. *See also* argumentation
   as capitalism balance, 475. *See also* capitalism
   coalitions, 128. *See also* coalitions
   controversy, 129–130. *See also* controversy
   definition, 127
   fallacies in argument, 156–158. *See also* argumentation; fallacies

framing messages, 154–155
harm principle, 581–588
Internet for, 656
ISO 14000 environmental protection, 655
issue statements, 130–132, 134. *See also* issues of public policy
leadership, 571–573. *See also* leadership
persuasion, 572, 573
policy networks, 132, 133, 572
prevention policy, 25, 158–159. *See also* prevention
resolution of issues, 132–134, 145–148, 193, 651
AEC. *See* U.S. Atomic Energy Commission
Afghanistan
   forced child labor, 452, 453
   life expectancy, 399
AFL-CIO
   AFL-CIO v. OSHA, 191–192
   American Federation of Labor (AFL), 93, 95, 97–98, 103, 609
   CDC reorganization, 297
   Congress of Industrial Organizations (CIO), 98
   formation of, 98, 609
   fraud in workers' compensation, 512
   ILO representatives, 654
   Industrial Union Department, AFL-CIO v. Hodgson, 178, 183, 186–187
   National Advisory Environmental Health Committee, 277
   NIOSH director Howard, 297
   OSHAct creation, 113, 115, 139, 140, 147, 279, 610
   as public health coalition, 616, 625
AFL-CIO v. OSHA (1992), 191–192
Africa
   agricultural workers, 414
   DBCP pesticide exposure, 454
   forced child labor, 453
   occupational injuries/diseases, 417, 418
afterdamp mine gas, 311, 312
agencies. *See* public health agencies
Agency for Toxic Substances and Disease Registry (ATSDR), 501
agency workers. *See* public health professionals
agenda setting and framing, 152–155
agreements. *See* Memorandums of Understanding (MOUs) with OSHA
Agricola, Georgius, 85, 336
agricultural workers. *See also* rollover protective structures (ROPS)
   agriculture standards, 171, 172
   Centers for Agricultural Disease and Injury Research, Education, and Prevention, 289
   child labor, 382
   deaths among, 21, 385–386, 387–388, 414, 586
   EPA vs. OSHA, 378–379
   exclusion from Commerce Clause, 111
   exclusion from NLRA, 381
   exclusion from OSHA, 21, 258, 658
   exclusion from workers' compensation, 483, 486, 492
   exemption for overtime pay, 382
   exemption for small farms, 182, 268, 384, 385
   Food and Agriculture Organization, 398, 414–415
   Haddon matrix, 26
   hazards to, 414–415
   master-servant contract, 56
   Migrant and Seasonal Agricultural Worker Protection Act, 383
   NIOSH program review, 292, 293–294
   NIOSH recommended standards, 264
   NORA research councils, 295
   OECD tractor certification, 419
   percentages by global region, 414
   pesticides, 378–379, 414–415, 452–455
   short-handled hoe, 586–587
   Standards Advisory Committee on Agriculture, 181–182
   U.S. Department of Agriculture, 42–43, 386
Air Quality Act (1967), 45
Air Transportation Safety and System Stabilization Act (2001), 500
airlines NLRA exclusion, 381
Alaska Fishermen's Fund, 93
Algeria asbestos imports, 439
Alien Tort Claims Act (1789), 57, 74–75
alliances. *See* coalitions
Allied Chemical Corporation, 46, 567
Alzheimer's disease costs, 471, 472
American Association of Industrial Physicians, 102
American Conference of Governmental Industrial Hygienists (ACGIH), 176, 273, 607
American Cyanamid Co., 211–212, 536
American Federation of Labor (AFL), 93, 95, 97–98, 103, 609
American Industrial Health Council (AIHC), 193
American Industrial Hygiene Association (AIHA), 29, 297
American Medical Association (AMA), 489–490
American National Standards Institute (ANSI)
   American Standard Method of Measuring and Recording Work Injury Experience, 265
   consensus standards for interim, 176, 177

formation of, 101
  hazard communication, 534, 537, 542
  Occupational Health and Safety Management Systems, 29
  OSHA and, 405–406
American Occupational Medical Association, 102
American Society for Testing and Materials, 176
American Society of Safety Engineers (ASSE), 297
American Standard Method of Measuring and Recording Work Injury Experience (ANSI), 265
American Standards Association, 100, 101
American Textile Manufacturers v. Donovan (1981), 183, 185, 188, 638
American University Experimental Station (BoM), 335–336
Americans With Disabilities Act (1990), 557
amphibole forms of asbestos, 439–440. *See also* asbestos
analysis. *See* policy analysis
analytic horizon, 509
Anderson, Jason, 366
Anderson, John F., 333
Anderson, Vernon Putz, 660
angiosarcoma, 38, 159, 186, 205, 519, 566, 568
annotated text of OSHAct, 671–726
annual report in OSHAct, 266
ANSI. *See* American National Standards Institute
Anthraco-Silicosis among Hard Coal Miners (USPHS), 342
anticipation of risk, 24
APA. *See* Administrative Procedures Act
appeals
  administrative law judges, 67
  agency approval of state plan, 226
  challenging standards, 179, 180, 186, 214–215
  Javits's amendment, 144, 146
  judicial prejudice, 555
  Mine Act (1977), 67, 323, 325, 330
  Mine Safety and Health Review Commission, 67, 323, 325, 330
  names of court cases, 65
  NTSB for FAA or USCG, 376
  OSHA rules, 64, 67, 179, 180, 186, 214–215
  OSHRC for citations/penalties, 213, 216, 217
  OSHRC rulings, 64, 67, 116, 216, 217
  workers' compensation, 485
applicability of OSHAct, 174, 369, 402
applied science
  antiscience arguments, 582, 583–588

  Challenger space shuttle, 591–593
  chrysotile and cancers, 440
  Collegium Ramazzini, 436–437
  consensus levels, 192
  data-driven science, 395
  Doubt Is Their Product (Michaels), 582
  evidence-based public health, 135
  expert testimony, 553–555
  Global Environmental and Occupational Health Sciences (GEOHealth), 396
  ICOH scientific objectivity, 436
  industrial safety movement, 99, 105, 106
  participation in policy, 654–656
  weight of evidence, 554–555
appropriations
  advocacy policy networks, 132, 133
  audits in OSHAct, 266
  CDC reorganization, 297
  congressional oversight, 60
  ergonomics standard, 627
  financial assistance for compliance, 267
  funding of research, 262
  Government Accountability Office, 60
  grants, 261, 262. *See also* grants
  Mine Act (1977), 323
  National Transportation Safety Board, 376
  Office of Management and Budget, 62 to OSHA, 200, 268
  OSHA appropriation riders, 384–385, 627
  OSHAct (Section 33), 268
  OSHAct (Sections 29–30), 267–268
  policy analysis, 606
  Social Security Act funding, 45, 88, 101, 272
  Treasury and General Government Appropriations Act, 71
  Unfunded Mandates Reform Act, 68, 70, 202, 613
  United Mine Workers Welfare and Retirement Fund, 343
  World Bank Group, 416
Arab Emirates life expectancy, 399
archives of *Industrial Hygiene Newsletter*, 276
Archter, Thorne G., 199
Argentina
  forced child labor, 453
  OSHA and, 403
argumentation
  argument for regulations, 603–606
  as claim, evidence, warrant, 129, 130, 134, 138
  claims, 129–134, 138, 145
  complex argument patterns, 145
  controversy for, 129–130. *See also* controversy
  convergent structure, 144, 145
  evidence, 129, 130, 134–136, 138. *See also* evidence

fallacies in argument, 156–158. *See also* fallacies
inductive reasoning, 149. *See also* abductive reasoning
inference, 129, 130, 134–136, 150
issue statements, 130–132, 134
narrative analysis, 627–637
parallel structure, 145, 147, 148
policy advanced by, 126–127, 129
policy analysis for, 130
resolution of issues, 132–134, 145–148, 193, 651
series structure, 140, 145
topoi of issues, 131
warrants, 129, 130, 134–136, 138, 604
Armenia asbestos use, 437
arsenic poisoning
in history of occupational health, 88, 89, 100
IPCS dangerous chemicals, 411
NIOSH recommended standards, 263
OSHA standard, 179
as reportable, 15, 269
artificial intelligence and precautionary principle, 150–151
asbestos
amphiboles vs. serpentine, 439–440
Asbestos and Other Natural Mineral Fibres (IPCS), 441
Asbestos Hazard Emergency Response Act, 38, 379, 380
asbestosis, 257–258, 438, 441, 583
avoid breathing, 533
chrysotile, 427, 440–443
Clean Air Act for abatement, 246–247
Corrosion Proof Fittings v. EPA (1991), 187, 644
cost of compliance, 204, 205
deaths from, 438, 439, 504, 584
Delaney Clause, 634
emergency standard, 179–180
Environmental Health Criteria 203: Chrysotile Asbestos (WHO), 443
exposure control, 37, 38
failure to warn, 505, 533
global pandemic, 437–445, 584, 648
history of occupational health, 89, 90, 158, 257–258, 659
industry antiscience, 583–584
industry coalitions, 437, 439–443, 583–584
IPCS dangerous chemicals, 411
IQA public health subversion, 72
judicial review, 182, 183, 186–187
latency of disease, 158, 180, 487
as leading work-related disease, 289, 438
litigation vs. regulation, 505
lung cancer, 20, 37, 89, 91, 205, 438, 440, 441, 583, 584
mesothelioma, 37, 89, 91, 205, 437, 438, 440, 441
NIOSH recommended standard, 263
number of workers exposed, 504
risk transfer to developing countries, 437–440
Rotterdam Convention, 427, 440
in schools, 380
smoking plus, 20
standard promulgated, 179
tort liability, 504–505
WTO dispute over ban, 444–445
Asbestos Hazard Emergency Response Act (AHERA; 1986), 38, 379, 380
Asbestos Information Association v. OSHA (1984), 179–180
Asbestos Worker Protection Rule (WPR), 380
Asbestos-in-Schools Rule, 380
Asheberle, Denise, 599
Asia
agricultural workers, 414
asbestos use, 437
occupational injuries/diseases, 417, 418
assaults, 20, 290
assessment techniques. *See also* research
environmental impact statements, 42
Program Assessment Rating Tool, 292
assumption of risk, 55, 102, 103
assurance. *See* enforcement
asthma
as leading work-related disease, 289, 291
miners' asthma, 341–342, 343–344
atomic energy
International Atomic Energy Agency (IAEA), 398, 412–414, 422
International Nuclear and Radiological Event Scale (INES), 413–414
Nuclear Weapons Cleanup Training Program, 547
nuclear worker programs, 372
OECD risk comparison, 419
reactor events, 414
U.S. Atomic Energy Commission (AEC), 160, 371, 518–519, 583
atomic weapon beryllium use, 284, 286
ATSDR. *See* Agency for Toxic Substances and Disease Registry
Attorney General. *See* U.S. Attorney General
attorneys
discovery and privacy, 548
subrogation and, 503
tort liability, 504
workers' compensation costs, 485, 497, 503, 517
workers' compensation fraud, 516, 518
audible warning devices, 27, 535
audits in OSHAct, 266

authority
  of agencies via OSHAct definitions, 173
  Atomic Energy Commission, 371
  Bureau of Mines, 108, 313, 316, 317, 318, 319, 320, 332, 338
  EPA pesticide authority, 378–379
  Mine Act (1977), 324, 325, 331–332
  Mine Act vs. OSHAct, 174, 331–332
  Mine Safety and Health Administration, 329
  NIOSH access to records, 299–300
  NIOSH broad authority, 258, 658
  NIOSH inspections, 213–214, 260, 278, 284, 300–301
  OMB over rule making, 184, 185, 190–191
  OSHA access to records, 299
  OSHA and state programs, 225
  OSHA inspections, 213–214, 300
  OSHA vs. NIOSH enforcement, 300
  OSHAct and other federal agencies, 174, 331–332, 367
  OSHAct applicability, 174, 369, 402
  OSHAct vs. Mine Act, 174, 331–332
  research (OSHAct Section 20), 259–260
  U.S. Coast Guard, 368–370
  USPHS pre-OSHAct, 269
autonomy
  removal of, 573
  respect for persons, 574, 576
  right-to-know moral rationale, 531
autopsies for CWP determination, 326, 501
avoid breathing the dust, 533
Ayers, William, 115, 142
Azerbaijan
  asbestos use, 437
  forced child labor, 453

B

Baier, Edward, 282, 284
Baird, William, 556
Ballenger, Cass, 622–625, 629–630, 660
Bangladesh
  factory hazards, 446–448
  forced child labor, 453
Barker, James, 87
Barrett, Robert, 354
Barry, Peter, 389–390
Basel Convention on Movements of Hazardous Wastes (1989), 422
Batson, Daniel, 570
BCOA. See Bituminous Coal Operators Association
begging the question fallacy, 157
behavioral economics and prospect theory, 154
behavioral strategies
  compliance analysis, 657
  health promotion, 19
  spectrum of prevention, 24, 648–649

Belarus asbestos use, 437
"Belmont Report" (1979), 530–531, 574
beneficence principle, 532, 574
benevolent societies, 92–93
Benin forced child labor, 452, 453
benzene
  claim of definition, 133
  definition of a standard, 173, 184
  IPCS dangerous chemicals, 411
  judicial review, 183, 184, 188–190, 657
  NIOSH recommended standard, 263
  OSHA cancer policy and, 185, 192–194, 611, 657
  risk assessment approach, 37, 638
  standard, 179, 611
Berkowitz, Deborah, 649
Bernoulli, Daniel, 506
beryllium
  industry antiscience, 583
  lung cancer, 284, 583
  Medical Advisory Committee on Beryllium, 275
  National Beryllium Registry, 89
  NIOSH recommended standards, 263, 284–285
  researcher Harriet L. Hardy, 89
Besant, Annie, 87
Bhopal (India)
  deaths from catastrophe, 220, 449–450
  HazCom Standard, 541
  worst industrial disaster, 245–246, 449–451
Bingham, Eula, 199, 287, 296–297, 610
birth defects 6, 450
Bituminous Coal Operators Association (BCOA), 344, 346, 355
Black Lung Association (BLA), 346–348
Black Lung Benefits Act (1969), 499, 500–501
Black Lung Benefits Reform Act (1977), 327
"black lung" term origins, 338–339. See also coal workers' pneumoconiosis
blackdamp mine gas, 311, 312, 333
bladder cancer, 587–588
blaming the victim, 515, 577–578. See also fault
blood lead concentrations. See lead
BLS. See Bureau of Labor Statistics
Blumenthal, Richard, 552
Board of Scientific Councilors (BSC), 288
Boden, Leslie I., 352, 353, 355
Boiler Inspection Act (1911), 373
Bolivia
  forced child labor, 453
  life expectancy, 399
Bolton, Frances Payne, 273
BoM. See Bureau of Mines
Bonilla, Henry, 630

Boone, Joel T., 343
Booth, Catherine, 87
Booth, William, 77, 87
Borel, Clarence, 504, 505
BOSH. *See* Bureau of Occupational Safety Health
Bouige, Daniel, 443
Boyle, W. A., 345–346, 348, 349–350
BP oil rig explosion, 365–366, 369, 590
brain cancer, 566, 568
Brandeis, Louis D., 108
Brazil
   asbestos mining, 439
   forced child labor, 453
   OSHA and, 403, 439
Bridbord, Kenneth, 395
Brown, Jerry, 586
Brown, Murray C., 277
Browne, K., 443
Bruner, Jerome, 627, 628, 632
Buff, Isadore, 344, 345, 346, 348
Bureau of Labor Act (1884), 107
Bureau of Labor Standards
   carbon tetrachloride, 137–138
   formation of, 106
Bureau of Labor Statistics (BLS)
   Census of Fatal Occupational Injuries, 288
   formation of, 105–106
   injuries survey in iron/steel, 106, 265
   public administration worker fatalities, 383
   statistics in OSHAct (Section 24), 265–266
   as surveillance, 3, 17
Bureau of Mines (BoM)
   authority for enforcement, 108, 313, 316, 317, 318, 319, 320, 332, 338
   creation of, 102, 107, 301, 313, 316, 333–334
   in DoC, 337
   in DoI, 269, 301, 337
   elimination of, 290, 301, 322, 327, 338
   explosives research, 334–335, 337
   gas mask production, 336
   mine rescue cars, 333–334
   Mining Enforcement and Safety Administration, 321, 329, 338, 354
   silicosis research, 269, 270, 334, 339–341
   World Wars, 335–336
Bureau of Occupational Safety Health (BOSH), 258, 262, 270, 278, 279, 609
Bureau of State Services, 274, 276
burial benefits, 490
Burkeen, Aaron Dale "Bubba," 366
Burkina Faso forced child labor, 452, 453
Burma forced child labor, 452, 453
Burton, Phillip, 114, 141
Bush, George H. W.
   coal dust sampling, 355
   musculoskeletal disorders, 195, 626, 632
   OSHA policies, 199
   Scannell under, 297
Bush, George W.
   agency operational guidance, 63
   ergonomics regulation, 196–197, 627, 632, 657
   NIOSH director Howard, 297–298
   OSHA policies, 199
Business Round Table, 128, 616
businesses. *See also* corporations; employers; small businesses
   business coalition, 128, 140, 195, 616
   business ethics, 575–576. *See also* ethics
   business school safety curriculum, 590–591
   co-determination laws, 655–656
   ergonomics regulations, 195, 626–627, 631, 642
   financial assistance for compliance, 267
   ISO 14000 environmental protection, 655
   Nixon worker protection, 142
   OSHA situational leadership, 588–591
   OSHA small business consultation, 260, 261, 590, 630
   OSHAct creation, 140–141, 610, 612
   Safety and Health Recognition and Achievement Program, 261–262
   training guidelines, 543, 545–546
   workers' compensation insurance pools, 495–496, 659
   workers' compensation owner exclusion, 486
Butler, Justice Pierce, 76
byssinosis disease, 105, 158, 205, 289, 517, 659

C

cadmium, 89, 179, 263, 411
caisson disease, 15, 88, 269
Califano, Joseph A., Jr., 284, 285, 286, 287
Cambodia
   factory hazards, 446, 448
   forced child labor, 453
Canada
   agricultural workers, 414
   asbestos dispute, 444–445
   asbestos export, 441–442, 443–444
   asbestos mining, 439
   common vs. civil law, 53
   harmonization of industrial classification, 402
   healthcare spending, 470
   NAFTA, 423, 424, 425
   public health policy, 18
   workers' compensation, 482, 483

cancers. *See also* leukemia; lung cancer; mesothelioma
    angiosarcoma, 38, 159, 186, 205, 519, 566, 568
    asbestos, 20, 37, 89, 91, 205, 438, 440, 441, 583, 584
    asbestos latency, 158, 180, 487
    benzene, 611
    benzene and OSHA standard, 185, 192–194, 611, 657
    bladder, 587–588
    brain cancer, 566, 568
    chimney sweeps, 86, 104
    Classes of suspect carcinogens, 193–194
    coke ovens, 91, 113, 659
    costs of, 471, 472
    Delaney Clause, 634
    dibromochloropropane (DBCP), 538
    diesel exhaust, 73, 283
    Evaluation of Carcinogenic Risks to Humans (IARC), 411
    formaldehyde, 169
    global DALYs, 401
    hexavalent chromium, 587
    history of occupational health, 86, 89, 90–91, 275
    International Agency for Research on Cancer, 398, 410–411, 440
    judicial review, 182, 183, 657
    as leading work-related disease, 5, 22, 289, 471
    life-years lost, 39
    lowest detectable level policy, 281
    National Cancer Institute, 270
    no safe carcinogen level, 182, 183
    OSHA standard, 43, 179, 185, 192–194, 611, 657
    risk assessment, 639
    significant risk, 133, 178, 183, 189–190, 194, 638–640
    steel mills, 91, 113, 659
    synthetic dyes, 587–588
    uranium mining, 90, 112, 160–161, 276, 371, 519
    vinyl chloride, 38, 159, 186, 205, 519, 566, 568
capitalism
    capital accumulation, 475–476
    capital mobility, 648, 649–650
    living wage contradiction, 476–477
    market allocation, 476
    planned economy versus, 475
    private vs. public sectors, 476
    public health vs. private gain, 540, 588, 649
    safety/health detractors, 475. *See also* greed

carbon dioxide mine gas, 312, 333
carbon monoxide mine gas, 312, 321, 333
cardiovascular disease
    costs of, 471, 472
    as leading work-related disease, 289, 471
    life-years lost, 39
    smoking ban and, 25
carpal tunnel syndrome. *See also* ergonomics
    Case Farm, 660–662
    computer workstations, 38
    ergonomic violations program, 231
Carson, Rachel, 37, 89
Carter, Jimmy
    agency operational guidance, 63
    Bingham under, 297, 610
    Califano under, 284
    cotton dust standard, 187, 204
    ergonomic standards, 625
    federal agency OSHA standards, 227
    lead standard, 182
    OSHA policy, 199
Case Farms, 660–662
"caution," 534–535
CBA. *See* cost-benefit analysis
CDC. *See* Centers for Disease Control and Prevention
CEA (cost-effectiveness analysis), 507, 641–645
Centers for Agricultural Disease and Injury Research, Education, and Prevention, 289
Centers for Disease Control and Prevention (CDC)
    constituencies of, 282
    as DHHS agency, 17, 62, 258, 262, 278
    mission of, 278
    Mortality and Morbidity Weekly Report, 15, 269, 387
    NIOSH reorganization, 282, 296–297
    NIOSH within, 17, 62, 258, 262, 278, 288
    notifiable diseases reported to, 15
CERCLA. *See* Comprehensive Environmental Response, Compensation, and Liability Act (1980)
certiorari, 64, 174
Chadwick, Edwin, 87
Chafee, John H., 390
Challenger space shuttle, 591–593
Chamber of Commerce. *See* U.S. Chamber of Commerce
Chaney, Lucian, 27
Chao v. Mallard Bay Drilling, Inc. (2002), 174
charts and flowcharts
    asbestos latency, 487
    asbestos policy and Canada, 442, 444
    bills of Gregg vs. Ballenger, 623
    bills of Kennedy vs. Ford, 618–620

burden globally of occupational injury, 400, 401, 417
burden nationally of occupational injury, 471, 472, 478
child/forced labor by country, 453
command-and-control process, 213
death rates, 4, 386, 605
disability costs by classification, 489
discrimination on age and gender, 511
healthcare spending by GDP, 470
IAEA standard development, 413
ILO recommendations, 408
injury rates, 5, 418
judicial review, 183–184
laws administrative, 68
laws from mine disasters, 315
laws on compensation, 500
laws on occupational safety/health, 107–108, 608
Mine Act (1977) authorities, 324
Mine Act (1977) titles and sections, 323
mining disasters → law, 316
NIOSH criteria documents, 263–265, 285
NIOSH offices, 280
OSHA egregious cases, 222–223, 224–225
OSHA emphasis programs, 228, 229
OSHA harmonized safety data sheets, 544
OSHA policies, 199, 611
OSHA situational leadership, 589
OSHA standards, 179, 183–184
OSHA structure, 200, 201
OSHAct legislation, 142
politics of policy making, 615
present value of earnings, 509, 511
regulatory politics framework, 608
Supreme Court decisions, 110–111
workers' compensation by state, 493
workers' compensation fraud, 514–515
workers' compensation laws, 500
Chávez, César, 571, 586, 609
Chemical Emergency Preparedness Program (EPA), 541
Chemical Industry Institute of Toxicology (CIIT), 169
Chemical Manufacturers Association, 128, 536–537
chemical safety. *See also* registries of toxic substances
 Bhopal leak origins, 220, 541
 cancer standard, 193–194
 Chemical Emergency Preparedness Program (EPA), 541
 Chemical Industry Institute of Toxicology, 169

Chemical Safety and Hazard Investigation Board, 40, 377
 criminal prosecution, 234–237
 endangerment crimes, 244–245
 European Chemical Agency, 434–435
 failure to warn, 505, 533
 Federal Hazardous Substances Labeling Act, 46, 539
 formaldehyde, 169–170
 Globally Harmonized System, 542–543
 Hazard Communication Standard, 202, 540
 Health Hazard Evaluations, 260, 287, 292, 293, 527–528, 538
 history of occupational health, 89
 Interagency Regulatory Liaison Group, 36, 42–43, 169
 International Bulk Chemical Code, 412
 IPCS International Chemical Safety Cards, 411
 NIOSH recommended standards, 263–265
 OECD guiding principles, 419
 Oil, Chemical, and Atomic Workers Union, 8–9, 212, 527, 538, 540, 609
 OSHA national emphasis programs, 228
 Pocket Guide to Chemical Hazards (NIOSH/OSHA), 282, 283
 Protecting the Health of Eighty Million Americans (USPHS), 139, 277–278, 609
 public health of chemical safety, 39–40
 Registration, Evaluation, Authorization, and Restriction of Chemicals (REACH), 431, 434–435
 releases of hazardous materials, 245–246, 540, 541, 547
 right-to-know laws, 8–9
 Rotterdam Convention, 426–427, 440
 standards promulgated, 179
 statutory law, 65
 TNT poisoning, 271, 273
 WHO dangerous chemicals, 411
 WHO International Programme on Chemical Safety (IPCS), 411
Chemical Safety and Hazard Investigation Board (CSB), 40, 377
Chemical Warfare Service, 336
Cheney, Dick, 606–607
Chernobyl (USSR) nuclear reactor event, 414
child labor
 agricultural employment, 382
 autonomy of employees, 531
 British law evolution, 104–105
 Child Labor Tax Act, 110
 chimney sweeping, 104
 code of conduct for multinationals, 76, 452
 DoL office of, 451–452, 453
 Employment Standards Administration, 198
 Fair Labor Standards Act, 88, 95, 376, 382

Federal Child Labor Act, 110
Findings on the Worst Forms of Child Labor (DoL), 451
international law, 57
labor movement, 95, 97, 99, 100
mining, 104–105
motor vehicle operation, 375–376
prohibition of products by, 452
quote by Hillary Clinton, 451
textile mills, 97, 104
worst forms of, 451–452, 453
Child Labor Tax Act (1919), 110
childbearing capacity. *See* reproductive disorders
Chile and OSHA, 403
China
   asbestos mining, 439
   factory hazards, 446
   forced child labor, 452, 453
   occupational injuries/diseases, 417, 418
   OSHA and, 404–405
chokedamp mine gas, 312
cholera and pump handle, 554
chronic obstructive pulmonary disease, 291, 401
chrysotile asbestos. *See also* asbestos
   labeling of, 427, 440
   safety of, 440–443, 445, 584
cigarettes. *See* smoking
CIPP approach to evaluation, 153–154
circular logic fallacy, 157
citations (references)
   OSHAct statute citation, 170
   regulation citation, 170–171
   United States Code citation, 170
citations (summons)
   access to records, 299
   appeals, 146, 216, 217
   coal dust sampling, 351, 352, 355
   in command-and-control process, 213
   consultation program for businesses, 261
   deadline for issuing, 239, 243
   general duty when standard exists, 233
   Mine Act (1977), 323, 324, 325
   mine disasters preceded by, 658
   MSHA authority, 329, 354
   OSHAct (Section 9), 215
   pesticide poisoning, 36
   posting by employer, 215, 220
   quotas on, 630
   reproductive disorders, 211–212
   for standards or general duty, 152, 219
   trade secrets, 219
   for violations, 152, 213, 215, 216
civil law
   common law versus, 53
   criminal law versus, 53
   as Napoleonic Code, 53
   settlements secret, 551–553
   weight of evidence, 554–555
civil liability in common law, 55
civil litigation representation, 218
civil penalties
   BoM authority, 108, 318, 338
   Coal Act (1969), 349
   coal dust sampling, 351
   Mine Improvement and New Emergency Response Act, 329
   MSHA authority, 329
   OSHAct (Section 17), 219–221
   pesticide regulations, 378
Civil Rights Act (1964), 111, 212, 248–249
claimant fraud, 513–515, 517
claims of advocacy
   in argumentation, 129, 130, 134, 138, 603–604
   authority placement, 146
   claims of definition, 131, 133
   claims of fact, 131, 134
   OSHAct conference committee, 145
   policy claims, 131–132, 134
   standards development, 145
   topoi of, 131
   value-based claims, 131, 134
Clarence Borel v. Fibreboard Paper Products Corporation, et al. (1973), 504, 505, 533
Clark, Donald, 366
class action suits, 503, 504
Clean Air Act (CAA; 1970)
   asbestos abatement, 246–247
   endangerment laws, 243–245
   felony convictions via, 240, 242, 243, 245
   history of occupational health, 610
   leaded gasoline, 38
   National Emission Standards for Hazardous Air Pollutants, 246–247
   negligence provision, 243
   OMB review of draft regulation, 62
   U.S. suing industries, 245
Clean Air Act Amendments (CAAA; 1990)
   Chemical Safety and Hazard Investigation Board (CSB), 40, 377
   polluters bear burden, 40, 175
   Process Safety Management of Highly Hazardous Chemicals (PSM) standard, 39
Clean Water Act (CWA; 1970)
   endangerment laws, 243–245
   felony convictions via, 241, 242
   oil spill, 366
   Water Pollution Control Act Amendments as, 46
Clinton, Bill
   agency administrators under, 297
   agency operational guidance, 63
   child labor, 452

coal dust sampling, 353
musculoskeletal disorders, 195, 627, 632
nuclear worker protection, 372
OSHA policies, 199, 617
"reinventing government," 296, 617–621, 625
veto of Republican bill, 622, 629
WTO perceptions, 419
Clinton, Hillary, 451
clock face painters, 90, 272
closure orders
  imminent danger, 324, 325, 328
  wages during, 325
Coal Mine Act (1947), 315, 316, 317–318
Coal Mine Health and Safety Act (Coal Act; 1969). *See also Federal Coal entries*
  BoM authority, 338
  coal dust sampling, 350–356
  Coal Mine Inspection and Investigation Act, 317
  CWP benefits, 320, 321, 326, 327, 349
  fatality reduction, 605
  history of occupational health, 91, 107, 108, 141, 610
  Mine Act (1977) amending, 321–322
  mine disasters (law), 141, 315, 316, 320–321
  passage of, 347–349
Coal Mine Inspection and Investigation Act (1941), 315, 316–317
coal workers. *See also* coal workers' pneumoconiosis; miners
  Bituminous Coal Operators Association, 344, 346, 355
  child labor, 104–105
  coal dust sampling, 350–356
  continuous mining, 90
  deaths among, 36, 99, 113, 314–321
  Federal Coal Mine Safety Act (1952), 108
  Federal Coal Mine Safety Board of Review, 318
  GAO report, 60
  mine explosions, 36, 113, 141, 311, 315–321, 320, 328, 332, 345, 348, 350
  mine gases, 311–312, 332–333
  miners' asthma, 341–342, 343–344
  MSHA Coal Mine Safety and Health, 329
  NIOSH recommended standards, 264, 265
  smoking by miners, 175
  UMWA Welfare and Retirement Fund, 342–344, 345–346
coal workers' pneumoconiosis (CWP; black lung)
  autopsies and X-rays, 326, 501
  "black lung" as term, 338–339
  Black Lung Benefits Act, 499, 500–501
  Black Lung Benefits Reform Act, 327

black lung movement, 113, 114, 141, 344–350
Coal Act benefits, 320, 321, 327
coal dust sampling, 350–356
compensation for, 344–350
GAO report, 60
Healthy People Objectives (2020), 20
history of occupational health, 17, 89, 90, 113, 275, 276, 588
as leading work-related disease, 289
Mine Act benefits, 323, 326, 327
miners' asthma, 341–342, 343–344
NIOSH miner programs, 279
coalitions
  American Industrial Health Council, 193
  asbestos industry, 437, 439–443, 583–584
  business coalition, 128, 140, 195, 616
  Chemical Industry Institute of Toxicology, 169
  Chemical Manufacturers Association, 128, 536–537
  ergonomics violations program, 231
  EU–U.S. occupational health and safety, 403–404
  Formaldehyde Institute, 169
  Interagency Regulatory Liaison Group, 36, 42–43, 169
  National Association of Manufacturers, 128, 142, 195, 616, 626
  National Civic Association, 103
  National Coalition on Ergonomics, 195, 626–627, 631, 642
  National Occupational Research Agenda, 290–291, 292, 294–295
  OSHAct passage, 113, 114–116, 582–583
  policy analysis, 606
  in public health, 25, 128, 572
  Society of Plastics Industry, 186
  spectrum of prevention, 25, 648–649
code of conduct for corporations, 76, 419, 452, 655
Code of Federal Regulations (*CFR*)
  codification of regulations, 170–171
  final regulation publication, 73
  regulation citation, 170–171
Code of Hammurabi, 51
Code of Safe Practice for Solid Bulk Cargoes (SOLAS), 412
Coffin, Lorenzo A., 88
coke ovens
  cancer, 91, 113, 659
  cost of compliance, 205
  judicial review, 182, 183
  NIOSH recommended standard, 263
  Standard on Coke Oven Emissions, 69, 179
Coleridge, Samuel Taylor, 608
collaborations. *See* coalitions; committees

collective bargaining, 98, 110, 609
Collegium Ramazzini, 398, 436–437, 442
Colombia
  forced child labor, 453
  OSHA and, 403
command-and-control approach
  flowchart of, 213
  history of, 29–30
  OSHA as, 2–3, 643
comment. *See* public comment
Commerce Clause of Constitution
  excluded industries, 111
  history of worker protection, 108–111
  NLRA jurisdiction, 381
  state vs. federal primacy, 140–141
  state-level standards, 226
  transportation industry sector, 372
  warrant in Sullivan bill, 138
Commercial Fishing Industry Vessel Safety Act (CFIVSA; 1988), 370, 391
committees. *See also* advisory committees
  conference committee, 60, 116, 144, 145–148
  of Congress, 59–60
  EU policy making, 430
  Federal Advisory Committee Act, 68, 69, 182
  ISO technical committees, 435
  Negotiated Rulemaking Act, 182
  OSHAct advisory committees, 180–182
common law
  British colonies, 53, 510
  civil liability, 55
  customary law, 52, 396
  discovery, 548–549, 552–553
  doctrine of judicial precedent, 53, 54–55, 64, 396–397
  Federal Rules of Civil Procedure, 548
  individual suing government, 74
  labor movement, 92
  in law hierarchy, 52
  for occupational injuries, 54–55, 102–103, 174, 454, 502
  tort law, 55. *See also* tort law
  tort liability, 501–505
  trial by judge, 553–555
Commons, John, 475
Commonwealth of Independent States
  asbestos use, 437
communicable diseases. *See* infectious diseases
communication. *See* hazard communication
community action level in spectrum of prevention, 24, 648–649
community right-to-know, 538, 540–541
compensating differential argument, 529–530
compensation. *See* wages; workers' compensation

compensation principle. *See also* workers' compensation
  compensation uniformity, 482, 518
  definition, 481
  hierarchy of controls, 27
competitions on lost-time injuries, 356–357
complaints
  in command-and-control process, 213
  complaint discrimination investigators, 200
  by Congress against NIOSH, 283
  employees filing with OSHA, 216. *See also* whistle-blowers
  ILO enforcement powers, 654
  NAFTA, 423–425
  OMB compliance reporting, 68, 71
  on-site inspection priority, 35–36, 203
  state program administration, 225–226
  trucking industry discrimination, 375
  WTO/GATT dispute settlement, 421
complex arguments, 140, 144, 145, 147, 148
compliance analysis, 657–658
compliance costs, 203–205, 481, 519–520, 649–650
compliance officers
  enforcement foundation, 212
  quotas on citations, 630
  training as focus, 545
Comprehensive Environmental Response, Compensation, and Liability Act (CERCLA; 1980), 242, 380–381
consensus standards, 176
conceptual frames for messages, 579, 580
conference committee, 60, 116, 144, 145–148
Conference on Occupational Safety, 106
confidence intervals, 151
confidentiality
  discovery and, 548, 553
  employee records, 490, 557–558
  NIOSH access to records, 299
  privacy rights, 555–558
  right to enter, 257–258, 269
  secret settlements, 551–553
  trade secrets, 219, 549–551
  vinyl chloride cover-up, 159, 565–568
confirmation bias, 573
congenital malformations, 6, 450
Congo forced child labor, 452, 453
Congress
  administrative agency creation, 66
  annual report in OSHAct, 266
  chambers of, 59, 60
  committees of, 59–60
  conference committee, 60, 116, 144, 145–148
  Congressional Accountability Act, 622
  Congressional Review Act, 68, 70–71, 196, 625

Freedom of Information Act, 67
Government Accountability Office, 60–61
judicial nominations, 64
law of nations, 56
as legislative branch, 58, 59
NIOSH director Howard, 297, 298
Office of Technology Assessment, 61
OSHA obstacles, 614
policy analysis, 606
Supreme Court, 64
Congress of Industrial Organizations (CIO), 98
Congressional Accountability Act (1995), 622
Congressional Review Act (CRA; 1996), 68, 70–71, 196, 625
consensus levels, 192
conspiracy around VCM, 159, 565–568, 569
constituencies of CDC and NIOSH, 282
constitutional law
   in law hierarchy, 52
   parliamentary system versus, 52–53
   safety movement impacted by, 108–111
Constitutional system
   checks and balances, 58–59
   executive branch, 58, 59, 62–63, 64. See also executive branch
   executive orders, 62–63
   federal system of government, 17, 57–58, 140–141
   Fourth Amendment and search warrants, 214
   Fourteenth Amendment and corporations, 75
   judicial branch, 58, 59, 64–65. See also judicial branch
   legislative branch, 58, 59–61. See also Congress
   parliamentary system versus, 52–53
   privacy rights, 556
   trade secret protection, 218
   unlawful agency actions, 214
construction industry
   asbestos, 380, 438
   Center for Construction Research and Training, 289
   construction standards, 171, 172
   deaths in self-employed vs. full-time, 386
   lead, 182, 185, 205, 206, 585
   multiple employers, 172, 232–233, 385
   NIOSH program review, 292, 293
   NIOSH recommended standards, 264
   NORA research councils, 295
Construction Safety Act (1969)
   Advisory Committee for Construction Safety and Health, 181, 182
   construction standards, 172, 176
   history of occupational safety, 108, 181

consultation program for businesses, 260, 261, 590, 630
Consumer Product Safety Act (1972), 45–46, 378
Consumer Product Safety Commission (CPSC)
   Federal Hazardous Substances Act, 377–378
   Interagency Regulatory Liaison Group, 42–43
   USPHS origins, 43, 45–46
containment of disease, 23–24
context, inputs, process, products (CIPP) of policy, 153–154
continental shelf workers OSHAct exclusion, 367, 368, 369–370
contingency theory, 571, 646–647, 655
continuous mining, 90
Contra Costa County v. KMGP Services Co. (2012), 238
contract law
   DBCP pesticide production, 454
   employment-at-will doctrine, 56
   GATT "contracting" parties, 420
   indentured workers, 96
   master-servant contracts, 55–56
   tort law from, 55
   workday length, 94
Contract With America, 621–625, 629
Contract With America Advancement Act (1996), 625
Contract Work Hours and Safety Standards Act (1936). See Walsh-Healey Public Contracts Act (1936)
Contract Work Hours and Safety Standards Act (1969). See Construction Safety Act (1969)
contributory negligence, 55, 102
control technology
   focus on, 287, 291, 604
   over PPE, 27, 182
controversy
   argument for regulations, 603–606
   argumentation, 129–131
   authority placement, 144, 146
   cancer standard, 193
   fetal vs. women's rights, 249
   "recognized" hazards, 152
   state vs. federal primacy, 140–141
conventions of ILO, 407
convergent arguments, 144, 145
Coolidge, Calvin, 336–337, 612
Corn, Morton, 199, 284, 610
corporations. See also businesses
   code of conduct for multinationals, 76, 419, 452, 655
   co-determination laws, 655–656
   ethics, 575–576. See also greed
   global standards, 448
   international law violation, 74–75

ISO 14000 environmental protection, 655
OSHA situational leadership, 588–591
personhood, 74, 75–76, 173, 235, 236
personhood criminal charges, 235, 236
risk transfer of asbestos, 437–440
risk transfer of factory hazards, 446–448
states sanction, 75
Corrosion Proof Fittings v. EPA (1991), 187, 644
Costa Rica
 DBCP pesticide exposure, 454
 OSHA and, 403
cost-benefit analysis (CBA)
 company-first volunteerism, 102
 cost analysis, 507
 cost of compliance, 203–205, 481, 519–520, 649–650
 cost savings of inspection, 247–248, 498–499, 659
 cost savings of prevention, 18, 204, 247–248, 410, 469–472, 480–481
 of draft regulation, 62–63
 economic policy analysis, 641–645
 greed as public health enemy, 158–159. *See also* greed
 judicial review, 183, 185, 187, 188
 OSHA feasibility, 519. *See also* feasibility
cost-effectiveness analysis (CEA), 507, 641–645
costs. *See also* direct costs; indirect costs; pain and suffering
 asbestos tort liability, 505
 capitalism contradiction, 477
 cost analysis, 505–512
 cost of compliance, 203–205, 481, 519–520, 649–650
 cost savings of inspection, 247–248, 498–499, 659
 cost savings of prevention, 18, 204, 247–248, 410, 469–472, 480–481
 environmental, 35
 explicit costs, 468
 externalizing costs, 477–480. *See also* externalizing costs
 fixed costs, 468
 formaldehyde cost per life saved, 644
 human life value, 509–512, 519–520
 implicit costs, 468
 of injuries, 471, 472, 510, 512
 intangible costs, 468
 opportunity costs, 474
 OSHA standards, 204–205, 481
 PPE paid for by workers, 660
 present value, 508, 509, 510, 511
 safety as cost of business, 175, 649–650
 tangible costs, 468
 tort liability cost, 472, 502, 503–504
 variable costs, 468
 workers' compensation costs, 492–493, 496–499
 workers' compensation disability levels, 489
cotton dust. *See* textile mills
Council of Occupational Safety and Health, 25
Council on Environmental Quality (CEQ), 41, 69
court of appeals
 judicial branch, 64, 65
 MSHRC rulings, 330
 NTSB for FAA or USCG, 376
 OSHRC rulings, 216, 217
 standards challenging, 179, 180
 state plan approval, 226
court records sealed, 551–553
court system. *See also* court of appeals; judicial review; Supreme Court of the United States
 administrative court of OSHRC, 217
 Alien Tort Claims Act (1789), 57, 74–75
 certiorari, 64, 174
 challenging temporary standards, 179
 coal dust sampling, 354
 common law origins, 54
 court records sealed, 551–553
 customary law evolution, 52, 56–57
 discovery, 548–549, 552–553
 doctrine of judicial precedent, 53, 54–55, 64
 doctrine of more convenient forum, 454
 expert testimony, 553–555
 Federal Rules of Civil Procedure, 548
 Freedom of Information Act, 67
 injunctions, 213, 218, 324
 injury recourse, 54–55
 International Court of Justice, 654
 judicial branch, 58, 59, 64–65. *See also* judicial branch
 judicial review, 64. *See also* judicial review
 labor suing for protection, 128–129
 litigation vs. regulation, 505
 matters of fact and law, 64, 72
 names of court cases, 65
 structure of, 64–65
 tort liability, 501–505
 trial by judge, 553–555
CPSC. *See* Consumer Product Safety Commission
CRA. *See* Congressional Review Act (1996)
Cranes and Derricks Negotiated Rulemaking Advisory Committee, 70, 182
criminal gross negligence, 235
criminal law vs. civil law, 53
criminal negligence, 235
criminal prosecution
 BP oil rig explosion, 366
 environmental law vs. criminal penalties, 239, 240
 government charging employer, 64

labor strikes, 96
manslaughter, 235, 366
Mine Act criminal penalties, 321, 325–326
Mine Improvement Act criminal penalties, 328–329
MSHA on coal dust sampling, 355–356
non-use of, 234–235, 658
number of cases, 223, 234
OSHAct criminal penalties, 223–225, 325
pesticide regulations, 378
process of, 221, 223
Severe Violator Enforcement Program, 232
state/local laws and OSHA, 234–239
Union Carbide India, 450
weight of evidence, 554
criminal recklessness, 235
criminal/willful violations, 215, 221, 223
critical thinking, 127, 130, 572
cross-examination of witnesses
ergonomics public hearings, 196
rule making under APA and OSHAct, 66, 178
Cullen, Mark R., 406
Cumming, Hugh S., 271
cumulative trauma disorders, 660
Current Intelligence Bulletins (NIOSH), 283
Curtis, Stephen Ray, 366
customary law
doctrinal perspective of, 396–397
international law basis, 52, 56–57, 396
CWP. *See* coal workers' pneumoconiosis
cybernetic feedback of regulation, 73

D

damps (mine gases), 311, 312, 332–333
dangerous conditions. *See* imminent dangers
Daniels, Domenick, 114, 116, 143–144
Darley, John, 570
Darrow, Clarence, 342
data. *See also* deaths; injuries (nonfatal); registries of toxic substances
BLS survey of iron/steel, 106, 265
Bureau of Labor Statistics (BLS), 3, 17, 265–266
carcinogen Classes, 193–194
data-driven science, 395
death certificates, 288
disability-adjusted life-years (DALYs), 400–401, 508
Eurofound, 432–433
expert testimony, 553–555
healthy worker effect, 342
human life value, 509–512, 519–520
ignorance as public health enemy, 159
Information Quality Act, 68, 71–73. *See also* information
international reporting systems, 399–400
National Beryllium Registry, 89
National Electronic Injury Surveillance System, 46
National Traumatic Occupational Fatality system, 288
OECD injury/disease among countries, 419
OSHA Data Initiative, 266
OSHAct (Section 24), 265–266
privacy, 557–558
quality-adjusted life-year (QALY), 508
scientific evidence objectivity, 135
security of, 558. *See also* confidentiality
state public employees, 383–384
surveillance-containment model, 498
Type I and II errors, 151–152
World Bank regions, 417
Database on Research into Safety of Manufactured Nanomaterials (OECD), 419
Daubert v. Merrell Dow Pharmaceuticals (1993), 554, 555, 631
Day, Jim, 353–354
day laborers employment-at-will, 56
days-away-from work, restricted work, or work transfer (DART), 227–228
DBCP. *See* dibromochloropropane
de minimis violations definition, 215
De Morbis Artificum Diatriba (Discourse on the Diseases of Workers; Ramazzini), 85–86
De Re Metallica (Agricola), 85, 336
deadlines
citation issuance, 239, 243, 325
employer contesting citation, 216
policy vs. applied science, 602
violation abatement, 213, 215
deafness. *See* noise-induced hearing loss
Dear, Joseph, 199, 290, 296
death certificates for data, 288
deaths
agricultural workers, 21, 385–386, 387–388, 414, 586
annually globally, 400, 401, 417
annually nationally, 3–5, 17, 22, 90, 91, 99, 102, 111–112, 139, 471, 605
asbestos, 438, 439, 504, 584
autopsies for CWP determination, 326, 501
average penalty for, 21
benzene, 611
carbon tetrachloride, 137–138
Census of Fatal Occupational Injuries (BLS), 288
Challenger space shuttle, 593
child textile mill workers, 97
coal workers, 36, 99, 113, 314–321
collapse of factories, 447, 448
court records sealed, 552
criminal penalties for, 221, 223, 225, 234, 239

criminal prosecution of, 236, 237–238, 238–239, 240–243
economic burden of, 471
endangerment prosecution, 243
ergonomics as cause, 625
Fatal Accident Circumstances and Epidemiology program (NIOSH), 288
felonies, 221, 223, 366, 658
fires in factories, 88, 446–447
formaldehyde rule, 644
global incidence, 400
Healthy People Objectives (2020), 20
history of occupational health, 86–87, 88, 89, 90, 91, 99, 102, 446
human life value, 509–512, 519–520
India agricultural workers, 414
India pesticide catastrophe, 220, 449–450, 541
injuries as cause, 6, 38–39
labor strikes, 95, 96, 98
leaded gasoline, 271, 585
Maximum Abbreviated Injury Scale, 512
Mine Act penalties, 326
mine inspectors, 321
miners, 36, 99, 113, 141, 311–312, 314–321, 328, 332–333, 340, 345, 371, 546
misdemeanors, 221, 223, 658
murder in workplace, 234–239, 608
National Traumatic Occupational Fatality system (NIOSH), 288
oil rig explosions, 365–366, 369, 590
opportunity costs of, 474
over span of OSHA history, 223
permanent total disability costs versus, 489
pesticide poisoning, 220, 414, 426, 449–450, 541
prosecution of, 21, 234
public administration workers, 383
railroad workers, 54, 99, 102
reduction with safety acts, 4, 200, 599, 600, 605
risk range, 640
self-employed workers, 385–386
settlements secret, 552
shipping vessel explosion, 411–412
significant vs. insignificant risk, 133, 178, 183, 189–190, 194, 638
silicosis, 197, 340
skull and crossbones, 542
smoke jumpers, 126
textile mills, 97
TNT poisoning, 271, 273
tractor overturns, 586
transportation industry, 4, 386
uranium miners, 371
vinyl chloride, 159, 519, 568
Worker Endangerment Initiative applied, 240–245

workers' compensation benefits, 489, 490, 513
workers' compensation incentive, 497
Debs, Eugene Victor, 92, 97
Deepwater Horizon explosion, 365–366, 369, 590
defendant in court case names, 65
definitions
  "adulteration," 539
  "caution," 534–535
  "danger," 534–535
  "designated" personnel, 543
  "economic and social," 431
  economics glossary, 468
  "employee," 385
  "employer," 173
  "eradication" vs. "elimination," 24
  "immediately dangerous," 282
  "incidents" vs. "accidents," 413–414
  levels of hazard warnings, 534–545
  "mislabeling," 539
  OSHAct (Section 3), 173
  "person," 75, 173
  "reasonably necessary or appropriate," 133, 173, 178, 189–190, 639
  "recognized hazard," 152, 175
  "should" vs. "shall," 177, 413, 534
  "significant risk," 133, 178, 183, 189–190, 194, 638–640
  "train" and "instruct," 543, 545
  "warning," 534–535
Delaney, James, 634
Delaney Clause (1958), 634
demand (economics), 468
Deming, W. Edward, 578
Denmark healthcare spending, 470
Department of Labor Act (1888), 105, 107
Departments of U.S. government. See U.S. Department entries
deposition, 548
dermatologic conditions. See skin diseases
derricks. See Cranes and Derricks Negotiated Rulemaking Advisory Committee
determinants of health, 18–20
"deviations" on event scale, 413
DHHS. See U.S. Department of Health and Human Services
DHS. See U.S. Department of Homeland Security
DI. See Social Security Disability Insurance
dibromochloropropane (DBCP), 452–455, 527–528, 535, 537–538, 610, 634, 659
diesel exhaust as carcinogen, 73, 283
dioxin substances, 411
direct costs
  definition, 468, 506
  health care, 469, 470, 471

human capital, 506
9/11 Victim Compensation Fund, 510
workers' compensation for, 485, 486, 488, 490
Directorates of OSHA, 200
disability
  Americans With Disabilities Act, 557
  Black Lung Disability Fund, 327
  classification of, 488–489, 496
  costs of, 471–472
  CWP and Coal Act (1969), 349
  disability-adjusted life-years (DALYs), 400–401, 508
  Guides to the Evaluation of Permanent Impairment (AMA), 489–490
  ILO skills and training program, 448
  from occupationally related diseases, 4
  second injury funds, 485
disability-adjusted life-years (DALYs), 400–401, 508
disasters. *See* asbestos; mine disasters
discounting (cost analysis), 508, 520
Discourse on the Diseases of Workers (Ramazzini), 85–86
discovery (law), 548–549, 552–553
discrimination
  Civil Rights Act (1964), 111
  employees filing complaints with MSHA, 325
  employees filing complaints with OSHA, 216. *See also* whistle-blowers
  lifetime earnings as basis, 510, 511
  OSHA complaint discrimination investigators, 200
  pregnancy discrimination, 248–249
  refusal to work, 216–217, 532–533, 558
  trucking industry complaints, 375
Disease Control Priorities in Developing Countries (World Bank), 416–417
diseases. *See also* infectious diseases; lung diseases; occupational diseases
  cardiovascular disease, 25, 39, 289, 471, 472
  "eradication" vs. "elimination," 24
  global incidence, 400, 401
  Haddon matrix, 25–26
  history of occupational health, 85–86
  latency of diseases, 486–488. *See also* latency of disease
  life-years lost, 39
  Public Health Service Act, 607
  skin diseases, 20, 272, 289, 488
  statutory law, 65
  surveillance–containment model, 23–24
  waterborne hazards, 25, 554
  workers' compensation coverage, 486–488
Diseases of Occupations (Hunter), 89

disincentives definition, 468
distance as public health enemy, 158
District of Columbia Workers' Compensation Act (1979), 499, 500
Division of Industrial Hygiene, 272, 273
Division of Industrial Hygiene and Medicine (DIHM), 270–271
Division of Occupational Health, 257, 276, 278, 279
DoC. *See* U.S. Department of Commerce
doctrine of employment at will, 55–56
doctrine of enterprise liability, 55
doctrine of judicial precedent
  common law adjudication, 53, 54–55, 64
  international lawmaking, 396
  matters of law, 64, 72
doctrine of more convenient forum, 454
doctrine of multiple employers, 232–233
doctrine of negligence, 502
doctrine of strict liability, 55, 502–503
Doe v. Bolton (1973), 557
DoI. *See* U.S. Department of the Interior
DoL. *See* U.S. Department of Labor
Dole, Elizabeth, 195, 626
Dole v. United Steelworkers of America (1990), 184, 191
domestic workers, 21, 483, 484, 486
Dominican Republic
  forced child labor, 453
  OSHA and, 403
Dominick, Peter, 144
Doubt Is Their Product (Michaels), 582
Douglas, Justice William O., 76, 556
Doyle, Henry N., 160, 276
Draper, Warren F., 343, 344
dusty trades
  avoid breathing, 533
  miners' asthma, 341–342, 343–344
  public health research, 271
  silicosis, 339–340. *See also* silicosis
duties
  common law obligation, 53
  employer–employee relationship, 52, 55, 367
  general duty clause, 152, 171, 175, 178, 211–212, 233
  OSHAct (Section 5), 175
  polluters bear burden, 40, 175
  standard of due care, 502
  standards compliance, 175
dyes, 587–588

E

earthquake (1989), 505
Eastman, Crystal, 88

Ebsen, Buddy, 534
Economic Policy Institute, 204–205
economics
　argument for regulations, 604
　behavioral economics, 154
　burden of externalities, 477–480
　burden of work disease/injury, 399–401, 417, 418, 469–472
　business cycle and injury rates, 90
　capital mobility, 648, 649–650
　capitalism, 475–477
　compensation principle, 27, 481–491, 518
　cost analysis, 505–512. *See also* cost-benefit analysis; costs
　cost of compliance, 22, 203–205, 481, 519–520, 649–650
　cost savings of prevention, 18, 410, 469–472, 480–481
　economic efficiency of incentives, 480–481
　environmental costs, 35
　Exclusive Economic Zone (EEZ), 368–370
　feasibility of hazard control, 178, 183, 187, 188
　Financial Action Task Force, 653
　glossary of terms, 468
　greed as public health enemy, 158–159. *See also* greed
　gross domestic product, 470, 471, 473
　healthcare spending by country, 470
　laissez-faire, 58
　major rule definition, 70
　mesoeconomics, 469, 472–481
　moral hazards, 480
　Organisation for Economic Co-operation and Development, 418–419
　perfect competition, 531–532
　policy analysis, 641–645
　private vs. public sectors, 476
　safety as cost of business, 175, 649–650
　scarce resource choices, 469, 615
　standards vs. economics, 647–654
　World Bank cost-effectiveness reports, 416–417
economies of scale, 468, 474
Ecuador
　forced child labor, 453
　OSHA and, 403
education
　BoM inspection authorization, 317
　business school safety curriculum, 590–591
　Center for Construction Research and Training, 289
　Centers for Agricultural Disease and Injury Research, Education, and Prevention, 289
　education and research centers (ERCs), 260–261, 284

　emergency responders, 261
　environmental impact statements, 42
　EU-OSHA, 433–434
　factory schools, 104
　grants for, 261, 374–375
　inspectors, 436
　Mine Act (1977), 323
　MSHA authority, 330
　National Mine Health and Safety Academy, 321, 327
　NIOSH conducting, 278
　OSHA emphasis programs, 228–229
　OSHA international agreements, 402–405
　OSHA mission, 198
　OSHA training institute, 198, 261
　OSHAct (Section 21), 260–262, 278
　as prevention intervention, 24–25, 102
　volunteer safety movement, 101
education and research centers (ERCs), 260–261, 284
effectiveness analysis, 658–659
The Effects of Arts, Trades, and Professions, and of Civic States and Habits of Living, on Health and Longevity (Thackrah), 86
egregious-case policy for civil penalties, 220–221, 222–223
EIS. *See* environmental impact statements
Eisenhower, Dwight
　Federal Radiation Council, 161
　industrial safety conferences, 106
　Sullivan hazardous materials bill, 138
Eisenstadt, Thomas, 556
Eisenstadt v. Baird (1972), 556
El Batawi, Mastafa A., 395–396, 410
El Salvador
　forced child labor, 453
　OSHA and, 403
electronic information
　HIPAA standard format, 557
　submission of, 68, 71, 557
"elimination" vs. "eradication" of disease, 24
emergency locator beacons, 268, 390
Emergency Planning and Community Right-to-Know Act (EPCRA; 1986)
　community right-to-know, 540
　Hazard Communication Standard origins, 38, 530, 535
　trade secret protection, 550–551
emergency preparedness
　Chemical Emergency Preparedness Program (EPA), 541
　current approach, 203
　International Nuclear and Radiological Event Scale, 413–414
　lessons learned, 404–405

Mine Improvement and New Emergency Response Act, 328
National Response Plan, 547–548
training grants for hazardous materials, 374–375
emergency responders
  in emergency response plans, 405
  Ground Zero, 291, 297–298, 500, 501
  NIEHS Worker Education and Training, 547–548
  public safety worker research, 384
  training, 261
  workers' compensation, 483, 487, 500, 501
  WTC Health Registry, 501
emergency temporary standards. *See also* temporary standards
  denied, 179–180, 183
  Mine Act (1977), 325
  overview, 604
  vinyl chloride, 186
emerging technologies
  analysis of, 640–641
  hazards of, 402
  NIOSH research priority, 290, 291
employees. *See also* exclusions; right-to-know; self-employed workers; whistle-blowers
  autonomy of, 531
  capital mobility versus, 648, 649–650
  claimant fraud, 513–515, 517
  co-determination laws, 655–656
  compensating differential argument, 529–530
  competitions on safety, 356–357
  compliance enforcement by employer, 175, 212
  confidentiality of records, 557–558
  deaths in self-employed vs. full-time, 385–386
  definition of employee, 385
  "designated" personnel, 543
  disabled, 485
  federal government, 173, 227, 367
  Health Hazard Evaluations, 260
  hearings for variances/exemptions, 219
  local government, 173, 226, 258, 383–384, 483, 657, 658
  master-servant relationship, 52, 55–56
  OSHAct as job killer, 247–248
  participation in policy, 654–656
  refusal to work, 216–217, 532–533, 558
  state government, 173, 383–384, 657
  Systematic Occupational Health and Safety Management, 655
  training, 260. *See also* training
  worker protection statutes, 381–383
  working and living environments, 415
  WTO labor standards, 421–422

employers. *See also* businesses; labor movement; workers' compensation
  appealing OSHRC rulings, 64
  appeals under Mine Act (1977), 67, 323, 325
  citation contesting, 146, 216, 217
  citation posting, 215, 220
  code of conduct for multinationals, 76, 419, 452, 655
  co-determination laws, 655–656
  common law defenses, 54–55, 102–103
  compensation principle, 27
  consultation program for, 260, 261, 590, 630
  criminal charges against, 64, 223, 239
  definition of employer, 173
  duty of care, 40, 52, 55, 152
  egregious-case policy for civil penalties, 220–221
  employee compliance enforcement, 175, 212
  employer liability emergence, 103
  employer not government duty, 40, 175
  employer premium fraud, 514, 515–516
  employment-at-will doctrine, 55–56
  ethics, 575–576. *See also* ethics
  general duty clause, 152, 171, 175, 178, 211–212, 233, 604, 658
  hazard communication, 535–536. *See also* hazard communication
  Hazard Communication Standard, 540
  health disparities, 21, 22
  Health Hazard Evaluations, 260
  master-servant relationship, 52, 55–56
  multiple employers, 172, 232–233, 385
  National Labor Relations Act, 381
  OSHA challenges, 610, 612
  OSHA situational leadership, 588–591
  OSHAct definition, 173
  participation in policy, 654–656
  personal protective equipment, 29
  posting citations, 215, 220
  posting injury records, 660
  recordkeeping, 173, 214, 266. *See also* recordkeeping
  Safety and Health Recognition and Achievement Program, 261–262
  Severe Violator Enforcement Program, 231–232
  small business impact of rules, 68, 69, 71
  standards as tax on employment, 653
  standards classifications, 171–172
  trade secrets, 219
  training, 260. *See also* training
  training guidelines, 543, 545–546
  variance application, 178, 180

voluntary protection program, 229–230
wages for refusal to work, 217
workers' compensation owner exclusion, 486
WTO labor standards, 421–422
Employment Standards Administration (ESA)
  Black Lung Benefits Act claims, 500–501
  child labor, 376, 382
  in DoL, 198, 376, 500
  Fair Labor Standards Act enforcement, 376, 382
  Longshore and Harbor Workers' Compensation Act enforcement, 383
  Walsh-Healey Public Contracts Act enforcement, 198
endangerment crimes, 243–245
Energy Employees Occupational Illness Compensation Program (2000), 372, 501
enforcement. *See also* citations (summons); judicial review; penalties; recordkeeping; whistle-blowers
  BoM authority, 108, 313, 316, 317, 318, 319, 320
  Bureau of Safety and Environmental Enforcement (MMS), 370
  Coal Act (1969), 320–321
  in command-and-control process, 213
  compliance officers, 212
  deadlines, 213, 215
  DoI of Coal Act, 141
  as DoL responsibility, 278
  employee compliance, 175
  ergonomic violations program, 231. *See also* ergonomics
  Hazardous Materials Transportation Act, 374–375
  inspection as first step, 213. *See also* inspections
  interference as criminal, 223
  International Labour Organization, 654
  international worker safety, 652–653
  Mine Act (1977), 322, 323, 324
  MSHA authority, 329, 356
  multiemployer doctrine, 232–233
  OSHA emphasis programs, 227–229
  OSHA vs. NIOSH authority, 300
  OSHAct (Section 10), 215–216
  "policy" and "police," 3
  in public health framework, 6, 7, 17
  Severe Violator Enforcement Program, 231–232
  of standards in *Federal Register*, 180
  standards vs. regulations, 214–215
  tax evasion laws for, 653
  voluntary protection program, 229–230
  Worker Endangerment Initiative, 239–247

engineering
  Challenger space shuttle, 591–593
  control technology focus, 287, 291, 604
  control technology over PPE, 27, 182
  engineer recruitment in history, 271, 335
  hazard control, 99, 171
  National Safety Council, 101
England. *See* Great Britain
environmental health
  chemical safety, 39–40. *See also* chemical safety
  code of conduct for multinationals, 76, 419
  common law rights, 53
  environmental impact statements, 41–42, 68–69
  EU environmental policy, 429, 431–433
  exporting hazards, 158, 417–418, 452–455
  Global Environmental and Occupational Health Sciences (GEOHealth), 396
  Haddon matrix, 25–26
  as health field, 18–19
  history of occupational health, 89, 99
  inspections of workplace, 35–36, 203, 214
  ISO 14000 environmental protection, 655
  National Environmental Policy Act, 41–42
  National Institute of Environmental Health Sciences, 287, 374
  NIEHS Worker Education and Training, 547–548
  protection agencies, 43–46
  protection legislation, 377–381
  public health of, 20, 37–39
  public health to protection agencies, 13, 43
  releases of hazardous materials, 245–246, 540, 541, 547
  as research priority, 291
  social environment, 20, 26, 52
  subversion by Information Quality Act, 71–73
  toxics use reduction, 40–41
  UN Environment Programme, 398, 415, 654, 655
  voluntary protection program, 229–230
Environmental Health Criteria 203: Chrysotile Asbestos (WHO), 443
environmental impact statements (EISs), 41–42, 68–69
environmental law
  common law rights, 53
  criminal penalties versus, 239, 240
  endangerment crimes, 243–245
  environmental justice, 396
  in law hierarchy, 52
  National Environmental Policy Act, 41–42
  protection legislation, 377–381
  unanticipated releases, 245–246
  Worker Endangerment Initiative, 239–247

EPA. *See* U.S. Environmental Protection Agency
EPCRA. *See* Emergency Planning and Community Right-to-Know Act (1986)
epidemiology
    Haddon matrix, 25–26
    NIOSH access to records, 299
    NIOSH leaders, 281, 287, 288
equivocation fallacy, 157
"eradication" vs. "elimination" of disease, 24
ERCs (education and research centers), 260–261, 284
ergonomics
    computer workstations, 38
    deaths from, 625
    ergonomic violations program, 231
    Healthy People Objectives (2020), 20
    labor specialization, 474–475
    National Coalition on Ergonomics, 195, 626–627, 631, 642
    policy analysis, 9, 625–627, 630–632, 642–643
    regulation thwarted, 1–2, 71, 128, 179, 194–197, 588, 614, 657
Erin Brockovich (movie), 129
errors
    false positives vs. negatives, 152
    fundamental attribution error, 515, 577
    Type I and II, 151–152
ESA. *See* Employment Standards Administration
Esch, John J., 107
ethics
    antiscience arguments, 582, 583–588. *See also* greed
    assessment of, 576
    "Belmont Report" (1979), 530–531, 574
    Bill Moyers on, 527
    business ethics, 575–576
    conspiracy definition, 569
    harm principle, 581–588
    morality foundations, 579–581
    public health ethics, 574–575
    right-to-know moral rationale, 530–531
    situational leadership, 588–591. *See also* situational attribution
    VCM hazard cover-up, 565–568
Ethyl Corporation, 567, 585
EU. *See* European Union
EU-OSHA (European Agency for Safety and Health at Work), 432, 433–434
Eurofound. *See* European Foundation for the Improvement of Living and Working Conditions
European Agency for Safety and Health at Work (EU-OSHA), 432, 433–434
European Foundation for the Improvement of Living and Working Conditions, 431–433
European Union (EU)
    agricultural workers, 414
    asbestos ban, 439, 443–445
    countries of, 428
    Economic and Social Committee of the Commission (EESC), 431
    "EU imperialism" of standards, 395
    European Agency for Safety and Health at Work, 432, 433–434
    European Chemical Agency, 434–435
    European Foundation for the Improvement of Living and Working Conditions, 431–433
    nation-states on worker safety, 651, 653
    origins of, 427–429
    OSHA and, 403–404
    policy making, 429–430
    precautionary principle, 429, 634–635, 646
    Registration, Evaluation, Authorization, and Restriction of Chemicals (REACH), 431, 434–435
    Single European Act (1987), 427–428, 430, 431
    strict liability, 503
    voluntary compliance, 430
evaluation. *See also* surveillance
    context, inputs, process, and expected products (CIPP), 153–154
    Evaluation of Carcinogenic Risks to Humans, 411
    Guides to the Evaluation of Permanent Impairment, 489–490
    Health Hazard Evaluations (HHE), 260, 287, 292–293, 527–528, 538
    Registration, Evaluation, Authorization, and Restriction of Chemicals (REACH), 431, 434–435
Evaluation of Carcinogenic Risks to Humans, 411
events, 413–414
evidence
    in argumentation, 129, 130, 134–136, 138, 603–604
    asbestos harm, 505
    carcinogen Classes, 193–194
    discovery (law), 548–549, 552–553
    evidence-based public health, 135, 409, 432–433
    expert testimony, 553–555
    Global Environmental and Occupational Health Sciences (GEOHealth), 396
    "junk science," 553–555, 631
    OSHRC administrative court, 217
    policy thwarted despite, 1–2, 72
    rulemaking, 66
    substantial evidence test, 177–178
    supporting claims, 134–136
    types of, 135–136

weight of evidence, 554–555
workplace torts, 502
exclusions
   agricultural workers, 21, 258, 658
   appropriation associated, 182, 268
   Commerce Clause exclusion, 111
   construction and lead, 182, 185, 205, 206, 585
   domestic workers, 21
   federal agencies and employees, 227
   firefighters, 226, 258, 658
   government not employer, 173, 367, 383–384, 657
   lead and construction, 182, 185, 205, 206
   liquid mining under Mine Act (1977), 321
   miners, 174, 318, 319
   NIOSH addressing, 258, 658
   NIOSH broad authority, 258–259
   NLRA jurisdiction, 381
   OSHAct (Section 16), 219
   other federal coverage, 174, 331–332, 367–372
   "records-check" inspection policy, 220
   self-employed workers, 367, 385–387, 657
   small businesses, 268, 384, 385
   small farms, 182, 268, 384, 385
   small mines, 318, 319
   workers' compensation, 483, 484, 486, 492
Exclusive Economic Zone (EEZ), 368–370
executive branch. *See also* Office of Management and Budget
   agency oversight, 60, 62–63, 66
   annual report in OSHAct, 266
   as branch of government, 58, 59, 62
   Federal Advisory Committee Act, 68, 69
   Federal Radiation Council, 371
   judicial appointments, 64, 67
   OSHAct creation, 112–113
   policy analysis, 606
executive orders
   agency operational guidance, 63
   Federal Radiation Council, 161
   Federal Register publication, 67
   force of law, 62
   OSHA precedents, 198
exemptions
   agricultural worker overtime pay, 382
   construction and lead, 182, 185, 205, 206, 585
   fishing industry, 268
   hearings for employee exemptions, 219
   hunting as work, 268
   oil industry from Mine Act (1977), 321
   small businesses, 268, 384, 385
   small farms, 182, 268, 384, 385
expert testimony, 553–555
explicit costs, 468

explosions
   BoM research, 334
   Challenger space shuttle, 591–593
   chemical safety, 36, 39–40
   criminal prosecution of, 238
   as energy transfer, 39
   Farmington, WV, mine explosion, 36, 113, 141, 315, 320, 345, 348
   mine explosions, 36, 102, 113, 141, 311, 315–321, 320, 328, 332, 345, 348, 350
   mine gases, 311–312, 332–333
   munitions plant, 274
   nuclear reactor events, 414
   oil refineries, 39–40, 245–246
   oil rigs, 365–366, 369, 590
   Organic Act (1910), 301
   shipping vessels, 411–412
   steam power, 84–85, 111
   volunteer safety movement, 101
exporting hazardous environments
   DBCP, 452–455
   distance as public health enemy, 158
   risk transfer of asbestos, 437–445, 584, 648
   risk transfer of factory hazards, 446–448
   World Bank Group, 417–418
externalizing costs
   argument for regulations, 604
   Bhopal (India) plant, 451
   cost externalization, 477–480
   employer premium fraud, 515
   moral hazard and, 480
   negative externalities, 468, 478–479
   offshore job hazards, 649–650
   positive externalities, 468, 478, 479, 658
   state workers' comp fraud, 518

F

FAA. *See* Federal Aviation Administration
failure to warn, 505, 533
failure-to-abate violations, 220, 221, 231–232
Fair Labor Standards Act (FLSA; 1938)
   child labor, 88, 95, 376, 382
   wages, 108, 382
   workday length, 108
fallacies
   ad hominem, 157, 582
   in argument, 156–158
   cost of compliance, 203–205, 481, 519–520, 649–650
   fundamental attribution error, 515
   OSHAct as job killer, 247–248
   straw man, 157, 631
   types of, 157
falling object protection structures (FOPS), 419
false positives and negatives, 149, 151–152

Family and Medical Leave Act (1993), 557
family members
    compensating differential argument, 529
    costs borne by, 479
    Family and Medical Leave Act, 557
    free trade and workers, 654
    of trapped miners, 328
    workers' compensation, 490
    work-related exposure, 258–259, 439
farm workers. *See* agricultural workers
Farmington, WV, mine explosion (1968), 36, 113, 141, 315, 320, 345, 348
Farr, William, 87
fatalities. *See* deaths
fault
    blaming the victim, 515, 577–578
    compensation principle, 481
    insurance claim denial, 517, 658, 660–661
    terrorism compensation act, 500
    workers' compensation, 102–103, 483, 484, 500, 502
FDA. *See* U.S. Food and Drug Administration
feasibility
    economic feasibility, 178, 183, 187, 188
    OSHA standards review, 481, 519
    phased approach, 190
    requirement of, 178, 183, 187, 188, 613
    technological feasibility, 178, 183, 184, 189, 481
    VCM standard, 519–520
FECA. *See* Federal Employees' Compensation Act (1916)
Federal Advisory Committee Act (FACA; 1973), 68, 69, 182
Federal Advisory Council on Occupational Safety and Health (FACOSH; 1971), 227
Federal Aviation Act (1958), 268
Federal Aviation Act (1975), 373–374
Federal Aviation Administration (FAA), 373–374, 376
Federal Caustic Poison Act (1927), 539
Federal Child Labor Act (1916), 110
Federal Coal Mine Health and Safety Act (1969). *See* Coal Mine Health and Safety Act (1969)
Federal Coal Mine Safety Act (1952), 108, 315, 316, 318, 338
Federal Coal Mine Safety Act (1966), 315, 316, 319
Federal Coal Mine Safety Board of Review, 318
federal employees
    occupational safety, 173, 227, 367
    workers' compensation, 486
Federal Employees' Compensation Act (FECA; 1916), 499, 500, 501
Federal Employers' Liability Act (1906), 110
Federal Employers' Liability Act (1908), 103, 499, 500

Federal Environmental Pesticide Control Act (1972), 378
Federal Food Quality Protection Act (1996), 379
Federal Hazardous Substances Act (1960), 377–378
Federal Hazardous Substances Labeling Act (1960), 46, 539
Federal Insecticide, Fungicide, and Rodenticide Act (FIFRA; 1947), 181, 378–379, 643–644
Federal Metal and Nonmetallic Mine Safety Act (1966), 108, 319, 321, 338
Federal Mine Safety and Health Act. *See* Mine Safety and Health Act (1977)
Federal Mine Safety and Health Review Commission. *See* Mine Safety and Health Review Commission
Federal Mine Safety Code, 317
Federal Motor Carrier Safety Administration (FMCSA), 375–376
Federal Pure Food and Drug Act (1906), 117
Federal Radiation Council, 161, 371
Federal Register
    "Belmont Report" (1979), 530–531, 574
    executive order publication, 67
    public comment, 66, 68, 177
    regulation publication, 62, 66, 73, 170–171
    standards issuance, 171, 177
    standards publication, 171, 179, 180
    state submitted plans, 225
    temporary standards, 179
Federal Rules of Civil Procedure, 548
federal system, 17, 57–58, 140–141
Federal Vocational Rehabilitation Act (1973), 490
Federal Water Quality Administration (FWQA), 45
Feehan, Francis, 332
Feinberg, Kenneth, 510
fellow-servant rule, 54–55, 102
felonies
    BP oil rig explosion, 366
    criminal violations as, 223
    deaths as, 221, 223, 366, 658
    environmental endangerment laws, 243
    felony prosecutions, 223–225
    Mine Act (1977), 325–326
    state prosecution, 235
figures. *See* charts and flowcharts
Financial Action Task Force, 653
financial assistance
    Mine Act compliance, 327, 328
    OSHAct compliance, 267
    second injury fund, 485
    World Bank Group, 416
financial incentives. *See* incentives
Findings on the Worst Forms of Child Labor (DoL), 451

Fingerhut, Marilyn, 406
Finklea, John, 282–287
fire
　criminal prosecution, 237–238
　factory fires, 88, 446–447, 624
　firefighter exclusion from OSHA, 226, 258, 658
　firefighter training, 261
　firefighters and workers' compensation, 483
　Great Fire of London (1666), 104
　Mine Act (1977), 323
　mine fires, 311–312, 328
　National Board of Fire Underwriters, 101
　National Fire Protection Association, 101
　Sunshine silver mine (1972), 321
　Triangle Shirtwaist Co. (1911), 88, 446
　wildfire blowup, 125–126, 130, 149, 579
firedamp mine gas, 311, 312
Firestone tire settlement, 552
first responders. *See* emergency responders
fishing industry
　agriculture standards, 172
　Alaska and workers' compensation, 93
　Commerce Clause exclusion, 111
　Commercial Fishing Industry Vessel Safety Act, 370, 391
　deaths among self-employed, 385–386
　emergency rescue equipment, 389–391
　Haddon matrix, 26
　IMO safety, 398, 411–412
　inspected vessels, 370
　local emphasis programs, 229
　NIOSH program review, 292, 293–294
　NORA research councils, 295
　OSHA exemption, 268
　OSHA partial coverage, 368
　SOLAS safety, 412
　uninspected vessels, 174, 368, 390
fixed costs, 468
flowcharts. *See* charts and flowcharts
Foege, William, 23
FOIA. *See* Freedom of Information Act (1966)
Food, Drugs, and Cosmetic Act (1938), 634
Food and Agriculture Organization (FAO), 398, 414–415
food safety
　Federal Pure Food and Drug Act, 117
　Food and Drug Administration, 42
　Food Safety and Inspection Service, 42
　Meat Inspection Act, 117
　statutory law for, 65
　Wholesome Meat Act, 117
　WTO agreement, 421
Food Safety and Inspection Service (FSIS), 42–43
food-borne disease statutory law, 65
forced labor DoL office, 451

Ford, Ford B., 354
Ford, Gerald, 63, 199, 610
Ford, William, 617–621, 622
Ford Motor Company, 519–520, 552
forestry
　agriculture standards, 172
　deaths among self-employed, 385–386
　logging operations, 177, 226, 263
　NIOSH program review, 292, 293–294
　NORA research councils, 295
formal rule making, 66–67, 177–178
formaldehyde
　cost per life saved, 644
　path from risk to standard, 169–170
　standard promulgation, 179
Formaldehyde Standards for Composite Wood Products Act (2010), 170
Foulke, Ewin G., Jr., 199, 404–405
Fourth Amendment and inspections, 214
fracking, 151
framing of messages
　agenda framing, 152–155
　conceptual frames, 579, 580
　fetal vs. women's rights, 249
　"prejudice against lead," 585
　scarcity principle, 573
　values before issues, 579
France
　asbestos ban, 443–445
　healthcare spending, 470
Frank, Peter, 29–30
fraud. *See also* greed
　coal dust sampling, 350–356
　workers' compensation, 512–519
free market. *See also* marketplace
　regulation and, 156, 473, 479, 582
　right-to-know and, 532
free trade. *See* North American Free Trade Agreement (1994)
Freedom of Information Act (FOIA; 1966), 67–68
Frost, Wade Hampton, 25
Frye, William W., 277, 278
"Frye Report." *See Protecting the Health of Eighty Million Americans* (USPHS)
Frye test (law), 553, 609
Frye v. United States (1923), 553
Fukushima (Japan) nuclear reactor event, 414
Fuller, Lon L., 51
fundamental attribution error, 515, 577
funding. *See* appropriations; grants

G

GAO. *See* U.S. Government Accountability Office
gasoline with lead, 38, 102, 271, 585–586, 643

GATT. *See* General Agreement on Tarrifs and Trade
GDP. *See* gross domestic product
General Agreement on Tarrifs and Trade (GATT)
    asbestos dispute, 444–445
    "contracting" parties, 420
    dispute settlement, 421
    escape clause, 651–653
    protection vs. protectionism, 420
general duty clause
    childbearing capacity, 211–212
    in command-and-control process, 213
    criminal violations, 223, 239
    employers must comply, 152, 171, 175, 604, 658
    ergonomic violations, 231
    Mine Act lacking, 175, 325
    no existing standard, 175, 178
    standard exists, 233
General Electric Co. v. Joiner (1997), 555
general industry standards, 171
generic standards
    HazCom Standard, 185
    OSHA cancer standard, 192–194
    permissible exposure limits, 185, 191–192
geographic bounds of OSHAct, 174, 369, 402
geographic coverage of OSHA offices, 201
Georgia (nation) asbestos use, 437
Gerberding, Julie, 296, 297, 298
germ theory, 339, 554
Germany
    healthcare spending, 470
    wergild ("man money"), 510
    workers' compensation, 482
GHS. *See* Globally Harmonized System
Gibbons v. Ogden (1824), 109
Gibbs, Graham W., 443
Ginsburg, Justice Ruth Bader, 75–76
Global Environmental and Occupational Health Sciences (GEOHealth), 396
global health and safety
    accountability, 654–656
    agricultural workers by region, 414
    asbestos, 437–445, 584, 648
    asthma DALYs, 401
    back pain DALYs, 401
    burden of disease/injury, 400, 401, 417, 418
    cancer DALYs, 401
    chronic obstructive pulmonary disease DALYs, 401
    corporation standards, 448, 655–656
    deaths annually, 400, 401, 417
    diseases incidence, 400, 401
    economics vs. standards, 647–654
    Global Environmental and Occupational Health Sciences (GEOHealth), 396
    global standards, 448
    Globally Harmonized System, 542–543, 544
    injuries (nonfatal), 400, 417, 418
    institutions for, 650–654
    international policy, 22–23, 645–656. *See also* international policy
    IPCS global poison centers, 411
    labor law, 647–649
    leukemia DALYs, 401
    lung cancer DALYs, 401
    NAFTA, 22, 422–426, 653
    noise-induced hearing loss DALYs, 401
    occupational diseases annually, 400, 401
    participation in policy, 654–656
    pesticide poisonings, 414–415. *See also* Bhopal (India)
    poverty, 647. *See also* poverty
    Systematic Occupational Health and Safety Management, 645–647, 655
    WHO Global Plan of Action, 410
global issues. *See* international policy
Globally Harmonized System (GHS) for Hazard Communication, 402, 542–543, 544
Gompers, Samuel, 93, 103, 609
Goodrich, B.F., 159, 186, 567, 568
goods (economics), 468
Gorsuch, Anne, 169
governance and scarce resources, 469, 615
Government Paperwork Elimination Act (1998), 68, 71
Government Performance and Results Act (1993), 292
Graham, Lindsay, 552
grants
    audits of grantees, 266
    Brookwood-Sago Mine Safety Grants, 328
    compliance with Mine Act, 327–328
    funding of research, 262
    hazardous materials training, 261, 374–375
    MSHA state programs, 546
    New Directions Grants for training, 261
    NIEHS Worker Education and Training, 547
    nongrant financial assistance, 267
    OSHAct (Section 23), 262
    Social Security Act funding, 272
    state motor carrier safety, 376
    for state OSHA programs, 262, 274
    training via Coal Act (1969), 321
    World Bank Group, 416
Great Britain
    Atlantic Charter, 406
    cholera outbreak (1854), 554
    common law, 53, 510
    healthcare spending, 470
    labor movement, 93, 102, 103
    Lloyd's of London, 505
    national legislation evolution, 103–105

public health movement origins, 84, 87, 89
workers' compensation, 482
Great Fire of London (1666), 104
Great Upheaval labor strike, 96
greed
    antiscience arguments, 582, 583–588
    asbestos, 158, 437–445
    coal dust sampling, 350–356
    elected officials against, 365
    lost-time injuries, 356–357
    lower wages, lower value, 418, 446–448, 647, 661
    public health vs. private gain, 540, 588, 649
    servitude practices, 451–452
    vinyl chloride, 159, 565–568
    workers' compensation fraud, 512–519
Greenspan, Alan, 258, 637
Gregg, Judd, 623, 624–625, 629–630
Griswold v. Connecticut (1965), 556
gross domestic product (GDP), 470, 471, 473
Ground Zero
    9/11 and NIOSH, 291, 297–298, 501
    9/11 Health and Compensation Act, 467, 500, 501
    9/11 Victim Compensation Fund, 467, 510, 511
    NIOSH director Howard, 291, 297–298
    World Trade Center Programs, 298, 501
    WTC Health Registry, 501
Guatemala
    forced child labor, 453
    immigrant workers, 661
    OSHA and, 403
Guenther, George, 199
Guides to the Evaluation of Permanent Impairment (AMA), 489–490

H

Haddon, William, Jr., 25–26, 28, 44
Haddon matrix, 25–26
hairspray hazards, 566, 567
Haley, Jack, 534
Hamilton, Alice, 88–89, 100, 265, 584
Hamilton, Margaret, 534
Hammurabi Code, 51
Hardesty, John F., 112, 277, 609
Hardesty, Robert, 112
Harding, Warren G., 98, 336
Hardy, Harriet L., 89, 585
harm principle, 581–588, 634
harmonization of systems
    hazard communication, 402, 542–543, 544
    industrial classification, 402
    International Organization for Standardization (ISO), 435–436
    Single European Act (1987), 427

WHO International Programme on Chemical Safety (IPCS), 411
Harwood, Susan, 261
hazard communication. *See also* Hazard Communication Standard (1983); right-to-know
    asbestos labeling, 440
    DBCP pesticide labeling, 454
    failure to warn, 533
    Globally Harmonized System, 402, 542–543, 544
    harmonization of systems, 402, 542–543, 544
    in hierarchy of controls, 171
    incident command system, 404
    International Nuclear and Radiological Event Scale (INES), 413–414
    IPCS International Chemical Safety Cards, 411
    labeling chemicals, 440, 454, 534, 539–540, 542–543
    levels of hazard warnings, 534–535
    OSHAct (Section 6), 528
    "poison" label, 534, 539, 542
    scraped off drums, 236
    trade name use, 536, 550
    trade secrets and, 550–551
    vinyl chloride cover-up, 159, 565–568
    warnings, 533–535
Hazard Communication Standard (HazCom Standard; 1983)
    CPSC regulations and, 378
    Emergency Planning and Community Right-to-Know Act from, 38, 530, 658
    GAO reports, 61
    generic standard, 465
    history, 535–539, 657–658
    judicial review, 184, 185, 191
    labeling law, 539–540
    MSDSs required, 540
    policy focus, 9
    promulgation, 179, 202
    state/local laws versus, 202, 540
    trade secrets, 550–551
    training, 543, 545–546
Hazardous Liquids Pipeline Safety Act (1979), 375
Hazardous Materials Safety Act, 138–139
Hazardous Materials Transportation Act (HMTA; 1975), 374–375
Hazardous Materials Transportation Uniform Safety Act (1990), 374–375
Hazardous Substances Labeling Act (1960), 46, 539
hazardous waste
    Basel Convention on Movements of, 422
    CERCLA worker protection, 381

NIEHS Worker Education and Training, 547–548
U.S.-Mexico Border Industrial Program, 422–423
hazards. *See also* exporting hazardous environments; hazard communication
  agricultural workers, 414–415
  assumption of risk, 55, 102, 103
  child labor and, 88, 382
  classified in *Diseases of Occupations*, 89
  code of conduct for multinationals, 76, 419
  Commerce Clause protection, 108–111
  congressional reports, 61
  control failure aftermath, 450–451
  emergency responder training, 261
  employers protect workers, 40
  engineers controlling, 99
  feasibility to control, 178. *See also* feasibility
  Federal Hazardous Substances Act, 377–378
  general duty clause, 152, 171, 175, 178, 211–212, 233
  Hazardous Substances Labeling Act, 46, 539
  hazardous waste, 381, 422–423, 547–548
  Health Hazard Evaluations, 260
  hierarchy of controls, 26–29, 171, 187
  "immediately dangerous," 282
  levels of hazard warnings, 534–535
  long latency hazards, 487, 646. *See also* latency of disease
  minor workers banned, 88, 382
  moral hazards, 480
  NIEHS Worker Education and Training, 547–548
  NIOSH recommended standards, 263–265
  Protecting the Health of Eighty Million Americans (USPHS), 139, 277–278, 609
  RCRA and hazardous wastes, 244
  "recognized hazards," 152, 175
  refusal to work, 216–217, 532–533, 558
  Rotterdam Convention, 426–427, 440
  statutory law, 65
  training for control, 29
health care
  disparities, 21–23
  as health field, 18–19
health definition per WHO, 3
health departments in public health, 17
health fields model, 18–20
Health Hazard Evaluations (HHEs)
  by CDC Epidemic Intelligence Officers, 287
  DBCP plant, 527–528, 538
  NIOSH conducting, 227
  NIOSH program review, 292, 293
  OSHAct (Section 20), 260
Health Insurance Portability and Accountability Act (HIPAA; 1996), 557–558

health metrics
  disability-adjusted life-years (DALYs), 400–401, 508
  quality-adjusted life-year (QALY), 508
Health Security Act, 500
Health Service and Mental Health Administration (HSMHA), 282
healthcare workers
  advocacy by, 127–137
  healthcare provider fraud, 514–515, 517–518
  infection prevention policies, 25
  spectrum of prevention, 24–25, 648–649
  vaccinations, 19
Healthy People (USPHS), 20
healthy worker effect, 342
hearing loss. *See* noise-induced hearing loss
hearings
  administrative law judges, 67
  CIPP approach to evaluation, 153
  employer citation appeals, 216
  employer variance from standard, 180
  ergonomics public hearings, 196
  field hearings, 142, 196
  formal vs. informal rule making, 66
  GATT escape clause, 651–652
  OSHRC administrative court, 217
  standards rule making, 177, 178
  variances and exemptions, 219
heart disease. *See* cardiovascular disease
heavy metals. *See* metal poisoning
Heckler, Ken, 347–350
Heckler, Margaret, 349
Heilbroner, Robert, 601
Heinrich, Herbert W., 106
Henshaw, John, 199
Hernandez, John, 169–170
hexavalent chromium
  industry antiscience, 587
  labor suing for protection, 128–129
  lung cancer, 587
  national emphasis programs, 228
  NIOSH recommended standard, 263
  OSHA standard, 179, 185, 587
HHEs. *See* Health Hazard Evaluations
hierarchy of controls
  as prevention model, 26–29
  standards writing by OSHA, 171, 187
  warnings, 534
HIPAA. *See* Health Insurance Portability and Accountability Act (1996)
Hippocrates, 85, 149, 582, 634
Hippocratic Corpus, 149, 582, 634
history. *See also* labor movement
  asbestosis and right of entry, 257–258
  British national legislation, 103–105
  Daniels bill, 114, 116, 142, 143–144

death reduction with safety acts, 4, 200, 223, 599, 600, 605
deaths over OSHA history, 223
global repetition of, 648
importance of, 84
Johnson worker protection, 112, 138–141, 142, 197, 198, 278, 609, 617
legislation charts, 68, 107–108, 315, 500, 608
legislation flowcharts, 142, 316
Mine Act early statutes, 314–321
mutual aid societies, 92–93
national program origins, 88–89
Nixon OSHAct proposal, 115, 141–144, 610
Nixon OSHAct signing, 91, 116, 147, 170, 198, 599, 610
OSHA precedents, 197–198
pioneers, 84–89
policy transitions, 606–614
public health agencies, 269–278
rates of injury and fatality, 90–91, 99, 102
Sullivan Hazardous Materials Safety Act, 137–139
U.S. national legislation, 105–111
workday length, 93–95, 108, 271, 341
World Wars, 270–278, 335–336, 418
Hodgson, Geoffrey M., 650
Hodgson, James D., 141, 147
Hoffman, Frederick L., 339–340
Holaday, Duncan A., 160, 161
Holmes, Joseph A., 332–333, 546
homicides, 20, 290. *See also* murder
Honduras
　DBCP pesticide exposure, 454
　OSHA and, 403
Hoover, Herbert C., 301, 336–337
horizon analytic, 509
hospitals
　infection prevention policies, 25
　National Electronic Injury Surveillance System, 46
Hotchkiss, Samuel C., 334
House of Representatives in Congress, 59
Howard, John, 285, 291–294
Hueper, William C., 89
human biology as health field, 18–19
human capital, 468, 506
human life value, 509–512, 519–520
human trafficking DoL office, 451
Humphrey, Hubert, 106, 197–198
Hungary life expectancy, 399
Hunter, Donald, 89
hunting exemption, 268
hybrid rule making
　APA and OSHAct, 66–67, 147
　OSHAct, 177–178
hydrogen sulfide mine gas, 312

hypothesis generation. *See* abductive reasoning

I

IAEA. *See* International Atomic Energy Agency
IARC. *See* International Agency for Research on Cancer
Iceland asbestos ban, 443
ICOH. *See* International Commission on Occupational Health
ignorance
　moral hazards, 480
　as public health enemy, 159
　radiation "gag rule," 160–161
illegal immigrant health disparities, 21
Illinois v. Chicago Magnet Wire Corp. (1985), 235–236
Illinois v. Film Recovery Systems Inc. et al. (1985), 236
illnesses. *See* infectious diseases; occupational diseases
illustrations. *See* charts and flowcharts
ILO Encyclopaedia of Occpational Health and Safety, 407–408. *See also* International Labour Organization (ILO)
"immediately dangerous," 282
immigrants. *See also* agricultural workers
　health disparities, 21
　history of factory safety, 446
　informal economy of, 23
　OSHA international policy, 402–403
　sweating system, 105
　Triangle Shirtwaist fire, 88
　as whistle-blowers, 21
　worker population shift to, 661
　World Trade Center compensation, 467
imminent dangers
　in command-and-control process, 213
　Federal Coal Mine Safety Act (1952), 108, 338
　Mine Act (1977), 323, 324, 325
　OSHAct (Section 13), 218
　OSHAct conference committee, 147
　priority of response, 203
IMO. *See* International Maritime Organization
implementation analysis, 656–657
implicit costs, 468
incentives
　compensation laws as, 102–103, 493, 495, 497–499
　definition, 468
　economic efficiency of, 480–481
　fraud in workers' compensation, 512
　lost-time injuries, 356–357
　Systematic Occupational Health and Safety Management, 646

tort liability as, 502, 504
transactional leadership, 571
"incidents" on event scale, 413
Independent Safety Board Act (1974), 376
India
   agricultural workers, 414
   asbestos importing, 439
   asbestos mining, 439
   Bhopal deaths from catastrophe, 220, 449–450
   Bhopal worst industrial disaster, 245–246, 449–451, 541
   forced child labor, 452, 453
   occupational injuries/diseases, 417, 418
indirect costs
   definition, 468, 506
   employer costs, 471
   human capital, 506
   inability to work, 469, 470, 471–472, 486, 506
   9/11 Victim Compensation Fund, 510
   U.S. health care costs, 471
   workers' compensation for, 485, 486, 488, 490
individual action level in spectrum of prevention, 24, 648–649
"individual" vs. "person," 74–75
Indonesia
   asbestos importing, 439
   forced child labor, 453
Indoor Radon Abatement Act (1988), 37
inductive reasoning, 127, 149, 150
Industrial Accident Prevention: A Scientific Approach (Heinrich), 106
industrial hygiene
   American Conference of Governmental Industrial Hygienists, 176, 273
   hierarchy of controls, 28–29
   numbers of hygienists increasing, 198, 288
   Patty's Industrial Hygiene and Toxicology, 337
   Pocket Guide to Chemical Hazards, 282
   Social Security Act funding, 45, 88, 101, 272
   spectrum of prevention, 24, 648–649
Industrial Hygiene Newsletter, 274, 276
Industrial Medical Association, 102
industrial medicine
   "father" Bernardino Ramazzini, 85–86, 437
   first physician Alice Hamilton, 88, 584
Industrial Revolution. *See also* labor movement
   corporation personhood, 75
   worker protection, 84–85, 98–99
   workers' compensation system, 54–55
Industrial Toxicology (Hamilton & Hardy), 89
Industrial Union Department, AFL-CIO v. American Petroleum Institute (1980), 638

Industrial Union Department, AFL-CIO v. Hodgson (1974), 178, 183, 186–187
Industrial Union Department v. American Petroleum Institute (1980), 178, 179–180, 183, 188–190
Industrial Workers of the World (Wobblies), 97, 98, 103
industry sectors
   deaths among self-employed, 385–386
   deaths annually, 4
   deaths from injury, 22
   generic approach to PELs, 191–192
   industrial classification, 402
   informal sector definition, 22
   manual rates, 493–494
   NLRA jurisdiction, 381
   NORA and OSHAct (Section 20), 294–295
   OSHA exclusions, 21, 367–376. *See also* exclusions
   policy focus, 9
   regulation by, 612
   standards classifications, 171–172
infectious diseases
   germ theory, 339, 554
   Haddon matrix, 25–26
   NORA research councils, 295
   as notifiable diseases, 15
   Public Health Service Act, 607
   as research priority, 291
   statutory law, 65
   surveillance–containment model, 23–24
   World Wars and public health, 270, 272, 273
inference
   abductive reasoning as, 150
   in argumentation, 129, 130, 134–136
   types of, 135
inflation (cost analysis), 509
informal leadership, 572
informal rule making
   APA rule making, 66–67
   Negotiated Rulemaking Act, 68, 69–70
informal sector, 22, 23
information. *See also* education; hazard communication; right-to-know; training
   agricultural community, 386
   BoM inspection authorization, 317
   business school safety curriculum, 590–591
   categories of information transfer, 530
   Collegium Ramazzini, 437
   in command-and-control process, 213
   correcting inaccurate governmental, 557
   electronic submission of, 68, 71
   EU-OSHA, 433–434
   expert testimony in court, 553–555
   forum for inspectors, 436
   Information Quality Act, 68, 71–73, 627

International Commission on Occupational Health, 436, 442, 443
Internet for federal agencies, 68
Internet for worker safety, 656
legal restrictions of disclosure, 549–555
NIOSH mission, 278
OSHA emphasis programs, 228–229
OSHA international policy, 402
pesticide labeling, 378, 379
requests for information from public, 68, 70
trade secrets, 218–219. *See also* confidentiality
UMWA Welfare and Retirement Fund, 344
Information Quality Act (IQA; 2000), 68, 71–73, 627
informed consent, 531, 534
injunctions
  imminent dangers, 213, 218
  Mine Act (1977), 324
injuries (nonfatal). *See also* musculoskeletal disorders
  annually globally, 400, 417, 418
  annually nationally, 3, 4–6, 17, 22, 90, 91, 102, 111–112, 139, 471
  back injuries, 195, 401
  BLS survey of iron/steel, 106, 265
  collapse of factories, 447
  common law as recourse, 54–55, 102–103, 174, 454, 502
  costs of, 471, 472, 510, 512
  criminal penalties for, 223
  CWP after Mine Act, 350
  definition, 39
  disease vs. injury compensation, 487
  economic burden of, 399–401, 417, 418, 469–472
  endangerment prosecution, 243
  epidemiology of, 288
  GAO reports, 61
  global incidence, 400
  Haddon matrix, 25–26
  Healthy People Objectives (2020), 20
  history of occupational safety, 87–88, 90–91, 99, 102
  incentives against, 356–357
  India agricultural workers, 414
  India pesticide catastrophe, 449, 450
  life-years lost, 39
  Mondays, 517
  National Electronic Injury Surveillance System, 46
  national emphasis programs, 227–228
  needlestick, 290
  OECD rates among countries, 419
  oil rig explosion, 365, 369
  opportunity costs of, 474
  OSHA reductions, 200
  posting records of, 660
  prevention as public health, 38–39
  records requirement, 173
  repetitive trauma, 195
  shipping vessel explosion, 411–412
  traumatic injuries, 289, 291, 292, 293
  Worker Endangerment Initiative applied, 240–243
  workers' compensation incentive, 497–498
injury pyramid, 106
insecticides. *See* pesticides
Insecticides Act (1910), 539
insignificant risk, 178, 183, 189, 638
inspected fishing vessels, 370
inspections
  asbestos, 380
  Bangladesh factories, 447, 448
  British mines, 103, 105
  Bureau of Mines, 108, 313, 316, 317, 319
  Coal Act (1969), 320
  Coal Mine Act (1952), 338
  in command-and-control process, 213
  confidentiality agreements, 257–258, 269
  consultation program, 261, 590, 630
  cost savings of, 247–248, 498–499, 659
  deaths of inspectors, 321
  enforcement's first step, 213
  ergonomics, 231
  Food Safety and Inspection Service, 42
  Health Hazard Evaluations, 260, 287, 292, 293, 527–528, 538
  industrial military establishments, 273
  International Association of Labour Inspection, 436
  Mine Act (1977), 322, 323, 324, 325
  MSHA authority, 329
  NIOSH authority, 213–214, 260, 278, 284, 300–301
  NIOSH mine investigations, 279
  number of federal and state (2011), 226
  OSHA authority, 213–214, 300
  OSHA on-site priority, 35–36
  of records, 173, 213–214, 299–300
  "records-check" inspection policy, 220
  search warrants, 147, 214, 223
  Severe Violator Enforcement Program, 231
  state regulations, 99, 100
  steamboats, 111
  targeted approach, 203, 266
  trade secrets, 218–219
  U.S. mines, 107, 108
  vessels via SOLAS, 412
  voluntary protection program, 229–230
Institute of Medicine (IOM)
  framework of public health, 6, 7, 16–17
  goal of public health, 15
  NIOSH program review, 292

institutions
    EU occupational safety/health, 430–435
    global worker safety, 650–654
    harm principle, 582
    institutional capitalism, 476
    norms changing via law, 398
    as social rule systems, 650
insurer fraud, 514, 517
intangible costs, 468
Interagency Regulatory Liaison Group (IRLG), 36, 42–43, 169
interim standards
    in command-and-control process, 213
    definitions in OSHAct, 173
    employer compliance, 171
    Mine Act (1977), 324, 326
    overview, 175–177, 604
    PELs as, 191
    vinyl chloride, 186
International Agency for Research on Cancer (IARC), 398, 410–411, 440
International Association of Labour Inspection, 436
International Atomic Energy Agency (IAEA), 398, 412–414, 422
International Bulk Chemical Code (IMO), 412
International Commission on Occupational Health (ICOH), 436, 442, 443
International Convention for Safety of Life at Sea (SOLAS), 411–412
International Journal of Occupational and Environmental Health (ICOH), 436
International Labour Organization (ILO)
    asbestos global ban, 440, 584
    Bangladesh garment factories, 447–448
    conventions, 407, 408
    enforcement powers, 654
    global worker safety, 650–654, 656
    ILO Encyclopaedia of Occpational Health and Safety, 407–408
    recommendations, 407, 408
    as UN agency, 397–398, 406–408, 410
international law. *See also* international policy; international trade
    civil vs. common law, 53
    codes of conduct for businesses, 76, 398
    customary law basis, 52, 56–57, 396
    foreigners suing in federal court, 57, 74–75
    IAEA safety standards, 412
    Islamic law, 53
    labor law, 57, 648–649
    in law hierarchy, 52
    law of nations, 56–57
    NAFTA, 22, 422–426, 653
    norms changing via law, 396, 397, 398
    perspectives of, 396–397, 448

International Maritime Organization (IMO), 398, 411–412
International Monetary Fund, 653
International Nuclear and Radiological Event Scale (INES), 413–414
International Organization for Standardization (ISO)
    asbestos in cement products, 444
    Globally Harmonized System, 543
    ISO 14000 environmental protection, 655
    as nongovernmental, 398, 435–436
international policy. *See also* global health and safety; international law
    Collegium Ramazzini, 398, 436–437
    exporting hazardous environments, 158, 417–418. *See also* exporting hazardous environments
    Food and Agriculture Organization, 398, 414–415
    Global Environmental and Occupational Health Sciences (GEOHealth), 396
    global occupational health, 22–23
    incidence of work disease/injury, 399–401
    labor law, 648–649
    life expectancy, 399
    NAFTA, 22, 422–426, 653
    OSHA, 402–406, 645
    policy analysis, 645–656
    questions to ask, 396–397
    UN Environment Programme, 398, 415, 654, 655
    World Health Organization, 398, 409–411. *See also* World Health Organization
International Programme on Chemical Safety (IPCS)
    Asbestos and Other Natural Mineral Fibres, 441
    asbestos working groups, 441–443, 584
    chemical safety, 411
    NIOSH and chrysotile, 442
International Register of Potentially Toxic Chemicals, 415
International Social Security Association (ISSA), 408–409
international trade
    Basel Convention, 422
    chrysotile asbestos, 440
    domestic safety policies vs. multinational, 651–654
    European Union, 427–435
    GATT "contracting" parties, 420
    ISO 14000 environmental protection, 655
    NAFTA, 22, 422–426, 653
    OECD tractor certification, 419
    Rotterdam Convention, 426–427, 440
    Trade and Development Act, 451

World Trade Organization, 397, 419, 420–422. *See also* World Trade Organization
International Training and Research in Environmental and Occupational Health program (NIH), 395
International Union, United Automobile, Aerospace and Agricultural Implement Workers of America v. General Dynamics Land Systems Division (1987), 233
International Union of Mine, Mill, and Smelter Workers (Mine-Mill), 318–319
Internet
  web presence of federal agencies, 68
  worker safety information, 656
interrogatories, 548
Interstate Commerce Clause. *See* Commerce Clause of Constitution
intervention
  as capitalism balance, 475
  cost analysis, 505–512
  as direct cost, 470
  disaster (law), 313, 315, 316, 328
  effectiveness as research priority, 291
  health fields model, 19–20
  Healthy People (USPHS), 20
  for prevention of disease or injury, 17–18, 23
  social discount rate, 508, 520
intuition
  intuitive primacy principle, 579
  precautionary principle, 149
  wildfire blowup, 126, 149, 579
investigations. *See also* inspections
  number conducted (2009), 21
  right of entry, 257–258
IOM. *See* Institute of Medicine
IPCS. *See* International Programme on Chemical Safety
IQA. *See* Information Quality Act
iron industry
  injury data, 106, 265
  NIOSH recommended standard, 264
  OSHAct opposition, 113
  volunteer safety movement, 101
Islamic law, 53
ISO. *See also* International Organization for Standardization (ISO)
issues of public policy; controversy
  asbestos globally, 437–445
  cancer standard, 193
  conceptual framing, 579, 580
  framing of, 152–155, 579–580
  hazard communication, 536
  issue statements, 130–132, 134
  mine disaster (law), 313, 315, 316, 328
  OSHAct, 137–148

policy analysis for, 130
policy networks for, 132
salience, 606
topoi of claims, 131
values before issues, 579, 580

J

Jackson, Andrew, 84–85
Japan
  healthcare spending, 470
  strict liability, 503
Javits, Jacob
  Javits amendment, 116, 144, 146
  on NIOSH, 278
  Nixon bill, 115, 142
Johnson, Lyndon B.
  automobile and highway safety, 44
  coal mine health and safety, 347, 348
  "Great Society," 607
  Volunteers in Service to America (VISTA), 346
  Wholesome Meat Act (1967), 117
  worker protection, 112, 138–141, 142, 197, 198, 278, 609, 617
joint employers, 232
joint-and-several liability, 503
Jones, Gordon, 366
Jones Act (Merchant Marine Act; 1917), 499, 500
Joseph A. Holmes Safety Association (MSHA), 546–547
Journal of Occupational Medicine, 102
judicial branch. *See also* judicial review; Supreme Court of the United States
  as branch of government, 58, 59, 64–65
  coal dust sampling, 354
  court records sealed, 551–553
  discovery, 548–549, 552–553
  expert testimony, 553–555
  Federal Rules of Civil Procedure, 548
  judicial appointments, 64, 67
  judicial decisions and international norms, 398
  litigation vs. regulation, 505
  statutory vs. common law, 65
  tort liability, 501–505
  trial by judge, 553–555
judicial notice, 64, 72
judicial precedent. *See* doctrine of judicial precedent
judicial review
  appealing OSHRC rulings, 64
  in command-and-control process, 213
  Federal Mine Safety and Health Review Commission, 330

judicial branch duty, 66
Mine Act (1977), 323, 324
OSHA standards overturned, 201, 611
OSHAct (Section 11), 216–217
precedence setting, 182–197
risk assessment approach, 37, 133, 638
The Jungle (Sinclair), 95, 116–117, 539
jurisdiction of OSHAct, 174, 369, 402

K

Kazakhstan
  asbestos labeling, 427
  asbestos mining, 439
  asbestos use, 437
  forced child labor, 453
Kehoe, Robert A., 102
Kemp, Roy Wyatt, 366
Kennedy, Justice Anthony, 75
Kennedy, Edward, 617–621
Kennedy, John F., 198
Kepone insecticide, 35–36, 46, 263
Kerr, Lorin E., 344, 346, 348, 609
Key, Marcus M., 278, 279, 281–282, 285, 296
King Coal (Sinclair), 116
Kleppinger, Karl, Jr., 366
knowledge. *See* education; information; training
Kohl, Herb, 552
Kravit, Daniel, 114
Krug, Julius Albert, 317
Kumho Tire Co. v. Carmichael (1999), 555
Kyrgyzstan
  asbestos labeling, 427
  asbestos use, 437
  forced child labor, 453

L

labeling. *See* hazard communication
labor law. *See also* labor movement
  applicable to Congress, 622
  child labor, 57. *See also* child labor
  code of conduct for multinationals, 76, 419, 452, 655
  international, 57, 648–649
  in law hierarchy, 52
  NAFTA, 423, 653
  National Labor Relations Act (1935), 98, 107, 381–382
  National Labor Relations Act (1947), 107
  statutory law, 65
  worker protection statutes, 381–383
  WTO labor standards, 421–422
labor movement. *See also* unions
  birth of, 91–92
  Great Upheaval, 96
  mutual aid societies, 92–93
  National Labor Relations Act (1935), 98, 107, 381–382
  National Labor Relations Act (1947), 107
  safety movement, 98–103
  trade unions legitimized, 97–98
  wage slavery, 95–98
  workday length, 93–95, 108, 341
Labor Policy Association, 626
Laborers International Union, 661
Lalonde, Marc, 18
LaMonica, Joseph A., 354–355
Landrigan, Philip J., 443
Landrum-Griffin Act (1959), 107
language
  "adulteration," 539
  "caution," 534–535
  "danger," 534–535
  "designated" personnel, 543
  "economic and social," 431
  economics glossary, 468
  "employee," 385
  "employer," 173
  "eradication" vs. "elimination," 24
  framing issues, 154
  "immediately dangerous," 282
  "incidents" vs. "accidents," 413–414
  levels of hazard warnings, 534–545
  "mislabeling," 539
  "person," 75, 173
  "reasonably necessary or appropriate," 133, 173, 178, 189–190, 639
  "recognized hazard," 152, 175
  "should" vs. "shall," 177, 413, 534
  "significant risk," 133, 178, 183, 189–190, 194, 638–640
  "train" and "instruct," 543, 545
  "warning," 534–535
Lanza, Anthony J., 269, 270, 271, 273, 335, 340
latency of disease
  asbestos, 158, 180, 487
  Bhopal catastrophe, 449
  cumulative trauma disorders, 660
  as externalized cost, 480
  OSHAct (Section 2), 259
  silent epidemics, 90–91, 350
  Systematic Occupational Health and Safety Management, 646
  undercounting, 4–5
  vinyl chloride, 159
  workers' compensation, 486–488
Latin America
  agricultural workers, 414
  asbestos use, 437
  DBCP pesticide exposure, 454
  occupational injuries/diseases, 417, 418
  OSHA and, 403

law. *See also* common law; Constitutional system; international law
  as behavior governed by norms, 51
  Code of Federal Regulations, 73
  deaths as felonies, 221, 223, 366, 658
  deaths as manslaughter, 235, 366
  deaths as misdemeanors, 221, 223, 658
  deposition, 548
  disaster (law), 313, 315, 316, 328
  discovery, 548–549, 552–553
  environmental law cost awareness, 35
  expert testimony, 553–555
  Federal Rules of Civil Procedure, 548
  hierarchy of, 52–53
  ILO recommendations, 407
  information disclosure restrictions, 549–555
  interrogatories, 548
  law of nations, 56–57. *See also* international law
  "person" vs. "individual," 74–75
  policy and, 599
  private property recognition, 555
  prosecution of workplace deaths, 21
  request for production, 549
  request of admission, 549
  Solicitor's Office, 606
  training as legal requirement, 29
  trial by judge, 553–555
  unlawful agency actions, 214
  workers' compensation statutes, 499–501
law of nations, 56–57. *See also* international law
lead
  air level testing, 129
  exempting construction, 182, 185, 205, 206, 585
  Healthy People Objectives (2020), 20
  history of occupational health, 85, 89, 90, 100, 265
  industry antiscience, 584–586
  IPCS dangerous chemicals, 411
  judicial review, 183, 184, 190
  lead paint, 205–206, 584–585
  leaded gasoline, 38, 102, 271, 585–586, 643
  National Emission Standards for Hazardous Air Pollutants, 246
  national emphasis programs, 228
  NIOSH recommended standards, 263, 264
  notifiable disease, 271
  prophylactic chelation, 283
  standards promulgated, 179, 205–206, 585
Lead Based Paint Poisoning Prevention Act (1971), 585
leadership
  advocacy and, 571–573
  contingency theory, 571, 646–647, 655
  effectiveness, 576
  ethical assessment of, 576. *See also* ethics
  informal leadership, 572
  the liking principle, 573
  NIOSH Marcus Key, 278, 279, 281–282, 285, 296
  NIOSH John Finklea, 282–287
  NIOSH Anthony Robbins, 285, 287–288, 296
  NIOSH J. Donald Millar, 285, 288–289, 296, 387, 389
  NIOSH Linda Rosenstock, 285, 290–291, 296, 406
  NIOSH John Howard, 285, 291–294
  OSHA administrators by president, 199
  OSHA directorates, 200
  persuasion, 573
  public health, 571–573, 576
  servant leadership, 571, 575
  situational leadership, 588–591. *See also* situational attribution
  social proof, 573
  transactional leadership, 571, 575
  transformational leadership, 571, 572, 575–576
Leahy, Patrick, 552
Leake, James P., 272
legislation. *See also* history
  conference committee, 60, 116, 144, 145–148
  Daniels bill, 114, 116, 142, 143–144
  energy workers, 372
  environmental protection, 377–381
  Exclusive Economic Zone (EEZ), 368–370
  Johnson worker protection, 112, 138–141, 142, 197, 198, 278, 609, 617
  legislation charts, 68, 107–108, 315, 500, 608
  legislation flowcharts, 142, 316
  mine disasters → law, 314–321, 328
  Nixon OSHAct proposal, 115, 141–144, 610
  Nixon OSHAct signing, 91, 116, 147, 170, 198, 599, 610
  originating statutes, 66
  OSHAct flowchart, 142
  regulation, 73
  spectrum of prevention, 25, 648–649
  as statutory law, 52
  Sullivan Hazardous Materials Safety Act, 137–139
  trade secret protection, 218
  transportation industry, 372–376
  United States Code (U.S.C.), 170
legislative branch. *See* Congress
Lemen, Richard, 442–443, 565–566
Letters of Agreement. *See* Memorandums of Understanding (MOUs) with OSHA
leukemia
  benzene, 136, 189, 190, 611
  global DALYs, 401
  work related, 22, 289
Lewis, John L., 314, 317, 337, 343, 344, 345

liability
    blaming the victim, 515, 577, 578
    DBCP pesticide, 454
    doctrine of enterprise liability, 55
    employer liability emergence, 103
    insurance for, 483
    joint-and-several, 503
    negligence vs. strict liability, 502
    no-fault workers' compensation, 103.
        See also fault
    as obstacle to safety, 447
    silicosis, 341
    strict liability, 55, 502-503
    tort liability, 501-505
    VCM in hairspray, 566
    warnings and, 534
life expectancy
    averages by country, 399
    U.S. residents, 599
lifestyle health as health field, 18-19
the liking principle, 573
Lincoln, Abraham, 548, 581-582
liquid natural gas (LNG) facilities, 375
Lloyd's of London, 505
local emphasis programs (LEPs), 228-229
local governments
    criminal prosecutions and OSHA, 234-239
    emergency response coordination, 405
    employees excluded, 173, 226, 258, 383-384, 483, 657, 658
    excluded as employer, 173, 367, 383-384
    Freedom of Information Act (FOIA), 67-68
    HazCom Standard, 202, 540
    in public health organization, 17
    state government creations, 57
locator beacons, 268, 390
Lochner v. New York (1905), 109, 110
logging operations
    NIOSH recommended standard, 263
    permanent standards, 177
    state standards, 226
Longshore and Harbor Workers' Compensation Act (1927), 172, 176, 383, 500
Louisiana Chemical Association v. Bingham (1981), 214
Louttit, Henry, 332
lowest detectable level policy, 281
Lowry, Mike, 390
lung cancer
    asbestos, 20, 37, 89, 91, 205, 438, 440, 441, 583, 584
    beryllium, 284, 583
    chrysotile, 440
    global DALYs, 401
    hexavalent chromium, 587
    as leading work-related disease, 289
    uranium mining, 90, 112, 160-161, 276, 371, 519
lung diseases. *See also* asbestos; coal workers' pneumoconiosis; lung cancer; silicosis
    byssinosis disease, 105, 158, 205, 289, 517, 659
    chronic obstructive pulmonary disease, 291, 401
    history of occupational health, 89, 90-91
    as leading work-related disease, 289
    national emphasis programs, 228
    NIOSH program review, 292, 294
    as notifiable diseases, 5, 15
    occupational disease, 17, 488
    standard promulgation, 179

M

Maastricht Treaty, 428-429
macroeconomics, 468, 473
mad hatter's disease, 38, 90, 272
Magnuson, Harold J., 160-161, 276
Main, Joseph A., 356
Maloney, Carolyn, 297-298
Maltoni, Cesare, 437, 566
mandatory standards "shall," 177, 413, 534
Manning, Van H., 335
manslaughter, 235, 366
Manuel, Keith Blair, 366
manufacturing
    Commerce Clause exclusion, 111
    deaths in self-employed vs. full-time, 386
    failure to warn, 533
    nanomaterials database, 419
    NORA research councils, 295
Manufacturing Chemists Association, 567
maritime standards, 171, 172
maritime workers and workers' comp, 486
marketplace
    compensating differential argument, 529-530
    cost analysis and, 506
    environmental law and, 35
    externalities, 477-480. *See also* externalizing costs
    free market and regulation, 156, 473, 479, 582
    free market and right-to-know, 532
    global worker safety, 651
    market justice, 155, 158-159, 491, 574, 577, 582, 588
    opportunities of regulation, 600
    perfect competition, 531-532
    public good and, 476, 652
    scarcity principle, 573, 615
    tort liability and, 502

willingness to pay, 468, 507
workers' comp monopoly versus, 482, 484, 485
Markey, Ed, 553
Markowitz, Gerald, 568
Marshall, George C., 418
Marshall, Ray, 187–188, 286
Marshall v. Barlow's Inc. (1978), 214, 300
Martin, Lynn, 355
Marx, Karl, 475
matches and phossy jaw, 65, 77–78, 87, 107, 269
matching fund state program grants, 262
material impairment
 air contaminants, 184
 asbestos, 187
 benzene, 184, 188–190, 657
 cotton dust, 187–188
 lead in blood, 183, 184, 190
 no employee will suffer, 133, 177, 178, 187–188, 189–190, 639
material safety data sheets (MSDSs)
 Emergency Planning and Community Right-to-Know Act, 541
 failure to warn response, 533
 Globally Harmonized System, 542–543, 544
 hazard communication issues, 536, 540
 trade secrets, 550
matter of fact, 64, 72
matter of law, 64, 72
Mauritania life expectancy, 399
Maximum Abbreviated Injury Scale, 510, 512
Mazzocchi, Tony, 609
McAteer, J. Davitt, 296, 346, 353
McCulloch v. Maryland (1819), 109
McDonald, Corbett, 441
McNamara, Robert, 415
McNamara-O'Hara Public Service Contract Act (1965), 106, 108, 174
McQuiggen, Howard, 610
McWane Corporation, 240–243
Meany, George, 113, 140, 147, 609
Meat Inspection Act (1906), 117, 539
medical mills, 517–518
medical records. *See also* recordkeeping
 access standard, 179
 NIOSH access to records, 300
 privacy rights, 557–558
 workers' compensation, 490
Medicare and Medicaid
 annual coverage amount, 479
 as externalized cost, 472, 477–478
 Social Security Disability Act (1956), 500
 state workers' comp fraud, 518
Meek, M. E., 441, 442, 443
Memorandums of Understanding (MOUs) with OSHA

 Department of Agriculture Extension Service, 386
 Department of Energy, 371–372
 Environmental Protection Agency, 379
 Federal Aviation Administration, 373–374
 international, 402–405
 Mine Safety and Health Administration, 331–332
 U.S. Coast Guard, 368
Merchant, James A., 387
Merchant Marine Act (Jones Act; 1917), 499, 500
mercury
 criminal prosecution, 236–237
 history of occupational health, 89, 100, 272
 IPCS dangerous chemicals, 411
 mad hatter's disease, 38, 90, 272
 NIOSH recommended standard, 263
MESA. *See* Mining Enforcement and Safety Administration
mesoeconomics, 469, 472, 473
mesothelioma
 asbestos related, 37, 89, 91, 205, 437, 438, 440, 441
 chrysotile related, 440
 history of occupational health, 89, 91
 as leading work-related disease, 289, 438
message framing. *See* framing of messages
metal and nonmetal MSHA activities, 329
Metal and Nonmetallic Mines Act (1961), 318–319, 341
metal poisoning. *See also* beryllium; hexavalent chromium; lead; mercury
 cadmium, 89, 179, 263, 411
 criminal prosecution, 236–237
 Healthy People Objectives (2020), 20
 history of occupational health, 85, 88, 89, 90, 100
 national emphasis programs, 228
 NIOSH recommended standard, 263
 as notifiable diseases, 6, 15, 269
 prophylactic chelation, 283
 standard promulgation, 179
metanarratives, 628–630
methane mine gas, 312, 334
metrics
 disability-adjusted life-years (DALYs), 400–401, 508
 quality-adjusted life-year (QALY), 508
Mexico
 agricultural workers, 414, 661
 asbestos importing, 439
 forced child labor, 453
 harmonization of industrial classification, 402
 NAFTA, 423, 424, 425
 OSHA and, 402–403

U.S.-Mexico Border Industrial Program, 422–423
World Trade Center compensation, 467
Michaels, David, 72, 199, 297, 402, 582
microeconomics, 468, 473
Middle East
  agricultural workers, 414
  life expectancy, 399
  occupational injuries/diseases, 417, 418
Migrant and Seasonal Agricultural Worker Protection Act (1983), 383
Milberg, William, 601
Milgram, Stanley, 569–570
Mill, John Stuart, 582
Millar, J. Donald, 285, 288–289, 296, 387, 389
Miller, Seward E., 275–276
mills. *See* steel industry; textile mills
mine disasters. *See also* miners
  BoM research into explosions, 102
  citations preceding, 658
  coal dust sampling, 350–356
  damps, 311–312, 332–333
  deaths of workers, 36, 99, 113, 141, 311–312, 314–321, 328, 332–333
  disaster (law), 313, 315, 316, 328
  Farmington, WV, explosion (1968), 36, 113, 141, 315, 320, 345, 348
  mine explosions, 36, 102, 113, 141, 311, 315–321, 320, 328, 332, 345, 348, 350
  mine gases, 311–312, 332–333
  Scofield, UT, explosion (1900), 311
  self-contained self-rescue (SCSR) devices, 312, 328
  Wilberg Mine, UT, fire (1984), 311–312
Mine Improvement and New Emergency Response Act (2006), 315, 316, 328–329
mine rescue teams, 324, 328
Mine Safety and Health Act (Mine Act; 1977)
  amending Coal Act (1969), 321–322
  appeals, 67, 323, 325, 330
  authorities flowchart, 324, 325
  CWP benefits, 323, 326, 327
  deaths reduction, 605
  general duty clause lack, 175, 325
  history of disaster → law, 313, 315, 316, 321–322
  history of early statutes, 314–321
  mine rescue teams, 324
  Mine Safety and Health Review Commission, 67, 325, 330
  NIOSH funding of research, 262, 279, 290
  OSHAct versus, 174, 331–332
  precedence over APA, 66
  titles and sections of, 322–328, 329, 330
Mine Safety and Health Administration (MSHA)
  authority of, 329
  certification by, 546
  coal dust sampling, 350–356
  Coal Mine Safety and Health program, 329
  creation of, 323, 324, 329, 354
  deaths of inspectors, 321
  in DoL, 67, 329
  employer/employee responsibilities, 175
  grants to states for compliance, 327–328
  IQA public health subversion, 72–73
  Joseph A. Holmes Safety Association, 546–547
  Metal and Nonmetal Mine Safety and Health, 329
  NIOSH miner programs, 279
  NIOSH recommended standards, 324
  OSHA versus, 174, 331–332
  Small Mine Office, 546
  structure of, 329–330
  training, 546–547
Mine Safety and Health Research Advisory Committee, 325
Mine Safety and Health Review Commission (MSHRC), 67, 325, 330, 355
Mine Safety Board Report (1963), 319
Mine-Mill. *See* International Union of Mine, Mill, and Smelter Workers
Minerals Management Service (MMS), 369, 370
miners. *See also* Bureau of Mines; coal workers; mine disasters; uranium mining
  asbestos deaths, 438
  child labor, 104–105
  China mine safety forum, 404
  Coal Act, 91, 107, 141. *See also* Coal Mine Health and Safety Act (1969)
  coal dust sampling, 350–356
  Commerce Clause exclusion, 111
  continuous mining, 90
  damps, 311–312, 332–333
  deaths of workers, 36, 99, 113, 141, 311–312, 314–321, 328, 332–333, 340, 345, 371, 546
  exclusion from OSHA, 174
  Federal Metal and Nonmetallic Mine Safety Act, 108
  in Great Britain, 103
  history of early statutes, 314–321
  history of occupational health, 85, 88, 90, 99, 275, 276
  inspection, 107, 108
  IQA public health subversion, 72–73
  Mine Act, 66, 67. *See also* Mine Safety and Health Act (1977)
  mine gases, 311–312, 332–333
  mine rescue teams, 324, 328
  Mine Safety Board Report (1963), 319
  miners' asthma, 341–342, 343–344
  Mining Safety in North America, 423
  mutual aid societies, 92–93

National Mine Health and Safety
  Academy, 321, 327, 330
NIOSH miner programs, 279
NIOSH program review, 292, 294
NIOSH recommended standards, 264, 265, 324
NORA research councils, 295
OSHAct creation, 113
radiation poisoning, 160–161. See also radiation poisoning
small mine exemption, 318, 319
statutory law, 65, 315
United Mine Workers Welfare and Retirement Fund, 342–344, 345–346
volunteer safety movement, 101
wage slavery, 95–96
workday length, 94, 104, 341
miners' asthma, 341–342, 343–344
minimum wage, 95, 108, 382
Mining Enforcement and Safety Administration (MESA)
  coal dust sampling, 354
  independence from BoM, 321, 338
  MSHA origins, 329, 354
misdemeanors
  deaths as, 221, 223, 658
  Mine Act (1977), 325–326
mission
  of CDC, 278
  of NIOSH, 278
  of OSHA, 198, 200–201, 259, 277, 600
  of OSHRC, 217
Mitchell, James, 138
Mitchell, John, 341
MMS. See Minerals Management Service
Moldova asbestos use, 437
Mondays and injuries, 517
moral hazards, 480
moral values
  ethical assessment of leader, 576
  ethics foundations, 579–581
  Hippocratic Corpus, 149, 582
  transformational leaders, 571
Mortality and Morbidity Weekly Report (CDC)
  notifiable diseases, 15, 269
  ROPS injury prevention, 387
Motor Carrier Safety Improvement Act (1999), 375–376
Moyers, Bill, 527, 565–568
MSD. See musculoskeletal disorders
MSDS. See material safety data sheets
MSHA. See Mine Safety and Health Administration
MSHRC. See Mine Safety and Health Review Commission
multiple employers, 172, 232–233, 385
munitions production, 270–271, 273–274

murder
  definition, 235
  UMWA candidate Yablonski, 349–350
  in workplace, 234–239, 608
Murray, H. Montague, 257
musculoskeletal disorders (MSDs). See also ergonomics
  Case Farms, 660–662
  costs of, 471, 472
  economic burden of, 194, 195, 627
  ergonomic violations program, 231
  global back pain DALYs, 401
  labor specialization, 475
  as leading work-related injury, 289, 471, 626
  A Proposed National Strategy for the Prevention of Musculoskeletal Injuries (NIOSH), 626
  as research priority, 291
  short-handled hoe, 586
  traumatogens, 660, 661
  workstation redesign, 38
mutual aid
  mutual aid societies, 92–93
  workers' compensation, 103

N

NAALC. See North American Agreement on Labor Cooperation
Nader, Ralph
  black lung movement, 113, 114, 141, 346
  Center for the Study of Responsive Law, 43–44, 45
  Johnson worker protection, 140
  Public Citizen, 128, 537
  Unsafe at Any Speed, 44
Nadler, Jerrold, 297, 552, 553
NAFTA. See North American Free Trade Agreement
nanomaterials safety database, 419
Napoleonic Code, 53
narrative analysis
  analytic narratives, 632–633
  metanarratives, 628–630
  narrative vs. paradigmatic thought, 628
  policy change theories, 630–632
  precautionary principle analysis, 633–637
NASA. See National Aeronautics and Space Administration
National Academy of Sciences, 292–294, 627
National Advisory Committee for Occupational Safety and Health (NACOSH), 180–181
National Advisory Committee on Ergonomics, 231
National Advisory Environmental Health Committee, 277

National Aeronautics and Space
    Administration (NASA), 591–593
National Association of Manufacturers
    in business coalition, 128, 195, 616
    ergonomics standard, 195, 626
    OSHAct creation, 142
National Board of Fire Underwriters, 101
National Bureau of Standards, 101
National Cancer Institute, 270
National Civic Association (NCA), 103
National Coalition on Ergonomics (NCE), 195,
    626–627, 631, 642
National Commission on State Workmen's
    Compensation Laws, 266–267,
    491–493
National Commission on the BP Deepwater
    Horizon Oil Spill and Offshore Drilling, 365,
    369, 590
National Council for Occupational Safety and
    Health, 617
national defense
    AEC workers' comp fraud, 518–519
    beryllium in atomic weapons, 284, 286
    federal control of coal mines, 317, 343
    variances and exemptions, 219
National Electrical Code, 176
National Electronic Injury Surveillance
    System, 46
National Emission Standards for Hazardous Air
    Pollutants (NESHAP), 246–247
national emphasis programs (NEPs), 227–228
National Environmental Policy Act (NEPA;
    1969), 41–42, 68–69
National Federation of Independent
    Business, 626
National Fire Protection Association, 101, 176
National Foundation on Arts and
    Humanities Act (1965), 106–107, 176
national government in public health organiza-
    tion, 17. See also United States (U.S.)
National Highway Traffic Safety
    Administration (NHTSA), 43, 44, 375
National Industrial Recovery Act (1935), 110
National Institute for Occupational Safety and
    Health (NIOSH)
    access to records authority, 299–300
    authority beyond OSHA, 258–259, 658
    beryllium exposure, 583
    Board of Scientific Councilors, 288
    BoM elimination, 290, 301, 322, 327, 338
    in CDC, 17, 62, 258, 262, 278, 288
    CDC reorganization, 282, 296–297
    congressional oversight, 60
    consensus standards organizations, 537
    constituencies of, 282
    creation of, 258, 262, 268, 270, 278
    Current Intelligence Bulletins, 283

CWP autopsies and X-rays, 326, 501
DBCP HHE, 538
director Marcus Key, 278, 279, 281–282,
    285, 296
director John Finklea, 282–287
director Anthony Robbins, 285, 287–288,
    296
director J. Donald Millar, 285, 288–289, 296,
    387, 389
director Linda Rosenstock, 285, 290–291,
    296, 406
director John Howard, 285, 291–294
education and research centers (ERCs),
    260–261, 284
emerging technologies, 290, 291
epidemiology approach, 281, 287, 288
ergonomics standard, 1, 195, 626
excluded workers coverage, 258, 658
executive branch oversight, 62–63
Ground Zero at WTC, 291, 297–298, 501
hazard communication, 535–537
Health Hazard Evaluations, 227, 538.
    See also Health Hazard Evaluations
inspection authority, 213–214, 260, 278, 284,
    300–301
IPCS and chrysotile, 442–443
Mine Act safety research, 262, 279, 290, 322,
    324–325, 326, 327
Mine Improvement and New Emergency
    Response Act, 328
National Occupational Hazard Survey, 281,
    550
National Occupational Research Agenda,
    290–291, 292, 294–295
Occupational Energy Research
    Program, 372
Office of Industrial Hygiene origins, 107
OMB interfering with, 606
as OSHAct creation, 17, 45, 115, 278, 281
Pocket Guide to Chemical Hazards (NIOSH/
    OSHA), 282, 283
Program Assessment Rating Tool, 292–294
Project MINERVA, 590–591
*A Proposed National Strategy for the Preven-
    tion of Musculoskeletal Injuries*, 626
public safety workers, 384
recommended standards, 213, 262,
    263–265, 281, 285, 610, 657
record access authority, 299–300
recordkeeping requirement, 260
Registry of Toxic Effects of Chemical Sub-
    stances, 37
research mission, 115, 278–279. *See also*
    research
research via Mine Act, 262, 279
respirator certification, 293, 299,
    326, 600

rollover protective structures (ROPS), 387–389
structure of, 279, 280
Total Worker Health™ program, 298
vinyl chloride, 568
National Institute of the Environmental Health Sciences (NIEHS), 287, 547
National Institutes of Health (NIH), 272, 274, 282, 374, 547
National Labor Relations Act (1935; NLRA), 98, 107, 110, 381–382, 532, 549
National Labor Relations Act (1947), 107
National Labor Relations Board (NLRB), 381, 549
National Mine Health and Safety Academy, 321, 327, 330
National Occupational Hazard Survey, 281, 550
National Occupational Research Agenda (NORA), 290–291, 292, 294–295
National Research Council, 292, 637
National Response Plan, 547–548
National Safety Council, 101, 480
National Toxicology Program (NIEHS), 287
National Traffic and Motor Vehicle Safety Act (1966), 44
National Traffic Safety Bureau, 44
National Transportation Safety Board (NTSB), 376, 390
Natural Gas Pipeline Safety Act (1968), 375
NCE. *See* National Coalition on Ergonomics
Needleman, Herbert, 585
needlestick injuries, 290
needs (economics), 468, 469, 575
needs assessment data, 131
negative externalities, 468, 478–479
negligence, 243, 366
Negotiated Rulemaking Act (RegNeg; 1990), 68, 69–70, 182
Nelson, Norton, 277–278
NEPA. *See* National Environmental Policy Act
Nepal forced child labor, 452, 453
New Directions Grants for training, 261
New York Bakeshop Act (1895), 110
news frames in messages, 155
NGOs. *See* nongovernmental organizations
Nicaragua
 DBCP pesticide exposure, 454–455
 forced child labor, 453
 OSHA and, 403
NIEHS. *See* National Institute of the Environmental Health Sciences
NIH. *See* National Institutes of Health
9/11 Health and Compensation Act (2010). *See also* terrorist attacks
 compensation, 510, 511
 overview, 467, 500, 501
NIOSH. *See* National Institute for Occupational Safety and Health

Nixon, Richard
 cancer cure, 192
 coal mine health and safety, 311, 348, 349
 EPA origins, 45
 federal employee occupational safety, 227
 lead paint, 585
 National Commission on State Workmen's Compensation Laws, 266
 OMB creation, 615
 OSHA policy, 199
 OSHAct proposal, 115, 141–144, 610
 OSHAct signing, 91, 116, 147, 170, 198, 599, 610
 "Quality of Life" review, 62
 workers' compensation, 491
NLRA. *See* National Labor Relations Act (1935)
no material impairment. *See* material impairment
no-fault. *See* fault
noise-induced hearing loss
 global DALYs, 401
 Healthy People Objectives (2020), 20
 history of occupational health, 88, 276
 judicial review, 184
 as leading work-related injury, 289
 Mine Act (1977), 326
 NIOSH program review, 292, 294
 NIOSH recommended standards, 263, 265
 OECD tractor certification, 419
 as research priority, 291
 standard promulgated, 179
 textile mill new equipment, 204
 workers' compensation, 488
non sequitur fallacy, 157
noneconomic damages, 503
nonfatal illnesses. *See* diseases; infectious diseases; occupational diseases
nonfatal injuries. *See* injuries
nongovernmental organizations (NGOs)
 Clean Clothes Campaign, 447
 Collegium Ramazzini, 398, 436–437
 definition, 435
 International Association of Labour Inspection, 436
 International Commission on Occupational Health (ICOH), 436
 International Organization for Standardization (ISO), 398, 435–436
nonprofit organizations
 NIEHS Worker Education and Training grants, 547
 Regulatory Flexibility Act, 68, 69
NORA. *See* National Occupational Research Agenda
North American Agreement on Labor Cooperation (NAALC), 423, 424, 426

North American Free Trade Agreement (NAFTA; 1994)
  complaints, 423–425
  enforcing global worker safety, 653
  health and safety language, 22, 426
  Mining Safety in North America, 423
  origins of, 422–423
North American Industry Classification System, 402
North Carolina v. Emmett Roe (1992), 237–238
Norway life expectancy, 399
notifiable diseases and injuries
  examples of, 5–6, 15, 269
  reported to CDC, 15
  workers' compensation, 485
Novello, Antonia C., 272
NTSB. *See* National Transportation Safety Board
nuclear energy
  International Atomic Energy Agency (IAEA), 398, 412–414, 422
  International Nuclear and Radiological Event Scale (INES), 413–414
  Nuclear Weapons Cleanup Training Program, 547
  nuclear worker programs, 372
  OECD risk comparison, 419
  reactor events, 414
  U.S. Atomic Energy Commission (AEC), 160, 371, 518–519, 583
nudges regulatory approach, 532

O

Obama, Barack
  agency operational guidance, 63
  drilling rig explosion, 365, 369
  enforcement, 212
  fishing vessel safety, 370
  MSHA director Main, 356
  NIOSH director Howard, 298
  OSHA administrator Michaels, 582
  OSHA policies, 199
  protecting citizens, 467
"Objectives for the Nation" (USPHS), 20
OCAW. *See* Oil, Chemical, and Atomic Workers Union
occupational diseases. *See also* asbestos; coal workers' pneumoconiosis; infectious diseases; lung diseases; metal poisoning; reproductive disorders; silicosis
  annually globally, 400, 401
  annually nationally, 3, 4–6, 17, 22, 471
  costs of, 471, 472
  definition, 5
  disability from, 4
  economic burden of, 399–401, 417, 418, 469–472
  GAO reports, 61
  Haddon matrix, 25–26
  history of, 85–89
  injury vs. disease compensation, 487
  judicial review, 182–185
  latency of diseases, 486–488. *See also* latency of disease
  leukemia, 22, 136, 189, 190, 289, 401, 611
  lifestyle affect on, 20
  Mortality and Morbidity Weekly Report, 269
  NAFTA labor principles, 423, 653
  NORA research councils, 295
  notifiable diseases, 5–6, 15, 269, 485
  OECD rates by country, 419
  opportunity costs of, 474
  public health achievements, 599
  public health ethic, 575
  Public Health Service Act, 607
  records requirement, 173. *See also* recordkeeping
  significant risk definition, 178, 638
  Total Worker Health™ program, 298
  USPHS authority, 317
  Voluntary Protection Program, 229–230, 590, 647, 659–660
  waterborne hazards, 25, 554
  workers' compensation, 486–488. *See also* workers' compensation
occupational health
  agencies other than OSHA, 367
  argument for regulations, 603–606
  asbestos as worst disaster, 504. *See also* asbestos
  code of conduct for multinationals, 76, 419, 655
  compliance analysis, 657–658
  congressional reports, 61
  effectiveness analysis, 658–659
  enforcement globally, 652–653
  implementation analysis, 656–657
  International Commission on Occupational Health, 436
  Internet for, 656
  judicial review, 182–185. *See also* judicial review
  OSHAct emergence, 111–116. *See also* history
  protection agencies, 13, 43–46
  public health achievements, 599–600
  public health ethic, 575
  public health of, 37–39, 269–270
  Social Security Act funding, 45, 88, 101, 272

INDEX | 767

standards promulgated, 179. *See also* standards
Systematic Occupational Health and Safety Management, 645–647, 655
waterborne hazards, 25, 554
Occupational Health and Safety Management Systems (ANSI/AIHA), 29
Occupational Health Program, 276
occupational injuries. *See* injuries
occupational medicine
"father" Bernardino Ramazzini, 85–86, 437
first physician Alice Hamilton, 88, 584
Occupational Mortality Supplement by the Registrar General, 87
occupational safety
agencies other than OSHA, 367
code of conduct for multinationals, 76, 419, 655
common law rights, 53
compliance analysis, 657–658
Conference on Occupational Safety, 106
Constitutional impact, 108–111
consumer safety from, 37–38
definition, 16
doctrine of enterprise liability, 55
effectiveness analysis, 658–659
enforcement globally, 652–653
GAO report, 61
general duty clause, 152, 171, 175, 178, 211–212, 233
history of, 87–88, 98–103. *See also* history; labor movement
implementation analysis, 656–657
injury pyramid, 106
Internet for, 656
judicial review, 182–185. *See also* judicial review
NAFTA labor principles, 423, 653
national emphasis programs, 228
national legislation evolution, 105–111
NORA research councils, 295
OSHAct emergence, 111–116. *See also* history
public health achievements, 599–600
public health ethic, 575
Safety First movement, 99
safety movement birth, 92, 98–99, 101
standards promulgated, 179. *See also* standards
Systematic Occupational Health and Safety Management, 645–647, 655
Total Worker Health™ program, 298
voluntary protection program, 229–230
waterborne hazards, 25, 554
Occupational Safety and Health Act (OSHAct; 1970)
annotated text of, 671–726

APA precedence, 66, 177
applicability of, 174, 369, 402
challenging rules of, 64, 67, 179, 180, 186, 214–215
command-and-control process flowchart, 213
conference committee, 145–148
congressional oversight, 60
creation of, 2, 45, 91, 111–116
criminal charges against employers, 64
definitions, 173
employers protect workers, 40, 175
enacted, 172–173, 198, 268
Frye report, 277
funding of, 200, 268, 384–385, 627
general duty clause, 152. *See also* general duty clause
goal of, 198, 200–201, 259, 277
hybrid rule making under, 66–67
as job killer, 247–248
judicial oversight, 64, 66, 182–197, 201, 216–217
jurisdiction of, 174, 369, 402
legislation flowchart, 142. *See also* history
Mine Act versus, 174, 331–332
OSHAct, 671–726
OSHAct (Section 1), 172
OSHAct (Section 2), 173, 185, 188, 259, 277
OSHAct (Section 3), 133, 173, 177, 189–190, 227, 232, 639
OSHAct (Section 4), 174–175, 233–234, 367, 368, 369, 372, 379, 491
OSHAct (Section 5), 175, 283, 604
OSHAct (Section 6), 133, 145, 146, 175–180, 186, 187–188, 189–190, 191, 205, 212, 214, 281, 528, 550, 610, 611, 639
OSHAct (Section 7), 180–182
OSHAct (Section 8), 213–215, 260, 266, 299, 300, 630
OSHAct (Section 9), 215
OSHAct (Section 10), 215–216
OSHAct (Section 11), 216–217, 232, 368, 375, 558
OSHAct (Section 12), 216, 217–218
OSHAct (Section 13), 218
OSHAct (Section 14), 218
OSHAct (Section 15), 218–219
OSHAct (Section 16), 219
OSHAct (Section 17), 219–225
OSHAct (Section 18), 225–226, 262
OSHAct (Section 19), 227
OSHAct (Section 20), 259–260, 262, 278, 294, 299
OSHAct (Section 21), 260–262, 278, 630
OSHAct (Section 22), 262, 278, 281
OSHAct (Section 23), 262
OSHAct (Section 24), 265–266

OSHAct (Sections 25–26), 266
OSHAct (Section 27), 266–267, 491
OSHAct (Section 28), 267
OSHAct (Sections 29–30), 267–268
OSHAct (Sections 31–34), 268
other federal agencies and, 174, 331–332, 367
paid employment as object of protection, 469
"person" definition, 75, 173
promise of, 600
right to refuse work, 216–217, 532–533, 558
text of, 671–726
Total Worker Health program, 298
United States Code citation, 170
variance from standards, 178, 180, 219
workman's compensation, 491
Occupational Safety and Health Administration (OSHA)
 ad hoc advisory committees, 69
 administrators of, 199, 200
 challenging rules of, 64, 67, 179, 180, 186, 214–215
 congressional oversight, 60
 congressional reports, 60–61
 creation of, 2, 17, 106, 173, 197–198, 267–268
 in DoL, 17, 45, 62, 67, 198
 environmental impact statements (EISs), 68–69
 ergonomics standard, 1–2, 71, 128, 179, 194–197, 588, 614, 657
 executive branch oversight, 62–63
 Hazardous Materials Transportation Act (HMTA; 1975), 374–375
 inspected vessels, 174, 368, 370
 inspection authority, 213–214, 300
 Interagency Regulatory Liaison Group, 36, 42–43, 169
 international policy, 402–406
 Memorandums of Understanding (MOUs), 331–332, 368, 371–372, 373–374, 379, 386, 402
 mission and resources gap, 624–625
 mission of, 198, 200–201, 259, 277, 600
 MSHA versus, 174, 331–332
 on-site inspection priority, 36
 penalties for violations, 21. *See also* penalties
 Pocket Guide to Chemical Hazards (NIOSH/OSHA), 282, 283
 policies by president, 199
 precedents of OSHA, 197–198
 reducing deaths and injuries, 200
 regional offices, 201
 situational leadership, 588–591. *See also* leadership
 strategic plan, 227–232
 structure of, 200–201, 225–226, 267–268
 training, 198, 260–262, 261, 278, 543, 545–546
 USPHS origins, 43, 45
Occupational Safety and Health Council. *See* Council of Occupational Safety and Health
Occupational Safety and Health Review Commission (OSHRC)
 appealing citations and penalties, 213, 216, 217
 appealing rulings, 64, 67, 116, 216, 217
 childbearing capacity, 211–212
 establishment of, 146, 268
 general duty when standard exists, 233
 joint enforcement actions, 243
 mission of, 217
 OSHAct (Section 12), 217–218
Occupational Tumors and Allied Diseases (Hueper), 89
OECD. *See* Organisation for Economic Co-operation and Development
Office of Dermatoses Investigations, 272
Office of Industrial Hygiene and Sanitation, 107, 270, 271, 272, 334
Office of Management and Budget (OMB)
 agency oversight, 62–63, 66, 68, 292, 606
 authority over rule making, 184, 185, 190–191
 creation by Richard Nixon, 615
 examiner, 133
 Information Quality Act, 68, 71–73
 interfering with NIOSH, 606
 Paperwork Reduction Act, 68, 70, 184, 190–191
 policy analysis, 606
 Program Assessment Rating Tool, 292
 requests for information from public, 68, 70
Office of Personnel Management, 67
Office of Technology Assessment (OTA)
 cost and feasibility of OSHA standards, 481, 641
 cost of VCM rule, 204
 ergonomics, 626
 issue analysis, 61
 Preventing Illness and Injury in the Workplace, 626
offices of OSHA geographic coverage, 201
offshore oil rigs, 365–370, 590
O'Hara, James, 140, 141, 144
Oil, Chemical, and Atomic Workers Union (OCAW), 8–9, 212, 527, 538, 540, 609
oil industry
 deaths among workers, 365–366, 369, 590
 drilling rig explosion, 365–366, 369, 590
 exclusion from OSHAct, 367, 368, 369–370

exemption from Mine Act (1977), 321
fracking, 151
history of occupational health, 90–91
Industrial Union Department v. American Petroleum Institute (1980), 178
NORA research councils, 295
offshore oil rigs, 365–370, 590
oil spills, 36, 365, 505
refinery explosions, 39–40, 245–246
O'Leary, Hazel R., 371
opportunity costs, 474
opportunity vs. threat framing, 154–155
ordnance production, 270–271, 273–274
Organic Act (1910), 107, 301, 313, 315–316
Organisation for Economic Co-operation and Development (OECD)
    code of conduct for businesses, 76, 419, 452, 655
    enforcing global worker safety, 653
    global worker safety, 650–654, 655
    hierarchy of controls, 27
    nuclear power risks, 419
    occupational health/safety role, 398, 418–419
organizational practices in spectrum of prevention, 25, 648–649
organized labor. *See* unions
Organized Migrants in Community Action, Inc. v. Brennan (1975), 378–379
OSHA. *See* Occupational Safety and Health Administration
OSHAct. *See* Occupational Safety and Health Act
OSHRC. *See* Occupational Safety and Health Review Commission
other-than-serious violations, 215, 221
Outer Continental Shelf Lands Act (1953), 368–369
oversight
    agencies by administrative law judges, 67
    agencies by GAO, 60
    agencies by OMB, 62–63, 66, 68, 292
    appropriations by Congress, 60
    audits in OSHAct, 266
    Federal Advisory Committee Act, 68, 69, 182
    Freedom of Information Act (FOIA), 67–68
    judicial, 64, 66, 182–185
    NIOSH program review, 292–294
    OSHA standards cost review, 481
    rule making under APA and OSHAct, 66–67
oxygen deficiency in mines, 312

P

paid employment as analysis factor, 468–469
pain and suffering
    externalities, 477–478
    human capital, 468, 506
    opportunity costs, 474
    tort liability, 472, 504
    willingness to pay, 468, 507
paint with lead, 205–206, 584–585
painters of clock faces, 90, 272
Pakistan forced child labor, 452, 453
Pan American Health Organization (PAHO), 409
Paperwork Reduction Act (PRA; 1995), 68, 70, 184, 190–191, 202, 613
paradigmatic analysis
    economic analysis, 641–645
    narrative vs. paradigmatic thought, 628
    prospective analysis, 640–641
    risk assessment, 637–640
parallel arguments, 145, 147, 148
paramedic training, 261. *See also* emergency responders
parliamentary system, 52–53
participation in policy, 654–656
partnerships. *See* coalitions
Patient Protection and Affordable Care Act (2010), 499
Patty, Frank A., 337
Patty's Industrial Hygiene and Toxicology, 337
Pelosi, Nancy, 627
PELs. *See* permissible exposure limits
penalties
    average (2009), 21
    BP oil rig explosion, 366
    Bureau of Mines authorization, 108, 318, 338
    citation not posted, 220
    civil penalties, 219–221, 329, 349, 351, 378
    Coal Act (1969), 349
    coal dust sampling, 351
    in command-and-control process, 213
    criminal penalties, 221, 223–225, 239, 378. *See also* criminal prosecution
    egregious-case policy for civil, 220–221, 222–223
    fishing vessel safety, 370
    Javits's amendment, 144, 146
    maximum civil, 219, 220
    Mine Act (1977), 323, 324, 325
    MSHA authority, 329, 354
    NAFTA, 423, 653
    pesticides, 36, 378, 450
    serious violations, 21, 219
    WTO dispute settlements, 421
Pendergrass, John A., 199, 235
People of the State of New York v. William Pymm, et al. (1987), 236–237
perfect competition, 531–532
Perkins, Carl, 320, 338
Perkins, Frances, 88, 197

permanent standards
  in command-and-control process, 213
  employer compliance, 171
  overview, 177–179, 604
  for temporary standards, 179, 186
permissible exposure limits (PELs)
  benzene, 189, 611
  generic rule making, 185, 191, 611–612
  as interim standards, 191
  lead, 205, 206
  lowest detectable level policy, 281
  Standards Completion Program (SCP), 281–282
"person" and corporations, 74, 75–76, 173, 235, 236
"person" vs. "individual," 74–75
personal protective equipment (PPE)
  blamed for death, 449
  BoM gas mask production, 336
  consumer safety occupational origins, 37
  control technology over PPE, 27, 182
  DBCP pesticide production, 454
  failure to warn, 533
  last line of defense, 28–29, 171, 187
  market for, 600
  National Response Plan, 548
  NIOSH miner programs, 279
  NIOSH program review, 292, 293
  self-contained self-rescue (SCSR) devices, 312, 328
  workers pay for, 660
persuasion, 572, 573
Peru
  forced child labor, 453
  OSHA and, 403
pesticides
  applicator examinations, 378
  Bhopal (India) disaster, 220, 245–246, 449–451, 541
  deaths annually, 426
  deaths in India, 414
  Delaney Clause, 634
  in developing economies, 22
  dibromochloropropane (DBCP), 452–455, 527–528, 535, 537–538, 610, 634, 659
  Federal Insecticide, Fungicide, and Rodenticide Act, 181, 378–379, 643–644
  global poisonings, 414–415
  history of occupational health, 89, 588
  IPCS dangerous chemicals, 411
  Kepone insecticide, 35–36, 46, 263
  labeling containers, 378, 379
  as notifiable disease, 6, 15
  Oil, Chemical, and Atomic Workers Union, 8–9, 212, 527, 538, 540, 609
  Rotterdam Convention, 426–427
  Silent Spring, 37

Standards Advisory Committee on Agriculture, 181–182
Peterson, Esther, 138, 610
petrochemical industry. *See* oil industry
PHI. *See* protected health information
Philippines
  DBCP pesticide exposure, 454
  forced child labor, 453
  OSHA and, 405
phosgene leaks, 449
phosphorus necrosis ("phossy jaw"), 77–78, 87, 107, 269, 607
phthisis, 339
pictogram of skull and crossbones, 542
Pipeline Safety Improvement Act (2002), 375
plaintiff in court case names, 65
Plinius Secundus (Pliny the Elder), 85
pneumoconiosis. *See* coal workers' pneumoconiosis
Pocket Guide to Chemical Hazards (NIOSH/OSHA), 282, 283
Poison Prevention Packaging Act (1970), 46
poisons. *See also* hazard communication
  IPCS global poison centers, 411
  notifiable diseases, 6, 15
  "poison" label, 534, 539, 542
policy advocacy. *See* advocacy
policy analysis
  accountability, 654–656
  argument for regulations, 603–606
  bills of Gregg vs. Ballenger, 622–625, 629–630
  bills of Kennedy vs. Ford, 617–621
  compliance analysis, 657–658
  Contract With America, 621–625
  cost analysis, 505–512. *See also* costs
  definition of analysis, 601
  definition of policy, 3, 600
  definition of policy analysis, 602
  economic analysis, 641–645
  effectiveness analysis, 658–659
  ergonomics, 625–627, 630–632, 642–643. *See also* ergonomics
  global policy, 645–656
  implementation analysis, 656–657
  law and policy, 599
  mobility of capital, 648, 649–650
  moral foundations, 580
  narrative analysis, 627–637
  paid employment as factor, 468–469
  paradigmatic analysis, 628, 637–645
  participation in policy, 654–656
  "policy" and "police," 3
  politics and, 614–627. *See also* politics
  precautionary principle, 633–637. *See also* precautionary principle

for public health advocates, 130
transitions in policy, 606–614
policy making
  complexity of, 9, 614, 615
  context, inputs, process, products (CIPP), 153–154
  cost analysis, 505–512. See also costs
  cost-benefit analysis, 507, 642. See also cost-benefit analysis
  economic efficiency of incentives, 480–481. See also incentives
  European Union, 429–430
  history's importance, 84
  ICOH scientific objectivity, 436
  judicial review importance, 64, 182–184
  OSHA policies by president, 199
  prevention policy fallacies, 156–158
  spectrum of prevention, 25, 648–649
  stages of, 153
  values before issues, 579, 580
policy networks, 132, 133, 572
politics
  bills of Gregg vs. Ballenger, 622–625, 629–630
  bills of Kennedy vs. Ford, 618–621
  chrysotile asbestos safety, 440–443, 445, 584
  as coalition of human activity, 114
  Contract With America, 621–625
  cost-benefit analysis neutrality, 507
  ergonomics standard, 194–197
  explanatory perspective of policy, 397
  intuitive primacy principle, 580
  policy analysis, 606, 614–627
  as policy-making stage, 153
  public health as, 3, 128
  regulatory politics framework, 608
  of right-to-know, 532–533
"polluter pays" principle
  employer not government duty, 40, 175
  EU environmental policy, 429
  hierarchy of controls, 27
Pollution Prevention Act (PPA; 1990), 41
polyvinyl chloride (PVC), 566
positive externalities, 468, 478, 479, 658
Pott, Percival, 86
poverty
  global prevalence, 647
  jobs to escape, 249, 446–448, 468, 647, 649
  War on Poverty, 346
  World Bank, 415, 416
PPE. See personal protective equipment
precautionary principle
  abductive reasoning at core, 127, 149, 151
  artificial intelligence and, 150–151
  blaming the victim versus, 578
  definition, 149, 633, 634
  EU policy, 429, 634–635, 646

  as narrative analysis approach, 634
  policy analysis, 633–637
  REACH risk assessment, 434–435
  right-to-know as, 528
  scientific uncertainty, 148–149
  sustainable world economic growth, 422
  Systematic Occupational Health and Safety Management, 646
  Wisconsin Industrial Commission Act (1911), 152
precedence. See also judicial review
  common law adjudication, 53, 54–55, 64
  federal agencies and OSHAct, 174
  international law perspective, 396–397
  matters of law, 64, 72
  "no material impairment," 187
  OSHAct over APA, 66, 177
  over general industry standards, 171
  unlawful agency actions, 214
Pregnancy Discrimination Act (1978), 211–212, 248–249
present value, 508, 509, 510, 511
Preventing Illness and Injury in the Workplace (OTA), 626
prevention
  Collegium Ramazzini, 437
  compensation laws as incentives, 493, 495, 497–498
  compliance analysis, 657–658
  cost savings of, 18, 204, 247–248, 410, 469–472, 480–481
  as direct cost, 470
  doctrine of enterprise liability, 55
  effectiveness analysis, 658–659
  efficiency and, 642–643
  enemies of, 158–159
  EPA Gold Book challenged, 72
  fallacies of, 156–158
  financial incentives for, 102–103
  Haddon matrix, 25–26
  hidden successes of, 606–607
  hierarchy of controls, 26–29
  implementation analysis, 656–657
  intervention for, 17–18, 23, 102
  levels of, 17–18
  long latency hazards, 486–487, 646. See also latency of disease
  models of, 23–29
  "Objectives for the Nation" (USPHS), 20
  recognized hazards as preventable, 175
  spectrum of prevention, 24–25, 648–649
  surveillance-containment model, 23–24
  Systematic Occupational Health and Safety Management, 646–647
primary prevention
  public health intervention, 17–18, 659
  WHO Global Plan of Action, 410

prime contractors and subcontractors,
    232–233
principle of beneficence, 532, 574
privacy
    discovery and, 548, 553
    medical records, 490
    NIOSH access to records, 299
    Privacy Act (1974), 557
    Privacy Rule (DHHS), 557–558
    protected health information, 557–558
    right of, 555–558
    right to enter, 257–258, 269
    secret settlements, 551–553
    trade secrets, 219, 549–551
    zone of privacy, 556–557
private property legal recognition, 555
Process Safety Management of Highly Hazardous Chemicals (PSM) standard (1992),
    39–40
professionals. See healthcare workers
Program Assessment Rating Tool (PART),
    292–294
"Prohibition of Acquition of Products Produced by Forced or Indentured Child Labor" (1999),
    452
Project MINERVA (NIOSH), 590–591
prosecution. See criminal prosecution
protected health information (PHI), 557–558
Protecting the Health of Eighty Million Americans (USPHS), 139, 277–278, 609
protection agencies, 13, 43–46
providers. See healthcare workers; hospitals
Proxmire, William, 181
psychology. See also situational attribution
    confirmation bias, 573
    contingency theory, 571, 646–647, 655
    fundamental attribution error, 515, 577
    the liking principle, 573
    market justice, 155, 158–159, 491, 574, 577,
        582, 588
    persuasion, 572, 573
    reciprocity, 573
    scarcity principle, 573, 615
    social proof, 573
Public Citizen, 128, 537
public comment. See also hearings
    EIS recommendations, 69
    ergonomic standard, 196
    Federal Register, 66, 68, 177
    Regulatory Fairness Program, 71
    Regulatory Flexibility Act, 68, 69
    rule making, 66
    state submitted plans, 225
public health. See also public health agencies
    achievements of, 599–600
    advocates, 127–137. See also advocacy
    argument for regulations, 603–606

"Belmont Report" (1979), 530–531, 574
    coalitions within, 25, 128, 572
    compliance analysis, 657–658
    controversy, 129–130. See also
        controversy
    cost analysis, 505–512. See also costs
    economic analysis, 641–645. See also
        economics
    economic expertise versus, 651
    effectiveness analysis, 658–659
    ethics, 574–575
    evidence based, 135
    federal involvement expansion, 109
    framework per IOM, 6, 7, 16–17
    goal per IOM, 15
    health fields model, 18–20
    hidden successes of, 606–607
    implementation analysis, 656–657
    Internet for advocacy, 656
    leadership, 571–573, 576. See also
        leadership
    morality foundations, 581
    movement origins, 87
    occupational health as, 37–39, 269–270
    occupational safety as, 599–600
    policy determinants, 16
    as politics, 3, 128
    prevention models, 23–29. See also prevention
    private gain versus, 540, 588, 649
    protection agencies, 13, 43–46
    Public Health Service Act (1912), 107,
        269–270
    sealed court records, 552
    statutory authority to protect, 65
    subversion by Information Quality Act,
        71–73
    U.S. Public Health Service formation,
        15, 107
public health agencies
    authority via OSHAct definitions, 173
    early agencies, 269–278
    levels of organization, 17
    movement to protection agencies, 13, 43
    oversight of, 60, 62–63, 66, 67, 68
    unlawful actions, 214
Public Health and Marine-Hospital Service, 333
public health law in law hierarchy, 52
public health professionals as advocates,
    127–137
Public Health Service Act (1912), 107, 269–270,
    607
public hearings. See hearings
public safety worker NIOSH research, 384
pump handle cholera control, 554
Pure Food and Drug Act (1906), 539
PVC (polyvinyl chloride), 566

Q

Quality of Life initiative, 112
quality-adjusted life-year (QALY), 508

R

r2p (research-to-practice), 291, 295
Radiation Exposure Compensation Act (1990), 499, 500, 501, 519
radiation poisoning
  airport security, 38
  clock face painters, 90, 272
  Energy Employees Occupational Illness Compensation Program, 501
  Federal Radiation Council, 161, 371
  history of occupational health, 89
  lung cancer, 90, 112, 160–161
  NIOSH Occupational Energy Research Program, 372
  as notifiable disease, 6
  Radiation Exposure Compensation Act (1990), 519
  uranium mining, 160–161, 518–519
radioactive material
  IAEA agreement, 422
  International Atomic Energy Agency, 398, 412–414
  International Nuclear and Radiological Event Scale (INES), 413–414
radon
  Indoor Radon Abatement Act, 37
  mining radiation poisoning, 37, 90, 160, 371, 519
  NIOSH recommended standards, 264
Rail Safety Act (1970), 373
railroads
  "coupler bill," 87–88, 107, 111, 373
  deaths of workers, 54, 99, 102
  mutual aid societies, 92
  NLRA exclusion, 381
  Railway Labor Act, 107
  volunteer safety movement, 101
  wage slavery, 96–97
  workers' compensation, 486
Railway Labor Act (1926), 107
Railway Safety Appliance Act (1893), 87–88, 107, 111, 373
Ramazzini, Bernardino, 85–86, 437
Rasmussen, Donald L., 345, 346, 348
Rau, Wolfgang Thomas, 29
REACH. See Registration, Evaluation, Authorization, and Restriction of Chemicals
Reagan, Ronald
  agency operational guidance, 63
  asbestos regulation, 380

egregious-case policy for civil penalties, 220
Exclusive Economic Zone (EEZ), 368–370
formaldehyde EPA draft notice, 169–170
hazard communication, 535, 537
HHS secretary Schweiker, 288
IRLG disbanded, 43
OSHA policy, 199
regulation elimination, 9, 202, 354, 608, 612
short-handled hoe, 586
trust but verify, 211
reasonably necessary or appropriate standards, 133, 173, 178, 189–190, 639
reasoning
  abductive reasoning, 127, 149–152
  as critical thinking, 127
  inductive reasoning, 127, 149, 150
  intuitive primacy principle, 579
  Type I and II errors, 151–152
reciprocity, 573
"recognized hazards," 152, 175
recommended standards
  in command-and-control process, 213
  International Labour Organization, 407
  Mine Act (1977), 324
  MSHA action required, 324
  number of by NIOSH directors, 285
  OSHAct (Section 22), 262, 281
  "should," 177, 413, 534
  submitted to OSHA/MSHA, 263–265, 610, 657
recordkeeping. See also medical records
  American Standard Method of Measuring and Recording Work Injury Experience (ANSI), 265
  ergonomics violations, 231
  inspection of, 173, 213–214, 299–300
  Mine Act (1977), 323
  national emphasis programs, 228
  OSHA mission, 259, 265–266
  OSHAct (Section 20), 260
  OSHAct (Section 24), 265–266
  "records-check" inspection policy, 220
  requirement to maintain, 173, 214, 266
  standards vs. regulations, 215
red herring fallacy, 157
red phosphorus matches, 77, 87
reference citations
  OSHAct statute citation, 170
  regulation citation, 170–171
  United States Code citation, 170
refinery explosions, 39–40, 245–246
Refrigerator Safety Act (1956), 46
refusal to work, 216–217, 532–533, 558
Refuse Act (1899), 46
regional offices of OSHA, 201

Registration, Evaluation, Authorization, and Restriction of Chemicals (REACH), 431, 434–435
registries of toxic substances. *See* Agency for Toxic Substances and Disease Registry; International Register of Potentially Toxic Chemicals; Registration, Evaluation, Authorization, and Restriction of Chemicals (REACH); Registry of Toxic Effects of Chemical Substances; Toxics Release Inventory
Registry of Toxic Effects of Chemical Substances (RTECS), 37, 260
RegNeg. *See* Negotiated Rulemaking Act (1990)
regulations
    Administrative Procedures Act, 65, 66
    argument for, 603–606
    Code of Federal Regulations codification, 73, 170–171
    Congressional Review Act, 68, 70–71, 625
    cost-benefit analysis, 507
    CPSC vs. OSHA, 378
    cybernetics feedback loop, 73
    EU policies, 429–430
    Federal Register publication, 62, 66, 73
    free market and, 156, 473, 479, 582
    global worker safety, 652–653
    judicial review, 182–197
    litigation vs. regulation, 505
    as market opportunities, 600
    as mesoeconomics, 473
    MSHA authority, 329
    NAFTA, 423, 653
    negative externalities, 478–479
    nudges, 532
    OSHA hybrid regulatory-voluntary, 647
    path from risk to standard, 169–170
    Regulatory Fairness Program, 71
    Regulatory Flexibility Act, 68, 69
    regulatory procedure vs. APA, 66, 67
    standards versus, 214–215
    state regulations in history, 99–100
Regulatory Flexibility Act (1980), 68, 69, 202, 613
rehabilitation
    as tertiary prevention, 18, 659
    workers' compensation, 488, 490
Rehnquist, Associate Justice William, 76
Reich, Robert, 630
Reid, Harry, 205–206
releases of hazardous materials, 245–246, 540, 541, 547
repeated violations
    civil penalties for, 221
    definition, 215, 221
    maximum civil penalties, 220

Severe Violator Enforcement Program, 231–232
repetitive motion disorders
    See also ergonomics
    Case Farm, 660–662
    occupational disease, 488
    trauma disorders of, 195, 660
reportable diseases and injuries. *See* notifiable diseases and injuries
reporting on safety/health. *See* recordkeeping
reproductive disorders
    American Cyanamid, 211–212
    Bhopal pesticide catastrophe, 450
    blood lead levels, 248–249
    congenital malformations, 6, 450
    dibromochloropropane (DBCP), 452–455, 527–528, 535, 537–538
    as leading work-related diseases, 289
    Oil, Chemical, and Atomic Workers Union, 8–9, 212, 527, 538, 540, 609
    OTA reports, 61
    privacy rights, 557
    as research priority, 291
request for production, 549
request of admission, 549
research. *See also* recordkeeping
    "Belmont Report" (1979), 530–531, 574
    Bureau of Mines, 102, 107, 334–335, 337
    Coal Act (1969), 349
    Collegium Ramazzini, 436–437
    Department of Health, Education, and Welfare, 112
    ethical, 530–531, 574
    EU-OSHA, 433–434
    funding of, 262
    ignorance as driver of, 159
    methods as research priority, 291
    Mine Act (1977), 322, 323, 324, 325
    Mine Safety and Health Research Advisory Committee, 325
    Mine Safety Board Report (1963), 319
    miner health standards, 320
    National Occupational Research Agenda, 290–291, 292, 294–295
    NIOSH conducting, 115, 278–279, 281–282
    NIOSH director Marcus Key, 278, 279, 281–282, 285, 296
    NIOSH director John Finklea, 282–287
    NIOSH director Anthony Robbins, 285, 287–288, 296
    NIOSH director J. Donald Millar, 285, 288–289, 296, 387, 389
    NIOSH director Linda Rosenstock, 285, 290–291, 296, 406
    NIOSH director John Howard, 285, 291–294
    NIOSH inspection authority, 213–214, 260, 278, 300–301

NIOSH Mine Act safety research, 262, 279, 290
NIOSH Occupational Energy Research Program, 372
NIOSH on public safety workers, 384
norms changing via law, 398
OSHA mission, 259
OSHAct (Section 20), 259–260, 278
in public health framework, 6, 7, 16–17
research-to-practice (r2p), 291, 295
self-contained self-rescue devices, 312
silicosis, 269, 339–341
Social Security Act funding, 272
training program for, 395
World Health Organization, 409
during World Wars, 270–278
Research Councils, 294–295
research-to-practice (r2p), 291, 295
Residential Lead-Based Paint Hazard Reduction Act (1992), 205–206
resolution of issues
advocacy, 132–134
cancer standard, 193
institutional legitimacy, 651
OSHAct conference committee, 145–148
Resource Conservation and Recovery Act (RCRA; 1976), 241, 243–245, 246
respirators
asbestos, 180
BoM military research, 336
certification of, 293, 299, 326, 600
coal dust, 348
lead, 190
National Response Plan, 548
Personal Protective Technology (PPT) program, 293
vinyl chloride, 186
respiratory protection standard promulgation, 179. *See also* lung cancer; lung diseases
Revette, Dewey A., 366
Richardson, Elliot, 279
right-of-entry
NIOSH inspections, 213–214, 260, 278, 284, 300–301
OSHA inspections, 213–214
rights and duties
doctrine of judicial precedent, 53, 54–55, 64
employer–employee relationship, 52, 530
international worker rights, 402–405
market justice, 155, 158–159, 491, 574, 577, 582, 588
privacy rights, 555–558
refusal to work, 216–217, 532–533, 558
right-to-know. *See also* hazard communication; information
Bhopal (India) catastrophe, 451, 541
community right-to-know, 538, 540–541

compensating differential argument, 529–530
discovery (law), 548–549, 552–553
economic rationale, 531–532
Emergency Planning and Community Right-to-Know Act, 38, 530, 535, 540, 550–551
failure to warn, 533
hazard communication, 535–540. *See also* hazard communication
moral rationale, 530–531
NIOSH leader Anthony Robbins, 287
origin of, 8–9, 527–528, 538
political rationale, 532–533
precautionary principle, 528
warnings, 533–535
risk. *See also* uncertainty
assessment methods as research priority, 291
assumption of risk, 55, 102, 103
beneficence principle, 532
citations grouped by, 215
classification of occupations, 494
code of conduct for multinationals, 76
Collegium Ramazzini, 437
externalizing, 451
framing as threat vs. opportunity, 154
hazard communication, 535. *See also* hazard communication
hierarchy of controls, 26–29, 171, 187
intervention as primary prevention, 17–18
judgment of risk management, 258
moral hazard, 480
Process Safety Management of Highly Hazardous Chemicals standard, 39–40
risk assessment approach, 37, 133, 637–641
risk transfer of asbestos, 437–440
risk transfer of factory hazards, 446–448
Sentinel Event Notification System for Occupational Risk program (NIOSH), 288
significant risk, 133, 178, 183, 189–190, 194, 638–640
violation categories, 215
Robbins, Anthony, 285, 287–288, 296
Roche, Josephine, 343
Roe v. Wade (1972), 557
Roland, Robert E., 199
rollover protective structures (ROPS)
deaths from overturns, 586
industry antiscience, 586
NIOSH report (1993), 387–389
OECD tractor certification, 419
policy synergism, 38
Standards Advisory Committee on Agriculture, 181
Roosevelt, Franklin D.
Atlantic Charter, 406

Federal Interdepartmental Safety Council, 198
National Industrial Recovery Act, 110
New Deal, 607
Roche and national health insurance, 343
union elections, 98
Roosevelt, Theodore
 BoM establishment, 333
 lauds occupational safety/health, 100
 miners' asthma, 341
 Square Deal, 607
ROPS. *See* rollover protective structures
Rosenstock, Linda, 285, 290–291, 296, 406
Roshto, Shane M., 366
Rosner, David, 566, 568
Ross, Dan, 566, 568
Rotterdam Convention (1998), 426–427, 440
Rucker, W. Colby, 333
rule making
 APA formal and informal, 66–67, 178
 carcinogens, 192–193
 challenging rules of OSHAct, 64, 67, 179, 180, 186, 214–215
 Congressional Review Act, 68, 70–71, 625
 ergonomics standard, 196
 Mine Act (1977), 324–325
 Negotiated Rulemaking Act, 68, 69–70, 182
 OMB authority, 184, 185, 190–191
 OSHAct conference committee, 147
 path from risk to enforcement, 213
 path from risk to standard, 169–170
 public information strategies as, 72
 questions to ask, 605
 Regulatory Flexibility Act, 68, 69
 risk assessment requirement, 133
 slowdown of, 201–202
 standards, 176, 177–178, 213
 standards vs. regulations, 214–215
Russia
 asbestos labeling, 427, 440
 asbestos mining, 439
 asbestos use, 437
 forced child labor, 453
 life expectancy, 399

S

Safeguards Agreement in GATT, 651–653
safety. *See* occupational safety
Safety and Health Recognition and Achievement Program (SHARP), 261–262
Safety Appliance Act (1893). *See* Railway Safety Appliance Act (1893)
safety data sheets (SDSs). *See* material safety data sheets (MSDSs)
Safety First movement, 99
safety movement birth, 92, 98–99, 101. *See also* history
Safety of Life at Sea (SOLAS), 411–412
Salazar, Ken, 370
salience of issues, 606
Salvation Army matches, 77, 87
San Francisco City and County v. Digital Pre-Press International (2012), 238–239
The Sanitary Condition of the Labouring Population of Britain (Chadwick), 87
Sayers, Royd R., 272, 335, 337, 343
Scalia, Eugene, 631, 642
Scannell, Gerald, 199, 296–297
scapegoating fallacy, 157
scarcity principle, 573, 615
Schereschewsky, Joseph W., 270
school asbestos exposure, 380, 439
Schwartz, Louis, 272
Schweiker, Richard, 287–288
science. *See* applied science
scope of OSHAct, 174
SDS. *See* material safety data sheets (MSDSs)
sealed court records, 551–553
seamen and USCG vs. OSHA, 368, 370
search warrants for inspections, 147, 214, 223
seat belts, 28, 387, 388
Sebelius, Kathleen, 298
secondary prevention, 18, 659
secret settlements, 551–553
self-contained self-rescue (SCSR) devices, 312, 328
self-employed workers
 deaths among, 385–386
 exclusion from OSHAct, 367, 385–387, 657
 exclusion from workers' compensation, 486
 multiple employers, 172, 232–233, 385
 National Traumatic Occupational Fatality system, 288
 NIOSH program review, 294
 NORA research councils, 295
 unincorporated vs. incorporated, 386
Selikoff, Irving J., 89, 140, 437, 565, 583–584
Sellers, Gary, 113, 141, 346
Senate in Congress, 59, 64
Sensor, David, 282, 283, 284
Sentencing Reform Act (1984), 223, 225
Sentinel Event Notification System for Occupational Risk program (NIOSH), 288
September 11. *See* terrorist attacks
series argument, 140, 145
serious violations
 civil penalties for, 221
 definition, 215, 221
 maximum civil penalties, 220
serpentine asbestos, 439–440. *See also* asbestos

INDEX

servant leadership, 571, 575
services (economics), 468
settlements as secret, 551–553
Severe Violator Enforcement Program, 231–232
Sewell, Marilyn, 365
Shalala, Donna, 290
"shall" vs. "should," 177, 413, 534
Sharp, Gerald, 352, 354
Sheehan, Jack, 114, 115, 279, 609, 610
shipping vessels, 411–412
short-handled hoe, 586–587
"should" vs. "shall," 177, 413, 534
significance of errors, 151
significant risk, 133, 178, 183, 189–190, 194, 638–640
Silent Spring (Carson), 37, 89
silicosis
    BoM research, 269, 270, 334, 339–341
    coal dust limits, 356
    germ theory, 339–340
    Hawks Nest Tunnel, WV, 197
    history of occupational health, 17, 90, 276, 588
    as leading work-related disease, 289
    Metal and Nonmetallic Mines Act, 319
    Mine Act (1977), 326
    National Conference on Silicosis, 197
    NIOSH recommended standard, 263
    as notifiable disease, 15, 269
    sand blasting media, 158
Sinclair, Upton, 95, 116–117, 539
Single European Act (SEA; 1987), 427–428, 430, 431
situational attribution
    contingency theory, 571, 646–647, 655
    Deepwater Horizon as, 590
    explanation, 569–570
    fundamental attribution error, 515, 577
    situational leadership, 588–591
    well-meaning people harming, 603
skill training. *See* education
skin diseases, 20, 272, 289, 488
skull and crossbones, 542
slavery and forced child labor, 451–452, 453
slippery slope fallacy, 157
Small Business Act (1958), 267, 328
Small Business Regulatory Enforcement Fairness Act (1996), 68, 71, 196, 202, 613
Small Business Survival Committee, 626
small businesses. *See also* employers
    exemptions from OSHA, 268, 384, 385
    financial assistance, 267
    impact of rules, 68, 69, 71
    Mine Act compliance financial assistance, 327, 328
    OSHA consultation program, 260, 261, 590, 630

OSHAct (Section 28), 267
Safety and Health Recognition and Achievement Program (SHARP), 261–262
small farm exemption, 182, 268, 384, 385
small mine exemption, 318, 319
Small Mine Office of MSHA, 546
training guidelines, 543, 545–546
workers' compensation, 486, 492
workers' compensation insurance pools, 495–496, 659
smallpox
    eradication of, 24
    statutory law, 65
    surveillance–containment model, 23–24
Smith, Adam, 476, 529, 531
Smith, George Otis, 333
smoking
    banning and heart attacks, 25
    cancers from asbestos plus, 20
    MSHA citing miners, 175
    OTA report, 61
    secondhand smoke, 38, 588
Snow, John, 554
social discount rate, 508, 520
social environment, 20, 26, 52
social proof, 573
Social Security Act (1935), 45, 88, 101, 272
Social Security Disability Act (1956), 500
Social Security Disability Insurance (DI), 472, 479–480, 518
social security internationally. *See* International Social Security Association
Society of Plastics Industry, Inc. v. OSHA (1975), 183, 185–186
SOHSM. *See* Systematic Occupational Health and Safety Management
SOLAS. *See* International Convention for Safety of Life at Sea
Solicitor's Office, 606
Sotomayor, Justice Sonia, 75
South Korea
    asbestos importing, 439
    life expectancy, 399
Southern Pacific Railroad v. State of California (1886), 75
sovereign immunity, 74
space shuttle Challenger, 591–593
spectrum of prevention, 24–25, 648–649
stakeholders
    constituencies, 282
    National Occupational Research Agenda (NORA), 290–291
    workers' compensation, 496–498
Standard Industrial Classification system, 402
Standards. *See also* emergency temporary standards; judicial review; permanent

standards; recommended standards; temporary standards
advisory, 177, 413, 534
agriculture, 171, 172
American National Standards Institute (ANSI), 101, 176, 405–406
American Standards Association, 100
asbestos, 380. *See also* asbestos
benzene, 179, 611
cancer standard, 43, 179, 185, 192–194, 611, 657
challenging, 179, 180, 186, 214–215
Coal Act (1969), 349, 350
codes of conduct for businesses, 76, 398
command-and-control process, 213
construction, 171, 172
cost of compliance, 203–205, 481, 519–520, 649–650
CPSC vs. OSHA, 378
criminal violations, 223, 239
definitions in OSHAct, 173
development time line, 201–202, 613
as DoL responsibility, 278
economics versus, 647–654
employment standards statutes, 381–383
Federal Metal and Nonmetallic Mine Safety Act, 319
Federal Register publication, 171, 179
Federal Register submission, 171, 177
GAO report, 61
general duty when standard exists, 233
general industry, 171
generic, 185, 465
global standards, 448
Hazard Communication, 9. *See also* Hazard Communication Standard (1983)
hierarchy of controls, 171, 187
interim, 171, 173, 175–177, 186, 191, 213, 324, 326
International Atomic Energy Agency, 412–413
International Labour Organization, 407
International Organization for Standardization (ISO), 435–436, 444
international standards, 405–406
international trade, 420–421
mandatory, 177, 413, 534
maritime, 171, 172
mining, 317, 322, 323, 324, 325, 326–327
MSHA authority, 329, 356
NAFTA, 423, 653
National Safety Council, 101
OSHA standards overturned, 201, 611
OSHAct standards development, 145, 146
path from risk to enforcement, 213
path from risk to standard, 169–170
pesticides, 379
polluters bear burden, 40, 175
promulgation, 178–179, 657
in public health framework, 6, 7, 17
radon exposure, 371
reasonably necessary or appropriate, 133, 173, 178, 189–190, 639
regulations versus, 214–215, 604
science in development of, 655
Standards Completion Program, 281–282
states vs. federal, 178, 225–226
Threshold Limit Values, 176
time to develop, 201–202, 613
variance from, 178, 180
for vehicles, 375–376
vinyl chloride, 179, 519–520, 568, 643
World Bank gradient approach, 417
World Health Organization, 409
Standards Advisory Committee on Agriculture (SACA), 181–182
Standards Completion Program (SCP), 281–282
State Department. *See* U.S. Department of State
state governments
BoM enforcement authority, 317
business consultation program, 261, 590
corporations sanctioned by, 75
criminal prosecutions and OSHA, 234–239
employees, 173, 383–384, 657
excluded as employer, 173, 367, 383–384
federal system of government, 17, 57–58
Freedom of Information Act, 67–68
grants for compliance with Mine Act, 327–328
grants for programs, 262, 274
HazCom Standard, 202, 540
mining programs, 322, 323, 327
motor carrier safety regulations, 375–376
MSHA grants for programs, 546
National Commission on State Workmen's Compensation Laws, 491–493
NIOSH first state-based, 287
prohibited from impeding federal, 109
in public health organization, 17, 57
state programs and OSHA, 225–226, 383–384
state regulations in history, 99–100
state standards exceeding federal, 178, 226
state vs. federal primacy, 140–141
Submerged Lands Act, 369
trade secret protection, 218
Wisconsin Industrial Commission Act, 152
workers' compensation fraud, 518–519
workers' compensation laws, 103, 266–267, 482, 483–485, 491–496
workers' compensation uniformity, 482, 518
state jurisdictions
local emphasis programs, 228–229
NIOSH offices, 280

OSHA regional offices, 201
OSHAct (Section 18), 225–226
Severe Violator Enforcement Program, 232
states with approved plans, 225, 226, 232
state offices of OSHA, 201
statistics
   disability-adjusted life-years (DALYs), 400–401, 508
   Eurofound, 432–433
   healthy worker effect, 342
   human life value, 509–512, 519–520
   OSHAct (Section 24), 265–266
   quality-adjusted life-year (QALY), 508
   risk assessment, 639
   significance, 151
   silicosis in dusty trades, 339–340
   Type I and II errors, 151–152
statutory law. *See also* judicial review; legislation
   common law and, 65
   customary law and, 56
   employment standards statutes, 381–383
   environmental protection, 377–381
   executive orders, 62–63
   in law hierarchy, 52
   legislative branch of government, 58, 59–61, 65
   mine disasters → law, 314–321
   originating statute, 66
   privacy rights, 556–558
   process of, 60, 62
   regulatory procedure vs. APA, 66, 67
   transportation industry, 372–376
   United States Code (U.S.C.), 170
   unlawful agency actions, 214
   workers' compensation statutes, 499–501
Steamboat Act (1852), 111
Steamboat Inspection Act (1838), 111
steel industry
   cancers, 91, 113
   early research, 269
   injury data, 106, 265
   judicial review, 182, 183
   NIOSH recommended standards, 263, 264
   OSHAct creation, 113
   Standard on Coke Oven Emissions, 69, 179
   volunteer safety movement, 101
Steiger, William A., 114, 115, 116, 144
Stender, John H., 199
Stern, Robert, 512
Stewart, Justice Potter, 217
Stewart, William H., 278
stinkdamp mine gas, 312
stories. *See* narrative analysis
Stowe, Harriet Beecher, 83–84
strategic plan of OSHA, 227–232

straw man fallacy, 157, 631
stress, 20
strict liability
   doctrine of enterprise liability, 55
   negligence versus, 502–503
strikes. *See* labor movement
Strunk, Dorothy, 626
Studds, Gerry E., 390
subcontractors and prime contractors, 232–233
Submerged Lands Act (1953), 369
subpoena power, 299
subrogation, 503
substantial evidence test, 177–178
suffering. *See* pain and suffering
Sullivan, Leonor K., 137–139, 148
Sunshine in Litigation Act, 552–553
Superfund Amendments and Reauthorization Act (1986), 380–381, 541, 547
supply (economics), 468
Supreme Court of the United States
   agency approval of state plan, 226
   Alien Tort Claims Act, 74–75
   benzene standard, 611
   civil litigation representation, 218
   corporations as persons, 74, 75–76
   cost-benefit of worker health, 505
   expert testimony, 554–555
   in judicial branch of government, 58, 64
   law of nations, 56
   number of justices, 64
   OSHA jurisdiction, 174
   "person" vs. "individual," 74–75
   Pregnancy Discrimination Act, 211–212, 248–249
   privacy rights, 556–557
   refusal to work, 216–217, 559
   risk assessment approach, 37, 133, 638
   safety movement impact, 108–111
   writ of certiorari, 64
Surface Transportation Act (1982), 375
Surgeon General
   Burney, Luther L., 43
   Cumming, Hugh S., 271
   Novello, Antonia C., 272
   Rucker, W. Colby, 333
   Scheele, Leonard A., 275
   Stewart, William H., 278
   Wyman, Walter, 333
surveillance
   asbestos, 380
   coal dust samples, 350–356
   industrial hygiene process, 24
   methods as research priority, 291
   Mine Act (1977), 322
   MSHA directorate, 330
   in public health framework, 6, 7, 17

surveillance-containment model, 23–24, 498–499
workers' compensation for, 498–499
surveillance-containment model, 23–24
Susan Harwood Training Grants program, 261
sustainability, 395–396, 422
Sutherland, William H., 354–355
sweating (labor), 105
Sweden
    healthcare spending, 470
    tractor rollovers, 389, 586
Swift, Marshall, 24
Symms, Steve, 2
synthetic dyes, 587–588
Systematic Occupational Health and Safety Management (SOHSM), 645–647, 655

T

tables. *See* charts and flowcharts
Taft, Helen, 97
Taft, William Howard, 77–78, 333
Taft-Hartley Act (1947). *See* National Labor Relations Act (1947)
Tajikistan
    asbestos use, 437
    forced child labor, 452, 453
tangible costs, 468
Taylor, George, 277, 279, 609
technology
    continuous mining, 90
    control technology focus, 287, 291
    control technology over PPE, 27, 182
    data-driven science, 395
    developed vs. developing countries, 450
    electronic information, 68, 71, 557
    emerging technologies, 290, 291, 402, 640–641
    fracking, 151
    Office of Technology Assessment (OTA), 61, 204, 481, 626, 641
    prospective analysis for emerging, 640–641
    technological feasibility, 178, 183, 184, 189, 481
    warning devices, 27, 535
    Watson abductive reasoning, 150–151
temporal aspects. *See* time
temporary standards
    in command-and-control process, 213
    emergency temporary denied, 179–180, 183
    employer compliance, 171
    Mine Act (1977), 325
    overview, 179–180, 604
    vinyl chloride, 186
termination notice, 56

terrorist attacks
    emergency preparedness, 203
    National Response Plan, 547–548
    9/11 and NIOSH, 291, 297–298, 501
    9/11 Health and Compensation Act, 500, 501
    9/11 Victim Compensation Fund, 467, 510, 511
    WTC Health Registry, 501
tertiary prevention, 18, 659
text of OSHAct, 671–726
textile mills
    byssinosis disease, 105, 158, 205, 289, 517, 659
    child labor, 97, 104
    cost of compliance, 204, 205
    cotton dust standard, 179, 588, 638
    judicial review, 183, 185, 187–188
    NIOSH recommended standard, 263
    wage slavery, 97
    workday length, 93, 94
Thackrah, Charles Turner, 86–87
Thailand
    asbestos importing, 439
    forced child labor, 453
Théry, Nicolas, 395
Thompson, Lewis R., 271–272
Thompson, Tommy G., 291, 296–297
threat vs. opportunity framing, 154–155
Three Mile Island, PA, nuclear reactor event, 414
Threshold Limit Values (TLVs), 176
time
    cost analysis, 508–509
    development of standards, 201–202, 613
    policy vs. applied science, 602
    as public health enemy, 158
    time-value of money, 508
TNT poisoning, 271, 273
tolerances, 219
topoi of issue statements, 131
tort law
    aftermath of hazard control failure, 451
    Alien Tort Claims Act, 57, 74–75
    asbestos torts, 504–505
    assumption of risk elimination, 103
    class action suits, 503
    Coal Act lacking, 349
    contract law origins, 55
    court records sealed, 551–553
    DBCP pesticide exposure, 454
    discovery, 548–549, 552–553
    doctrine of enterprise liability, 55
    Federal Rules of Civil Procedure, 548
    history of occupational safety, 102

as incentives, 502, 504
negligence vs. strict liability, 502–503
no-fault workers' compensation, 103
noneconomic damages, 503
subrogation, 503
Tort Claims Act, 74
tort definition, 55
tort liability, 501–505
tort liability cost, 472, 502, 503–504
trial by judge, 553–555
workers' compensation replacing, 607
Total Quality Management (TQM), 578, 655
Total Worker Health program, 298
Townsend, James E., 273
toxic substance registries. *See* Agency for Toxic Substances and Disease Registry; International Register of Potentially Toxic Chemicals; Registration, Evaluation, Authorization, and Restriction of Chemicals (REACH); Registry of Toxic Effects of Chemical Substances; Toxics Release Inventory
Toxic Substances Control Act (TSCA; 1976)
asbestos amendments, 379, 380
cost-benefit criteria, 643–644
cross-examination in rule making, 66
formaldehyde regulation, 169–170
hazardous substance tracking, 379
occupational exposures, 37
Registration, Evaluation, Authorization, and Restriction of Chemicals, 431, 434–435
Toxics Release Inventory (TRI), 540
TQM. *See* Total Quality Management
tractors, 419. *See also* rollover protective structures (ROPS)
trade. *See* international trade
Trade and Development Act (2000), 451
trade name use, 536
trade secrets
legal restrictions of, 549–551
OSHAct (Section 15), 218–219
"Trade Secrets: A Moyers Report," 565–568
Trade Secrets Act (1948), 218
training. *See also* education; information
agricultural workers and pesticides, 379
business school safety curriculum, 590–591
Center for Construction Research and Training, 289
Centers for Agricultural Disease and Injury Research, Education, and Prevention, 289
Coal Act (1969), 321
Coal Mine Safety and Health (MSHA), 329
"designated" personnel, 543
education and research centers (ERCs), 260–261, 284
emergency responders, 261

environmental and criminal investigation, 243
grants for, 261, 374–375
Hazard Communication Standard, 540, 543, 545–546
as hazard control, 29
of immigrants, 402
inspectors, 436
international OSHA agreements, 402–405
International Training and Research in Environmental and Occupational Health program (NIH), 395
as legal requirement, 29
local emphasis programs, 229
Mine Act (1977), 322, 323, 324, 325, 327–328
MSHA conducting, 330, 546–547
National Mine Health and Safety Academy, 321, 327, 330
NIEHS conducting, 547–548
NIOSH conducting, 115, 260–261, 278
OSHA mission, 259
OSHA Outreach Training Program, 546, 590
OSHA training guidelines, 543, 545–546
OSHA training institute, 198, 261, 546
OSHAct (Section 21), 260–262, 278
personal protective equipment, 29
rehabilitation, 490
self-contained self-rescue devices, 312
understandable language, 543, 545
voluntary protection program, 229
transactional leadership, 572, 575
transcripts in rule making, 178
transformational leadership, 571, 572, 575–576
transparency
acceptable risk determination, 635
conscience while watched, 580
ILO power over violators, 656
Internet for worker safety, 656
offshore operations, 649, 650
transportation industry
deaths in, 4, 386
International Maritime Organization, 398, 411–412
National Highway Traffic Safety Administration, 43, 44, 375
National Transportation Safety Board, 376
NLRA exclusion, 381
OSHA jurisdiction, 659
radioactive material, 413
shipping vessels, 411–412
worker safety legislation, 372–376
traumatic injuries
examples of, 289
as leading work-related injuries, 289
NIOSH program review, 292, 293
as research priority, 291
traumatogens, 660, 661

treaty obligations, 398, 407
trial by judge, 553–555
Triangle Shirtwaist Co. fire (1911), 88, 446
Truman, Harry S., 106, 198, 317, 343
TSCA. *See* Toxic Substances Control Act (1976)
tuberculosis in statutory law, 65
Turkey forced child labor, 453
Turkmenistan
   asbestos use, 437
   forced child labor, 453
Type I and II errors, 151–152

U

Ukraine
   asbestos use, 437
   forced child labor, 453
UN. *See* United Nations
unanticipated releases, 245–246, 540, 541, 547
uncertainty. *See also* risk
   abductive reasoning and, 150
   advocacy under, 127–128, 129, 149
   complexity and polarization driving, 629
   intuitive primacy principle, 579
   policy maker actions, 258, 637
   precautionary principle, 148–149, 634
   risk assessment for temporary standards, 179–180
   scarce resource choices, 469
   scientific certainty not required, 190
Uncle Tom's Cabin (Stowe), 83–84
Unfunded Mandates Reform Act (1995), 68, 70, 202, 613
Uninspected Commercial Fishing Vessels (NTSB; 1987), 390
uninspected fishing vessels, 174, 368, 390
Union Carbide Corporation
   egregious-case civil penalty policy, 220, 451
   right-to-know policies, 451, 541
   settlement for catastrophe, 450
   vinyl chloride cover-up, 567
   worst industrial disaster, 245–246, 449–451
unions. *See also* labor movement; United Mine Workers of America; United Steelworkers of America
   AFL-CIO formation, 98, 609. *See also* AFL-CIO
   American Federation of Labor (AFL), 93, 95, 97–98
   Bangladesh, 447, 448
   as capitalism balance, 475
   co-determination laws, 655–656
   collective bargaining, 609
   global worker safety, 653, 655–656
   hazard communication, 537, 539
   Industrial Workers of the World (Wobblies), 97, 98, 103
   International Union of Mine, Mill, and Smelter Workers (Mine-Mill), 318–319
   Laborers International Union, 661
   Landrum-Griffin Act, 107
   leader, 133
   mutual aid societies, 92–93
   National Labor Relations Act (1935), 98, 107, 381–382
   National Labor Relations Act (1947), 107
   as NGO, 435
   NIOSH director Howard, 297
   Oil, Chemical, and Atomic Workers Union (OCAW), 8–9, 212, 527, 538, 540, 609
   OSHA challenges, 610–611
   OSHAct creation, 113, 115, 139, 140
   as public health coalition, 128–129, 143, 616
   state regulations for safety, 99–100
   toxic exposure in Union Carbide India, 449
   United Automobile Workers, 656
   United Farm Workers, 571, 586
   United Food and Commercial Workers, 649
   voluntary protection program, 230
   wage slavery, 95–98
   workday length, 93–95, 341
   WTO labor standards, 421–422
United Automobile Workers, 656
United Farm Workers, 571, 586
United Food and Commercial Workers, 649
United Kingdom. *See* Great Britain
United Mine Workers of America (UMWA)
   CWP recognition, 344, 346–347
   discontent against, 344, 345, 347, 348
   early statutes, 113, 143, 317
   mine gas, 332
   miners' asthma, 341, 342
   Sayers as BoM director, 337
   Welfare and Retirement Fund, 342–344, 345–346
   Yablonski murder, 349–350
United Nations (UN)
   agencies of occupational health/safety, 398, 406
   Food and Agriculture Organization, 398, 414–415
   harmonization, 542
   International Atomic Energy Agency, 398, 412–414, 422
   International Labour Organization, 397–398, 406–408. *See also* International Labour Organization
   International Maritime Organization, 398, 411–412
   norms changing via law, 398
   UN Charter, 406
   UN Environment Programme, 398, 415, 654, 655

INDEX | 783

Universal Declaration of Human Rights, 406
World Health Organization, 398, 409–411.
 See also World Health Organization
United Nations Environment
 Programme (UNEP)
 global worker safety, 654
 ISO 14000 environmental protection, 655
 as UN agency, 398, 415
United States (U.S.). *See also* Constitutional
  system; Supreme Court of the
  United States
 agricultural workers, 414
 common vs. civil law, 53–54
 employment-at-will doctrine, 56
 excluded as employer, 173
 Exclusive Economic Zone (EEZ), 368–370
 harmonization of industrial
  classification, 402
 healthcare spending, 470–472
 ILO representatives, 654
 law of nations, 56–57
 life expectancy, 399, 599
 NAFTA, 423, 424, 425
 protection legislation evolution,
  105–111
 regulatory approach, 52
 suing industries via CAA, 245
 suits by foreigners, 57, 74–75
 suits by individuals, 74
 United States Code (U.S.C.), 170
 U.S.-Mexico Border Industrial Program,
  422–423
 workers' compensation, 482–491. *See also*
  workers' compensation
United States Code (U.S.C.), 170
United States v. Atlantic States Cast Iron Pipe Co.,
 et al. (2006), 241–242, 243
United States v. BP Products North America
 (2007), 245–246
United States v. Company B and Two Individuals
 (1987), 244
United States v. Elias (2001), 244
United States v. Motiva Enterprises LLC, et al.
 (2003), 244–245
U.S. Atomic Energy Commission (AEC)
 beryllium standard, 583
 radiation "gag rule," 160
 radon exposure standard, 371
 workers' compensation fraud, 518–519
U.S. Attorney General, 218, 235
U.S. Coast Guard (USCG)
 continental shelf, 368, 369
 in DHS, 372
 fishing vessel safety, 370, 389–390
 inspected vessels, 370
 NTSB as "court of appeals," 372
 uninspected vessels, 174, 368

U.S. Department of Agriculture (USDA)
 Interagency Regulatory Liaison Group,
  42–43
 MOU with OSHA, 386
U.S. Department of Commerce (DoC)
 BoM transferred to, 336–337
 National Bureau of Standards within, 101
 National Traffic Safety Bureau, 44
 sanction authority, 651
U.S. Department of Energy (DoE)
 Hazardous Materials Transportation Act
  (HMTA; 1975), 374–375
 NIOSH Occupational Energy Research
  Program, 372
 Nuclear Weapons Cleanup Training Program,
  547
 oversight transferred to OSHA, 371–372
U.S. Department of Health, Education, and
 Welfare (DHEW), 112
U.S. Department of Health and Human Services
 (DHHS)
 CDC within, 17, 62, 258, 262, 278
 interfering with NIOSH, 606
 NIH within, 17
 in public health organization, 17
U.S. Department of Homeland Security (DHS)
 forced child labor products, 452, 453
 National Response Plan, 547–548
 USCG within, 372
U.S. Department of Labor (DoL)
 archives of *Industrial Hygiene*
  Newsletter, 276
 child labor worst forms, 451–452
 CWP benefits from Coal Act, 320
 ESA within, 198, 376, 500
 forced child labor products, 452, 453
 MSHA within, 67, 329
 OSHA reporting to Secretary of, 606
 OSHA within, 17, 45, 62, 67, 198
 responsibilities for standards and
  enforcement, 278
 Worker Endangerment Initiative,
  239–247
U.S. Department of State
 asbestos industry and IPCS, 443
 forced child labor products, 452, 453
U.S. Department of the Interior (DoI)
 BoM within, 269, 301, 316, 337
 Coal Act enforcement, 141
 Deepwater Horizon aftermath, 590
 Federal Water Quality Administration, 45
 GAO report, 61
 Mine Safety Board Report (1963), 319
 Minerals Management Service in, 369, 370
U.S. Department of Transportation (DoT)
 Maximum Abbreviated Injury Scale, 510, 512
 safety statutes, 372–376

standards for vehicles, 375–376
USCG transferred from, 372
U.S. Environmental Protection Agency (EPA)
    administrative law judges in, 218
    asbestos ban, 441, 442
    chemical bans since TSCA, 644
    Chemical Emergency Preparedness Program, 541
    dibromochloropropane (DBCP), 453
    Emergency Planning and Community Right-to-Know Act, 38
    environmental impact statements, 42
    formaldehyde, 169–170
    Hazardous Materials Transportation Act (HMTA; 1975), 374–375
    as health protection agency, 17
    hexavalent chromium, 587
    human life value, 519
    Interagency Regulatory Liaison Group, 42–43
    IQA public health subversion, 72
    lead paint, 585
    OMB review of draft regulation, 62
    pesticide authority, 378–379
    Registry of Toxic Effects of Chemical Substances, 37
    USPHS origins, 43, 45
U.S. Food and Drug Administration (FDA)
    Delaney Clause, 634
    dibromochloropropane (DBCP), 452–453
    Interagency Regulatory Liaison Group, 42–43
U.S. Geologic Survey (USGS), 316, 332–333
U.S. Government Accountability Office (GAO)
    coal dust sampling, 351–352, 353
    independent congressional agency, 60–61
    rate of issuing standards, 286
U.S. Nuclear Regulatory Commission, 374
U.S. Public Health Service (USPHS)
    authority pre-OSHAct, 269
    Coat Act research authority, 320
    Division of Occupational Health, 257, 276, 278, 279
    Healthy People, 20
    notifiable diseases and injuries, 5–6, 15, 269
    Protecting the Health of Eighty Million Americans, 139, 277–278, 609
    protection agencies, 43–46
    Public Health and Marine-Hospital Service origins, 333
    Public Health Service Act (1912), 107, 269–270
    Social Security Act funding, 101, 272
    in Treasury Department, 269, 343
U.S. Treasury Department, 269, 343

United Steelworkers of America
    early statutes, 113, 143, 609
    fluorides, 275
    hazard communication, 539
    Mine-Mill merger, 319
    OSHAct promotion, 279
United Steelworkers of America v. Marshall and Bingham (1980), 183, 190
Universal Declaration of Human Rights (UN), 406
unlawful agency actions, 214
Unsafe at Any Speed (Nader), 44
uranium mining
    early research, 274, 276
    early standards, 277
    Energy Employees Occupational Illness Compensation Program, 501
    lung cancer, 90, 112, 160–161, 276, 371, 519
    Radiation Exposure Compensation Act, 519
    radiation poisoning, 160–161, 518–519
    radon progeny emissions, 37, 90, 160, 371, 519
    workers' compensation fraud, 518–519
Uruguay life expectancy, 399
U.S. Chamber of Commerce
    in business coalition, 128, 195, 616
    ergonomics standard, 195
    OSHAct creation, 142, 144, 147
U.S. Council for International Business, 654
USDA. *See* U.S. Department of Agriculture
USPHS. *See* U.S. Public Health Service
Uzbekistan
    asbestos use, 437
    forced child labor, 452, 453

V

vaccinations, 18, 19, 23–24
Valic, Fedor, 441, 443
Van Buren, Martin, 93
variable costs, 468
variance from standards
    employer application for, 178, 180
    Mine Safety and Health Review Commission, 325
    OSHAct (Section 16), 219
VCM. *See* vinyl chloride monomer
Venezuela and OSHA, 403
vessels
    inspected vessels, 370, 412
    shipping vessel Code of Safe Practice, 412
    uninspected vessels, 174, 368
Vietnam
    asbestos labeling, 427

factory hazards, 446
forced child labor, 453
vinyl chloride monomer (VCM)
  angiosarcoma, 38, 159, 186, 205, 519, 566, 568
  cost of compliance, 204, 205, 519–520
  deaths, 159, 519, 568
  greedy cover-up, 159, 565–568
  judicial review, 182, 183, 185–186
  NIOSH recommended standard, 263
  OSHA standard, 179, 519–520, 568, 643
Viola, Publio L., 566
violations
  average penalty for serious violation, 21
  BoM authority, 108, 318, 319, 338
  categories of, 215
  civil, 220–221, 222–223
  Coal Act (1969), 321, 349
  coal dust sampling, 351
  criminal, 221, 223–225
  ergonomic violations program, 231
  failure to correct versus, 114
  fishing vessel safety, 370
  global worker safety, 652–653
  ILO power in transparency, 656
  Mine Act (1977), 324, 325
  Mine Improvement Act, 328–329
  NAFTA, 423, 653
  number of inspections (2009), 21
  OSHA citations for, 152, 213, 215, 216
  Severe Violator Enforcement Program, 231–232
  for standards not general duty, 223, 239
  for standards or general duty, 152, 219
  trade secrets, 219
  WTO dispute settlements, 421
visual warning devices, 27, 535
Voluntary Protection Program (VPP), 229–230, 590, 647, 659–660
volunteer safety movement, 101–102, 138, 480
volunteers exclusion from workers' compensation, 486
Volunteers in Service to America (VISTA), 346

W

wages
  agricultural workers, 382, 383
  capitalism contradiction, 476–477
  closure order of mine, 325
  collective bargaining, 609
  compensating differential argument, 529–530
  Fair Labor Standards Act, 108, 382
  global poverty, 647
  immigrants, 403
  lower wages, lower value, 418, 446–448, 647, 661
  minimum wage, 95, 108, 382
  present value of earnings discrimination, 510, 511
  present value of future earnings, 508, 509
  quote by Adam Smith, 529
  refusal to work, 217
  Social Security Disability Insurance (DI), 479
  sweating, 105
  wage slavery, 95–98, 108
  whistle-blower back pay, 375
  workday length and, 94–95, 108, 382
  workers' compensation, 486, 489
Wagner, Robert R., 381
Wagner Act (1935). *See* National Labor Relations Act (1935)
Waite, Chief Justice Morrison, 75
Walsh-Healey Public Contracts Act (1936)
  application restrictions, 89, 95, 101
  federal standards for interim, 176
  occupational safety and health foundation, 88–89, 91, 110, 198, 607
  radon exposure standard, 371
  subsumed by OSHAct, 174
  uranium mining, 161, 277
  workday length, 95, 108
wants (economics), 468, 469, 575
"warning," 534–535
warnings, 27, 533–535
warrants
  in argumentation, 129, 130, 134–136, 138, 604
  search warrants for inspections, 147, 214, 223
Water Pollution Control Act (1948), 45
Water Pollution Control Act Amendments (1972), 46
Water Quality Act (1965), 45
waterborne commerce. *See* maritime standards
waterborne hazards, 25, 554
Watkins, James A., 269
Watson computer and precautionary principle, 150–151
The Wealth of Nations (Smith), 529, 531
web presence of federal agencies, 68
weight of evidence, 554–555
Weil, Andrew, 540
Weinberger, Caspar, 283
Weise, Adam, 366
Wells, Hawey, 345, 346, 348
What Is a Life Worth? (Feinberg), 510
Whirlpool Corp. v. Marshall (1980), 216, 559
whistle-blowers

arresting, 661
back pay for, 375
global worker safety, 653
Mine Act (1977), 325
rights of, 203, 216, 217, 559
Systematic Occupational Health and Safety Management, 655
whistle-blower program, 230–231
white lead, 408, 584–585. *See also* lead
white phosphorus matches, 65, 77–78, 87, 107, 269
White Phosphorus Matches Prohibition Act (1912), 65, 77, 107, 111, 269
whitedamp mine gas, 312, 333
Whitehouse, Sheldon, 552
WHO. *See* World Health Organization
WHO International Programme on Chemical Safety (IPCS), 411, 441–443, 442, 584
Wholesome Meat Act (1967), 117
willful violations
 civil penalties for, 221
 Coal Act criminal penalties, 321
 criminal prosecution, 221, 223, 225, 239
 definition, 215, 221
 maximum civil penalties, 220
 Severe Violator Enforcement Program, 231–232
Williams, Harrison, 114, 116, 141, 143, 348
Williams, R. C., 335
Williams-Steiger Occupational Safety and Health Act (1970). *See* Occupational Safety and Health Act
willingness to pay (WTP), 468, 507
Wilson, Woodrow, 336
Wirth, Timothy, 443
Wirtz, Willard W., 138, 140, 161, 371
Wisconsin Industrial Commission Act (1911), 152
The Wizard of Oz (movie), 534
Wobblies (Industrial Workers of the World), 97, 98, 103
women workers
 autonomy of employees, 531
 childbearing capacity, 211–212, 248–249
 fetal vs. women's rights, 249
 labor movement, 95, 99, 100
 mining, 104–105
 phosphorus necrosis, 77
 radiation poisoning, 90, 272
 statutory law protecting, 65
 textile mills, 97
 Triangle Shirtwaist fire, 88
work
 average hours per year, 21
 developed vs. developing countries, 647–648, 649
 economics of, 468–469, 647–648

 informal sector definition, 22
 poverty escape, 249, 446–448, 468, 647, 649
 right to refuse work, 216–217, 532–533, 558
 workday length, 93–95, 108, 271, 341
Work-Accidents and the Law (Eastman), 88
Worker Endangerment Initiative, 239–247
Worker Protection Standard (WPS) for pesticides, 379
workers. *See* employees
workers' compensation. *See also* pain and suffering
 administration, 485
 aftermath of hazard control failure, 451
 Alaska fishers, 93
 argument for regulations, 604
 attorney fees, 485, 503, 517
 back injuries, 195
 benefits, 488–491, 513
 benefits annually, 479
 compensating differential argument, 529–530
 compensation principle, 27, 481, 482, 518
 compulsory vs. elective, 483, 484
 costs of, 485, 496–499, 503, 517
 coverage, 486
 coverage shortfall, 478
 CWP compensation, 344–350, 349
 DBCP pesticide exposure, 454–455
 employer costs, 492–493
 Employment Standards Administration, 198
 excluded owners, 486
 excluded workers, 483, 484, 486, 492
 experience modification, 493, 494–495
 externalized costs of, 477–480
 fault, 102–103, 483, 484, 500, 502
 federal laws that provide, 499–501
 fraud in, 512–519
 Guides to the Evaluation of Permanent Impairment (AMA), 489–490
 health care disparities, 21
 health care reform, 499
 history of compensation, 54, 481–484
 history of occupational safety, 88, 102–103, 607
 as incentive, 493, 495, 497–498, 498–499
 injury vs. disease, 487
 insurance claim denial, 517, 658, 660–661
 insurance pools, 495–496, 659
 longshore and harbor workers, 383
 manual rate, 492–493, 493–494
 Mine Act (1977), 328
 miners' asthma, 342
 monopoly vs. market-driven, 482, 484, 485
 NAFTA, 423
 National Commission on State Workmen's Compensation Laws, 491–493

as no-fault, 102–103, 483, 484, 500, 502
nuclear workers, 372
occupational diseases, 486–488
OSHAct (Section 27), 266–267
OSHAct nonaffecting, 174
other compensation statutes, 499–501
physician selection, 490
process, 485
qualification requirements, 488
rehabilitation, 488, 490
second injury funds, 485
self-insurance, 486, 495
Social Security disability and, 479
state laws, 103, 266–267, 483–485
unfiled claims, 513
universal vs. variable services, 483, 484
Working Conditions Services (WCS), 270
World Bank Group
  establishment, 415
  global burden of disease/injury, 417, 418
  occupational health/safety role, 398
  organization of, 415–416
World Development Report 1993: Investing in Health (World Bank), 417
World Health Organization (WHO)
  asbestos global ban, 440
  DALYs in metrics, 400–401, 508
  Environmental Health Criteria 203: Chrysotile Asbestos, 443
  "health" definition, 3
  International Programme on Chemical Safety, 411, 441–443, 442, 584
  smallpox eradication, 24
  sustainability, 395–396
  UN public health arm, 398, 409–411
World Trade Center (WTC) attack
  9/11 and NIOSH, 291, 297–298, 501

9/11 Health and Compensation Act, 500, 501
9/11 Victim Compensation Fund, 467, 510, 511
World Trade Center Programs, 298, 501
WTC Health Registry, 501
World Trade Organization (WTO)
  Canada asbestos dispute, 397, 444–445
  dispute settlement, 420, 421, 444–445
  enforcing global worker safety, 653
  global worker safety, 650–654
  international trade, 420–422
  labor standards, 421–422
  perceptions of, 419
  standards and protectionism, 421
World Wars
  Bureau of Mines and, 335–336
  Organisation for Economic Co-operation and Development, 418
  public health and, 270–278
Worley, J. F., 335
writ of certiorari, 64, 174
WTC. *See* World Trade Center (WTC) attack

Y

Yablonski, Joseph A., 346, 349–350
Yarborough, Ralph, 140

Z

Zimbabwe
  asbestos labeling, 427
  asbestos mining, 439
Zimbardo, Philip, 570
zone of privacy, 556–557
zoonotic diseases in statutory law, 65

Barrett Library
Allen College Campus
Waterloo, Iowa 50703